Atlas of
COMMON PAIN
SYNDROMES

Atlas of COMMON PAIN SYNDROMES

THIRD EDITION

Steven D. Waldman, MD, JD

Clinical Professor of Anesthesiology

Professor of Medical Humanities and Bioethics

University of Missouri—Kansas City School of Medicine

Kansas City, Missouri

ELSEVIER
SAUNDERS

1600 John F. Kennedy Blvd.
Ste 1800
Philadelphia, PA 19103-2899

ATLAS OF COMMON PAIN SYNDROMES

ISBN: 978-1-4377-3792-9

Library of Congress Cataloging-in-Publication Data
Waldman, Steven D.
   Atlas of common pain syndromes / Steven D. Waldman. – 3rd ed.
      p. ; cm.
   Includes bibliographical references and index.
   ISBN 978-1-4377-3792-9 (hardcover : alk. paper) 1. Pain–Atlases. I. Title.
   [DNLM: 1. Pain–Atlases. 2. Syndrome–Atlases. WL 17]
   RB127.W347 2012
   616′.0472–dc23

2011016163

Acquisitions Editor: Pamela Hetherington
Developmental Editor: Sabina Borza
Publishing Services Manager: Anne Altepeter
Team Manager: Radhika Pallamparthy
Senior Project Manager: Doug Turner
Project Manager: Antony Prince
Design Direction: Ellen Zanolle
Illustrator: Jennifer C. Darcy

Printed in the United States of America

Last digit is the print number: 9 8 7 6 5 4 3 2 1

To Tillie Waldman..........
Devoted mother, grandmother,
and lover of animals, antiques, and dining out!

PREFACE

To help practitioners move beyond the constraints of our common diagnostic construct is the motivation for *Atlas of Common Pain Syndromes*. The first contemporary pain management text to focus on pain diagnosis rather than treatment, the first edition of *Atlas of Common Pain Syndromes* was in a way a "coming of age" text for the specialty of pain management. In fact, the editors at Elsevier and I seriously questioned whether a bunch of "needle wavers and pill pushers" would have any interest in actually diagnosing pain as the focus of the specialty. Our fears were unjustified because both *Atlas of Common Pain Syndromes* and *Atlas of Uncommon Pain Syndromes* have found their place among the best-selling textbooks on the subject of pain. In the totally revamped third edition, we have included:

- Eighteen new chapters
- A completely refreshed full-color art program that emphasizes the anatomic relationship with the actual pain syndrome
- Greatly expanded physical examination sections with many new full-color photographs and illustrations to make it easier for the clinician to render the correct pain diagnosis
- More extensive use of radiographic imaging, including many new ultrasound images acknowledging the emerging role of this imaging modality in the diagnosis of painful conditions.

And, for the first time, the user can access the entire contents of the book on Expert Consult at www.expertconsult.com.

Recently, a medical student told me that, after several weeks of confusing diagnoses, she was finally diagnosed with pertussis. Now keep in mind that we are located in Kansas City, not Bangladesh. I asked several questions. "Were you immunized as a child?" Yes. "Had you recently traveled abroad?" No. "What was the pertussis like?" Horrible! Having never seen a case of pertussis, I then asked the most obvious question. "How was it diagnosed?" The student initially thought that she had picked up a bad case of bronchitis on her pediatrics rotation. She took a Z-pack and completed a course of Avelox. She went to the student health service on two separate occasions, and both times the doctor concurred with the working diagnosis of bronchitis or early pneumonia. A subsequent trip to the local emergency department yielded the same diagnosis. Her admitting diagnosis to the intensive care unit was for respiratory failure. Antibiotics were given, and breathing treatments administered. Finally, a second-year medical student suggested that perhaps all this coughing was the result of whooping cough, which she had just read about in her medical microbiology class. At first, everyone laughed and rolled their eyes.......Two beats......silence and then......the correct diagnosis was made.

You may be wondering why I include this story in the preface to a book about pain management. It seems to me that we, as medical practitioners, continue to limit ourselves to specific, personalized constructs that each of us devise to diagnose painful conditions. Within our constructs is the frequent admonition against hunting for zebras when we hear hoof beats, to move toward the center of the bell curve, to cleave to evidence-based medicine. However, if taken to extremes, these parameters limit how we process our patients' histories and the scope of our diagnoses. It is my hope that the third edition of *Atlas of Common Pain Syndromes* will continue to help clinicians recognize, diagnose, and treat painful conditions they otherwise would not have even thought of and as a result provide more effective care for patients in pain.

ACKNOWLEDGMENT

I want to give a special thanks to my editors at Elsevier, Pamela Hetherington and Sabina Borza, for their keen insights, great advice, and amazing work ethic.

Steven D. Waldman, MD, JD

CONTENTS

SECTION 1 • **Headache Pain Syndromes**

1 ACUTE HERPES ZOSTER OF THE FIRST DIVISION OF THE TRIGEMINAL NERVE   1

2 MIGRAINE HEADACHE   5

3 TENSION-TYPE HEADACHE   8

4 CLUSTER HEADACHE   11

5 SWIMMER'S HEADACHE   14

6 ANALGESIC REBOUND HEADACHE   17

7 OCCIPITAL NEURALGIA   19

8 PSEUDOTUMOR CEREBRI   22

9 INTRACRANIAL SUBARACHNOID HEMORRHAGE   25

SECTION 2 • **Facial Pain Syndromes**

10 TRIGEMINAL NEURALGIA   29

11 TEMPOROMANDIBULAR JOINT DYSFUNCTION   33

12 ATYPICAL FACIAL PAIN   36

13 HYOID SYNDROME   39

14 REFLEX SYMPATHETIC DYSTROPHY OF THE FACE   42

SECTION 3 • **Neck and Brachial Plexus Pain Syndromes**

15 CERVICAL FACET SYNDROME   45

16 CERVICAL RADICULOPATHY   48

17 FIBROMYALGIA OF THE CERVICAL MUSCULATURE   52

18 CERVICAL STRAIN   55

19 LONGUS COLLI TENDINITIS   58

20 RETROPHARYNGEAL ABSCESS   61

21 CERVICOTHORACIC INTERSPINOUS BURSITIS   65

22 BRACHIAL PLEXOPATHY   68

23 PANCOAST'S TUMOR SYNDROME   72

24 THORACIC OUTLET SYNDROME   77

SECTION 4 • **Shoulder Pain Syndromes**

25 ARTHRITIS PAIN OF THE SHOULDER   80

26 ACROMIOCLAVICULAR JOINT PAIN   82

27 SUBDELTOID BURSITIS   85

28 BICIPITAL TENDINITIS   88

29 AVASCULAR NECROSIS OF THE GLENOHUMERAL JOINT   91

30 ADHESIVE CAPSULITIS   94

31 BICEPS TENDON TEAR   98

32 SUPRASPINATUS SYNDROME   102

33 ROTATOR CUFF TEAR   105

34 DELTOID SYNDROME   109

35 TERES MAJOR SYNDROME   113

36 SCAPULOCOSTAL SYNDROME   117

SECTION 5 • **Elbow Pain Syndromes**

37 ARTHRITIS PAIN OF THE ELBOW   120

38 TENNIS ELBOW   123

39 GOLFER'S ELBOW   126

40 DISTAL BICEPS TENDON TEAR   129

41 THROWER'S ELBOW   132

42 ANCONEUS SYNDROME   137

43 SUPINATOR SYNDROME   140

44 BRACHIORADIALIS SYNDROME   143

45 ULNAR NERVE ENTRAPMENT AT THE ELBOW   146

46 LATERAL ANTEBRACHIAL CUTANEOUS NERVE ENTRAPMENT AT THE ELBOW   149

47 OSTEOCHONDRITIS DISSECANS OF THE ELBOW   151

48 OLECRANON BURSITIS   154

SECTION 6 • **Wrist Pain Syndromes**

49 ARTHRITIS PAIN OF THE WRIST   157

50 CARPAL TUNNEL SYNDROME   160

51 de QUERVAIN'S TENOSYNOVITIS   164

52 ARTHRITIS PAIN AT THE CARPOMETACARPAL JOINTS   167

53 GANGLION CYSTS OF THE WRIST   170

SECTION 7 • **Hand Pain Syndromes**

54 TRIGGER THUMB   175

55 TRIGGER FINGER   178

56 SESAMOIDITIS OF THE HAND   181

57 PLASTIC BAG PALSY   183

58 CARPAL BOSS SYNDROME   185

59 DUPUYTREN'S CONTRACTURE   188

SECTION 8 • **Chest Wall Pain Syndromes**

60 COSTOSTERNAL SYNDROME   191

61 MANUBRIOSTERNAL SYNDROME   194

62 INTERCOSTAL NEURALGIA   197

63 DIABETIC TRUNCAL NEUROPATHY   200

64 TIETZE'S SYNDROME   203

65 PRECORDIAL CATCH SYNDROME   206

66 FRACTURED RIBS   209

67 POSTTHORACOTOMY PAIN SYNDROME   212

SECTION 9 • **Thoracic Spine Pain Syndromes**

68 ACUTE HERPES ZOSTER OF THE THORACIC DERMATOMES   215

69 COSTOVERTEBRAL JOINT SYNDROME   218

70 POSTHERPETIC NEURALGIA   221

71 THORACIC VERTEBRAL COMPRESSION FRACTURE   224

SECTION 10 • **Abdominal and Groin Pain Syndromes**

72 ACUTE PANCREATITIS   227

73 CHRONIC PANCREATITIS   230

74 ILIOINGUINAL NEURALGIA   233

75 GENITOFEMORAL NEURALGIA   235

SECTION 11 • **Lumbar Spine and Sacroiliac Joint Pain Syndromes**

76 LUMBAR RADICULOPATHY   238

77 LATISSIMUS DORSI SYNDROME   242

78 SPINAL STENOSIS   245

79 ARACHNOIDITIS   248

80 DISKITIS   252

81 SACROILIAC JOINT PAIN   256

SECTION 12 • **Pelvic Pain Syndromes**

82 OSTEITIS PUBIS   260

83 GLUTEUS MAXIMUS SYNDROME   263

84 PIRIFORMIS SYNDROME   266

85 ISCHIOGLUTEAL BURSITIS   269

86 LEVATOR ANI SYNDROME   271

87 COCCYDYNIA   275

SECTION 13 • **Hip and Lower Extremity Pain Syndromes**

88 ARTHRITIS PAIN OF THE HIP   279

89 SNAPPING HIP SYNDROME   282

90 ILIOPECTINEAL BURSITIS   285

91 ISCHIAL BURSITIS   288

92 MERALGIA PARESTHETICA   291

93 PHANTOM LIMB PAIN   294

94 TROCHANTERIC BURSITIS   297

SECTION 14 • **Knee and Distal Lower Extremity Pain Syndromes**

95 ARTHRITIS PAIN OF THE KNEE   300

96 AVASCULAR NECROSIS OF THE KNEE JOINT   303

97 MEDIAL COLLATERAL LIGAMENT SYNDROME   306

98 MEDIAL MENISCAL TEAR   309

99 ANTERIOR CRUCIATE LIGAMENT SYNDROME   313

100 JUMPER'S KNEE   317

101 RUNNER'S KNEE   321

102 SUPRAPATELLAR BURSITIS   325

103 PREPATELLAR BURSITIS   328

104 SUPERFICIAL INFRAPATELLAR BURSITIS   331

105 DEEP INFRAPATELLAR BURSITIS   334

106 OSGOOD-SCHLATTER DISEASE   337

107 BAKER'S CYST OF THE KNEE   341

108 PES ANSERINE BURSITIS   344

109 TENNIS LEG   347

SECTION 15 • **Ankle Pain Syndromes**

110 ARTHRITIS PAIN OF THE ANKLE   349

111 ARTHRITIS OF THE MIDTARSAL JOINTS   351

112 DELTOID LIGAMENT STRAIN   353

113 ANTERIOR TARSAL TUNNEL SYNDROME   356

114 POSTERIOR TARSAL TUNNEL SYNDROME   359

115 ACHILLES TENDINITIS   362

116 ACHILLES TENDON RUPTURE   365

SECTION 16 • **Foot Pain Syndromes**

117 ARTHRITIS PAIN OF THE TOES   368

118 BUNION PAIN   370

119 MORTON'S NEUROMA   372

120 FREIBERG'S DISEASE   374

121 PLANTAR FASCIITIS   377

122 CALCANEAL SPUR SYNDROME   380

123 MALLET TOE   383

124 HAMMER TOE   385

Chapter **1**

ACUTE HERPES ZOSTER OF THE FIRST DIVISION OF THE TRIGEMINAL NERVE

ICD-9 CODE `053.12`

ICD-10 CODE `B02.22`

THE CLINICAL SYNDROME

Herpes zoster is an infectious disease caused by the varicella-zoster virus (VZV). Primary infection with VZV in a nonimmune host manifests clinically as the childhood disease chickenpox (varicella). Investigators have postulated that during the course of this primary infection, the virus migrates to the dorsal root or cranial ganglia, where it remains dormant and produces no clinically evident disease. In some individuals, the virus reactivates and travels along the sensory pathways of the first division of the trigeminal nerve, where it produces the characteristic pain and skin lesions of herpes zoster, or shingles.

Why reactivation occurs in some individuals but not in others is not fully understood, but investigators have theorized that a decrease in cell-mediated immunity may play an important role in the evolution of this disease by allowing the virus to multiply in the ganglia, spread to the corresponding sensory nerves, and produce clinical disease. Patients who are suffering from malignant disease (particularly lymphoma) or chronic disease and those receiving immunosuppressive therapy (chemotherapy, steroids, radiation) are generally debilitated and thus are much more likely than the healthy population to develop acute herpes zoster. These patients all have in common a decreased cell-mediated immune response, which may also explain why the incidence of shingles increases dramatically in patients older than 60 years and is relatively uncommon in those younger than 20 years.

The first division of the trigeminal nerve is the second most common site for the development of acute herpes zoster, after the thoracic dermatomes. Rarely, the virus attacks the geniculate ganglion and results in hearing loss, vesicles in the ear, and pain (Fig. 1-1). This constellation of symptoms is called Ramsay Hunt syndrome and must be distinguished from acute herpes zoster involving the first division of the trigeminal nerve.

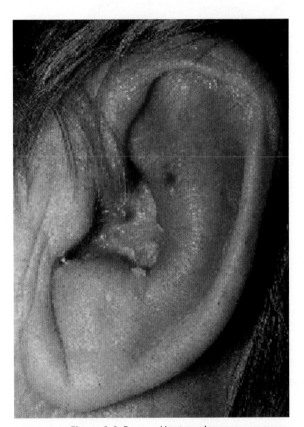

Figure 1-1 Ramsay Hunt syndrome.

SIGNS AND SYMPTOMS

As viral reactivation occurs, ganglionitis and peripheral neuritis cause pain that may be accompanied by flulike symptoms. The pain generally progresses from a dull, aching sensation to dysesthetic or neuritic pain in the distribution of the first division of the trigeminal nerve. In most patients, the pain of acute herpes zoster precedes the eruption of rash by 3 to 7 days, and this delay often leads to an erroneous diagnosis (see "Differential Diagnosis"). However, in most patients, the clinical diagnosis of shingles is readily made when the characteristic rash appears. As with chickenpox, the rash of herpes zoster appears in crops of macular lesions that rapidly progress to papules and then to vesicles (Fig. 1-2). Eventually, the vesicles coalesce, and crusting occurs. The affected area can be extremely painful, and the pain tends to be exacerbated by any movement or contact (e.g., with clothing or sheets). As the lesions heal, the crust falls away, leaving pink scars that gradually become hypopigmented and atrophic.

In most patients, the hyperesthesia and pain resolve as the skin lesions heal. In some patients, however, pain persists beyond lesion healing. This common and feared complication of acute herpes zoster is called postherpetic neuralgia, and older persons are affected at a higher rate than is the general population suffering from acute herpes zoster (Fig. 1-3). The symptoms of postherpetic neuralgia can vary from a mild, self-limited condition to a debilitating, constantly burning pain that is exacerbated by light touch,

movement, anxiety, or temperature change. This unremitting pain may be so severe that it completely devastates the patient's life; ultimately, it can lead to suicide. To avoid this disastrous sequela to a usually benign, self-limited disease, the clinician must use all possible therapeutic efforts in patients with acute herpes zoster of the trigeminal nerve.

TESTING

Although in most instances the diagnosis is easily made on clinical grounds, confirmatory testing is occasionally required. Such testing may be desirable in patients with other skin lesions that confuse the clinical picture, such as in patients with acquired immunodeficiency syndrome who are suffering from Kaposi's sarcoma. In such patients, the diagnosis of acute herpes zoster may be confirmed by obtaining a Tzanck smear from the base of a fresh vesicle; this smear reveals multinucleated giant cells and eosinophilic inclusions (Fig. 1-4). To differentiate acute herpes zoster from localized herpes simplex infection, the clinician can obtain fluid from a fresh vesicle and submit it for immunofluorescent testing.

DIFFERENTIAL DIAGNOSIS

A careful initial evaluation, including a thorough history and physical examination, is indicated in all patients suffering from acute herpes zoster of the trigeminal nerve. The goal is to rule out occult malignant or systemic disease that may be responsible for the patient's immunocompromised state. A prompt diagnosis allows early recognition of changes in clinical status that may presage the development of complications, including myelitis or dissemination of the disease. Other causes of pain in the distribution of the first division of the trigeminal nerve include trigeminal neuralgia, sinus disease, glaucoma, retro-orbital tumor, inflammatory disease (e.g., Tolosa-Hunt syndrome), and intracranial disease, including tumor.

TREATMENT

The therapeutic challenge in patients presenting with acute herpes zoster of the trigeminal nerve is twofold: (1) the immediate relief of acute pain and symptoms and (2) the prevention of complications, including postherpetic neuralgia. Most pain specialists agree that the earlier treatment is initiated, the less likely it is that

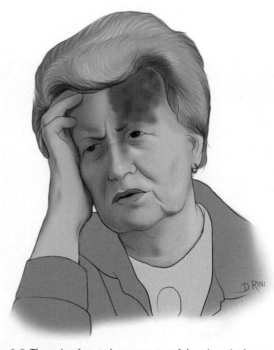

Figure 1-2 The pain of acute herpes zoster of the trigeminal nerve often precedes the characteristic vesicular rash.

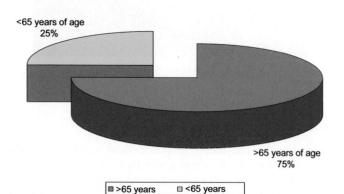

Figure 1-3 Age of patients suffering from acute herpes zoster.

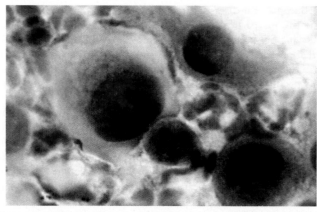

Figure 1-4 Tzanck smear showing giant multinucleated cell. *(Courtesy of Dr. John Minarcik.)*

postherpetic neuralgia will develop. Further, because older individuals are at the highest risk for developing postherpetic neuralgia, early and aggressive treatment of this group of patients is mandatory.

Nerve Block

Sympathetic neural blockade with local anesthetic and steroid through stellate ganglion block is the treatment of choice to relieve the symptoms of acute herpes zoster of the trigeminal nerve, as well as to prevent postherpetic neuralgia. As vesicular crusting occurs, the steroid may also reduce neural scarring. Sympathetic nerve block is thought to achieve these goals by blocking the profound sympathetic stimulation caused by viral inflammation of the nerve and gasserian ganglion. If untreated, this sympathetic hyperactivity can cause ischemia secondary to decreased blood flow of the intraneural capillary bed. If this ischemia is allowed to persist, endoneural edema forms, thus increasing endoneural pressure and causing a further reduction in endoneural blood flow, with irreversible nerve damage.

These sympathetic blocks should be continued aggressively until the patient is pain free and should be reimplemented if the pain returns. Failure to use sympathetic neural blockade immediately and aggressively, especially in older patients, may sentence the patient to a lifetime of suffering from postherpetic neuralgia. Occasionally, some patients do not experience pain relief from stellate ganglion block but do respond to blockade of the trigeminal nerve.

Opioid Analgesics

Opioid analgesics can be useful to relieve the aching pain that is common during the acute stages of herpes zoster, while sympathetic nerve blocks are being implemented. Opioids are less effective in relieving neuritic pain, which is also common. Careful administration of potent, long-acting opioid analgesics (e.g., oral morphine elixir, methadone) on a time-contingent rather than an as-needed basis may be a beneficial adjunct to the pain relief provided by sympathetic neural blockade. Because many patients suffering from acute herpes zoster are older or have severe multisystem disease, close monitoring for the potential side effects of potent opioid analgesics (e.g., confusion or dizziness, which may cause a patient to fall) is warranted. Daily dietary fiber supplementation and Milk of Magnesia should be started along with opioid analgesics to prevent constipation.

Adjuvant Analgesics

The anticonvulsant gabapentin represents a first-line treatment for the neuritic pain of acute herpes zoster of the trigeminal nerve. Studies suggest that gabapentin may also help prevent postherpetic neuralgia. Treatment with gabapentin should begin early in the course of the disease; this drug may be used concurrently with neural blockade, opioid analgesics, and other adjuvant analgesics, including antidepressants, if care is taken to avoid central nervous system side effects. Gabapentin is started at a bedtime dose of 300 mg and is titrated upward in 300-mg increments to a maximum of 3600 mg given in divided doses, as side effects allow. Pregabalin represents a reasonable alternative to gabapentin and is better tolerated in some patients. Pregabalin is started at 50 mg three times a day and may be titrated upward to 100 mg three times a day as side effects allow. Because pregabalin is excreted primarily by the kidneys, the dosage should be decreased in patients with compromised renal function.

Carbamazepine should be considered in patients suffering from severe neuritic pain who fail to respond to nerve blocks and gabapentin. If this drug is used, strict monitoring of hematologic parameters is indicated, especially in patients receiving chemotherapy or radiation therapy. Phenytoin may also be beneficial to treat neuritic pain, but it should not be used in patients with lymphoma; the drug may induce a pseudolymphoma-like state that is difficult to distinguish from the actual lymphoma.

Antidepressants may also be useful adjuncts in the initial treatment of patients suffering from acute herpes zoster. On a short-term basis, these drugs help alleviate the significant sleep disturbance that is commonly seen. In addition, antidepressants may be valuable in ameliorating the neuritic component of the pain, which is treated less effectively with opioid analgesics. After several weeks of treatment, antidepressants may exert a mood-elevating effect, which may be desirable in some patients. Care must be taken to observe closely for central nervous system side effects in this patient population. In addition, these drugs may cause urinary retention and constipation, which may mistakenly be attributed to herpes zoster myelitis.

Antiviral Agents

A few antiviral agents, including valacyclovir, famciclovir, and acyclovir, can shorten the course of acute herpes zoster and may even help prevent the development of postherpetic neuralgia. They are probably useful in attenuating the disease in immunosuppressed patients. These antiviral agents can be used in conjunction with the aforementioned treatment modalities. Careful monitoring for side effects is mandatory.

Adjunctive Treatments

The application of ice packs to the lesions of acute herpes zoster may provide relief in some patients. Application of heat increases pain in most patients, presumably because of the increased conduction of small fibers; however, it is beneficial in an occasional patient and may be worth trying if the application of cold is ineffective. Transcutaneous electrical nerve stimulation and vibration may also be effective in a limited number of patients. The favorable risk-to-benefit ratio of these modalities makes them reasonable alternatives for patients who cannot or will not undergo sympathetic neural blockade or cannot tolerate pharmacologic interventions.

Topical application of aluminum sulfate as a tepid soak provides excellent drying of the crusting and weeping lesions of acute herpes zoster, and most patients find these soaks soothing. Zinc oxide ointment may also be used as a protective agent, especially during the healing phase, when temperature sensitivity is a problem. Disposable diapers can be used as absorbent padding to protect healing lesions from contact with clothing and sheets.

COMPLICATIONS AND PITFALLS

In most patients, acute herpes zoster of the trigeminal nerve is a self-limited disease. In older patients and in immunosuppressed patients, however, complications may occur. Cutaneous and visceral dissemination may range from a mild rash resembling chickenpox to an overwhelming, life-threatening infection in those already suffering from severe multisystem disease. Myelitis may cause bowel, bladder, and lower extremity paresis. Ocular complications of trigeminal nerve involvement may range from severe photophobia to keratitis with loss of sight.

Clinical Pearls

Because the pain of herpes zoster usually precedes the eruption of skin lesions by 3 to 7 days, some other painful condition (e.g., trigeminal neuralgia, glaucoma) may erroneously be diagnosed. In this setting, an astute clinician should advise the patient to call immediately if a rash appears, because acute herpes zoster is a possibility. Some pain specialists believe that in a few immunocompetent patients, when reactivation of VZV occurs, a rapid immune response attenuates the natural course of the disease, and the characteristic rash of acute herpes zoster may not appear. In this case, pain in the distribution of the first division of the trigeminal nerve without an associated rash is called zoster sine herpete and is, by necessity, a diagnosis of exclusion. Therefore, other causes of head pain must be ruled out before this diagnosis is invoked.

SUGGESTED READINGS

Dworkin RH, Nagasako EM, Johnson RW, et al: Acute pain in herpes zoster: the famciclovir database project, *Pain* 94(1):113–119, 2001.

Easton HG: Zoster sine herpete causing acute trigeminal neuralgia, *Lancet* 2(7682):1065–1066, 1970.

Waldman SD: Postherpetic neuralgia. In *Pain review*, Philadelphia, 2009, Saunders, pp 365–366.

Waldman SD: Acute herpes zoster and postherpetic neuralgia. *Pain management*, Philadelphia, 2007, Saunders, pp 279–282.

Chapter 2

MIGRAINE HEADACHE

ICD-9 CODE **346.00**

ICD-10 CODE **G43.109**

THE CLINICAL SYNDROME

Migraine headache is a periodic unilateral headache that may begin in childhood but almost always develops before age 30 years. Attacks occur with variable frequency, ranging from every few days to once every several months. More frequent migraine headaches are often associated with a phenomenon called analgesic rebound. Between 60% and 70% of patients who suffer from migraine are female, and many report a family history of migraine headache. The personality type of migraineurs has been described as meticulous, neat, compulsive, and often rigid. They tend to be obsessive in their daily routines and often find it hard to cope with the stresses of everyday life. Migraine headache may be triggered by changes in sleep patterns or diet or by the ingestion of tyramine-containing foods, monosodium glutamate, nitrates, chocolate, or citrus fruits. Changes in endogenous and exogenous hormones, such as with the use of birth control pills, can also trigger migraine headache. Approximately 20% of patients suffering from migraine headache also experience a neurologic event before the onset of pain called an aura. The aura most often takes the form of a visual disturbance, but it may also manifest as an alteration in smell or hearing; these are called olfactory and auditory auras, respectively.

SIGNS AND SYMPTOMS

Migraine headache is, by definition, a unilateral headache. Although the headache may change sides with each episode, the headache is never bilateral. The pain of migraine headache is usually periorbital or retro-orbital. It is pounding, and its intensity is severe. The time from onset to peak of migraine pain is short, ranging from 20 minutes to 1 hour. In contradistinction to tension-type headache, migraine headache is often associated with systemic symptoms, including nausea and vomiting, photophobia, and sonophobia, as well as alterations in appetite, mood, and libido. Menstruation is a common trigger of migraine headache.

As mentioned, in approximately 20% of patients, migraine headache is preceded by an aura (called migraine with aura). The aura is thought to be the result of ischemia of specific regions of the cerebral cortex. A visual aura often occurs 30 to 60 minutes before the onset of headache pain; this may take the form of blind spots, called scotoma, or a zigzag disruption of the visual field, called fortification spectrum. Occasionally, patients with migraine lose an entire visual field during the aura. Auditory auras usually take the form of hypersensitivity to sound, but other alterations of hearing, such as sounds perceived as farther away than they

actually are, have also been reported. Olfactory auras may take the form of strong odors of substances that are not actually present or extreme hypersensitivity to otherwise normal odors, such as coffee or copy machine toner. Migraine that manifests without other neurologic symptoms is called migraine without aura.

Rarely, patients who suffer from migraine experience prolonged neurologic dysfunction associated with the headache pain. Such neurologic dysfunction may last for more than 24 hours and is termed migraine with prolonged aura. These patients are at risk for the development of permanent neurologic deficit, and risk factors such as hypertension, smoking, and oral contraceptives must be addressed. Even less common than migraine with prolonged aura is migraine with complex aura. Patients suffering from migraine with complex aura experience significant neurologic dysfunction that may include aphasia or hemiplegia. As with migraine with prolonged aura, patients suffering from migraine with complex aura may develop permanent neurologic deficits.

Patients suffering from all forms of migraine headache appear systemically ill (Fig. 2-1). Pallor, tremulousness, diaphoresis, and

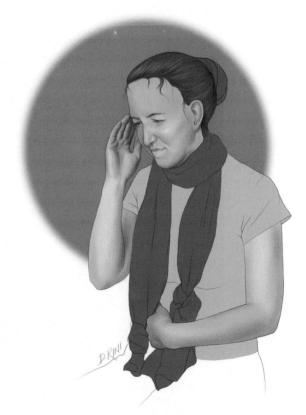

Figure 2-1 Migraine headache is an episodic, unilateral headache that occurs more commonly in female patients.

light sensitivity are common physical findings. The temporal artery and the surrounding area may be tender. If an aura is present, results of the neurologic examination will be abnormal; the neurologic examination is usually within normal limits before, during, and after migraine without aura.

TESTING

No specific test exists for migraine headache. Testing is aimed primarily at identifying occult pathologic processes or other diseases that may mimic migraine headache (see "Differential Diagnosis"). All patients with a recent onset of headache thought to be migraine should undergo magnetic resonance imaging (MRI) of the brain. If neurologic dysfunction accompanies the patient's headache symptoms, MRI should be performed with and without gadolinium contrast medium (Fig. 2-2); magnetic resonance angiography should be considered as well. MRI should also be performed in patients with previously stable migraine headaches who experience an inexplicable change in symptoms. Screening laboratory tests, including an erythrocyte sedimentation rate, complete blood count, and automated blood chemistry, should be performed if the diagnosis of migraine is in question. Ophthalmologic evaluation is indicated in patients who experience significant ocular symptoms.

DIFFERENTIAL DIAGNOSIS

The diagnosis of migraine headache is usually made on clinical grounds by obtaining a targeted headache history. Tension-type headache is often confused with migraine headache, and this misdiagnosis can lead to illogical treatment plans because these two headache syndromes are managed quite differently. Table 2-1 distinguishes migraine headache from tension-type headache and should help clarify the diagnosis.

Diseases of the eyes, ears, nose, and sinuses may also mimic migraine headache. The targeted history and physical examination, combined with appropriate testing, should allow the clinician to identify and properly treat any underlying diseases of these organ systems. The following conditions may all mimic migraine and must be considered when treating patients with headache: glaucoma; temporal arteritis; sinusitis; intracranial disease, including chronic subdural hematoma, tumor (see Fig. 2-2), brain abscess, hydrocephalus, and pseudotumor cerebri; and inflammatory conditions, including sarcoidosis.

TABLE 2-1

Comparison of Migraine Headache and Tension-Type Headache

	Migraine Headache	Tension-Type Headache
Onset-to-peak interval	Minutes to 1 hr	Hours to days
Frequency	Rarely >1/wk	Often daily or continuous
Location	Temporal	Nuchal or circumferential
Character	Pounding	Aching, pressure, bandlike
Laterality	Always unilateral	Usually bilateral
Aura	May be present	Never present
Nausea and vomiting	Common	Rare
Duration	Usually <24 hr	Often days

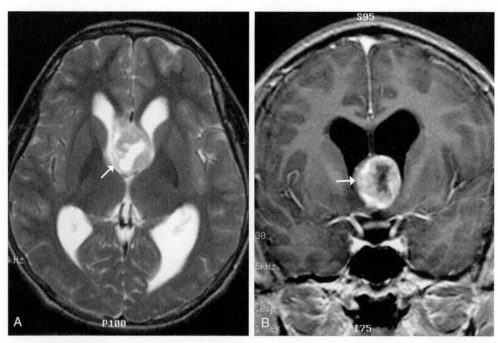

Figure 2-2 Glioblastoma multiforme involving the septum pellucidum. **A,** Axial T2-weighted magnetic resonance imaging (MRI) through the inferior aspect of the frontal horns of the lateral ventricles. An ovoid, heterogeneously hyperintense mass *(arrow)* arising from the inferior aspect of the septum pellucidum indents and partially occludes the frontal horns bilaterally. Note the irregularly marginated intratumoral hyperintensity, suggesting central necrosis. **B,** Following intravenous administration of gadolinium, coronal T1-weighted MRI demonstrates intense contrast enhancement *(arrow)* of the thick peripheral rind, with nonenhancement of the central cavity. *(From Haaga JR, Lanzieri CF, Gilkeson RC, editors: CT and MR imaging of the whole body, ed 4, Philadelphia, 2003, Mosby, p 140.)*

TREATMENT

When deciding how best to treat a patient suffering from migraine, the clinician should consider the frequency and severity of the headaches, their effect on the patient's lifestyle, the presence of focal or prolonged neurologic disturbances, the results of previous testing and treatment, any history of previous drug abuse or misuse, and the presence of other systemic diseases (e.g., peripheral vascular or coronary artery disease) that may preclude the use of certain treatment modalities.

If the patient's migraine headaches occur infrequently, a trial of abortive therapy may be warranted. However, if the headaches occur with greater frequency or cause the patient to miss work or be hospitalized, prophylactic therapy is warranted.

Abortive Therapy

For abortive therapy to be effective, it must be initiated at the first sign of headache. This is often difficult because of the short interval between the onset and peak of migraine headache, coupled with the problem that migraine sufferers often experience nausea and vomiting that may limit the use of oral medications. By altering the route of administration to parenteral or transmucosal, this situation can be avoided.

Abortive medications that can be considered in patients with migraine headache include compounds that contain isomethepene mucate (e.g., Midrin), the nonsteroidal antiinflammatory drug (NSAID) naproxen, ergot alkaloids, the triptans including sumatriptan, and intravenous lidocaine combined with antiemetic compounds. The inhalation of 100% oxygen may abort migraine headache, and sphenopalatine ganglion block with local anesthetic may be effective. Caffeine-containing preparations, barbiturates, ergotamines, triptans, and opioids have a propensity to cause a phenomenon called analgesic rebound headache, which may ultimately be more difficult to treat than the original migraine. The ergotamines and triptans should not be used in patients with coexistent peripheral vascular disease, coronary artery disease, or hypertension.

Prophylactic Therapy

For most patients with migraine headache, prophylactic therapy is a better option than abortive therapy. The mainstay of prophylactic therapy is β-blocking agents. Propranolol and most other drugs in this class can control or decrease the frequency and intensity of migraine headache and help prevent auras. An 80-mg daily dose of the long-acting formulation is a reasonable starting point for most patients with migraine. Propranolol should not be used in patients with asthma or other reactive airway diseases.

Valproic acid, calcium channel blockers (e.g., verapamil), clonidine, tricyclic antidepressants, and NSAIDs have also been used for the prophylaxis of migraine headache. Each of these drugs has advantages and disadvantages, and the clinician should tailor a treatment plan that best meets the needs of the individual patient.

COMPLICATIONS AND PITFALLS

In most patients, migraine headache is a painful but not life-threatening disease. However, patients who suffer from migraine with prolonged aura or migraine with complex aura are at risk for the development of permanent neurologic deficits. Such patients are best treated by headache specialists who are familiar with these unique risks and are better equipped to deal with them. Occasionally, prolonged nausea and vomiting associated with severe migraine headache may result in dehydration that necessitates hospitalization and treatment with intravenous fluids.

Clinical Pearls

The most common reason for a patient's lack of response to traditional treatment for migraine headache is that the patient is actually suffering from tension-type headache, analgesic rebound headache, or a combination of headache syndromes. The clinician must be sure that the patient is not taking significant doses of over-the-counter headache preparations containing caffeine or other vasoactive drugs such as barbiturates, ergots, or triptans that may cause analgesic rebound headache. Until these drugs are withdrawn, the patient's headache will not improve.

SUGGESTED READINGS

Abel M: Migraine headaches: diagnosis and management, *Optometry* 80(3):138–148, 2009.

Aurora SK: Pathophysiology of migraine and cluster headaches, *Semin Pain Med* 2(2):62–71, 2004.

Chang M, Rapoport AM: Acute treatment of migraine headache, *Tech Reg Anesth Pain Manag* 13(1):9–15, 2009.

Evans RW: Diagnostic testing for migraine and other primary headaches, *Neurol Clin* 27(2):393–415, 2009.

Diamond S, Nissan G: Acute headache. In Waldman SD, editor: *Pain management*, Philadelphia, 2007, Saunders, pp 2262–2267.

Waldman SD: Migraine headache. In *Pain review*, Philadelphia, 2009, Saunders, pp 213–215.

Chapter 3

TENSION-TYPE HEADACHE

ICD-9 CODE 307.81

ICD-10 CODE G44.209

THE CLINICAL SYNDROME

Tension-type headache, formerly known as muscle contraction headache, is the most common type of headache that afflicts humankind. It can be episodic or chronic, and it may or may not be related to muscle contraction. Significant sleep disturbance usually occurs. Patients with tension-type headache are often characterized as having multiple unresolved conflicts surrounding work, marriage, social relationships, and psychosexual difficulties. Testing with the Minnesota Multiphasic Personality Inventory in large groups of patients with tension-type headache revealed not only borderline depression but somatization as well. Most researchers believe that this somatization takes the form of abnormal muscle contraction in some patients; in others, it results in simple headache.

SIGNS AND SYMPTOMS

Tension-type headache is usually bilateral but can be unilateral, and it often involves the frontal, temporal, and occipital regions (Fig. 3-1). It may present as a bandlike, nonpulsatile ache or tightness in the aforementioned anatomic areas. Associated neck symptoms are common. Tension-type headache evolves over a period of hours or days and then tends to remain constant, without progression. It has no associated aura, but significant sleep disturbance is usually present. This disturbance may manifest as difficulty falling asleep, frequent awakening at night, or early awakening. These headaches most frequently occur between 4 and 8 AM and 4 and 8 PM. Although both sexes are affected, female patients predominate. No hereditary pattern to tension-type headache has no hereditary pattern, but this type of headache may occur in family clusters because children mimic and learn the pain behavior of their parents.

The triggering event for acute, episodic tension-type headache is invariably either physical or psychological stress. This may take the form of a fight with a coworker or spouse or an exceptionally heavy workload. Physical stress such as a long drive, working with the neck in a strained position, acute cervical spine injury resulting from whiplash, or prolonged exposure to the glare from a cathode ray tube may precipitate a headache. A worsening of preexisting degenerative cervical spine conditions, such as cervical spondylosis, can also trigger a tension-type headache. The pathologic process responsible for the development of tension-type headache can produce temporomandibular joint dysfunction as well.

TESTING

No specific test exists for tension-type headache. Testing is aimed primarily at identifying an occult pathologic process or other diseases that may mimic tension-type headache (see "Differential Diagnosis"). All patients with the recent onset of headache that is thought to be tension type should undergo

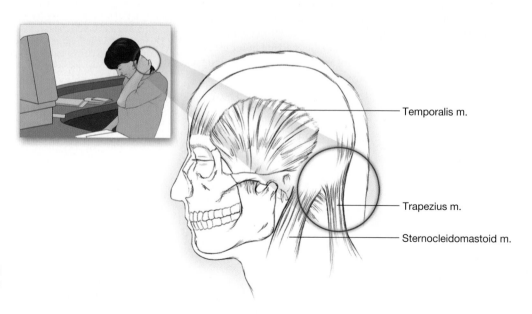

Temporalis m.

Trapezius m.

Sternocleidomastoid m.

Figure 3-1 Mental or physical stress is often the precipitating factor in tension-type headache.

magnetic resonance imaging (MRI) of the brain and, if significant occipital or nuchal symptoms are present, of the cervical spine. MRI should also be performed in patients with previously stable tension-type headaches who have experienced a recent change in symptoms. Screening laboratory tests consisting of a complete blood count, erythrocyte sedimentation rate, and automated blood chemistry should be performed if the diagnosis of tension-type headache is in question.

DIFFERENTIAL DIAGNOSIS

Tension-type headache is usually diagnosed on clinical grounds by obtaining a targeted headache history. Despite their obvious differences, tension-type headache is often incorrectly diagnosed as migraine headache. Such misdiagnosis can lead to illogical treatment plans and poor control of headache symptoms. Table 3-1 helps distinguish tension-type headache from migraine headache and should aid the clinician in making the correct diagnosis.

Diseases of the cervical spine and surrounding soft tissues may also mimic tension-type headache. Arnold-Chiari malformations may manifest clinically as tension-type headache, but these malformations can be easily identified on images of the posterior fossa and cervical spine (Fig. 3-2). Occasionally, frontal sinusitis is confused with tension-type headache, although individuals with acute frontal sinusitis appear systemically ill. Temporal arteritis, chronic subdural hematoma, and other intracranial disease such as tumor may be incorrectly diagnosed as tension-type headache.

TREATMENT

Abortive Therapy

In determining the best treatment, the physician must consider the frequency and severity of the headaches, their effect on the patient's lifestyle, the results of any previous therapy, and any prior drug misuse or abuse. If the patient suffers an attack of tension-type headache only once every 1 or 2 months, the condition can often be managed by teaching the patient to reduce or avoid stress. Analgesics or nonsteroidal antiinflammatory drugs (NSAIDs) can provide symptomatic relief during acute attacks. Combination analgesic drugs used concomitantly with barbiturates or opioid analgesics have no place in the management of patients with headache. The risk of abuse and dependence more than outweighs any theoretical benefit. The physician should also avoid an abortive treatment approach in patients with a prior history of drug misuse or abuse. Many drugs, including simple analgesics and NSAIDs, can produce serious consequences if they are abused.

TABLE 3-1		
Comparison of Tension-Type Headache and Migraine Headache		
	Tension-Type Headache	**Migraine Headache**
Onset-to-peak interval	Hours to days	Minutes to 1 hr
Frequency	Often daily or continuous	Rarely >1/wk
Location	Nuchal or circumferential	Temporal
Character	Aching, pressure, bandlike	Pounding
Laterality	Usually bilateral	Always unilateral
Aura	Never present	May be present
Nausea and vomiting	Rare	Common
Duration	Often days	Usually <24 hr

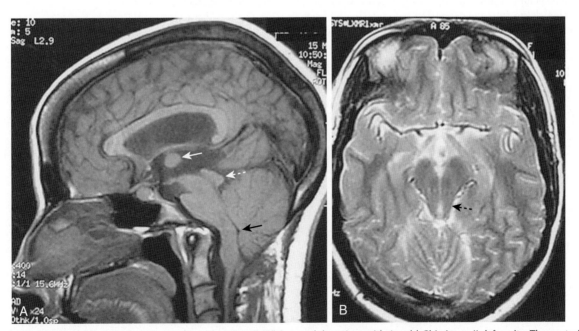

Figure 3-2 **A,** Sagittal T1-weighted magnetic resonance imaging (MRI) in an adult patient with Arnold-Chiari type II deformity. The posterior fossa is small with a widened foramen magnum. Inferior displacement of the cerebellum and medulla with elongation of the pons and fourth ventricle *(black arrow)* is evident. The brainstem is kinked as it passes over the back of the odontoid. An enlarged massa with intermedia *(white arrow)* and beaking of the tectum *(broken white arrow)* are visible. **B,** Axial T2-weighted MRI shows the small posterior fossa with beaking of the tectum *(broken black arrow)*. *(From Waldman SD, Campbell RSD:* Imaging of pain, *Philadelphia, 2011, Saunders, p 30.)*

Prophylactic Therapy

If the headaches occur more frequently than once every 1 or 2 months or are so severe that the patient repeatedly misses work or social engagements, prophylactic therapy is indicated.

Antidepressants

Antidepressants are generally the drugs of choice for the prophylactic treatment of tension-type headache. These drugs not only help decrease the frequency and intensity of headaches but also normalize sleep patterns and treat any underlying depression. Patients should be educated about the potential side effects of this class of drugs, including sedation, dry mouth, blurred vision, constipation, and urinary retention. Patients should also be told that relief of headache pain generally takes 3 to 4 weeks. However, normalization of sleep occurs immediately, and this may be enough to provide a noticeable improvement in headache symptoms.

Amitriptyline, started at a single bedtime dose of 25 mg, is a reasonable initial choice. The dose may be increased in 25-mg increments as side effects allow. Other drugs that can be considered if the patient does not tolerate the sedative and anticholinergic effects of amitriptyline include trazodone (75 to 300 mg at bedtime) or fluoxetine (20 to 40 mg at lunchtime). Because of the sedating nature of these drugs (with the exception of fluoxetine), they must be used with caution in older patients and in others who are at risk for falling. Care should also be exercised when using these drugs in patients who are prone to cardiac arrhythmias, because these drugs may be arrhythmogenic. Simple analgesics or longer-acting NSAIDs may be used with antidepressant compounds to treat exacerbations of headache pain.

Biofeedback

Monitored relaxation training combined with patient education about coping strategies and stress-reduction techniques may be of value in some tension-type headache sufferers who are adequately motivated. Patient selection is of paramount importance if good results are to be achieved. If the patient is significantly depressed, it may be beneficial to treat the depression before trying biofeedback. The use of biofeedback may allow the patient to control the headaches while avoiding the side effects of medications.

Cervical Epidural Nerve Block

Multiple studies have demonstrated the efficacy of cervical epidural nerve block with steroid in providing long-term relief of tension-type headaches in patients for whom all other treatment modalities have failed. This treatment can also be used while waiting for antidepressant compounds to become effective. Cervical epidural nerve block can be performed on a daily to weekly basis, depending on clinical symptoms.

COMPLICATIONS AND PITFALLS

A few patients with tension-type headache have major depression or uncontrolled anxiety states in addition to a chemical dependence on opioid analgesics, barbiturates, minor tranquilizers, or alcohol. Attempts to treat these patients in the outpatient setting is disappointing and frustrating. Inpatient treatment in a specialized headache unit or psychiatric setting results in more rapid amelioration of the underlying and coexisting problems and allows the concurrent treatment of headache. Monoamine oxidase inhibitors can often reduce the frequency and severity of tension-type headache in this subset of patients. Phenelzine, at a dosage of 15 mg three times a day, is usually effective. After 2 to 3 weeks, the dosage is tapered to an appropriate maintenance dose of 5 to 10 mg three times a day. Monoamine oxidase inhibitors can produce life-threatening hypertensive crises if special diets are not followed or if these drugs are combined with some commonly used prescription or over-the-counter medications. Therefore, their use should be limited to highly reliable and compliant patients. Physicians prescribing this potentially dangerous group of drugs should be well versed in how to use them safely.

Clinical Pearls

> Although tension-type (muscle contraction) headache occurs frequently, it is commonly misdiagnosed as migraine headache. By obtaining a targeted headache history and performing a targeted physical examination, the physician can make a diagnosis with a high degree of certainty. The avoidance of addicting medications, coupled with the appropriate use of pharmacologic and nonpharmacologic therapies, should result in excellent palliation and long-term control of pain in most patients suffering from this headache syndrome.

SUGGESTED READINGS

Ashina S, Bendtsen L, Jensen R: Analgesic effect of amitriptyline in chronic tension-type headache is not directly related to serotonin reuptake inhibition, *Pain* 108(1–2):108–114, 2004.

Bendtsen L, Jensen R: Tension-type headache, *Neurol Clin* 27(2):525–535, 2009.

Diamond S, Nissan G: Acute headache. In Waldman SD, editor: *Pain management*, Philadelphia, 2007, Saunders, pp 2262–2267.

Evans RW: Diagnostic testing for migraine and other primary headaches, *Neurol Clin* 27(2):393–415, 2009.

McGeeney BE: Tension-type headache, *Tech Reg Anesth Pain Manag* 13(1):16–19, 2009.

Waldman SD: Cervical epidural block: translaminar approach. In *Atlas of interventional pain management*, ed 3, Philadelphia, 2009, Saunders, p 174.

Waldman SD: Tension-type headache. In *Pain review*, Philadelphia, 2009, Saunders, pp 209–210.

Chapter 4

CLUSTER HEADACHE

ICD-9 CODE **339.00**

ICD-10 CODE **G44.009**

THE CLINICAL SYNDROME

Cluster headache derives its name from the headache pattern—that is, headaches occur in clusters, followed by headache-free remission periods. Unlike other common headache disorders that affect primarily female patients, cluster headache is much more common in male patients, with a male-to-female ratio of 5:1. Much less common than tension-type headache or migraine headache, cluster headache is thought to affect approximately 0.5% of the male population. Cluster headache is most often confused with migraine by clinicians who are unfamiliar with the syndrome; however, a targeted headache history allows the clinician to distinguish between these two distinct headache types easily (Table 4-1).

The onset of cluster headache occurs in the late third or early fourth decade of life, in contradistinction to migraine, which almost always manifests by the early second decade. Unlike migraine, cluster headache does not appear to run in families, and cluster headache sufferers do not experience auras. Attacks generally occur approximately 90 minutes after the patient falls asleep. This association with sleep is reportedly maintained when a shift worker changes from nighttime to daytime hours of sleep. Cluster headache also appears to follow a distinct chronobiologic pattern that coincides with seasonal changes in the length of the day. This pattern results in an increased frequency of cluster headache in the spring and fall.

During a cluster period, attacks occur two or three times a day and last for 45 minutes to 1 hour. Cluster periods usually last for 8 to 12 weeks, interrupted by remission periods of less than 2 years. In rare patients, the remission periods become shorter and shorter, and the frequency may increase up to 10-fold. This situation is termed chronic cluster headache and differs from the more common episodic cluster headache described earlier.

SIGNS AND SYMPTOMS

Cluster headache is characterized as a unilateral headache that is retro-orbital and temporal in location. The pain has a deep burning or boring quality. Physical findings during an attack of cluster headache may include Horner's syndrome, consisting of ptosis, abnormal pupil constriction, facial flushing, and conjunctival injection (Fig. 4-1). Additionally, profuse lacrimation and rhinorrhea are often present. The ocular changes may become permanent with repeated attacks. Peau d'orange skin over the malar region, deeply furrowed glabellar folds, and telangiectasia may be observed.

Attacks of cluster headache may be provoked by small amounts of alcohol, nitrates, histamines, and other vasoactive substances, as well as occasionally by high altitude. When the attack is in progress, the patient may be unable to lie still and may pace or rock back and forth in a chair. This behavior contrasts with that characterizing other headache syndromes, during which patients seek relief by lying down in a dark, quiet room.

TABLE 4-1		
Comparison of Cluster Headache and Migraine Headache		
	Cluster Headache	**Migraine Headache**
Gender	Male 5:1	Female 2:1
Age of onset	Late 30s to early 40s	Menarche to early 20s
Family history	No	Yes
Aura	Never	May be present (20% of the time)
Chronobiologic pattern	Yes	No
Onset-to-peak interval	Seconds to minutes	Minutes to 1 hr
Frequency	2 or 3/day	Rarely >1/wk
Duration	45 min	Usually <24 hr

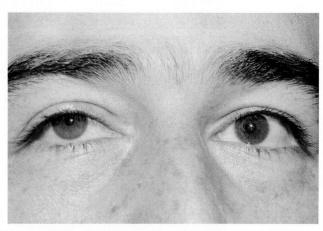

Figure 4-1 Horner's eye findings. Classic clinical eye findings are demonstrated in this patient with a right Horner syndrome (ptosis of the upper eyelid, elevation of the lower eyelid, and miosis). *(From Reede DL, Garcon E, Smoker WR, Kardon R: Horner's syndrome: clinical and radiographic evaluation,* Neuroimaging Clin N Am *18[2]:369–385, 2008.)*

The pain of cluster headache is said to be among the worst pain a human being can suffer. Because of the severity of the pain, the clinician must watch closely for medication overuse or misuse. Suicide has been associated with prolonged, unrelieved attacks of cluster headache.

TESTING

No specific test exists for cluster headache. Testing is aimed primarily at identifying an occult pathologic process or other diseases that may mimic cluster headache (see "Differential Diagnosis"). All patients with a recent onset of headache thought to be cluster headache should undergo magnetic resonance imaging (MRI) of the brain. If neurologic dysfunction accompanies the patient's headache symptoms, MRI should be performed with and without gadolinium contrast medium (Fig. 4-2); magnetic resonance angiography should be considered as well. MRI should also be performed in patients with previously stable cluster headache who experience an inexplicable change in symptoms. Screening laboratory tests, including an erythrocyte sedimentation rate, complete blood count, and automated blood chemistry, should

be performed if the diagnosis of cluster headache is in question. Ophthalmologic evaluation, including measurement of intraocular pressures, is indicated in patients who experience significant ocular symptoms.

DIFFERENTIAL DIAGNOSIS

Cluster headache is usually diagnosed on clinical grounds by obtaining a targeted headache history. Migraine headache is often confused with cluster headache, and this misdiagnosis can lead to illogical treatment plans because the management of these two headache syndromes is quite different. Table 4-1 distinguishes cluster headache from migraine headache and should help clarify the diagnosis.

Diseases of the eyes, ears, nose, and sinuses may also mimic cluster headache. The targeted history and physical examination, combined with appropriate testing, should help an astute clinician identify and properly treat any underlying diseases of these organ systems. The following conditions may all mimic cluster headache and must be considered in patients with headache: glaucoma; temporal arteritis; sinusitis (see Fig. 4-2; intracranial disease, including

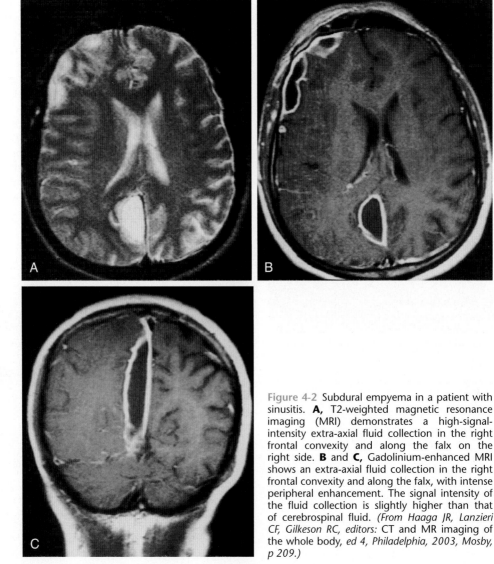

Figure 4-2 Subdural empyema in a patient with sinusitis. **A,** T2-weighted magnetic resonance imaging (MRI) demonstrates a high-signal-intensity extra-axial fluid collection in the right frontal convexity and along the falx on the right side. **B** and **C,** Gadolinium-enhanced MRI shows an extra-axial fluid collection in the right frontal convexity and along the falx, with intense peripheral enhancement. The signal intensity of the fluid collection is slightly higher than that of cerebrospinal fluid. *(From Haaga JR, Lanzieri CF, Gilkeson RC, editors: CT and MR imaging of the whole body, ed 4, Philadelphia, 2003, Mosby, p 209.)*

chronic subdural hematoma, tumor, brain abscess, hydrocephalus, and pseudotumor cerebri; and inflammatory conditions, including sarcoidosis.

TREATMENT

Whereas most patients with migraine headache experience improvement with β-blocker therapy, patients suffering from cluster headache usually require more individualized therapy. Initial treatment is commonly prednisone combined with daily sphenopalatine ganglion blocks with local anesthetic. A reasonable starting dose of prednisone is 80 mg given in divided doses and tapered by 10 mg/dose per day. If headaches are not rapidly brought under control, inhalation of 100% oxygen through a close-fitting mask is added.

If headaches persist and the diagnosis of cluster headache is not in question, a trial of lithium carbonate may be considered. The therapeutic window of lithium carbonate is small, however, and this drug should be used with caution. A starting dose of 300 mg at bedtime may be increased after 48 hours to 300 mg twice a day. If no side effects are noted after 48 hours, the dose may be increased again to 300 mg three times a day. The patient should stay at this dosage for a total of 10 days, after which the drug should be tapered over a 1-week period. Other medications that can be considered if these treatments are ineffective include methysergide and sumatriptan and sumatriptan-like drugs.

In rare patients, the aforementioned treatments are ineffective. In this setting, given the severity of the pain of cluster headache and the risk of suicide, more aggressive treatment is indicated. Destruction of the gasserian ganglion either by injection of glycerol or by radiofrequency lesioning may be a reasonable next step. Case studies suggest that deep brain stimulation may play a role in the treatment of intractable cluster headache.

COMPLICATIONS AND PITFALLS

The major risk in patients suffering from uncontrolled cluster headache is that they may become despondent owing to the unremitting, severe pain and commit suicide. Therefore, if the clinician has difficulty controlling the patient's pain, hospitalization should be considered.

Clinical Pearls

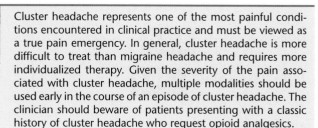

Cluster headache represents one of the most painful conditions encountered in clinical practice and must be viewed as a true pain emergency. In general, cluster headache is more difficult to treat than migraine headache and requires more individualized therapy. Given the severity of the pain associated with cluster headache, multiple modalities should be used early in the course of an episode of cluster headache. The clinician should beware of patients presenting with a classic history of cluster headache who request opioid analgesics.

SUGGESTED READINGS

Aurora SK: Pathophysiology of migraine and cluster headaches, *Semin Pain Med* 2(2):62–71, 2004.

Benitez-Rosario MA, McDarby G, Doyle R, et al: Chronic cluster-like headache secondary to prolactinoma: uncommon cephalalgia in association with brain tumors, *J Pain Symptom Manage* 37(2):271–276, 2009.

Grover PJ, Pereira EA, Green AL, et al: Deep brain stimulation for cluster headache, *J Clin Neurosci* 16(7):861–866, 2009.

Russell MB: Epidemiology and genetics of cluster headache, *Lancet Neurol* 3(5):279–283, 2004.

Waldman SD: Cluster headache. In *Pain review,* Philadelphia, 2009, Saunders, pp 216–217.

Waldman SD: Sphenopalatine ganglion block: transnasal approach. In *Atlas of interventional pain management,* ed 3, Philadelphia, 2009, pp 12–15.

Chapter 5

SWIMMER'S HEADACHE

ICD-9 CODE **350.8**

ICD-10 CODE **G50.8**

THE CLINICAL SYNDROME

Swimmer's headache is seen with increasing frequency owing to the growing number of people who are swimming as part of a balanced program of physical fitness. Although an individual suffering from swimmer's headache most often complains of a unilateral frontal headache that occurs shortly after he or she begins to swim, this painful condition is more correctly characterized as a compressive mononeuropathy. Swim goggles that are either too large or too tight compress the supraorbital nerve as it exits the supraorbital foramen and cause swimmer's headache (Fig. 5-1). The onset of symptoms is insidious in most patients, usually after the patient has been swimming for a while, and is caused by prolonged compression of the supraorbital nerve. The several reported cases of acute-onset swimmer's headache have a common history of the patient's suddenly tightening one side of the goggles after experiencing a leak during his or her swim. In most cases, symptoms abate after use of the offending goggles is discontinued. However, with chronic compression of the supraorbital nerve, permanent nerve damage may result.

SIGNS AND SYMPTOMS

Swimmer's headache is usually unilateral and involves the skin and scalp subserved by the supraorbital nerve (Fig. 5-2). Swimmer's headache usually manifests as cutaneous sensitivity above the affected supraorbital nerve that radiates into the ipsilateral forehead and scalp. This sensitivity may progress to unpleasant dysesthesias and allodynia, and the patient often complains that his or her hair hurts. With prolonged compression of the supraorbital nerve, a "woody" or anesthetized feeling of the supraorbital region and forehead may occur. Physical examination may reveal allodynia in the distribution of the compressed supraorbital nerve or, rarely, anesthesia. An occasional patient may present with edema of the eyelid resulting from compression of the soft tissues by the tight goggles. Rarely, purpura may be present, secondary to damage to the fragile blood vessels in the loose areolar tissue of the eyelid.

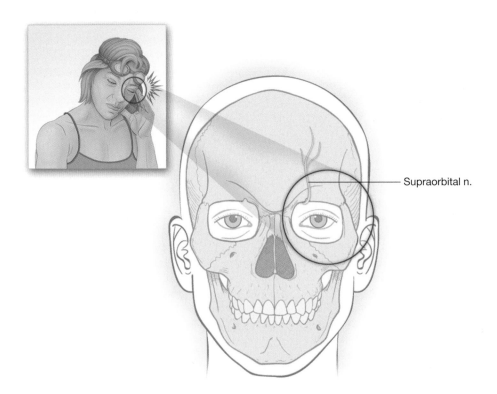

Supraorbital n.

Figure 5-1 Swim goggles that are too tight can compress the supraorbital nerve and cause swimmer's headache.

TESTING

No specific test exists for swimmer's headache. Testing is aimed primarily at identifying an occult pathologic process or other diseases that may mimic swimmer's headache (see "Differential Diagnosis"). All patients with the recent onset of headache thought to be swimmer's headache should undergo magnetic resonance imaging (MRI) of the brain, and strong consideration should be given to obtaining computed tomography (CT) scanning of the sinuses, with special attention to the frontal sinuses, given the frequency of sinusitis in swimmers. Screening laboratory tests consisting of a complete blood count, erythrocyte sedimentation rate, and automated blood chemistry should be performed if the diagnosis of swimmer's headache is in question.

DIFFERENTIAL DIAGNOSIS

Swimmer's headache is usually diagnosed on clinical grounds by obtaining a targeted headache history. Despite their obvious differences, swimmer's headache is often misdiagnosed as migraine headache. Such misdiagnosis leads to illogical treatment plans and poor control of headache symptoms. Table 5-1 distinguishes swimmer's headache from migraine headache and should aid the clinician in making the correct diagnosis.

As mentioned earlier, diseases of the frontal sinuses may mimic swimmer's headache and can be differentiated with MRI and CT scanning. Rarely, temporal arteritis may be confused with swimmer's headache, although individuals with temporal arteritis appear systemically ill. Intracranial disease such as tumor may also be incorrectly diagnosed as swimmer's headache (Fig. 5-3).

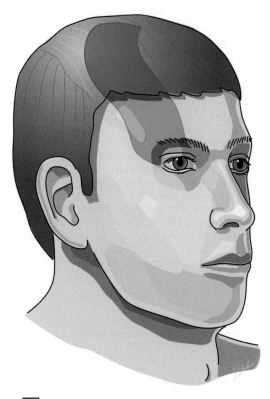

■ Sensory distribution of supraorbital nerve

Figure 5-2 Sensory distribution of the supraorbital nerve. (*From Waldman SD: Atlas of interventional pain management, ed 2, Philadelphia, 2004, Saunders, p 40.*)

TREATMENT

The mainstay of treatment of swimmer's headache is removal of the offending goggles. Often, simply substituting a new pair of goggles made of softer rubber does the trick, but occasionally, custom-fitted goggles that do not compress the supraorbital nerve but are large enough to avoid compressing the globe may be required. Analgesics or nonsteroidal antiinflammatory drugs can provide symptomatic relief. However, even these drugs can lead to serious consequences if they are abused.

If the symptoms persist after removal of the offending goggles, gabapentin may be considered. Baseline blood tests should be obtained before starting therapy with 300 mg of gabapentin at bedtime for 2 nights. The patient should be cautioned about potential side effects, including dizziness, sedation, confusion, and rash. The drug is then increased, as side effects allow, in 300-mg increments given in equally divided doses over 2 days, until pain relief is obtained or a total dose of 2400 mg/day is reached. At this point, if the patient has experienced partial pain relief, blood values are measured, and the drug is carefully titrated upward using 100-mg tablets. Rarely is more than 3600 mg/day required. If significant sleep disturbance is present, amitriptyline at an initial bedtime dose of 25 mg and titrated upward, as side effects allow, may be beneficial.

In rare patients with persistent symptoms, supraorbital nerve block with local anesthetic and steroid may be a reasonable next step. To perform supraorbital nerve block, the patient is placed supine with the head in the neutral position. The skin is prepared with povidone-iodine solution, with care taken to avoid spilling solution into the eye. The supraorbital notch is identified by palpation. A 1½-inch, 25-gauge needle is advanced perpendicularly to the skin at the level of the supraorbital notch. Then, 3 to 4 mL

TABLE 5-1		
Comparison of Swimmer's Headache and Migraine Headache		
	Swimmer's Headache	**Migraine Headache**
Onset-to-peak interval	Minutes	Minutes to 1 hr
Frequency	With swimming	Rarely >1/wk
Localization	Supraorbital radiating into the ipsilateral forehead and scalp	Temporal
Character	Cutaneous and scalp sensitivity progressing to painful dysesthesias and numbness	Pounding
Laterality	Usually unilateral	Always unilateral
Aura	Never present	May be present
Nausea and vomiting	Rare	Common
Duration	Usually subsides with removal of goggles, but may become chronic	Usually <24 hr

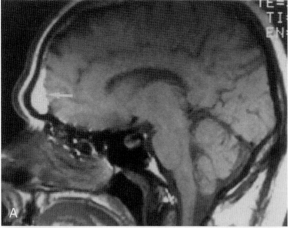

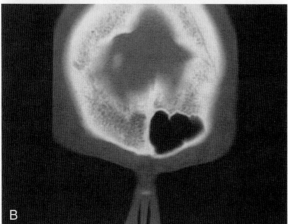

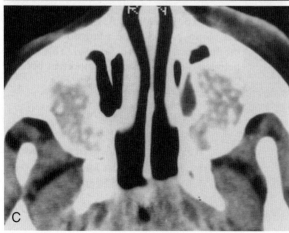

Figure 5-3 Intracranial disease that may mimic swimmer's headache. **A,** Sagittal T1-weighted (TR 500, TE 32) magnetic resonance image in the midline. Increased signal is seen overlying the frontal sinus *(arrow)*. This may represent fat, hemorrhage, or a paramagnetic substance in a metastatic tumor such as melanoma. **B,** Accompanying coronal computed tomography (CT) scan shows a nonpneumatized and nondeveloped right frontal sinus. The marrow signal from this right frontal sinus was thought to produce the abnormal signal in the study in **A. C,** Non–contrast-enhanced axial CT scan through the maxillary sinuses in a patient with sickle cell disease. The speckled pattern overlying the maxillary sinuses proved to be hyperactive marrow. *(From Haaga JR, Lanzieri CF, Gilkeson RC, editors: CT and MR imaging of the whole body, ed 4, Philadelphia, 2003, Mosby, p 565.)*

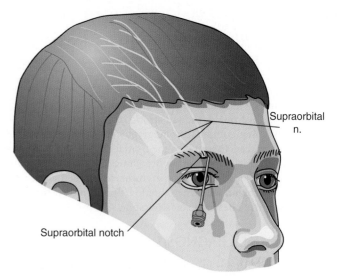

Figure 5-4 Correct needle placement for supraorbital nerve block. *(From Waldman SD:* Atlas of interventional pain management, *ed 2, Philadelphia, 2004, Saunders, p 40.)*

of preservative-free local anesthetic and 40 mg of depot methylprednisolone are injected in a fan configuration to anesthetize the peripheral branches of the nerve (Fig. 5-4). To block the supratrochlear nerve, the needle is directed medially from the supraorbital notch toward the apex of the nose. Paresthesias are occasionally elicited.

COMPLICATIONS AND PITFALLS

In most cases, swimmer's headache is a painful but self-limited condition that is easily managed once it is diagnosed. Failure to remove the offending goggles promptly may result in permanent nerve damage with associated dysesthesias and numbness. Failure to recognize coexistent intracranial disease or systemic diseases such as frontal sinusitis or tumor can have disastrous results.

Clinical Pearls

Although swimmer's headache is occurring with greater frequency owing to the increased interest in physical fitness, it is often misdiagnosed as sinus headache or occasionally migraine. By obtaining a targeted headache history and performing a targeted physical examination, the physician can make a diagnosis with a high degree of certainty. Avoidance of potentially addictive medications, coupled with the appropriate use of pharmacologic and nonpharmacologic therapies, should result in excellent palliation and long-term control of pain in most patients suffering from this headache syndrome.

SUGGESTED READINGS

Levin M: Nerve blocks and nerve stimulation in headache disorders, *Tech Reg Anesth Pain Manag* 13(1):42–49, 2009.

Sharma RR, Pawar SJ, Lad SD, et al: Frontal intraosseous cryptic hemangioma presenting with supraorbital neuralgia, *Clin Neurol Neurosurg* 101(3):215–219, 1999.

Waldman SD: Supraorbital nerve block. In *Atlas of interventional pain management,* ed 3, Philadelphia, 2009, Saunders, pp 59–62.

Chapter 6

ANALGESIC REBOUND HEADACHE

ICD-9 CODE `784.0`

ICD-10 CODE `G44.10`

THE CLINICAL SYNDROME

Analgesic rebound headache is a recently identified headache syndrome that occurs in headache sufferers who overuse abortive medications to treat their symptoms. The overuse of these medications results in increasingly frequent headaches that become unresponsive to both abortive and prophylactic medications. Over a period of weeks, the patient's episodic migraine or tension-type headache becomes more frequent and transforms into a chronic daily headache. This daily headache becomes increasingly unresponsive to analgesics and other medications, and the patient notes an exacerbation of headache symptoms if abortive or prophylactic analgesic medications are missed or delayed (Fig. 6-1). Analgesic rebound headache is probably underdiagnosed by health care professionals, and its frequency is on the rise owing to the heavy advertising of over-the-counter headache medications containing caffeine.

SIGNS AND SYMPTOMS

Clinically, analgesic rebound headache manifests as a transformed migraine or tension-type headache and may assume the characteristics of both these common headache types, thus blurring their distinctive features and making diagnosis difficult. Common to all analgesic rebound headaches is the excessive use of any of the following medications: simple analgesics, such as acetaminophen; sinus medications, including simple analgesics; combinations of aspirin, caffeine, and butalbital (Fiorinal); nonsteroidal antiinflammatory drugs; opioid analgesics; ergotamines; and triptans, such as sumatriptan (Table 6-1). As with migraine and tension-type headache, the physical examination is usually within normal limits.

TESTING

No specific test exists for analgesic rebound headache. Testing is aimed primarily at identifying an occult pathologic process or other diseases that may mimic tension-type or migraine headaches (see "Differential Diagnosis"). All patients with the recent onset of chronic daily headaches thought to be analgesic rebound headaches should undergo magnetic resonance imaging (MRI) of the brain and, if significant occipital or nuchal symptoms are present, of the cervical spine. MRI should also be performed in patients with previously stable tension-type or migraine headaches who have experienced a recent change in headache symptoms.

Screening laboratory tests consisting of a complete blood count, erythrocyte sedimentation rate, and automated blood chemistry should be performed if the diagnosis of analgesic rebound headache is in question.

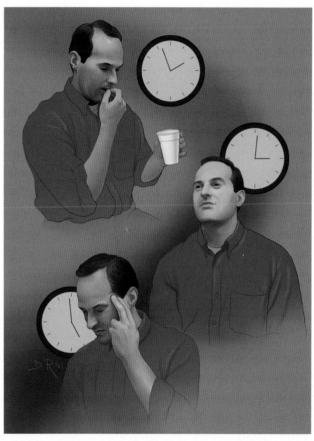

Figure 6-1 Classic temporal relationship between the taking of abortive medications and the onset of analgesic rebound headache.

TABLE 6-1
Drugs Implicated in Analgesic Rebound Headache
Simple analgesics
Nonsteroidal antiinflammatory drugs
Opioid analgesics
Sinus medications
Ergotamines
Combination headache medications that include butalbital
Triptans (e.g., sumatriptan)

DIFFERENTIAL DIAGNOSIS

Analgesic rebound headache is usually diagnosed on clinical grounds by obtaining a targeted headache history. Because analgesic rebound headache assumes many of the characteristics of the underlying primary headache, diagnosis can be confusing in the absence of a careful medication history, including specific questions regarding over-the-counter headache medications and analgesics. Any change in a previously stable headache pattern needs to be taken seriously and should not automatically be attributed to analgesic overuse without a careful reevaluation of the patient.

TREATMENT

Treatment of analgesic rebound headache consists of discontinuation of the overused or abused drugs and complete abstention for at least 3 months. Many patients cannot tolerate outpatient discontinuation of these medications and ultimately require hospitalization in a specialized headache unit. If outpatient treatment is being considered, the following points should be carefully explained to the patient:

- The headaches and associated symptoms will get worse before they get better.
- Any use, no matter how small, of the offending medications will result in continued analgesic rebound headaches.
- The patient cannot self-medicate with over-the-counter drugs.
- The significant overuse of opioids or combination medications containing butalbital or ergotamine can result in physical dependence, and discontinuation of such drugs must be done under the supervision of a physician familiar with the treatment of physical dependencies.
- If the patient follows the physician's orders regarding discontinuation of the offending medications, he or she can expect the headaches to improve.

COMPLICATIONS AND PITFALLS

Patients who overuse or abuse medications, including opioids, ergotamines, and butalbital, develop a physical dependence on these drugs, and their abrupt cessation results in a drug abstinence syndrome that can be life-threatening if it is not properly treated. Therefore, most of these patients require inpatient tapering in a controlled setting.

Clinical Pearls

Analgesic rebound headache occurs much more commonly than was previously thought. The occurrence of analgesic rebound headache is a direct result of the overprescribing of abortive headache medications in patients for whom they are inappropriate. When in doubt, the clinician should avoid abortive medications altogether and treat most headache sufferers prophylactically.

SUGGESTED READINGS

Calabresi P, Cupini LM: Medication-overuse headache: similarities with drug addiction, *Trends Pharmacol Sci* 26(2):62–68, 2005.

Diener H-C, Limmroth V: Medication-overuse headache: a worldwide problem, *Lancet Neurol* 3(8):475–483, 2004.

Michultka DM, Blanchard EB, Appelbaum KA, et al: The refractory headache patient. II. High medication consumption (analgesic rebound) headache, *Behav Res Ther* 27(4):411–420, 1989.

Waldman SD: Analgesic rebound headache. In *Pain review,* Philadelphia, 2009, Saunders, pp 219–220.

Ward TN: Medication overuse headache, *Prim Care* 31(2):369–380, 2004.

Chapter 7

OCCIPITAL NEURALGIA

ICD-9 CODE `723.8`

ICD-10 CODE `M53.82`

THE CLINICAL SYNDROME

Occipital neuralgia is usually the result of blunt trauma to the greater and lesser occipital nerves (Fig. 7-1). The greater occipital nerve arises from fibers of the dorsal primary ramus of the second cervical nerve and, to a lesser extent, from fibers of the third cervical nerve. The greater occipital nerve pierces the fascia just below the superior nuchal ridge, along with the occipital artery. It supplies the medial portion of the posterior scalp as far anterior as the vertex. The lesser occipital nerve arises from the ventral primary rami of the second and third cervical nerves. The lesser occipital nerve passes superiorly along the posterior border of the sternocleidomastoid muscle and divides into cutaneous branches that innervate the lateral portion of the posterior scalp and the cranial surface of the pinna of the ear.

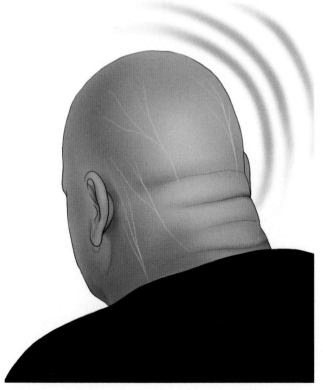

Figure 7-1 Occipital neuralgia is caused by trauma to the greater and lesser occipital nerves.

Less commonly, repetitive microtrauma from working with the neck hyperextended (e.g., painting ceilings) or looking for prolonged periods at a computer monitor whose focal point is too high, thus extending the cervical spine, may also cause occipital neuralgia. Occipital neuralgia is characterized by persistent pain at the base of the skull with occasional sudden, shocklike paresthesias in the distribution of the greater and lesser occipital nerves. Tension-type headache, which is much more common, occasionally mimics the pain of occipital neuralgia.

SIGNS AND SYMPTOMS

A patient suffering from occipital neuralgia experiences neuritic pain in the distribution of the greater and lesser occipital nerves when the nerves are palpated at the level of the nuchal ridge. Some patients can elicit pain with rotation or lateral bending of the cervical spine.

TESTING

No specific test exists for occipital neuralgia. Testing is aimed primarily at identifying an occult pathologic process or other diseases that may mimic occipital neuralgia (see "Differential Diagnosis"). All patients with the recent onset of headache thought to be occipital neuralgia should undergo magnetic resonance imaging (MRI) of the brain and cervical spine. MRI should also be performed in patients with previously stable occipital neuralgia who have experienced a recent change in headache symptoms. Computed tomography scanning of the brain and cervical spine may also be useful in identifying intracranial disease that may mimic the symptoms of occipital neuralgia (Fig. 7-2). Screening laboratory tests consisting of a complete blood count, erythrocyte sedimentation rate, and automated blood chemistry should be performed if the diagnosis of occipital neuralgia is in question.

Neural blockade of the greater and lesser occipital nerves can help confirm the diagnosis and distinguish occipital neuralgia from tension-type headache. The greater and lesser occipital nerves can easily be blocked at the nuchal ridge.

DIFFERENTIAL DIAGNOSIS

Occipital neuralgia is an infrequent cause of headache and rarely occurs in the absence of trauma to the greater and lesser occipital nerves. More often, patients with headaches involving the occipital region are suffering from tension-type headache. Tension-type headache does not respond to occipital nerve blocks but is amenable to treatment with antidepressants such as amitriptyline, in conjunction with cervical epidural nerve block. Therefore, the clinician should reconsider the diagnosis of occipital neuralgia

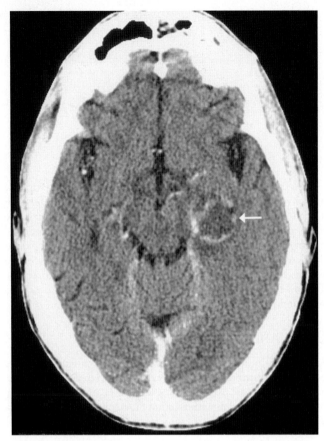

Figure 7-2 Supratentorial ependymoma. Axial computed tomography scan after intravenous contrast demonstrates a cystic-appearing, hypodense mass with irregular, rimlike contrast enhancement *(arrow)* in the medial aspect of the left temporal lobe. *(From Haaga JR, Lanzieri CF, Gilkeson RC, editors:* CT and MR imaging of the whole body, *ed 4, Philadelphia, 2003, Mosby, p 149.)*

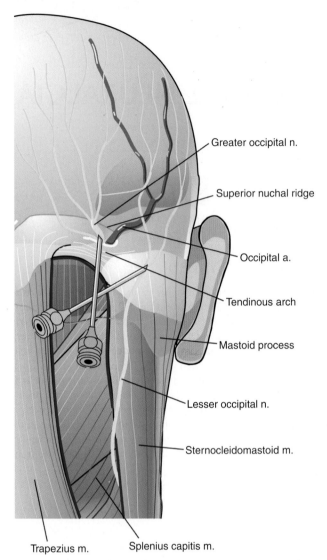

Figure 7-3 Proper needle placement for greater and lesser occipital nerve block. *(From Waldman SD:* Atlas of interventional pain management, *ed 2, Philadelphia, 2004, Saunders, p 25.)*

in patients whose symptoms are consistent with occipital neuralgia but who fail to respond to greater and lesser occipital nerve blocks.

TREATMENT

The treatment of occipital neuralgia consists primarily of neural blockade with local anesthetic and steroid, combined with the judicious use of nonsteroidal antiinflammatory drugs, muscle relaxants, tricyclic antidepressants, and physical therapy.

To perform neural blockade of the greater and lesser occipital nerves, the patient is placed in a sitting position with the cervical spine flexed and the forehead on a padded bedside table. A total of 8 mL of local anesthetic is drawn up in a 12-mL sterile syringe. For treatment of occipital neuralgia or other painful conditions involving the greater and lesser occipital nerves, a total of 80 mg methylprednisolone is added to the local anesthetic with the first block, and 40 mg of depot steroid is added with subsequent blocks. The occipital artery is palpated at the level of the superior nuchal ridge. After the skin is prepared with antiseptic solution, a 1½-inch, 22-gauge needle is inserted just medial to the artery and

is advanced perpendicularly until the needle approaches the periosteum of the underlying occipital bone. Paresthesias may be elicited, and the patient should be warned of this possibility. The needle is then redirected superiorly, and after gentle aspiration, 5 mL of solution is injected in a fanlike distribution, with care taken to avoid the foramen magnum, which is located medially (Fig. 7-3). The lesser occipital nerve and several superficial branches of the greater occipital nerve are then blocked by directing the needle laterally and slightly inferiorly. After gentle aspiration, an additional 3 to 4 mL of solution is injected (see Fig. 7-3). Should the patient experience a recurrence of symptoms after initial relief from a trial of occipital nerve blocks, radiofrequency lesioning of the affected occipital nerves is a reasonable next step (Fig. 7-4). For patients suffering from occipital neuralgia that fails to respond to the foregoing treatment modalities, a trail of occipital nerve stimulation should be considered (Fig. 7-5).

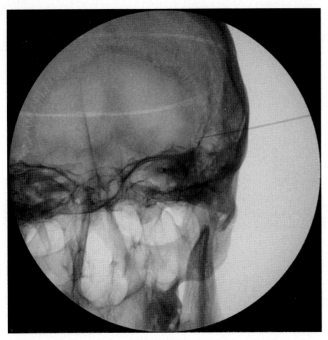

Figure 7-4 Radiofrequency lesioning of the greater occipital nerve.

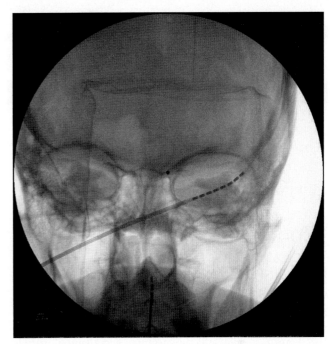

Figure 7-5 Occipital nerve stimulator lead in correct position.

COMPLICATIONS AND PITFALLS

The scalp is highly vascular. This vascularity, coupled with the close proximity to arteries of both the greater and lesser occipital nerves, means that the clinician must carefully calculate the total dose of local anesthetic that can be safely given, especially if bilateral nerve blocks are being performed. This vascularity and the proximity to the arterial supply give rise to an increased incidence of postblock ecchymosis and hematoma formation. These complications can be decreased if manual pressure is applied to the area of the block immediately after injection. Application of cold packs for 20 minutes after the block can also decrease the amount of pain and bleeding. Care must be taken to avoid inadvertent needle placement into the foramen magnum, because the subarachnoid administration of local anesthetic in this region results in immediate total spinal anesthesia.

As with other headache syndromes, the clinician must be sure that the diagnosis is correct and that the patient has no coexistent intracranial disease or disease of the cervical spine that may be erroneously attributed to occipital neuralgia.

Clinical Pearls

The most common reason that greater and lesser occipital nerve blocks fail to relieve headache pain is that the patient has been misdiagnosed. Any patient with headaches so severe that they require neural blockade should undergo MRI of the head to rule out unsuspected intracranial disease. Further, cervical spine radiographs should be considered to rule out congenital abnormalities such as Arnold-Chiari malformations that may be the hidden cause of the patient's occipital headaches.

SUGGESTED READINGS

Levin M: Nerve blocks and nerve stimulation in headache disorders, *Tech Reg Anesth Pain Manag* 13(1):42–49, 2009.

Vallejo R, Benyamin R, Kramer J: Neuromodulation of the occipital nerve in pain management, *Tech Reg Anesth Pain Manag* 10(1):12–15, 2006.

Waldman SD: Occipital nerve block. In *Atlas of interventional pain management*, ed 3, Philadelphia, 2009, Saunders, pp 24–28.

Waldman SD: Occipital neuralgia. In *Pain review,* Philadelphia, 2009, Saunders, pp 234–235.

Chapter 8

PSEUDOTUMOR CEREBRI

ICD-9 CODE `348.2`

ICD-10 CODE `G93.2`

THE CLINICAL SYNDROME

An often missed diagnosis, pseudotumor cerebri is a relatively common cause of headache. It has an incidence of 2.2 per 100,000 patients, approximately the same incidence as cluster headache. Also known as idiopathic intracranial hypertension, pseudotumor cerebri is seen most frequently in overweight women between the ages of 20 and 45 years. If epidemiologic studies look only at obese women, the incidence increases to approximately 20 cases per 100,000 patients. An increased incidence of pseudotumor cerebri is also associated with pregnancy. The exact cause of pseudotumor cerebri has not been elucidated, but the common denominator appears to be a defect in the absorption of cerebrospinal fluid (CSF). Predisposing factors include ingestion of various medications including tetracycline, vitamin A, corticosteroids, and nalidixic acid (Table 8-1). Other implicating factors include blood dyscrasias, anemias, endocrinopathies, and chronic respiratory insufficiency. In many patients, however, the exact cause of pseudotumor cerebri remains unknown.

SIGNS AND SYMPTOMS

More than 90% of patients suffering from pseudotumor cerebri present with the complaint of headache, are female, and have headaches that increase with Valsalva's maneuver. Associated nonspecific central nervous system signs and symptoms such as dizziness, visual disturbance including diplopia, tinnitus, nausea and vomiting, and ocular pain can often obfuscate what should otherwise be a reasonably straightforward diagnosis, given that basically all patients suffering from pseudotumor cerebri (1) have papilledema on fundoscopic examination, (2) are female, and (3) are obese. The extent of papilledema varies from patient to patient and may be associated with subtle visual field defects including an enlarged blind spot and inferior nasal visual field defects (Fig. 8-1). If the condition is untreated, blindness may result (Fig. 8-2).

TESTING

By convention, the diagnosis of pseudotumor cerebri is made when four criteria are identified: (1) signs and symptoms suggestive of increased intracranial pressure including papilledema; (2) normal results of magnetic resonance imaging (MRI) or computed tomography (CT) of the brain; (3) increased CSF pressure documented by lumbar puncture; and (4) normal CSF chemistry, cultures, and

TABLE 8-1
Medications Reportedly Associated With Intracranial Hypertension
Vitamins
Vitamin A Retinol Retinoids
Antibiotics
Tetracycline and derivatives Nalidixic acid Nitrofurantoin Penicillin
Protein Kinase C Inhibitors
Lithium carbonate
Histamine (H₂)-Receptor Antagonists
Cimetidine
Steroids
Corticosteroid withdrawal Levonorgestrel Danazol Leuprolide acetate Tamoxifen Growth hormone Oxytocin Anabolic steroids
Nonsteroidal Antiinflammatory Drugs
Ketoprofen Indomethacin Rofecoxib
Antiarrhythmics
Amiodarone
Anticonvulsants
Phenytoin
Dopamine Precursors
Levodopa Carbidopa

cytology (Table 8-2). Urgent MRI and CT scanning of the brain with contrast media should be obtained on all patients suspected of having increased intracranial pressure, to rule out intracranial mass and infection, among other disorders. Patients suffering from pseudotumor cerebri have small to normal-sized ventricles on neuroimaging with an otherwise normal scan. Once the absence of space-occupying lesions of dilated ventricles is confirmed on neuroimaging, it is safe to proceed with lumbar puncture to measure CSF pressure and obtain fluid for chemistry, cultures, and cytology.

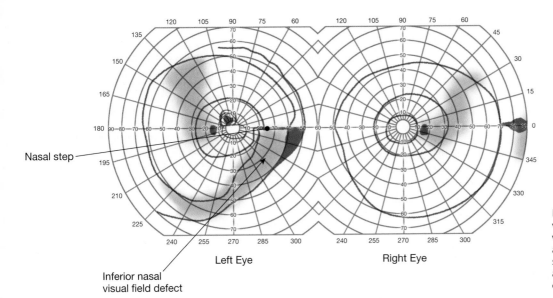

Nasal step

Inferior nasal
visual field defect

Left Eye

Right Eye

Figure 8-1 The most common
visual field defects associated
with pseudotumor cerebri are
an abnormally enlarged blind
spot and a nasal step defect
affecting the inferior quadrants
of the visual field.

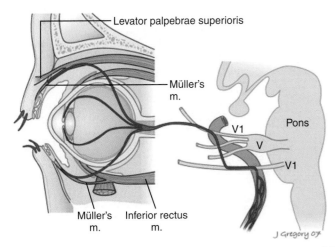

Figure 8-2 Müller's muscles. The Müller's muscle in the upper eyelid
arises from the undersurface of the levator palpebrae superioris muscle.
Interruptions of the sympathetic innervation to this muscle cause ptosis
of the upper eyelid. The Müller's muscle in the lower lid will elevate the
lower eyelid slightly in Horner's syndrome ("upside-down ptosis"). (From
Reede DL, Garcon E, Smoker WR, Kardon R: Horner's syndrome: clinical and
radiographic evaluation, Neuroimaging Clin N Am 18[2]:369–385, 2008.)

TABLE 8-2
Diagnostic Criteria for Pseudotumor Cerebri
1. Signs and symptoms suggestive of increased intracranial pressure including papilledema
2. Normal magnetic resonance imaging or computed tomography of the brain performed with and without contrast media
3. Increased cerebrospinal fluid pressure documented by lumbar puncture
4. Normal cerebrospinal fluid chemistry, cultures, and cytology

DIFFERENTIAL DIAGNOSIS

If a specific cause is found for a patient's intracranial hypertension,
it is by definition not idiopathic but rather is a specific secondary type of intracranial hypertension. Causes of secondary intracranial hypertension that should be considered before diagnosing
a patient with idiopathic intracranial hypertension are listed in

TABLE 8-3
Common Causes of Secondary Intracranial Hypertension
Intracranial Hemorrhage
Intraventricular hemorrhage Subarachnoid hemorrhage Intraparenchymal hemorrhage Subdural hematoma Epidural hematoma
Intracranial Tumor
Primary brain tumors Meningiomas Pineal tumors Pituitary tumors Posterior fossa tumors Hamartomas
Cranial or Cervical Spine Abnormalities
Arnold-Chiari Malformation Craniosynostosis Craniofacial dysostosis
Cerebral Venous Sinus Thrombosis
Abnormalities of the Ventricular System
Aqueductal stenosis Dandy-Walker syndrome
Intracranial Infections
Meningitis Encephalitis Intracranial abscess Intracranial parasites Epidural abscess
Intracranial Granulomas
Eosinophilic granuloma Wegener's granulomatosis Sarcoidosis
Lead Poisoning

Table 8-3. These include the various forms of intracranial hemorrhage, intracranial tumor, cranial or cervical spine abnormalities
such as Arnold-Chiari malformation, cerebral venous sinus thrombosis, abnormalities of the ventricular system, hepatic failure, and

intracranial infections. A failure to diagnosis a potentially treatable cause of intracranial hypertension may result in significant mortality and morbidity.

TREATMENT

A reasonable first step in the management of patients who exhibit all four criteria necessary for the diagnosis of pseudotumor cerebri is the initiation of oral acetazolamide. If poorly tolerated, the use of furosemide or chlorthalidone can be considered. A short course of systemic corticosteroids such as dexamethasone may also be used if the patient does not respond to diuretic therapy. For resistant cases, neurosurgical interventions including CSF shunt procedures are a reasonable next step. If papilledema persists, decompression procedures on the optic nerve sheath have been advocated.

COMPLICATIONS AND PITFALLS

As mentioned earlier, untreated pseudotumor cerebri can result in permanent visual loss and significant morbidity. Furthermore, a failure to diagnose and treat properly the secondary causes of increased intracranial hypertension can lead to disastrous results for the patient, including potentially avoidable death.

Clinical Pearls

Psuedotumor cerebri is predominately a disease that affects women. It is a relatively straightforward diagnosis if one thinks of it. Patients suffering from pseudotumor cerebri have papilledema on fundoscopic examination and are invariably obese. Visual field defects can be subtle and include an enlarged blind spot and associated inferior nasal visual field defects. Often, medications are found to be the causative agent in the evolution of this headache syndrome and should be diligently searched for. As with all headache syndromes, other causes of increased intracranial pressure, such as tumor or hemorrhage, must be ruled out.

SUGGESTED READINGS

Ball AK, Clarke CE: Idiopathic intracranial hypertension, *Lancet Neurol* 5(5):433–442, 2006.

Bynke G, Zemack G, Bynke H, et al: Ventriculoperitoneal shunting for idiopathic intracranial hypertension, *Am J Ophthalmol* 139(2):401–402, 2005.

Digre K: Papilledema and idiopathic intracranial hypertension. In *Neuro-ophthalmology, Blue books of neurology,* vol 32, New York, 2008, Elsevier, pp 280–311.

Donahue SP: Recurrence of idiopathic intracranial hypertension after weight loss: the carrot craver, *Am J Ophthalmol* 130(6):850–851, 2000.

Vargiami E, Zafeiriou DI, Gombakis NP, et al: Hemolytic anemia presenting with idiopathic intracranial hypertension, *Pediatr Neurol* 38(1):53–54, 2008.

Chapter 9

INTRACRANIAL SUBARACHNOID HEMORRHAGE

ICD-9 CODE `430`

ICD-10 CODE `160.9`

THE CLINICAL SYNDROME

Subarachnoid hemorrhage (SAH) represents one of the most neurologically devastating forms of cerebrovascular accident. Fewer than 60% of patients suffering from the malady will recover cognitively and functionally to their premorbid state. From 65% to 70% of all SAH results from rupture of intracranial berry aneurysms. Arteriovenous malformations, neoplasm, and angiomas are responsible for most of the remainder (Fig. 9-1). Berry aneurysms are prone to rupture because of their lack of a fully developed muscular media and collagen-elastic layer. Systemic diseases associated with an increased incidence of berry aneurysm include Marfan's syndrome, Ehlers-Danlos syndrome, sickle cell disease, coarctation of the aorta, polycystic kidney disease, fibromuscular vascular dysplasia, and pseudoxanthoma elasticum (Table 9-1). Hypertension, alcohol and cocaine use, and cerebral atherosclerosis increase the risk of SAH. Blacks are more than twice as likely to suffer SAH when compared with whites. Female patients are affected more often than male patients, and the mean age of patients suffering from SAH is 50 years. Even with modern treatment, the mortality associated with significant SAH is approximately 25%.

SIGNS AND SYMPTOMS

Massive SAH is often preceded by a warning in the form of what is known as a sentinel headache. This headache is thought to be the result of leakage from an aneurysm that is preparing to rupture. The sentinel headache is of sudden onset, with a temporal profile characterized by a rapid onset to peak in intensity. The sentinel headache may be associated with photophobia and nausea and vomiting. Ninety percent of patients with intracranial SAH will experience a sentinel headache within 3 months of significant SAH.

Patients with significant SAH experience the sudden onset of severe headache, which the patient often describes as the worst headache of his or her life (Fig. 9-2). This headache is usually associated with nausea and vomiting, photophobia, vertigo, lethargy, confusion, nuchal rigidity, and neck and back pain (Table 9-2). The patient experiencing acute SAH appears acutely ill, and up to 50% will lose

TABLE 9-1

Systemic Diseases Associated With an Increased Incidence of Berry Aneurysm

Marfan's syndrome
Ehlers-Danlos syndrome
Sickle cell disease
Polycystic kidneys
Coarctation of the aorta
Fibromuscular vascular dysplasia
Pseudoxanthoma elasticum

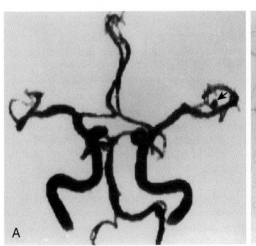
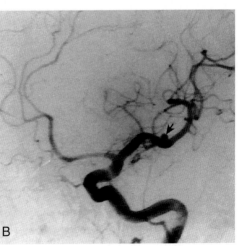

Figure 9-1 Berry aneurysm in a patient with autosomal dominant polycystic kidney disease. **A,** A three-dimensional time-of-flight magnetic resonance angiogram with a vessel-tracking postprocessing algorithm discloses a left middle cerebral artery bifurcation aneurysm *(arrow).* **B,** Catheter angiogram shows the same lesion *(arrow).* (From Edelman RR, Hesselink JR, Zlatkin MB, Crues JV, editors: Clinical magnetic resonance imaging, *ed 3, Philadelphia, 2006, Saunders, p 1420.)*

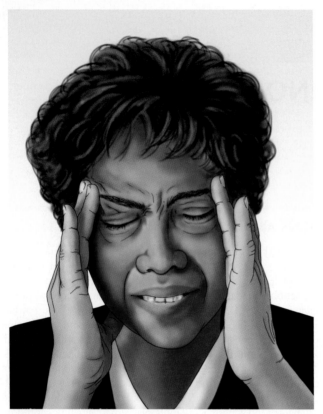

Figure 9-2 The headache associated with subarachnoid hemorrhage is often described as the worst headache the patient has ever experienced.

TABLE 9-2

Symptoms Associated With Subarachnoid Hemorrhage

Severe headache
Nausea and vomiting
Photophobia
Vertigo
Lethargy
Confusion
Nuchal rigidity
Neck and back pain

consciousness as the intracranial pressure rapidly rises in response to unabated hemorrhage. Cranial nerve palsy, especially of the abducens nerve, may also occur as a result of increased intracranial pressure. Focal neurologic signs, paresis, seizures, subretinal hemorrhages, and papilledema are often present on physical examination.

TESTING

Testing in patients suspected of suffering with SAH has two immediate goals: (1) to identify an occult intracranial pathologic process or other diseases that may mimic SAH and may be more amenable to treatment (see "Differential Diagnosis") and (2) to identify the presence of SAH. All patients with a recent onset of severe headache thought to be secondary to SAH should undergo emergency computed tomography (CT) scanning of the brain (Fig. 9-3). Modern multidetector CT scanners have a diagnostic accuracy approaching 100% for SAH if CT angiography of the cerebral

vessels is part of the scanning protocol. Cerebral angiography may also be required if surgical intervention is being considered and the site of bleeding cannot be accurately identified.

Magnetic resonance imaging (MRI) of the brain and magnetic resonance angiography may be useful if an aneurysm is not identified on CT studies and may be more accurate in the diagnosis of arteriovenous malformations (Fig. 9-4). Screening laboratory tests, including an erythrocyte sedimentation rate, complete blood count, coagulation studies, and automated blood chemistry, should be performed in patients suffering from SAH. Blood typing and crossmatching should be considered in any patient in whom surgery is being contemplated or who has preexisting anemia. Careful serial ophthalmologic examination should be performed on all patients suffering from SAH, to chart the course of papilledema.

Lumbar puncture may be useful in revealing blood in the spinal fluid, but its utility may be limited by the presence of increased intracranial pressure, which makes lumbar puncture too dangerous. Electrocardiographic abnormalities are common in patients suffering from SAH and are thought to result from abnormally high levels of circulating catecholamines and hypothalamic dysfunction.

DIFFERENTIAL DIAGNOSIS

For the most part, the differential diagnosis of SAH can be thought of as the diagnosis of the lesser of two evils because most of the diseases that mimic SAH are also associated with significant mortality and morbidity. Table 9-3 lists diseases that may be mistaken for SAH. Prominent among them are stroke, collagen vascular disease, infection, neoplasm, hypertensive crisis, spinal fluid leaks, and various more benign causes of headache.

TREATMENT

Medical Management

The treatment of SAH begins with careful acute medical management, with an eye to minimizing the sequelae of both the cerebral insult and the morbidity associated with a severe illness. Bed rest with the head of bed elevated to 30 to 35 degrees to promote good venous drainage is a reasonable first step in the management of the patient suffering from SAH. Accurate intake and output determinations, as well as careful management of hypertension and hypotension, are also essential during the initial management of SAH, and invasive cardiovascular monitoring should be considered sooner rather than later in this setting. Pulse oximetry and end-tidal carbon dioxide monitoring should be initiated early in the course of treatment to identify respiratory insufficiency. Avoidance of overuse of opioids and sedatives is important, to prevent hypoventilation with its attendant increase in intracranial pressure and cerebral ischemia. Seizure precautions and aggressive treatment of seizures are also required. Vomiting should be controlled to avoid the increase in intracranial pressure associated with the Valsalva maneuver. Prophylaxis of gastrointestinal bleeding, especially if steroids are used to treat increased intracranial pressure, and the use of pneumatic compression devices to avoid thrombophlebitis are also worth considering. If unconsciousness occurs, endotracheal intubation using techniques to avoid increases in intracranial pressure should be performed, and hyperventilation to decreased blood carbon dioxide levels should be considered.

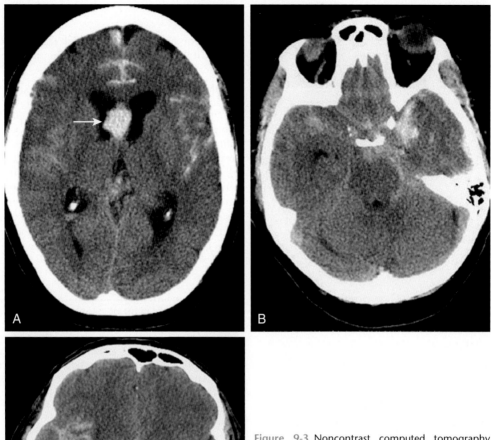

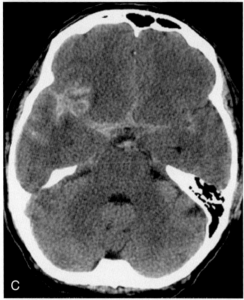

Figure 9-3 Noncontrast computed tomography images from different patients demonstrating that the particular location of thick clot can often help in predicting the location of ruptured aneurysm. **A,** Blood collection along the interhemispheric fissure from a ruptured anterior communicating artery aneurysm *(arrow).* **B,** Focal collection along the left side of the suprasellar cistern from a ruptured left posterior communicating artery aneurysm. **C,** Blood pooling in the right sylvian fissure from a ruptured middle cerebral artery aneurysm. Please note the lucent center representing the actual aneurysm. *(From Marshall SA, Kathuria S, Nyquist P, Gandhi D: Noninvasive imaging techniques in the diagnosis and management of aneurysmal subarachnoid hemorrhage,* Neurosurg Clin North Am *21[2]: 305–323, 2102.)*

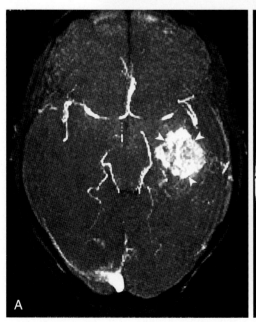

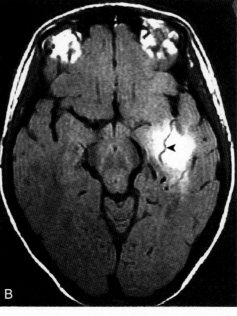

Figure 9-4 Left temporal hemorrhage from an arteriovenous malformation. **A,** On gradient-echo magnetic resonance imaging (MRI), the hematoma appears bright because of methemoglobin *(arrowheads),* and no abnormal vessel is visualized. **B,** On spin-echo MRI with flow presaturation below the section to be imaged, flow voids of abnormal vessels posterior to the hematoma and an abnormal vessel running through the hematoma *(arrowhead)* are visible. *(From Mattle H, Edelman RR, Atkinson DJ: Zerebrale Angiographie mittels Kernspintomographie,* Schweiz Med Wochenschr *122:323–333, 1992.)*

TABLE 9-3

Diseases That May Mimic Subarachnoid Hemorrhage

Stroke
  Hemorrhagic
  Ischemic
Neoplasm
Infection
  Meningitis
  Encephalitis
  Abscess
  Parasitic
Hypertensive crisis
Loss of spinal fluid
  Postdural puncture headache
  Spontaneous spinal fluid leak
Collagen vascular disease
  Lupus cerebritis
  Vasculitis
  Polymyositis
Headache
  Cluster headache
  Thunderclap headache
  Migraine
  Ice-pick headache
  Sexual headache

Treatment of increased intracranial pressure with dexamethasone, the osmotic agent mannitol, and furosemide may be required. Calcium channel blockers and magnesium may be beneficial to reduce cerebrovascular spasm and decrease the zone of ischemia. Studies showed that statins may also be useful in this setting. Antifibrinolytics, such as epsilon-aminocaproic acid, may be useful to decrease the incidence of rebleeding in selected patients.

Surgical Treatment

Surgical treatment of hydrocephalus with ventricular drainage may be required to treat highly elevated intracranial pressure, with the caveat that too rapid a decrease in intracranial pressure in this setting may result in an increased incidence of rebleeding. Surgical treatment with clipping of the aneurysm or interventional radiologic endovascular occlusive coil treatment of continued bleeding or rebleeding carries a high risk of morbidity and mortality, but it may be necessary if more conservative treatments fail.

COMPLICATIONS AND PITFALLS

Complications and pitfalls in the diagnosis and treatment of SAH generally fall into three categories. The first category involves the failure to recognize a sentinel hemorrhage and to evaluate and treat the patient before significant SAH occurs. The second category involves misdiagnosis, which results in treatment delays that ultimately cause an increase in mortality and morbidity. The third category involves less than optimal medical management, which results in avoidable mortality and morbidity. Examples are pulmonary embolus from thrombophlebitis and aspiration pneumonia from failure to protect the patient's airway.

Clinical Pearls

The identification of sentinel headache and subsequent aggressive treatment before significant SAH occurs give the patient his or her best chance of a happy outcome. Treatment of significant SAH is difficult, and ultimately results are disappointing. Careful attention to initial and ongoing medical management, with aggressive monitoring and treatment of associated hypertension and hypotension and respiratory abnormalities, is crucial to prevent avoidable complications.

SUGGESTED READINGS

Andersen T: Current and evolving management of subarachnoid hemorrhage, *Crit Care Nurs Clin North Am* 21(4):529–539, 2009.

Janardhan V, Biondi A, Riina HA, et al: Vasospasm in aneurysmal subarachnoid hemorrhage: diagnosis, prevention, and management, *Neuroimaging Clin N Am* 16(3):483–496, 2006.

Manno EM: Subarachnoid hemorrhage, *Neurol Clin* 22(2):347–366, 2004.

Newfield P: Intracranial aneurysms: vasospasm and other issues. In Atlee JL, editor: *Complications in anesthesia*, ed 2, Philadelphia, 2006, Saunders, pp 719–723.

Palestrant D, Connolly ES Jr: Subarachnoid hemorrhage. In Gilman S, editor: *Neurobiology of disease*, Burlington, Mass, 2007, Academic Press, pp 265–270.

Pouration N, Dumont AS, Kassell NF: Subarachnoid hemorrhage. In Alves WM, Skolnick BE, editors: *Handbook of neuroemergency clinical trials,* Burlington, Mass, 2005, Academic Press, pp 17–44.

Chapter **10**

TRIGEMINAL NEURALGIA

ICD-9 CODE **350.1**

ICD-10 CODE **G50.0**

THE CLINICAL SYNDROME

Trigeminal neuralgia occurs in many patients because of tortuous blood vessels that compress the trigeminal root as it exits the brainstem. Acoustic neuromas, cholesteatomas, aneurysms, angiomas, and bony abnormalities may also lead to compression of the nerve. The severity of the pain produced by trigeminal neuralgia is rivaled only by that of cluster headache. Uncontrolled pain has been associated with suicide and should therefore be treated as an emergency. Attacks can be triggered by daily activities involving contact with the face, such as brushing the teeth, shaving, and washing (Fig. 10-1). Pain can be controlled with medication in most patients. Approximately 2% to 3% of patients with trigeminal neuralgia also have multiple sclerosis. Trigeminal neuralgia is also called tic douloureux.

SIGNS AND SYMPTOMS

Trigeminal neuralgia causes episodic pain afflicting the areas of the face supplied by the trigeminal nerve. The pain is unilateral in 97% of cases; when it does occur bilaterally, the same division of

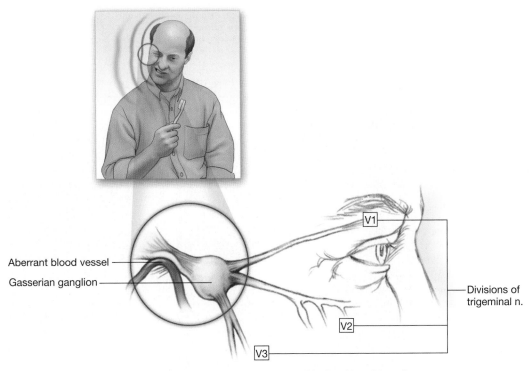

Aberrant blood vessel

Gasserian ganglion

V1

V2

V3

Divisions of trigeminal n.

Figure 10-1 Paroxysms of pain triggered by brushing the teeth.

the nerve is involved on both sides. The second or third division of the nerve is affected in most patients, and the first division is affected less than 5% of the time. The pain develops on the right side of the face in 57% of unilateral cases. The pain is characterized by paroxysms of electric shock–like pain lasting from several seconds to less than 2 minutes. The progression from onset to peak is essentially instantaneous.

Patients with trigeminal neuralgia go to great lengths to avoid any contact with trigger areas. In contrast, persons with other types of facial pain, such as temporomandibular joint dysfunction, tend to rub the affected area constantly or apply heat or cold to it. Patients with uncontrolled trigeminal neuralgia frequently require hospitalization for rapid control of pain. Between attacks, patients are relatively pain free. A dull ache remaining after the intense pain subsides may indicate persistent compression of the nerve by a structural lesion. This disease is hardly ever seen in persons younger than 30 years unless it is associated with multiple sclerosis.

Patients with trigeminal neuralgia often have severe depression (sometimes to the point of being suicidal), with high levels of superimposed anxiety during acute attacks. Both these problems may be exacerbated by the sleep deprivation that often accompanies painful episodes. Patients with coexisting multiple sclerosis may exhibit the euphoric dementia characteristic of that disease. Physicians should reassure persons with trigeminal neuralgia that the pain can almost always be controlled.

TESTING

All patients with a new diagnosis of trigeminal neuralgia should undergo magnetic resonance imaging (MRI) of the brain and brainstem, with and without gadolinium contrast medium, to rule out posterior fossa or brainstem lesions and demyelinating disease (Fig. 10-2). Magnetic resonance angiography is also useful to confirm vascular compression of the trigeminal nerve by aberrant blood vessels (Fig. 10-3). Additional imaging of the sinuses should be considered if occult or coexisting sinus disease is a possibility. If the first division of the trigeminal nerve is affected, ophthalmologic evaluation to measure intraocular pressure and

to rule out intraocular disease is indicated. Screening laboratory tests consisting of a complete blood count, erythrocyte sedimentation rate, and automated blood chemistry should be performed if the diagnosis of trigeminal neuralgia is in question. A complete blood count is required for baseline comparisons before starting treatment with carbamazepine (see "Treatment").

DIFFERENTIAL DIAGNOSIS

Trigeminal neuralgia is generally a straightforward clinical diagnosis that can be made on the basis of a targeted history and physical examination. Diseases of the eyes, ears, nose, throat, and teeth may all mimic trigeminal neuralgia or may coexist and confuse the diagnosis. Atypical facial pain is sometimes confused with trigeminal neuralgia, but it can be distinguished by the character of the

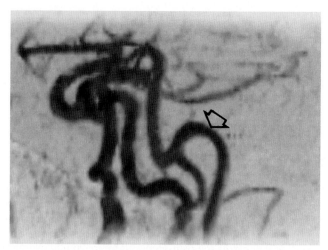

Figure 10-3 Vascular compression of the left trigeminal (fifth cranial) nerve in a 69-year-old man with trigeminal neuralgia. Three-dimensional time-of-flight magnetic resonance angiogram demonstrates that the compressive lesion is the markedly dominant right vertebral artery, which extends cephalad into the left cerebellopontine angle cistern *(open arrowhead)*. *(From Stark DD, Bradley WG Jr, editors:* Magnetic resonance imaging, *vol 3, ed 3, St Louis, 1999, Mosby, p 1214.)*

Figure 10-2 Cystic and solid schwannoma of the right trigeminal nerve and ganglion. **A,** Axial enhanced magnetic resonance imaging (MRI) showing a dumbbell-shaped tumor extending across the incisura from the posterior fossa into the medial portion of the right middle fossa. Note the heterogeneous enhancement of the tumor that suggests areas of decreased cellularity and cystic change and a more solid component. **B,** Axial magnetic resonance angiogram performed after the MRI examination showing near-homogeneous enhancement of the tumor because of the delay in imaging. Note the exquisite demonstration of the tumor in the skull base, including the displaced right petrous carotid artery. *(From Stark DD, Bradley WG Jr, editors:* Magnetic resonance imaging, *vol 3, ed 3, St Louis, 1999, Mosby, p 1218.)*

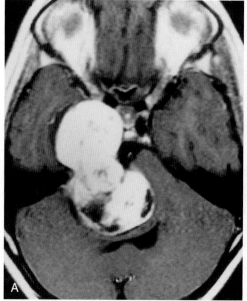

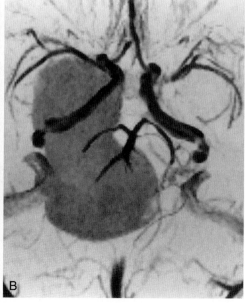

pain: atypical facial pain is dull and aching, whereas the pain of trigeminal neuralgia is sharp and neuritic. Additionally, the pain of trigeminal neuralgia occurs in the distribution of the divisions of the trigeminal nerve, whereas the pain of atypical facial pain does not follow any specific nerve distribution. Multiple sclerosis should be considered in all patients who present with trigeminal neuralgia before the fifth decade of life.

TREATMENT

Drug Therapy

Carbamazepine

Carbamazepine is considered first-line treatment for trigeminal neuralgia. In fact, a rapid response to this drug essentially confirms the clinical diagnosis. Despite the safety and efficacy of carbamazepine, some confusion and anxiety have surrounded its use. This medication, which may be the patient's best chance for pain control, is sometimes discontinued because of laboratory abnormalities erroneously attributed to it. Therefore, baseline measurements consisting of a complete blood count, urinalysis, and automated blood chemistry profile should be obtained before starting the drug.

Carbamazepine should be initiated slowly if the pain is not out of control, with a starting dose of 100 to 200 mg at bedtime for 2 nights. The patient should be cautioned about side effects, including dizziness, sedation, confusion, and rash. The drug is increased in 100- to 200-mg increments given in equally divided doses over 2 days, as side effects allow, until pain relief is obtained or a total dose of 1200 mg/day is reached. Careful monitoring of laboratory parameters is mandatory to avoid the rare possibility of a life-threatening blood dyscrasia. *At the first sign of blood count abnormality or rash, this drug should be discontinued.* Failure to monitor patients who are taking carbamazepine can be disastrous, because aplastic anemia can occur. When pain relief is obtained, the patient should be kept at that dosage of carbamazepine for at least 6 months before tapering of the medication is considered. The patient should be informed that under no circumstances should the drug dosage be changed or the drug refilled or discontinued without the physician's knowledge.

Gabapentin

In the uncommon event that carbamazepine does not adequately control a patient's pain, gabapentin may be considered. As with carbamazepine, baseline blood tests should be obtained before starting therapy, and the patient should be cautioned about potential side effects, including dizziness, sedation, confusion, and rash. The initial dose of gabapentin is 300 mg at bedtime for 2 nights. The drug is then increased in 300-mg increments given in equally divided doses over 2 days, as side effects allow, until pain relief is obtained or a total dose of 2400 mg/day is reached. At this point, if the patient has experienced only partial pain relief, blood values are measured, and the drug is carefully titrated upward using 100-mg tablets. Rarely is a dosage greater than 3600 mg/day required.

Baclofen

Baclofen may be of value in some patients who fail to obtain relief from carbamazepine or gabapentin. As with those drugs, baseline laboratory tests should be obtained before beginning baclofen therapy, and the patient should be warned about the same potential adverse effects. The patient starts with a 10-mg dose at bedtime for 2 nights; then, the drug is increased in 10-mg increments given in equally divided doses over 7 days, as side effects allow, until pain relief is obtained or a total dose of 100 mg/day is reached. This drug has significant hepatic and central nervous system side effects, including weakness and sedation. As with carbamazepine, careful monitoring of laboratory values is indicated when using baclofen.

When treating individuals with any of these drugs, the physician should make sure that the patient knows that premature tapering or discontinuation of the medication may lead to the recurrence of pain, which will be more difficult to control.

Invasive Therapy

Trigeminal Nerve Block

The use of trigeminal nerve block with local anesthetic and steroid is an excellent adjunct to drug treatment of trigeminal neuralgia. This technique rapidly relieves pain while medications are being titrated to effective levels. The initial block is carried out with preservative-free bupivacaine combined with methylprednisolone. Subsequent daily nerve blocks are performed in a similar manner, but using a lower dose of methylprednisolone. This approach may also be used to control breakthrough pain.

Retrogasserian Injection of Glycerol

The injection of small quantities of glycerol into the area of the gasserian ganglion can provide long-term relief for patients suffering from trigeminal neuralgia who have not responded to optimal drug therapy. This procedure should be performed only by a physician well versed in the problems and pitfalls associated with neurodestructive procedures (Fig. 10-4).

Radiofrequency Destruction of the Gasserian Ganglion

The gasserian ganglion can be destroyed by creating a radiofrequency lesion under biplanar fluoroscopic guidance. This procedure is reserved for patients in whom all the previously mentioned

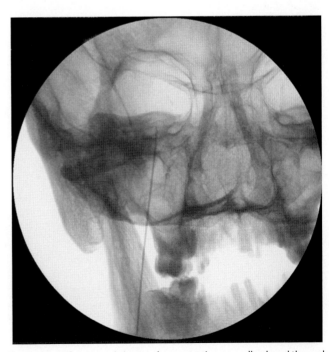

Figure 10-4 Fluoroscopic image demonstrating a needle placed through the foramen ovale into Meckel's cave.

treatments for intractable trigeminal neuralgia have failed and who are not candidates for microvascular decompression of the trigeminal root.

Balloon Compression of the Gasserian Ganglion

The insertion of a balloon by a needle placed through the foramen ovale into Meckel's cave under radiographic guidance is a straightforward technique. Once the balloon is in proximity to the gasserian ganglion, it is inflated to compress the ganglion. This technique has been shown to provide palliation of the pain of trigeminal neural in selected candidates in whom medication management has failed and who are not candidates for more invasive procedures.

Microvascular Decompression of the Trigeminal Root

This technique, which is also called Jannetta's procedure, is the major neurosurgical treatment of choice for intractable trigeminal neuralgia. It is based on the theory that trigeminal neuralgia is in fact a compressive mononeuropathy. The operation consists of identifying the trigeminal root close to the brainstem and isolating the compressing blood vessel. A sponge is then interposed between the vessel and the nerve, to relieve the compression and thus the pain.

COMPLICATIONS AND PITFALLS

The pain of trigeminal neuralgia is severe and can lead to suicide. Therefore, it must be considered a medical emergency, and strong consideration should be given to hospitalizing such patients. If a dull ache remains after the intense pain of trigeminal neuralgia subsides, this is highly suggestive of persistent compression of the nerve by a structural lesion such as a brainstem tumor or schwannoma. Trigeminal neuralgia is hardly ever seen in persons younger than 30 years unless it is associated with multiple sclerosis, and all such patients should undergo MRI to identify demyelinating disease.

Clinical Pearls

Trigeminal nerve block with local anesthetic and steroid is an excellent stopgap measure for patients suffering from the uncontrolled pain of trigeminal neuralgia while waiting for drug treatments to take effect. This technique may lead to the rapid control of pain and allow the patient to maintain adequate oral hydration and nutrition and avoid hospitalization.

SUGGESTED READINGS

Cheng W-C, Change C-N: Trigeminal neuralgia caused by contralateral supratentorial meningioma, *J Clin Neurosci* 15(10):1162–1163, 2008.

Cruccu G, Biasiotta A, Di Rezze S, et al: Trigeminal neuralgia and pain related to multiple sclerosis, *Pain* 143(3):186–191, 2009.

Goru SJ, Pemberton MN: Trigeminal neuralgia: the role of magnetic resonance imaging, *Br J Oral Maxillofac Surg* 47(3):228–229, 2009.

Toda K: Operative treatment of trigeminal neuralgia: review of current techniques, *Oral Surg Oral Med Oral Pathol Oral Radiol Endod* 106(6):788–805, 2008.

Waldman SD: Gasserian ganglion block. In *Atlas of interventional pain management,* ed 3, Philadelphia, 2009, Saunders, pp 32–37.

Waldman SD: Gasserian ganglion block: balloon compression technique. In *Atlas of interventional pain management,* ed 3, Philadelphia, 2009, Saunders, pp 43–46.

Waldman SD: Gasserian ganglion block: radiofrequency lesioning. In *Atlas of interventional pain management,* ed 3, Philadelphia, 2009, Saunders, pp 38–42.

Chapter 11

TEMPOROMANDIBULAR JOINT DYSFUNCTION

ICD-9 CODE `524.60`

ICD-10 CODE `M26.60`

THE CLINICAL SYNDROME

Temporomandibular joint (TMJ) dysfunction (also known as myofascial pain dysfunction of the muscles of mastication) is characterized by pain in the joint itself that radiates into the mandible, ear, neck, and tonsillar pillars. The TMJ is a true joint that is divided into upper and lower synovial cavities by a fibrous articular disk. Internal derangement of this disk may result in pain and TMJ dysfunction, but extracapsular causes of TMJ pain are much more common. The TMJ is innervated by branches of the mandibular nerve. The muscles involved in TMJ dysfunction often include the temporalis, masseter, and external and internal pterygoids; the trapezius and sternocleidomastoid may be involved as well.

SIGNS AND SYMPTOMS

Headache often accompanies the pain of TMJ dysfunction and is clinically indistinguishable from tension-type headache. Stress is often the precipitating factor or an exacerbating factor in the development of TMJ dysfunction (Fig. 11-1). Dental malocclusion may also play a role in its evolution. Internal derangement and arthritis of the TMJ may manifest as clicking or grating when the mouth is opened and closed. If the condition is untreated, the patient may experience increasing pain in the aforementioned areas, as well as limitation of jaw movement and mouth opening.

Trigger points may be identified when palpating the muscles involved in TMJ dysfunction. Crepitus on range of

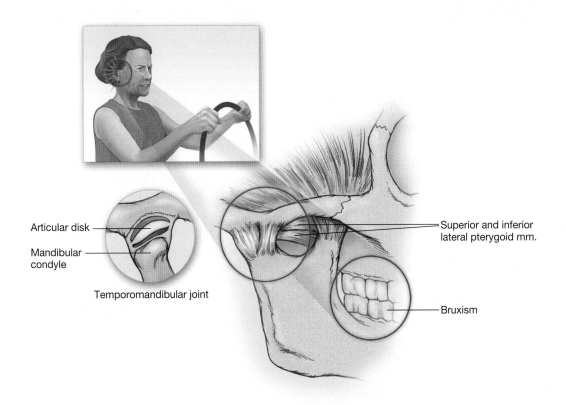

Articular disk

Mandibular condyle

Temporomandibular joint

Superior and inferior lateral pterygoid mm.

Bruxism

Figure 11-1 Stress is often a trigger for temporomandibular joint dysfunction.

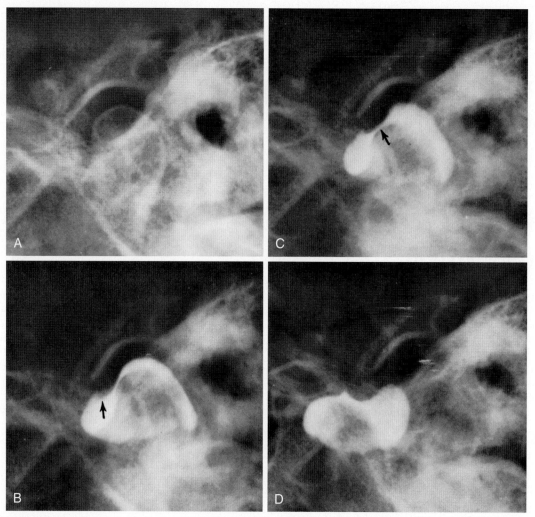

Figure 11-2 Arthrography of an abnormal temporomandibular joint showing disk dislocation with reduction in a 20-year-old woman with clicking and intermittent pain. **A,** Magnification transcranial radiograph with the mouth closed shows normal osseous anatomy and isocentric condyle position in the mandibular fossa. **B,** With the mouth closed, contrast agent fills the inferior joint space and outlines the undersurface of the disk. The posterior band of the disk is located anterior to the condyle *(arrow)* and bulges prominently in the anterior recess. This appearance is diagnostic of anterior dislocation of the disk. **C,** With the mouth half opened, contrast agent has been redistributed, and the condyle has moved onto the posterior band *(arrow),* which is now compressed between the condyle and the eminence. **D,** With the mouth fully opened, the condyle has translated anterior to the eminence; in so doing, it has crossed the prominent, thick posterior band and is causing a click. The posterior band is now in a normal position posterior to the condyle. *(From Resnick D: Diagnosis of bone and joint disorders, ed 4, Philadelphia, 2002, Saunders, p 1723.)*

motion of the joint suggests arthritis rather than dysfunction of myofascial origin. A history of bruxism or jaw clenching is often present.

TESTING

Radiographs of the TMJ are usually within normal limits in patients suffering from TMJ dysfunction, but they may be useful to help identify inflammatory or degenerative arthritis of the joint. Imaging of the joint can help the clinician identify derangement of the disk, as well as other abnormalities of the joint itself (Fig. 11-2). Magnetic resonance imaging may provide more detailed information regarding the condition of the disk and articular surface and should be considered in complicated cases. A complete blood count, erythrocyte sedimentation rate, and antinuclear antibody testing are indicated if inflammatory arthritis or temporal arteritis is suspected. Injection of the joint with small

amounts of local anesthetic can serve as a diagnostic maneuver to determine whether the TMJ is in fact the source of the patient's pain (Fig. 11-3).

DIFFERENTIAL DIAGNOSIS

The clinical symptoms of TMJ dysfunction may be confused with pain of dental or sinus origin or may be characterized as atypical facial pain. With careful questioning and physical examination, however, the clinician can usually distinguish these overlapping pain syndromes. Tumors of the zygoma and mandible, as well as retropharyngeal tumors, may produce ill-defined pain attributed to the TMJ, and these potentially life-threatening diseases must be excluded in any patient with facial pain. Reflex sympathetic dystrophy of the face should also be considered in any patient presenting with ill-defined facial pain after trauma, infection, or central nervous system injury. The pain of TMJ dysfunction is

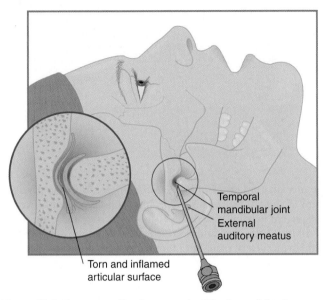

Figure 11-3 Correct needle placement for injections of the temporomandibular joint. *(From Waldman SD: Atlas of pain management injection techniques, Philadelphia, 2000, Saunders, p 5.)*

dull and aching, whereas the pain of reflex sympathetic dystrophy of the face is burning, with significant allodynia often present. Stellate ganglion block may help distinguish the two pain syndromes, because the pain of reflex sympathetic dystrophy of the face readily responds to this sympathetic nerve block, whereas the pain of TMJ dysfunction does not. In addition, the pain of TMJ dysfunction must be distinguished from the pain of jaw claudication associated with temporal arteritis.

TREATMENT

The mainstay of therapy is a combination of drug treatment with tricyclic antidepressants, physical modalities such as oral orthotic devices and physical therapy, and intraarticular injection of the joint with small amounts of local anesthetic and steroid. Antidepressant compounds such as nortriptyline at a single bedtime dose of 25 mg can help alleviate sleep disturbance and treat any underlying myofascial pain syndrome. Orthotic devices help the patient avoid jaw clenching and bruxism, which may exacerbate the clinical syndrome. Intraarticular injection is useful to palliate acute pain to allow physical therapy, as well as to treat joint arthritis that may contribute to the patient's pain and joint dysfunction. Rarely, surgical treatment of the displaced intraarticular disk is required to restore the joint to normal function and reduce pain.

For intraarticular injection of the TMJ, the patient is placed in the supine position with the cervical spine in the neutral position. The TMJ is identified by asking the patient to open and close the mouth several times and palpating the area just anterior and slightly inferior to the acoustic auditory meatus. After the joint is identified, the patient is asked to hold his or her mouth in the neutral position. A total of 0.5 mL of local anesthetic is drawn up in a 3-mL sterile syringe. When treating TMJ dysfunction, internal derangement of the TMJ, or arthritis or other painful conditions involving the TMJ, a total of 20 mg methylprednisolone is added to the local anesthetic with the first block; 10 mg methylprednisolone is added to the local anesthetic with subsequent blocks. After the skin overlying the TMJ is prepared with antiseptic solution, a 1-inch, 25-gauge styleted needle is inserted just below the zygomatic arch directly in the middle of the joint space. The needle is advanced approximately ¼ to ¾ inch in a plane perpendicular to the skull until a pop is felt, indicating that the joint space has been entered (see Fig. 11-3). After careful aspiration, 1 mL of solution is slowly injected. Injection of the joint may be repeated at 5- to 7-day intervals if symptoms persist.

COMPLICATIONS AND PITFALLS

The vascularity of the region and the proximity to major blood vessels lead to an increased incidence of postblock ecchymosis and hematoma formation, and the patient should be warned of this potential complication. Despite the region's vascularity, intraarticular injection can be performed safely (albeit with an increased risk of hematoma formation) in the presence of anticoagulation by using a 25- or 27-gauge needle, if the clinical situation indicates a favorable risk-to-benefit ratio. These complications can be decreased if manual pressure is applied to the area of the block immediately after injection. Application of cold packs for 20 minutes after the block also decreases the amount of postprocedural pain and bleeding. Another complication that occurs with some frequency is inadvertent block of the facial nerve, with associated facial weakness. When this occurs, protection of the cornea with sterile ophthalmic lubricant and patching is mandatory.

Clinical Pearls

Pain from TMJ dysfunction requires careful evaluation to design an appropriate treatment plan. Infection and inflammatory causes, including collagen vascular diseases, must be excluded. When TMJ pain occurs in older patients, it must be distinguished from the jaw claudication associated with temporal arteritis. Stress and anxiety often accompany TMJ dysfunction, and these factors must be addressed and managed. The myofascial pain component is best treated with tricyclic antidepressants, such as amitriptyline. Dental malocclusion and nighttime bruxism should be treated with an acrylic bite appliance. Opioid analgesics and benzodiazepines should be avoided in patients suffering from TMJ dysfunction.

SUGGESTED READINGS

Dimitroulis G: The role of surgery in the management of disorders of the temporomandibular joint: a critical review of the literature. Part 1, *Int J Oral Maxillofac Surg* 34(2):107–113, 2005.

Farina D, Bodin B, Gandolfi S, et al: TMJ disorders and pain: assessment by contrast-enhanced MRI, *Eur J Radiol* 70(1):25–30, 2009.

Lupoli TA, Lockey RF: Temporomandibular dysfunction: an often overlooked cause of chronic headaches, *Ann Allergy Asthma Immunol* 99(1):314–318, 2007.

Sano T, Otonari-Yamamoto M, Otonari T, et al: Osseous abnormalities related to the temporomandibular joint, *Semin Ultrasound CT MR* 28(3):213–221, 2007.

Sano T, Yamamoto M, Okano T, et al: Common abnormalities in temporomandibular joint imaging, *Curr Probl Diagn Radiol* 33(1):16–24, 2004.

Tomas X, Pomes J, Berenguer J, et al: Temporomandibular joint soft-tissue pathology. II. Nondisc abnormalities, *Semin Ultrasound CT MR* 28(3):205–212, 2007.

Chapter **12**

ATYPICAL FACIAL PAIN

ICD-9 CODE `350.2`

ICD-10 CODE `G50.1`

THE CLINICAL SYNDROME

Atypical facial pain (also known as atypical facial neuralgia) describes a heterogeneous group of pain syndromes that have in common the fact that the facial pain cannot be classified as trigeminal neuralgia. The pain is continuous but may vary in intensity. It is almost always unilateral and may be characterized as aching or cramping, rather than the shocklike neuritic pain typical of trigeminal neuralgia. Most patients suffering from atypical facial pain are female. The pain is felt in the distribution of the trigeminal nerve but invariably overlaps the divisions of the nerve (Fig. 12-1).

Headache often accompanies atypical facial pain and is clinically indistinguishable from tension-type headache. Stress is often the precipitating factor or an exacerbating factor in the development of atypical facial pain. Depression and sleep disturbance are also present in many patients. A history of facial trauma, infection, or tumor of the head and neck may be elicited in some patients with atypical facial pain, but in most cases, no precipitating event can be identified.

SIGNS AND SYMPTOMS

Table 12-1 compares atypical facial pain with trigeminal neuralgia. Unlike trigeminal neuralgia, which is characterized by sudden paroxysms of neuritic shocklike pain, atypical facial pain is constant and has a dull, aching quality, but it may vary in intensity. The pain of trigeminal neuralgia is always within the distribution of one division of the trigeminal nerve, whereas atypical facial pain always overlaps these divisional boundaries. The trigger areas characteristic of trigeminal neuralgia are absent in patients suffering from atypical facial pain.

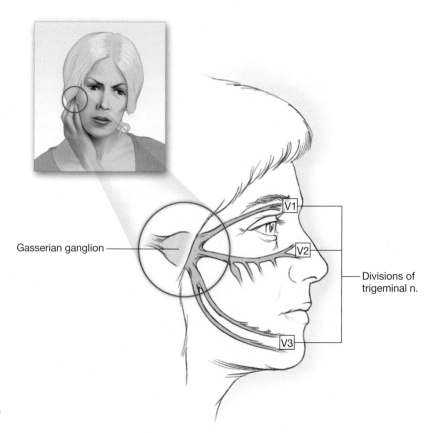

Gasserian ganglion

V1

V2

Divisions of trigeminal n.

V3

Figure 12-1 Patients with atypical facial pain often rub the affected area; those with trigeminal neuralgia do not.

TESTING

Radiographs of the head are usually within normal limits in patients suffering from atypical facial pain, but they may be useful to identify a tumor or bony abnormality (Fig. 12-2). Magnetic resonance imaging (MRI) of the brain and sinuses can help the clinician identify an intracranial disorder such as tumor, sinus disease, and infection. A complete blood count, erythrocyte sedimentation rate, and antinuclear antibody testing are indicated if inflammatory arthritis or temporal arteritis is suspected. Injection of the temporomandibular joint with small amounts of local anesthetic can serve as a diagnostic maneuver to determine whether the temporomandibular joint is the source of the patient's pain. MRI of the cervical spine is also indicated if the patient is experiencing significant occipital or nuchal pain.

DIFFERENTIAL DIAGNOSIS

The clinical symptoms of atypical facial pain may be confused with pain of dental or sinus origin or may be erroneously characterized as trigeminal neuralgia. Careful questioning and physical examination usually allow the clinician to distinguish these overlapping pain syndromes. Tumors of the zygoma and mandible, as well as posterior fossa and retropharyngeal tumors, may produce ill-defined pain that is attributed to atypical facial pain, and these potentially life-threatening diseases must be excluded in any patient with facial pain (Fig. 12-3). Reflex sympathetic dystrophy of the face should also be considered in any patient presenting with ill-defined facial pain after trauma, infection, or central nervous system injury. As noted, atypical facial pain is dull and aching, whereas reflex sympathetic dystrophy of the face causes burning pain, and significant allodynia is often present. Stellate ganglion block may help distinguish these two pain syndromes; the pain of reflex sympathetic dystrophy of the face readily responds to this sympathetic nerve block, whereas atypical facial pain does not. Atypical facial pain must also be distinguished from the pain of jaw claudication associated with temporal arteritis.

TABLE 12-1

Comparison of Trigeminal Neuralgia and Atypical Facial Pain

	Trigeminal Neuralgia	Atypical Facial Pain
Temporal pattern of pain	Sudden and intermittent	Constant
Character of pain	Shocklike and neuritic	Dull, cramping, aching
Pain-free intervals	Usual	Rare
Distribution of pain	One division of trigeminal nerve	Overlapping divisions of trigeminal nerve
Trigger areas	Present	Absent
Underlying psychopathology	Rare	Common

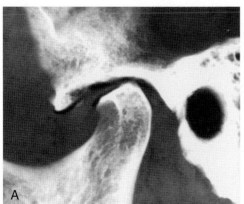
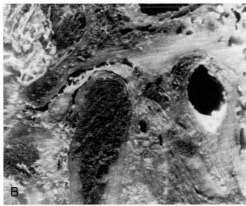

Figure 12-2 Osteoarthritis compared in a specimen radiograph **(A)** and a photograph **(B)** of a sagittally sectioned specimen. *(From Resnick D: Diagnosis of bone and joint disorders, ed 4, Philadelphia, 2002, Saunders, p 1739.)*

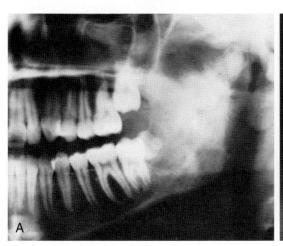
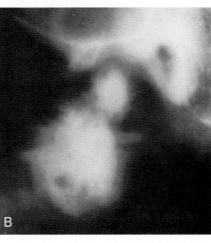

Figure 12-3 Osteosarcoma of the mandible **(A)** and the condylar head and neck **(B)** in a 12-year-old girl. *(From Resnick D: Diagnosis of bone and joint disorders, ed 4, Philadelphia, 2002, Saunders, p 1726.)*

TREATMENT

The mainstay of therapy is a combination of drug treatment with tricyclic antidepressants and physical modalities such as oral orthotic devices and physical therapy. Trigeminal nerve block and intraarticular injection of the temporomandibular joint with small amounts of local anesthetic and steroid may also be of value. Antidepressants such as nortriptyline, at a single bedtime dose of 25 mg, can help alleviate sleep disturbance and treat any underlying myofascial pain syndrome. Orthotic devices help the patient avoid jaw clenching and bruxism, which may exacerbate the clinical syndrome. Management of underlying depression and anxiety is also mandatory.

COMPLICATIONS AND PITFALLS

The major pitfall when caring for patients thought to be suffering from atypical facial pain is the failure to diagnose an underlying pathologic process that may be responsible for the patient's pain. Atypical facial pain is essentially a diagnosis of exclusion. If trigeminal nerve block or intraarticular injection of the temporomandibular joint is being considered as part of the treatment plan, the clinician must remember that the region's vascularity and proximity to major blood vessels can lead to an increased incidence of postblock ecchymosis and hematoma formation, and the patient should be warned of this potential complication.

Clinical Pearls

Atypical facial pain requires careful evaluation to design an appropriate treatment plan. Infection and inflammatory causes, including collagen vascular diseases, must be excluded. Stress and anxiety often accompany atypical facial pain, and these factors must be addressed and treated. The myofascial pain component of atypical facial pain is best treated with tricyclic antidepressants such as amitriptyline. Dental malocclusion and nighttime bruxism should be treated with an acrylic bite appliance. Opioid analgesics and benzodiazepines should be avoided in patients suffering from atypical facial pain.

SUGGESTED READINGS

Cook RJ, Sharif I, Escudier M: Meningioma as a cause of chronic orofacial pain: case reports, *Br J Oral Maxillofac Surg* 46(6):487–489, 2008.

Forssell H, Svensson P: Atypical facial pain and burning mouth syndrome, *Handb Clin Neurol* 81:597–608, 2006.

Koopman JS, Dieleman JP, Huygen FJ, et al: Incidence of facial pain in the general population, *Pain* 147(1–3):122–127, 2009.

McQuay HJ, Tramér M, Nye BA, et al: A systematic review of antidepressants in neuropathic pain, *Pain* 68(2–3):217–227, 1996.

Türp JC, Gobetti JP: Trigeminal neuralgia versus atypical facial pain: a review of the literature and case report, *Oral Surg Oral Med Oral Pathol Oral Radiol Endod* 81(4):424–432, 1996.

Waldman SD: Atypical facial pain. In *Pain review,* Philadelphia, 2009, Saunders, pp 233–234.

Chapter **13**

HYOID SYNDROME

ICD-9 CODE 727.82

ICD-10 CODE M65.20

THE CLINICAL SYNDROME

Hyoid syndrome is caused by calcification and inflammation of the attachment of the stylohyoid ligament to the hyoid bone. The styloid process extends in a caudal and ventral direction from the temporal bone from its origin just below the auditory meatus. The stylohyoid ligament's cephalad attachment is to the styloid process, and its caudad attachment is to the hyoid bone. In hyoid syndrome, the stylohyoid ligament becomes calcified at its caudad attachment to the hyoid bone (Fig. 13-1). Tendinitis of the other muscular attachments to the hyoid bone may contribute to this painful condition. Hyoid syndrome also may be seen in conjunction with Eagle's syndrome. Patient's suffering from diffuse idiopathic skeletal hyperostosis are thought to be prone to the development of hyoid syndrome because of the propensity for calcification of the stylohyoid ligament in this disease (Fig. 13-2).

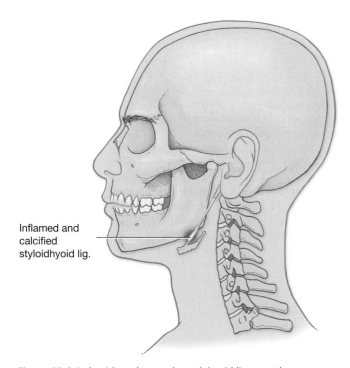

Inflamed and
calcified
styloidhyoid lig.

Figure 13-1 In hyoid syndrome, the stylohyoid ligament becomes calcified at its caudad attachment to the hyoid bone.

SIGNS AND SYMPTOMS

The pain of hyoid syndrome is sharp and stabbing and occurs with movement of the mandible, turning of the neck, or swallowing. The pain starts below the angle of the mandible and radiates into the anterolateral neck (Fig. 13-3); it is often referred to the ipsilateral ear. Some patients complain of a foreign body sensation in the pharynx. Injection of local anesthetic and steroid into the attachment of the stylohyoid ligament to the greater cornu of the hyoid bone is both a diagnostic and a therapeutic maneuver.

TESTING

No specific test exists for hyoid syndrome. Plain radiography, computed tomography, or magnetic resonance imaging of the neck may reveal calcification of the caudad attachment of the stylohyoid ligament at the hyoid bone. This calcification is highly suggestive of hyoid syndrome in patients suffering from the previously described constellation of symptoms. A complete blood count, erythrocyte sedimentation rate, and antinuclear antibody testing are indicated if inflammatory arthritis or temporal arteritis is suspected. As noted earlier, injection of small amounts of anesthetic into the attachment of the stylohyoid ligament to the hyoid bone can help determine whether this is the source of the patient's pain. If difficulty swallowing is a prominent feature of the clinical presentation, endoscopy of the esophagus, with special attention to the gastroesophageal junction, is mandatory to identify esophageal tumors or strictures resulting from gastric reflux.

DIFFERENTIAL DIAGNOSIS

The diagnosis of hyoid syndrome is one of exclusion, and the clinician must first rule out other conditions (Table 13-1). Retropharyngeal infection and tumor may produce ill-defined pain that mimics the pain and other symptoms of hyoid syndrome, and these potentially life-threatening diseases must be excluded (Fig. 13-4).

Osteomyelitis of the hyoid bone, especially in immunocompromised patients, may also mimic hyoid syndrome. Glossopharyngeal neuralgia is another painful condition that can be mistaken for hyoid syndrome. However, the pain of glossopharyngeal neuralgia is similar to the paroxysms of shocklike pain in trigeminal neuralgia, rather than the sharp, shooting pain with movement associated with hyoid syndrome. Because glossopharyngeal neuralgia may be associated with serious cardiac bradyarrhythmias and syncope, the clinician must distinguish between the two syndromes.

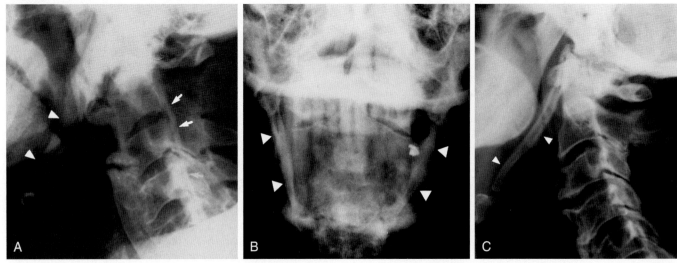

Figure 13-2 Cervical spine abnormalities in diffuse idiopathic skeletal hyperostosis (DISH). **A** and **B,** Radiographic abnormalities in this patient with DISH include extensive anterior bone formation, ossification of the posterior longitudinal ligament *(arrows),* and ossification of both stylohyoid ligaments *(arrowheads).* **C,** In another patient, note the extensive ossification of the stylohyoid ligament *(arrowheads)* and the changes caused by spinal DISH. *(From Resnick D:* Diagnosis of bone and joint disorders, *ed 4, Philadelphia, 2002, Saunders, p 1483.)*

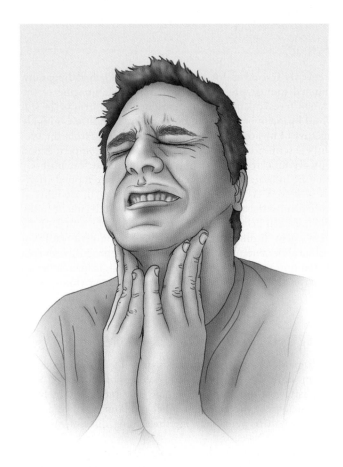

Figure 13-3 The pain of hyoid syndrome is sharp and stabbing and occurs with movement of the mandible, turning of the neck, or swallowing. The pain starts below the angle of the mandible and radiates to the anterolateral neck.

TABLE 13-1
Conditions That Can Mimic Hyoid Syndrome
Glossopharyngeal neuralgia
Retropharyngeal tumor
Retropharyngeal abscess
Osteomyelitis of the hyoid bone
Atypical facial pain
Mandibular tumor
Esophageal disease
Jaw claudication of temporal arteritis

TREATMENT

The pain of hyoid syndrome is best treated with local anesthetic and steroid injection of the attachment of the stylohyoid ligament. Owing to the vascularity of this area and the proximity to neural structures, this technique should be performed only by those familiar with the regional anatomy. A trial of nonsteroidal antiinflammatory agents may also be worthwhile in mild cases. Antidepressants such as nortriptyline, at a single bedtime dose of 25 mg, can help alleviate sleep disturbance and treat any underlying myofascial pain syndrome.

COMPLICATIONS AND PITFALLS

The major pitfall when caring for patients thought to be suffering from hyoid syndrome is the failure to diagnose some other underlying disease that may be responsible for the pain. If injection of the caudad attachment of the stylohyoid ligament is being considered as part of the treatment plan, the clinician should remember that the area's vascularity and proximity to major blood vessels can lead to an increased incidence of postblock ecchymosis and hematoma formation, and the patient should be warned of this potential complication.

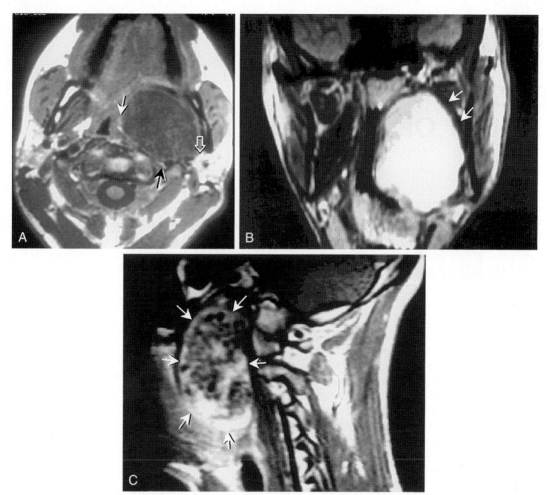

Figure 13-4 Pleomorphic adenoma. **A,** Nonenhanced, T1-weighted axial magnetic resonance imaging (MRI) demonstrates a well-defined mass of lower signal intensity than adjacent muscle. The mass is displacing the prestyloid parapharyngeal fat medially *(solid white arrow)* and the internal carotid artery posteriorly *(solid black arrow)*. No intact fat plane can be demonstrated between the lesion and the deep lobe of the parotid gland *(open arrow)*. **B,** Intermediate-weighted coronal MRI demonstrates a relatively homogeneous, well-defined mass of increased signal intensity relative to adjacent muscle and lymphoid tissue. The oropharyngeal mucosa is displaced medially. The left medial pterygoid muscle is compressed and displaced superolaterally *(arrows)*. **C,** Contrast-enhanced, T1-weighted sagittal MRI demonstrates a markedly heterogeneous mass *(arrows)*, with multiple low-signal-intensity regions that may represent areas of calcification or fibrosis. (*From Haaga JR, Lanzieri CF, Gilkeson RC, editors:* CT and MR imaging of the whole body, *ed 4, Philadelphia, 2003, Mosby, p 653.*)

Clinical Pearls

The clinician should always look for occult malignant disease in patients suffering from pain in this region. Tumors of the larynx, hypopharynx, and anterior triangle of the neck may manifest with clinical symptoms identical to those of hyoid syndrome. Given the low incidence of hyoid syndrome compared with pain secondary to malignant disease, hyoid syndrome must be considered a diagnosis of exclusion.

SUGGESTED READINGS

Carlson GW: The pharyngoesophageal region. In McCarthy JG, Galiano RD, Boutros SG, editors: *Current therapy in plastic surgery,* Philadelphia, 2005, Saunders, pp 172–175.

Ernest EA III, Salter G: Hyoid bone syndrome: a degenerative injury of the middle pharyngeal constrictor muscle with photomicroscopic evidence of insertion tendinosis, *J Prosthet Dent* 66(1):78–83, 1991.

Rubin MM, Sanfilippo RJ: Osteomyelitis of the hyoid caused by torulopsis glabrata in a patient with acquired immunodeficiency syndrome, *J Oral Maxillofac Surg* 48(11):1217–1219, 1990.

van der Westhuijzen AJ, van der Merwe J, Grotepass FW: Eagle's syndrome: lesser cornu amputation—an alternative surgical solution? *Int J Oral Maxillofac Surg* 28(5):335–337, 1999.

Chapter 14

REFLEX SYMPATHETIC DYSTROPHY OF THE FACE

ICD-9 CODE **337.29**

ICD-10 CODE **G90.59**

THE CLINICAL SYNDROME

Reflex sympathetic dystrophy (RSD) is an infrequent cause of face and neck pain. Also known as chronic regional pain syndrome type I, RSD of the face is a classic case in which the clinician must think of the diagnosis to make it. Although the symptom complex in this disorder is relatively constant from patient to patient, and although RSD of the face and neck closely parallels its presentation in the upper or lower extremity, the diagnosis is often missed. As a result, extensive diagnostic and therapeutic procedures may be performed in an effort to palliate the patient's facial pain. The common denominator in all patients suffering from RSD of the face is trauma (Fig. 14-1), which may take the following forms: actual injury to the soft tissues, dentition, or bones of the face; infection; cancer; arthritis; or insults to the central nervous system or cranial nerves.

SIGNS AND SYMPTOMS

The hallmark of RSD of the face is burning pain. The pain is frequently associated with cutaneous or mucosal allodynia and does not follow the path of either the cranial or the peripheral nerves. Trigger areas, especially in the oral mucosa, are common, as are trophic skin and mucosal changes in the area affected by RSD

(Fig. 14-2). Sudomotor and vasomotor changes may also be identified, but these are often less obvious than in patients suffering from RSD of the extremities. Often, patients with RSD of the face have evidence of previous dental extractions performed in an effort to achieve pain relief. These patients also frequently experience significant sleep disturbance and depression.

TESTING

Although no specific test exists for RSD, a presumptive diagnosis can be made if the patient experiences significant pain relief after stellate ganglion block with local anesthetic. Given the diverse nature of the tissue injury that can cause RSD of the face, however, the clinician must assiduously search for occult disease that may mimic or coexist with RSD (see "Differential Diagnosis"). All patients with a presumptive diagnosis of RSD of the face should undergo magnetic resonance imaging of the brain and, if significant occipital or nuchal symptoms are present, of the cervical spine. Screening laboratory tests consisting of a complete blood count, erythrocyte sedimentation rate, and automated blood chemistry should be performed to rule out infection or other inflammatory causes of tissue injury that may serve as a nidus for RSD.

DIFFERENTIAL DIAGNOSIS

The clinical symptoms of RSD of the face may be confused with pain of dental or sinus origin or may be erroneously characterized as atypical facial pain or trigeminal neuralgia (Table 14-1).

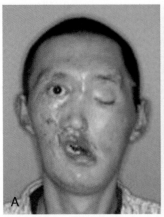
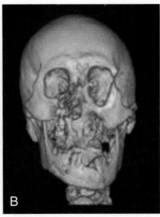
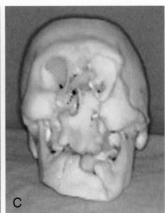

Figure 14-1 Example of severe facial deformity secondary to panfacial fractures before definitive treatment. **A,** Preoperative facial photograph. **B,** Three-dimensional computed tomography (CT) scan showing the mandibular fracture in the tooth-bearing region. The left side of the midface has severely displaced fractures, and the right side has bone defects. **C,** Stereolithic model based on CT data to assist in treatment planning. *(From He D, Zhang Y, Ellis E III: Panfacial fractures: analysis of 33 cases treated late,* J Oral Maxillofac Surg *65(12):2459–2465, 2007.)*

Careful questioning and physical examination usually allow the clinician to distinguish among these overlapping pain syndromes. Stellate ganglion block may help distinguish RSD from atypical facial pain, because RSD readily responds to sympathetic nerve block, whereas atypical facial pain does not. Tumors of the zygoma and mandible, as well as posterior fossa and retropharyngeal tumors, may produce ill-defined pain attributed to RSD of the face, and these potentially life-threatening diseases must be excluded in any patient with facial pain. RSD of the face must also be distinguished from the pain of jaw claudication associated with temporal arteritis.

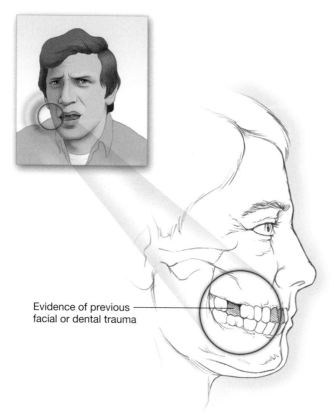

Evidence of previous facial or dental trauma

Figure 14-2 Reflex sympathetic dystrophy of the face frequently occurs following trauma, such as dental extractions.

TREATMENT

The successful treatment of RSD of the face requires two phases. First, any nidus of tissue trauma that is contributing to the ongoing sympathetic dysfunction responsible for the symptoms must be identified and removed. Second, interruption of the sympathetic innervation of the face by means of stellate ganglion block with local anesthetic must be implemented. This may require daily stellate ganglion block for a significant period. Occupational therapy consisting of tactile desensitization of the affected skin may also be of value. Underlying depression and sleep disturbance are best treated with a tricyclic antidepressant such as nortriptyline, given as a single 25-mg dose at bedtime. Gabapentin may help palliate any neuritic pain component and is best started slowly with a single bedtime dose of 300 mg, with dosage titration upward in divided doses to a maximum dose of 3600 mg per day. Pregabalin represents a reasonable alternative to gabapentin and is better tolerated in some patients. Pregabalin is started at 50 mg three times a day and may be titrated upward to 100 mg three times a day as side effects allow. Because pregabalin is excreted primarily by the kidneys, the dosage should be decreased in patients with compromised renal function.

Opioid analgesics and benzodiazepines should be avoided to prevent iatrogenic chemical dependence.

COMPLICATIONS AND PITFALLS

The main complications of RSD of the face are those associated with its misdiagnosis. In this case, chemical dependence, depression, and multiple failed therapeutic procedures are the rule rather than the exception. Stellate ganglion block is a safe and effective technique for pain management, but it is not without side effects and risks.

Clinical Pearls

The key to recognizing RSD of the face is a high index of clinical suspicion. RSD should be suspected in any patient who has burning pain or allodynia associated with antecedent trauma. Once the syndrome is recognized, blockade of the sympathetic nerves subserving the painful area confirms the diagnosis. Repeated sympathetic blockade, combined with adjunctive therapies, results in pain relief in most cases. The frequency and number of sympathetic blocks recommended to treat RSD vary among pain practitioners; however, early and aggressive neural blockade is believed to provide more rapid resolution of pain and disability.

TABLE 14-1

Differential Diagnosis of Reflex Sympathetic Dystrophy of the Face

	Trigeminal Neuralgia	Atypical Facial Pain	RSD of the Face
Temporal pattern of pain	Sudden and intermittent	Constant	Constant
Character of pain	Shocklike and neuritic	Dull, cramping, aching	Burning with allodynia
Pain-free intervals	Usual	Rare	Rare
Distribution of pain	One division of trigeminal nerve	Overlapping divisions of trigeminal nerve	Overlapping divisions of trigeminal nerve
Trigger areas	Present	Absent	Present
Underlying psychopathology	Rare	Common	Common
Trophic skin changes	Absent	Absent	Present
Sudomotor and vasomotor changes	Absent	Absent	Often present

RSD, reflex sympathetic dystrophy.

SUGGESTED READINGS

Jaeger B, Singer E, Kroening R: Reflex sympathetic dystrophy of the face: report of two cases and a review of the literature, *Arch Neurol* 43(7):693–695, 1986.

Waldman SD: Reflex sympathetic dystrophy of the face. In *Pain review,* Philadelphia, 2009, Saunders, pp 253–254.

Waldman SD: Stellate ganglion block: anterior approach. In *Atlas of interventional pain management,* ed 3, Philadelphia, 2009, Saunders, pp 131–134.

Waldman SD, Waldman K: Reflex sympathetic dystrophy of the face and neck: report of six patients treated with stellate ganglion block, *Reg Anesth Pain Med* 12(1):15–17, 1987.

Chapter **15**

CERVICAL FACET SYNDROME

ICD-9 CODE **721.0**

ICD-10 CODE **M47.812**

THE CLINICAL SYNDROME

Cervical facet syndrome is a constellation of symptoms consisting of neck, head, shoulder, and proximal upper extremity pain that radiates in a nondermatomal pattern. The pain is ill defined and dull. It may be unilateral or bilateral and is thought to be the result of a pathologic process of the facet joint. The pain of cervical facet syndrome is exacerbated by flexion, extension, and lateral bending of the cervical spine. It is often worse in the morning after physical activity. Each facet joint receives innervation from two spinal levels; it receives fibers from the dorsal ramus at the corresponding vertebral level and from the vertebra above. This pattern explains the ill-defined nature of facet-mediated pain and explains why the dorsal nerve from the vertebra above the offending level must often be blocked to provide complete pain relief.

SIGNS AND SYMPTOMS

Most patients with cervical facet syndrome have tenderness to deep palpation of the cervical paraspinous musculature; muscle spasm may also be present. Patients exhibit decreased range of motion of the cervical spine and usually complain of pain on flexion, extension, rotation, and lateral bending of the cervical spine (Fig. 15-1). No motor or sensory deficit is present unless the patient has coexisting radiculopathy, plexopathy, or entrapment neuropathy.

If the C1-2 facet joints are involved, the pain is referred to the posterior auricular and occipital region. If the C2-3 facet joints are involved, the pain may radiate to the forehead and eyes. Pain emanating from the C3-4 facet joints is referred superiorly to the suboccipital region and inferiorly to the posterolateral neck, and pain from the C4-5 facet joints radiates to the base of the neck. Pain from the C5-6 facet joints is referred to the shoulders and interscapular region, and pain from the C6-7 facet joints radiates to the supraspinous and infraspinous fossae.

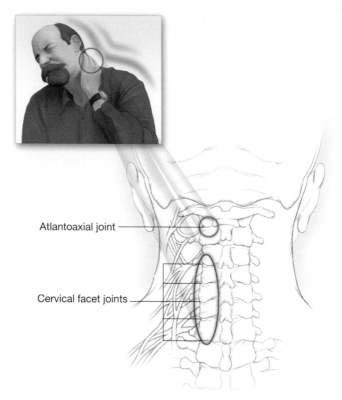

Atlantoaxial joint

Cervical facet joints

Figure 15-1 The pain of cervical facet syndrome is made worse by flexion, extension, and lateral bending of the cervical spine.

TESTING

By the fifth decade of life, almost all individuals exhibit some abnormality of the facet joints of the cervical spine on plain radiographs (Fig. 15-2). The clinical significance of these findings has long been debated by pain specialists, but it was not until the advent of computed tomography scanning and magnetic resonance imaging (MRI) that the relationship between these abnormal facet joints and the cervical nerve roots and other surrounding structures was clearly understood. MRI of the cervical spine should be performed in all patients suspected

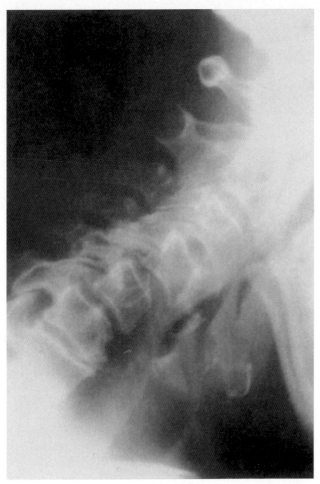

Figure 15-2 Lateral view of the cervical spine showing osteoarthritis of the apophyseal joints of the upper cervical spine, with resultant subluxation of C4 on C5. Additional findings are degenerative disk disease at C5-6 and C6-7, associated osteophyte formation at C6-7, and subluxation of C5 on C6. *(From Brower AC, Flemming DJ: Arthritis in black and white, ed 2, Philadelphia, 1997, Saunders, p 290.)*

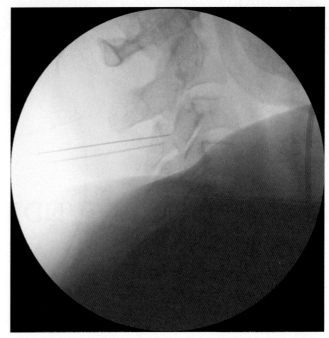

Figure 15-3 Fluoroscopic image of medial branch block for cervical facet syndrome.

TREATMENT

Cervical facet syndrome is best treated with a multimodality approach. Physical therapy consisting of heat modalities and deep sedative massage, combined with nonsteroidal antiinflammatory drugs and skeletal muscle relaxants, is a reasonable starting point. The addition of cervical facet blocks is a logical next step. For symptomatic relief, blockade of the medial branch of the dorsal ramus or intraarticular injection of the facet joint with local anesthetic and steroid is extremely effective (Fig. 15-3). Radiofrequency lesioning of the medial branches of the affect facet joints should be considered in patients who have experienced good, but temporary relief of their pain following facet block with local anesthetic and steroid. Underlying sleep disturbance and depression are best treated with a tricyclic antidepressant such as nortriptyline, which can be started at a single bedtime dose of 25 mg.

Cervical facet block is often combined with atlanto-occipital block for treatment of pain in this area. Although the atlanto-occipital joint is not a true facet joint in the anatomic sense, the technique is analogous to the facet joint block commonly used by pain practitioners and may be viewed as such.

COMPLICATIONS AND PITFALLS

The proximity to the spinal cord and exiting nerve roots makes it imperative that cervical facet block be carried out only by those familiar with the regional anatomy and experienced in interventional pain management techniques. The proximity to the vertebral artery, combined with the vascular nature of this region, makes the potential for intravascular injection high, and the injection of even a small amount of local anesthetic into the vertebral artery can result in seizures. Given the proximity of the brain and brainstem, ataxia resulting from vascular uptake of local anesthetic is not uncommon after cervical facet block. Many patients also complain of a transient increase in headache and cervicalgia after injection of the joint.

of suffering from cervical facet syndrome. However, any data gleaned from this sophisticated imaging technique can provide only a presumptive diagnosis. To prove that a specific facet joint is contributing to the patient's pain, a diagnostic intraarticular injection of that joint with local anesthetic is required. If the diagnosis of cervical facet syndrome is in doubt, screening laboratory tests consisting of a complete blood count, erythrocyte sedimentation rate, antinuclear antibody testing, human leukocyte antigen (HLA)-B27 antigen screening, and automated blood chemistry should be performed to rule out other causes of the patient's pain.

DIFFERENTIAL DIAGNOSIS

Cervical facet syndrome is a diagnosis of exclusion that is supported by a combination of clinical history, physical examination, radiography, MRI, and intraarticular injection of the suspect facet joint. Pain syndromes that may mimic cervical facet syndrome include cervicalgia, cervical bursitis, cervical fibromyositis, inflammatory arthritis, and disorders of the cervical spinal cord, roots, plexus, and nerves.

Clinical Pearls

Cervical facet syndrome is a common cause of neck, occipital, shoulder, and upper extremity pain. It is often confused with cervicalgia and cervical fibromyositis. Diagnostic intra-articular facet block can confirm the diagnosis. The clinician must take care to rule out diseases of the cervical spinal cord, such as syringomyelia, that may initially manifest in a similar manner. Ankylosing spondylitis may also manifest as cervical facet syndrome and must be correctly identified to avoid ongoing joint damage and functional disability.

Many pain specialists believe that cervical facet block and atlanto-occipital block are underused in the treatment of "post-whiplash" cervicalgia and cervicogenic headaches and that they should be considered whenever cervical epidural or occipital nerve blocks fail to provide palliation of headache and neck pain syndromes.

SUGGESTED READINGS

Kirpalani D, Mitra R: Cervical facet joint dysfunction: a review, *Arch Phys Med Rehabil* 89(4):770–774, 2008.

Uhrenholt L, Charles AV, Hauge E, et al: Pathoanatomy of the lower cervical spine facet joints in motor vehicle crash fatalities, *J Forensic Leg Med* 16(5):253–260, 2009.

Waldman SD: Cervical facet block: medial branch technique block. In *Atlas of interventional pain management*, ed 3, Philadelphia, 2009, Saunders, pp 157–160.

Waldman SD: Cervical facet joints. In *Pain review*, Philadelphia, 2009, Saunders, pp 58–59.

Waldman SD: Cervical facet syndrome. In *Pain review*, Philadelphia, 2009, Saunders, pp 241–243.

White K, Hudgins TH, Alleva JT: Cervical facet mediated pain, *Dis Month* 55(12):729–736, 2009.

Chapter 16

CERVICAL RADICULOPATHY

ICD-9 CODE **723.4**

ICD-10 CODE **M54.12**

THE CLINICAL SYNDROME

Cervical radiculopathy is a constellation of symptoms consisting of neurogenic neck and upper extremity pain emanating from the cervical nerve roots. In addition to pain, the patient may experience numbness, weakness, and loss of reflexes. The causes of cervical radiculopathy include herniated disk, foraminal stenosis, tumor, osteophyte formation, and, rarely, infection.

SIGNS AND SYMPTOMS

Patients suffering from cervical radiculopathy complain of pain, numbness, tingling, and paresthesias in the distribution of the affected nerve root or roots (Table 16-1). Patients may also note weakness and lack of coordination in the affected extremity. Muscle spasms and neck pain, as well as pain referred to the trapezius and interscapular region, are common. Decreased sensation, weakness, and reflex changes are demonstrated on physical examination. Patients with C7 radiculopathy commonly place the hand of the affected extremity on top of the head to obtain relief (Fig. 16-1). Occasionally, patients suffering from cervical radiculopathy experience compression of the cervical spinal cord, with resulting myelopathy. Cervical myelopathy is most commonly caused by a midline herniated cervical disk, spinal

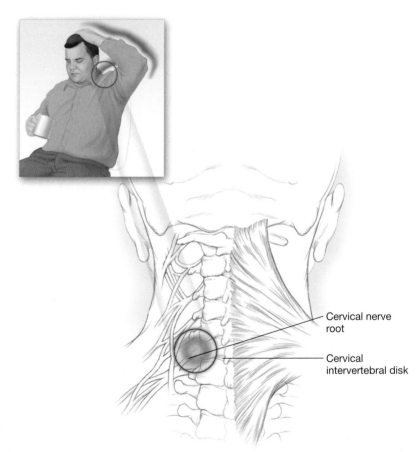

Cervical nerve root

Cervical intervertebral disk

Figure 16-1 Patients with C7 radiculopathy often place the hand of the affected extremity on the head to obtain relief.

TABLE 16-1

Clinical Features of Cervical Radiculopathy

Cervical Root	Pain	Sensory Changes	Weakness	Reflex Changes
C5	Neck, shoulder, anterolateral arm	Numbness in deltoid area	Deltoid and biceps	Biceps reflex
C6	Neck, shoulder, lateral aspect of arm	Dorsolateral aspect of thumb and index finger	Biceps, wrist extensors, pollicis longus	Brachioradialis reflex
C7	Neck, shoulder, lateral aspect of arm, dorsal forearm	Index and middle fingers and dorsum of hand	Triceps	Triceps reflex

stenosis, tumor, or, rarely, infection. Patients suffering from cervical myelopathy experience lower extremity weakness and bowel and bladder symptoms. This condition represents a neurosurgical emergency and should be treated as such.

TESTING

Magnetic resonance imaging (MRI) provides the best information regarding the cervical spine and its contents (Fig. 16-2). MRI is highly accurate and can identify abnormalities that may put the patient at risk for cervical myelopathy (Fig. 16-3). In patients who cannot undergo MRI, such as those with pacemakers, computed tomography or myelography is a reasonable alternative. Provocative diskography may also provide useful diagnostic information if the MRI findings are equivocal. Radionuclide bone scanning and plain radiography are indicated if fractures or bony abnormalities such as metastatic disease are being considered.

Although these tests provide the clinician with useful neuroanatomic information, electromyography and nerve conduction velocity testing furnish neurophysiologic information that can determine the actual status of each individual nerve root and the brachial plexus. Electromyography can also distinguish plexopathy from radiculopathy and can identify a coexistent entrapment neuropathy, such as carpal tunnel syndrome. Screening laboratory tests consisting of a complete blood count, erythrocyte sedimentation rate, antinuclear antibody testing, human leukocyte antigen (HLA)-B27 antigen screening, and automated blood chemistry should be performed if the diagnosis of cervical radiculopathy is in question.

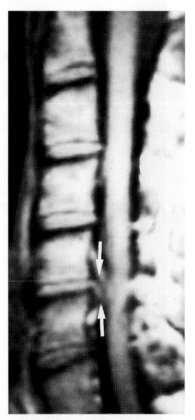

Figure 16-2 Disk herniation at the C5-6 level. Sagittal T1-weighted spin-echo magnetic resonance image showing a herniated fragment *(arrows)* extending below the disk space level. *(From Stark DD, Bradley WG Jr, editors: Magnetic resonance imaging, vol 3, ed 3, St Louis, 1999, Mosby, p 1848.)*

DIFFERENTIAL DIAGNOSIS

Cervical radiculopathy is a clinical diagnosis supported by a combination of clinical history, physical examination, radiography, and MRI. Pain syndromes that may mimic cervical radiculopathy include cervicalgia, cervical bursitis, cervical fibromyositis, inflammatory arthritis, and disorders of the cervical spinal cord, roots, plexus, and nerves.

TREATMENT

Cervical radiculopathy is best treated with a multimodality approach. Physical therapy, including heat modalities and deep sedative massage, combined with nonsteroidal antiinflammatory drugs and skeletal muscle relaxants, is a reasonable starting point. The addition of cervical epidural nerve blocks is a logical next step. Cervical epidural blocks with local anesthetic and steroid

are extremely effective in the treatment of cervical radiculopathy. Underlying sleep disturbance and depression are best treated with a tricyclic antidepressant such as nortriptyline, which can be started at a single bedtime dose of 25 mg. In patients who fail to respond to epidural steroid injections, a trial of spinal cord stimulation is a reasonable next step if definitive surgical treatment is not an option (Fig. 16-4).

COMPLICATIONS AND PITFALLS

Failure to diagnosis cervical radiculopathy accurately may put the patient at risk for the development of cervical myelopathy, which, if untreated, may progress to quadriparesis or quadriplegia.

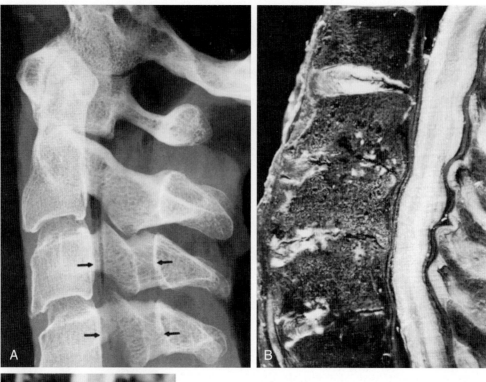

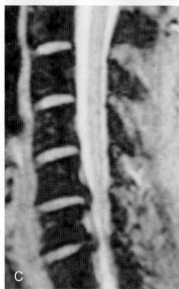

Figure 16-3 Cervical spinal stenosis. **A,** Measurement of the sagittal diameter of the spinal canal is accomplished by calculating the distance between the posterior surface of the vertebral body and the spinolaminar line *(between the arrows).* At the C4-7 levels, spinal cord compression is unlikely if the diameter of the canal is 13 mm or more. **B,** Photograph of a sagittal section of the cervical spine reveals stenosis of the central canal related to intervertebral (osteo)chondrosis and osteophytes anteriorly and ligamentous laxity and hypertrophy posteriorly. **C,** Sagittal multiple planar gradient recalled (MPGR) magnetic resonance image reveals stenosis of the lower cervical spine related to the presence of osteophytes arising from the posterior surface of the vertebral bodies. *(From Resnick D:* Diagnosis of bone and joint disorders, *ed 4, Philadelphia, 2002, Saunders, p 1655.)*

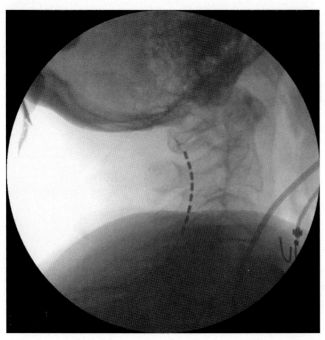

Figure 16-4 Spinal cord stimulator lead within the cervical epidural space.

Clinical Pearls

Carpal tunnel syndrome should be differentiated from cervical radiculopathy involving the cervical nerve roots, which may mimic median nerve compression. Further, cervical radiculopathy and median nerve entrapment may coexist in the double-crush syndrome, which is seen most commonly in patients with carpal tunnel syndrome.

SUGGESTED READINGS

Ellis H: The anatomy of the epidural space, *Anaesth Intensive Care Med* 10(11): 533–535, 2009.

Polston DW: Cervical radiculopathy, *Neurol Clin* 25(2):373–385, 2007.

Roth D, Mukai A, Thomas P, et al: Cervical radiculopathy, *Dis Month* 55(12): 737–756, 2009.

Waldman SD: Cervical epidural nerve block: the translaminar approach. In *Atlas of interventional pain management,* ed 3, Philadelphia, 2009, Saunders, pp 169–174.

Waldman SD: Cervical radiculopathy. In *Pain review,* Philadelphia, 2009, Saunders, pp 236–237.

Waldman SD: Cervical spinal cord stimulation: stage I trial stimulation. In *Atlas of interventional pain management,* ed 3, Philadelphia, 2009, Saunders, pp 659–652.

Chapter **17**

FIBROMYALGIA OF THE CERVICAL MUSCULATURE

ICD-9 CODE `729.1`

ICD-10 CODE `M79.7`

THE CLINICAL SYNDROME

Fibromyalgia is a chronic pain syndrome that affects a focal or regional portion of the body. Fibromyalgia of the cervical spine is one of the most common painful conditions encountered in clinical practice. The sine qua non for diagnosis is the finding of myofascial trigger points on physical examination. These trigger points are thought to be the result of microtrauma to the affected muscles. Stimulation of the myofascial trigger points reproduces or exacerbates the patient's pain. Although these trigger points are generally localized to the cervical paraspinous musculature, the trapezius, and other muscles of the neck, the pain is often referred to other areas. This referred pain may be misdiagnosed or attributed to other organ systems, thus leading to extensive evaluation and ineffective treatment.

The pathophysiology of the myofascial trigger points of fibromyalgia of the cervical spine remains unclear, but tissue trauma seems to be the common denominator. Acute trauma to muscle caused by overstretching commonly results in fibromyalgia. More subtle muscle injury in the form of repetitive microtrauma, damage to muscle fibers from exposure to extreme heat or cold, overuse, chronic deconditioning of the agonist and antagonist muscle unit, or other coexistent disease processes such as radiculopathy may also produce fibromyalgia of the cervical spine.

Various other factors seem to predispose patients to the development of fibromyalgia of the cervical spine. For example, a weekend athlete who subjects his or her body to unaccustomed physical activity may develop fibromyalgia. Poor posture while sitting at a computer or while watching television has also been implicated as a predisposing factor. In addition, previous injuries may result in abnormal muscle function and increase the risk of developing fibromyalgia. All these predisposing factors may be intensified if the patient also suffers from poor nutritional status or coexisting psychological abnormalities.

Often, stiffness and fatigue accompany the pain of fibromyalgia of the cervical spine. These symptoms increase the functional disability associated with this disease and complicate its treatment. Fibromyalgia may occur as a primary disease state or in conjunction with other painful conditions, including radiculopathy and chronic regional pain syndromes. Psychological or behavioral abnormalities, including depression, frequently coexist with the muscle abnormalities, and the management of these concurrent conditions must be an integral part of any successful treatment plan. Studies have suggested that an abnormality in the serotonin transport gene may predispose patients to the development of fibromyalgia as a result of abnormal pain processing.

SIGNS AND SYMPTOMS

As noted earlier, the sine qua non of fibromyalgia of the cervical spine is the myofascial trigger point. This trigger point represents the pathologic lesion and is characterized by a local point of exquisite tenderness in the affected muscle. Mechanical stimulation of the trigger point by palpation or stretching produces not only intense local pain but also referred pain. Taut bands of muscle fibers are often identified when myofascial trigger points are palpated. In addition, involuntary withdrawal of the stimulated muscle, called a jump sign, is often seen (Fig. 17-1). A positive jump sign is characteristic of fibromyalgia of the cervical spine, as are stiffness of the neck, pain on range of motion, and pain referred to the upper extremities in a nondermatomal pattern. Although this referred pain has been well studied and occurs in a characteristic pattern, it often leads to misdiagnosis.

TESTING

Biopsies of clinically identified trigger points have not revealed consistently abnormal histologic features. The muscle hosting the trigger points has been described either as "moth eaten" or as containing

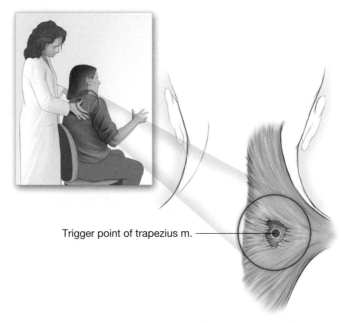

Trigger point of trapezius m.

Figure 17-1 Palpation of a trigger point results in a positive jump sign.

"waxy degeneration." Increased plasma myoglobin has been reported in some patients with fibromyalgia of the cervical spine, but other investigators have not corroborated this finding. Electrodiagnostic testing has revealed an increase in muscle tension in some patients, but again, this finding has not been reproducible. Thus, the diagnosis is based on the clinical findings of trigger points in the cervical paraspinous muscles and an associated jump sign, rather than on specific laboratory, electrodiagnostic, or radiographic testing.

DIFFERENTIAL DIAGNOSIS

The clinician must rule out other disease processes that may mimic fibromyalgia of the cervical spine, including primary inflammatory muscle disease, multiple sclerosis, Lyme disease, hypothyroid disease, and collagen vascular disease (Table 17-1). The judicious use of electrodiagnostic testing and radiography can identify coexisting disorders such as a herniated nucleus pulposus or rotator cuff tear. The clinician must also identify any psychological and behavioral abnormalities that may mask or exacerbate the symptoms associated with fibromyalgia or other pathologic processes.

TREATMENT

Treatment is focused on blocking the myofascial trigger and achieving prolonged relaxation of the affected muscle. Because the mechanism of action is poorly understood, an element of trial and error is often required when developing a treatment plan. Conservative therapy consisting of trigger point injections with local anesthetic or saline solution is the starting point. Because underlying depression and anxiety are present in many patients suffering from fibromyalgia of the cervical spine, the administration of antidepressants is an integral part of most treatment plans. Pregabalin and gabapentin have also been shown to provide some palliation of the symptoms associated with fibromyalgia.

TABLE 17-1

Medical Disorders That Mimic Symptoms of Fibromyalgia or Are Comorbid With Fibromyalgia

Medical Disorder	Differentiating Signs and Symptoms	Laboratory Tests
Rheumatoid arthritis	Predominant joint pain, joint swelling, and joint line tenderness	Positive rheumatoid factor in 80%–90% of patients, radiographic evidence of joint erosion
Systemic lupus erythematosus	Multisystem involvement, commonly arthritis, arthralgia, rash	Antinuclear antibody test, other autoantibodies
Polyarticular osteoarthritis	Multiple painful joints	Radiographic evidence of joint degeneration
Polymyalgia rheumatica	Proximal shoulder and hip girdle pain, more common in older persons	Elevation of erythrocyte sedimentation rate in ~80% of patients
Polymyositis or other myopathies	Symmetrical proximal muscle weakness	Elevated serum muscle enzymes (creatinine kinase, aldolase), abnormal EMG, abnormal muscle biopsy
Spondyloarthropathy	Localization of spinal pain to specific sites in the neck, midthoracic, anterior chest wall, or lumbar regions; objective limitation of spinal mobility resulting from pain and stiffness	Radiographic sacroiliitis, vertebral body radiographic changes
Osteomalacia	Diffuse bone pain, fractures, proximal myopathy, with muscle weakness	Low 25-hydroxyvitamin D levels, low phosphate levels, DEXA scan abnormalities
Lyme disease	Rash, arthritis, or arthralgia; occurs in areas of endemic disease	Positive Lyme serologic test results (ELISA, Western blot)
Hypothyroidism	Cold intolerance, mental slowing, constipation, weight gain, hair loss	Elevated thyroid stimulating level
Sleep apnea	Interrupted breathing during sleep, heavy snoring, excessive sleepiness during the day	Polysomnography abnormalities
Hepatitis C	Right upper quadrant pain, nausea, decreased appetite	Elevated liver enzymes (alanine aminotransferase), hepatitis C antibody, hepatitis C RNA
Hyperparathyroidism	Increased thirst and urination, kidney stones, nausea or vomiting, decreased appetite, thinning bones, constipation	Elevated serum calcium and parathyroid levels
Cushing's syndrome	Hypertension, diabetes, hirsutism, moon facies, weight gain	Elevated 24-hour urinary free cortisol level
Addison's disease	Postural hypotension, nausea, vomiting, skin pigmentation, weight loss	Blunted ACTH stimulation test
Multiple sclerosis	Visual changes (unilateral partial or complete loss, double vision), ascending numbness in a leg or bandlike truncal numbness, slurred speech (dysarthria)	Magnetic resonance imaging of brain or spinal cord, cerebrospinal fluid analysis for immunoglobulins, visual evoked potentials
Neuropathy	Shooting or burning pain, tingling, numbness	Tests to identify underlying cause (e.g., diabetes, herniated disk), EMG, nerve conduction study, nerve biopsy

ACTH, adrenocorticotropic hormone; *DEXA,* dual-energy x-ray absorptiometry; *ELISA,* enzyme-linked immunosorbent assay; *EMG,* electromyography.
Modified from Arnold LM: The pathophysiology, diagnosis and treatment of fibromyalgia, *Psychiatr Clin North Am* 33(2):375–408, 2010.

In addition, several adjuvant methods are available for the treatment of fibromyalgia of the cervical spine. The therapeutic use of heat and cold is often combined with trigger point injections and antidepressants to achieve pain relief. Some patients experience decreased pain with the application of transcutaneous nerve stimulation or electrical stimulation to fatigue the affected muscles. Exercise may also provide some palliation of symptoms and improve the fatigue associated with this disease. Although not currently approved by the Food and Drug Administration for this indication, the injection of minute quantities of botulinum toxin type A directly into trigger points has been used with success in patients who have not responded to traditional treatment modalities.

COMPLICATIONS AND PITFALLS

Trigger point injections are extremely safe if careful attention is paid to the clinically relevant anatomy. Sterile technique is required to prevent infection, as are universal precautions to minimize any risk to the operator. Most side effects of trigger point injection are related to needle-induced trauma at the injection site and in underlying tissues. The incidence of ecchymosis and hematoma formation can be decreased if pressure is applied to the injection site immediately after injection. The avoidance of overly long needles can decrease the incidence of trauma to underlying structures. Special care must be taken to avoid pneumothorax when injecting trigger points in proximity to the underlying pleural space.

Clinical Pearls

Fibromyalgia of the cervical spine is a common disorder that often coexists with various somatic and psychological disorders, yet it is often misdiagnosed. In patients suspected of suffering from fibromyalgia of the cervical spine, a careful evaluation is mandatory to identify any underlying disease processes. Treatment is focused on blocking the myofascial trigger to achieve pain relief. This is accomplished with trigger point injections with local anesthetic or saline solution, along with antidepressants to treat underlying depression. Physical therapy, therapeutic heat and cold, transcutaneous nerve stimulation, and electrical stimulation may be helpful in some cases. For patients who do not respond to traditional measures, consideration should be given to the use of botulinum toxin type A injection.

SUGGESTED READINGS

Ablin J, Neumann L, Buskila D: Pathogenesis of fibromyalgia: a review, *Joint Bone Spine* 75(3):273–279, 2008.

Arnold LM: The pathophysiology, diagnosis and treatment of fibromyalgia, *Psychiatr Clin North Am* 33(2):375–408, 2010.

Arnold LM: Strategies for managing fibromyalgia, *Am J Med* 122(12 Suppl 1):S31–S43, 2009.

Bradley LA: Pathophysiology of fibromyalgia, *Am J Med* 122(12 Suppl 1):S22–S30, 2009.

Chapter 18

CERVICAL STRAIN

ICD-9 CODE `847.0`

ICD-10 CODE `S13.4xxA`

THE CLINICAL SYNDROME

Acute cervical strain is a constellation of symptoms consisting of nonradicular neck pain that radiates in a nondermatomal pattern into the shoulders and interscapular region; headache often accompanies these symptoms. The trapezius is commonly affected, with resultant spasm and limited range of motion of the cervical spine. Cervical strain is usually the result of trauma to the cervical spine and associated soft tissues (Fig. 18-1), but it may occur without an obvious inciting incident. The pathologic lesions responsible for this clinical syndrome may emanate from the soft tissues, facet joints, or intervertebral disks.

SIGNS AND SYMPTOMS

Neck pain is the hallmark of cervical strain. It may begin in the occipital region and radiate in a nondermatomal pattern into the shoulders and interscapular region. The pain of cervical strain is often exacerbated by movement of the cervical spine and shoulders. Headaches often occur and may worsen with emotional stress. Sleep disturbance is common, as is difficulty concentrating on simple tasks. Depression may occur with prolonged symptoms.

On physical examination, tenderness is elicited on palpation; spasm of the paraspinous musculature and trapezius is often present. Decreased range of motion is invariably present, and pain is increased when this maneuver is attempted. The neurologic examination of the upper extremities is within normal limits, despite the frequent complaint of upper extremity pain.

TESTING

No specific test exists for cervical strain. Testing is aimed primarily at identifying an occult pathologic process or other diseases that may mimic cervical strain (see "Differential Diagnosis"). Plain radiographs can delineate any bony abnormality of the cervical spine, including arthritis, fracture, congenital abnormality (e.g., Arnold-Chiari malformation), and tumor. Straightening of the lordotic curve is frequently noted. All patients with the recent onset of cervical strain should undergo magnetic resonance imaging (MRI) of the cervical spine and, if significant occipital or headache symptoms are present, of the brain (Fig. 18-2). Screening laboratory tests consisting of a complete blood count, erythrocyte sedimentation rate, antinuclear antibody testing, human leukocyte antigen (HLA)-B27 antigen screening, and automated blood

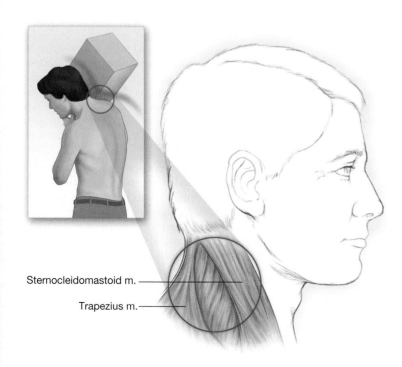

Sternocleidomastoid m.

Trapezius m.

Figure 18-1 Cervical strain is often caused by trauma to the cervical spine and adjacent soft tissues.

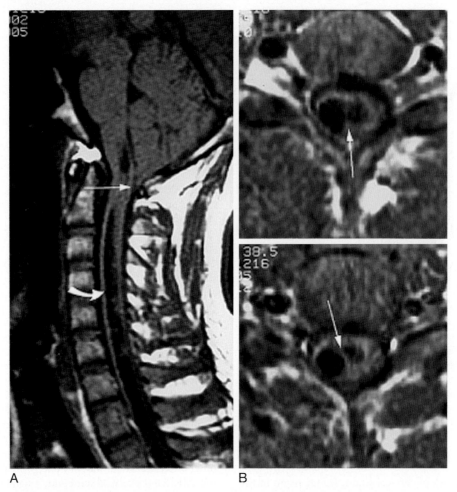

A   B

Figure 18-2 Syringohydromyelia. **A,** T1-weighted sagittal magnetic resonance imaging (MRI) of the cervical spine demonstrating a Chiari type I malformation with low-lying cerebellar tonsils *(straight arrow)* and a tight foramen magnum. A syrinx cavity is noted in the cervical spinal cord *(curved arrow).* **B,** T1-weighted axial MRI demonstrating the eccentric nature of the syrinx cavity, with internal septa or haustrations *(arrows). (From Edelman RR, Hesselink JR, Zlatkin MB, Crues JV, editors:* Clinical magnetic resonance imaging, *ed 3, Philadelphia, 2006, Saunders, p 2304.)*

chemistry should be performed to rule out occult inflammatory arthritis, infection, and tumor.

DIFFERENTIAL DIAGNOSIS

Cervical strain is a clinical diagnosis supported by a combination of clinical history, physical examination, radiography, and MRI. Pain syndromes that may mimic cervical strain include cervical bursitis, cervical fibromyositis, inflammatory arthritis, and disorders of the cervical spinal cord, roots, plexus, and nerves.

TREATMENT

Cervical strain is best treated with a multimodality approach. Physical therapy, including heat modalities and deep sedative massage, combined with nonsteroidal antiinflammatory drugs and skeletal muscle relaxants, is a reasonable starting point. For symptomatic relief, cervical epidural block, blockade of the medial branch of the dorsal ramus, or intraarticular injection of the facet joint with local anesthetic and steroid is extremely effective. Underlying sleep disturbance and depression are best treated

with a tricyclic antidepressant such as nortriptyline, which can be started at a single bedtime dose of 25 mg.

Cervical facet block is often combined with atlanto-occipital block when treating pain in this area. Although the atlanto-occipital joint is not a true facet joint in the anatomic sense, the technique is analogous to the facet joint block commonly used by pain practitioners and may be viewed as such.

COMPLICATIONS AND PITFALLS

The proximity to the spinal cord and exiting nerve roots makes it imperative that cervical epidural block and cervical facet block be carried out only by those familiar with the regional anatomy and experienced in interventional pain management techniques. The proximity to the vertebral artery, combined with the vascular nature of this region, makes the potential for intravascular injection high, and the injection of even a small amount of local anesthetic into the vertebral artery can result in seizures. Given the proximity of the brain and brainstem, ataxia resulting from vascular uptake of local anesthetic is not uncommon after cervical facet block. Many patients also complain of a transient increase in headache and cervicalgia after injection of the cervical facet joints.

Clinical Pearls

Cervical strain is a common cause of neck, occipital, shoulder, and upper extremity pain. It is often confused with cervical radiculopathy and cervical fibromyositis. The clinician must rule out diseases of the cervical spinal cord, such as syringomyelia, that may initially manifest in a manner similar to cervical strain. Ankylosing spondylitis may also manifest as cervical strain and must be correctly identified to avoid ongoing joint damage and functional disability.

Many pain specialists believe that cervical facet block and atlanto-occipital block are underused in the treatment of "post-whiplash" cervicalgia and cervicogenic headaches and that they should be considered whenever cervical epidural or occipital nerve blocks fail to provide palliation.

SUGGESTED READINGS

DeBritz JN, Wiesel SW: Treatment options for disorders of the cervical spine. In Nordin MN, Andersson GB, Pope MH, editors: *Musculoskeletal disorders in the workplace,* ed 2, Philadelphia, 2006, Mosby, pp 73–86.

Devereaux M: Neck pain, *Med Clin North Am* 93(2):273–284, 2009.

Jull G, Sterling M, Falla D, et al: Clinical assessment: physical examination of the cervical region. *Whiplash, headache, and neck pain,* Philadelphia, 2008, Churchill Livingstone, pp 155–187.

Moskovich R, Petrizzo A: Evaluation of the neck. In Nordin MN, Andersson GB, Pope MH, editors: *Musculoskeletal disorders in the workplace,* ed 2, Philadelphia, 2006, Mosby, pp 55–72.

White K, Hudgins TH, Alleva JT: Cervical sprain/strain definition, *Dis Month* 55(12):724–728, 2009.

Chapter 19

LONGUS COLLI TENDINITIS

ICD-9 CODE 727.82

ICD-10 CODE M65.20

THE CLINICAL SYNDROME

The tendons of the longus colli muscle are prone to the development of tendinitis. Longus colli tendinitis is usually caused either by repetitive trauma to the musculotendinous apparatus or by the deposition of calcium hydroxyapatite crystals. This crystal deposition usually occurs in the superior fibers of the musculotendinous apparatus and is easily identified on a lateral plain radiograph of the neck. The onset of longus colli tendinitis is generally acute, and it is often misdiagnosed as acute pharyngitis or retropharyngeal abscess because the acute onset of retropharyngeal pain is frequently accompanied by a mild elevation in temperature and leukocytosis. Longus colli tendinitis is most often seen in the third to sixth decades of life.

SIGNS AND SYMPTOMS

The pain of longus colli tendinitis is constant and severe and is localized to the retropharyngeal area. It is made worse by swallowing (Fig. 19-1). The patient may complain of acute anterior neck pain in addition to the pain on swallowing. A mild fever is often present, as is mild leukocytosis. Intraoral palpation of the superior attachment of the muscle usually reproduces the symptoms.

TESTING

Plain radiographs are indicated for all patients who present with retropharyngeal pain. Characteristic amorphous calcification of the superior attachment of the musculotendinous unit just below the anterior arch of atlas is highly suggestive of longus colli tendinitis (Fig. 19-2). Computed tomographic scanning may further delineate the problem (Fig. 19-3). The finding of a smooth, linear prevertebral fluid collection is considered pathognomonic for this disease (Fig. 19-4). Unlike in a retropharyngeal

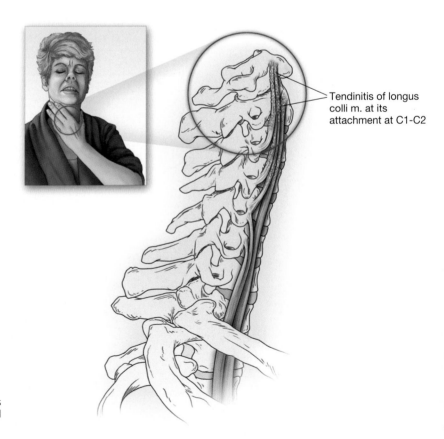

Tendinitis of longus colli m. at its attachment at C1-C2

Figure 19-1 The pain of longus colli tendinitis is constant, severe, made worse by swallowing, and localized to the retropharyngeal area.

or prevertebral abscess, the wall of the fluid-containing structure does not enhance. Additional testing may be indicated, including a complete blood count, erythrocyte sedimentation rate, and complete blood chemistry tests, in patients suspected of suffering from longus colli tendinitis.

DIFFERENTIAL DIAGNOSIS

Longus colli tendinitis is often misdiagnosed as acute pharyngitis or retropharyngeal abscess. Occasionally, the patient is diagnosed with an early peritonsillar abscess. This delay in diagnosis can often subject the patient to unnecessary antibiotic therapy and occasionally surgical drainage of the suspected "abscess." In some clinical situations, consideration should be given to primary or secondary tumors involving this anatomic region.

TREATMENT

Initial treatment of the pain and functional disability associated with longus colli tendinitis includes a combination of nonsteroidal antiinflammatory drugs (NSAIDs) or cyclooxygenase-2 inhibitors. Local application of heat and cold may also be beneficial. For patients who do not respond to these treatment modalities, injection of the superior portion of the tendon with local anesthetic and steroid is a reasonable next step. Such injection should be considered only if the clinician is certain that no occult infection in this anatomic region exists.

COMPLICATIONS AND PITFALLS

The main pitfalls in the treatment of longus colli tendinitis are failure to diagnose this painful condition in a timely manner and mistaking it for a disease requiring more intensive treatment (e.g., retropharyngeal abscess or peritonsillar abscess). Rapid institution of treatment

with NSAIDs and reassurance is often all that is required. For more recalcitrant cases, injection with local anesthetic and steroid almost always results in prompt resolution of symptoms. Use of this injection technique is safe if careful attention is paid to the clinically relevant anatomy. Sterile technique must be used to avoid infection, along with universal precautions to minimize any risk to the operator. The incidence of ecchymosis and hematoma formation can be decreased if pressure is applied to the injection site immediately after injection. Trauma to the tendon from the injection itself is also a possibility. Tendons that are highly inflamed or previously damaged are subject

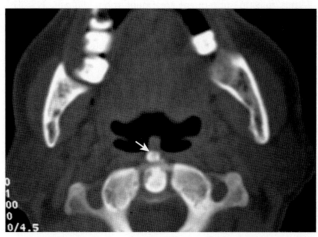

Figure 19-3 Computed tomography scan showing calcification of the superior aspect of the musculotendinous unit of the longus colli muscle *(arrow)*. Note the relationship with the anterior arch of the atlas. *(From Omezzine SJ, Hafsa C, Lahmar I, et al: Calcific tendinitis of the longus colli: diagnosis by CT, Joint Bone Spine 75[1]:90–91, 2008.)*

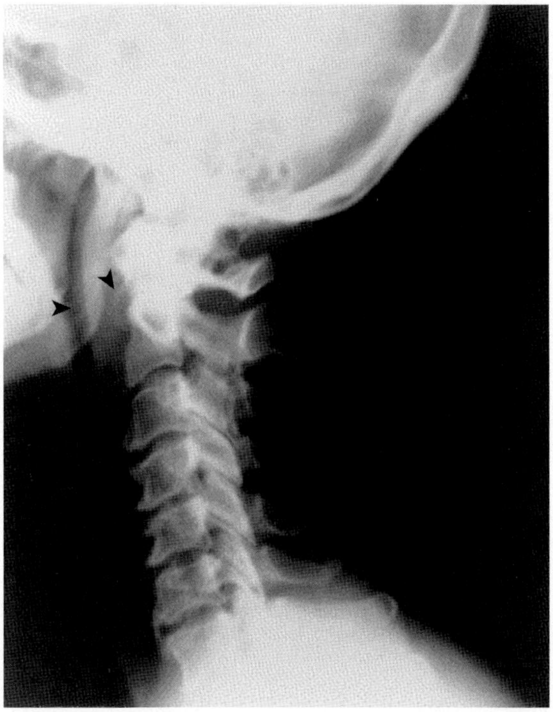

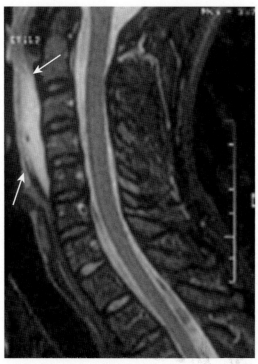

Figure 19-4 Magnetic resonance imaging of the neck demonstrating a fluid collection *(arrows)* measuring 5 × 0.7 cm anterior to the cervical spine at the C2-C5 vertebral bodies. *(From Benanti JC, Grambling O, Bulat PI, et al: Retropharyngeal calcific tendinitis: report of five cases and review of the literature, J Emerg Med 4[1]:15–24, 1986.)*

Figure 19-2 Lateral cervical spine x-ray study showing faint calcification anterior to the junction of C1-C2 *(arrow heads)*. *(From Guss DA, Jacoby IJ: Longus colli tendinitis causing acute neck pain, J Emerg Med 22[2]: 211–212, 2002.)*

to rupture if they are injected directly. This complication can often be avoided if the clinician uses a gentle technique and stops injecting immediately on encountering significant resistance. Approximately 25% of patients complain of a transient increase in pain after injection, and patients should be warned of this possibility.

Clinical Pearls

The musculotendinous unit of the longus colli muscle is susceptible to the development of tendinitis. Calcium hydroxyapatite deposition around the tendon may occur, thus making subsequent treatment more difficult. NSAIDs usually provide excellent palliation of the patient's pain. If they do not, properly performed injection of the inflamed musculotendinous unit with local anesthetic and steroid is a reasonable next step.

SUGGESTED READINGS

Benanti JC, Grambling O, Bulat PI, et al: Retropharyngeal calcific tendinitis: report of five cases and review of the literature, *J Emerg Med* 4(1):15–24, 1986.

Eastwood JD, Hudgins PA, Malone D: Retropharyngeal effusion in acute calcific prevertebral tendonitis: diagnosis with CT and MR imaging, *AJNR Am J Neuroradiol* 19(9):1789–1792, 1998.

Guss DA, Jacoby IJ: Longus colli tendinitis causing acute neck pain, *J Emerg Med* 22(2):211–212, 2002.

Hartley J: Acute cervical pain associated with retropharyngeal calcium deposit: a case report, *J Bone Joint Surg Am* 46:1753–1754, 1964.

Omezzine SJ, Hafsa C, Lahmar I, et al: Calcific tendinitis of the longus colli: diagnosis by CT, *Joint Bone Spine* 75(1):90–91, 2008.

Ring D, Vaccaro AR, Scuderi G, et al: Acute calcific retropharyngeal tendinitis: clinical presentation and pathological characterization, *J Bone Joint Surg Am* 76(11):1636–1642, 1994.

Chapter 20

RETROPHARYNGEAL ABSCESS

ICD-9 CODE 478.24

ICD-10 CODE J39.0

THE CLINICAL SYNDROME

Once a disease almost exclusively seen in children, retropharyngeal abscess is occurring more commonly in the adult population. It may occur as a sequela of upper respiratory tract infection, trauma to the posterior pharynx (e.g., difficult endotracheal intubation), or perforation from a foreign body, among other causes (Fig. 20-1). Often misdiagnosed, retropharyngeal abscess can result in life-threatening complications and, if untreated, death. The mortality and morbidity associated with retropharyngeal abscess are primarily the result of airway obstruction, mediastinitis, spread of infection to the epidural space, necrotizing fasciitis, erosion into the carotid artery, and, in immunocompromised patients, overwhelming sepsis. Lying posterior to the pharynx, the retropharyngeal space is bound by the prevertebral fascia posteriorly, the buccopharyngeal fascia anteriorly, and the carotid sheaths laterally. Extending from the base of the skull inferiorly to the mediastinum, the retropharyngeal space is susceptible to infection by aerobic organisms such as *Streptococcus, Staphylococcus,* and *Haemophilus* and anaerobic organisms such as *Bacteroides.* Rarely, fungal and mycobacterial infections of the retropharyngeal space have been reported in immunocompromised patients.

The patient suffering from retropharyngeal abscess initially presents with sore throat, neck pain, and painful and difficult swallowing (Fig. 20-2). This pain becomes more intense and localized as the abscess increases in size and compresses adjacent structures. Low-grade fever and vague constitutional symptoms including malaise and anorexia progress to frank sepsis with a high-grade fever, rigors, and chills. At this point, the mortality rate associated with retropharyngeal abscess rises dramatically, despite treatment with appropriate antibiotics and surgical drainage of the abscess.

SIGNS AND SYMPTOMS

The patient with retropharyngeal abscess initially presents with ill-defined pain in the general area of the infection. At this point, the patient may have mild pain on swallowing and range of motion

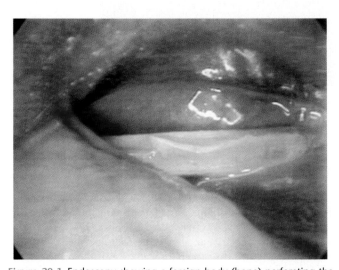

Figure 20-1 Endoscopy showing a foreign body (bone) perforating the cervical esophagus in a patient with a retropharyngeal abscess. *(From Poluri A, Singh B, Sperling N, et al: Retropharyngeal abscess secondary to penetrating foreign bodies,* J Craniomaxillofac Surg *28[4]:243–246, 2000.)*

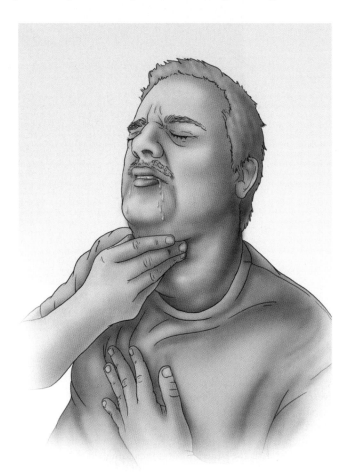

Figure 20-2 The patient suffering from retropharyngeal abscess appears acutely ill and exhibits drooling as swallowing becomes increasingly difficult.

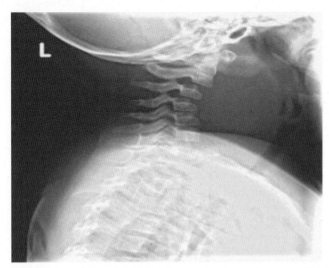

Figure 20-3 Lateral neck radiograph revealing a massive prevertebral swelling that caused cervical spine kyphosis. *(From Strovski E, Mickelson J-I, Ludemann JP: Minimally invasive drainage of a giant retropharyngeal abscess,* Int J Pediatr Otorhinolaryngol Extra *4[2]:92–95, 2009.)*

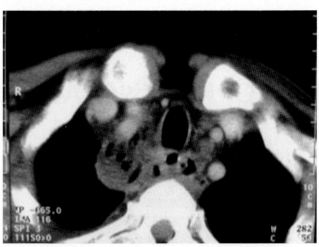

Figure 20-4 Computed tomography scan demonstrating multiple air-fluid collections in the upper mediastinum and the retropharyngeal and parapharyngeal spaces that represented the presence of abscess. *(From Abu Abeeleh M, Al Smady M, Qasem H, et al: Descending necrotising mediastinitis: a fatal disease to keep in mind,* Heart Lung Circ *19[4]: 254–256, 2010.)*

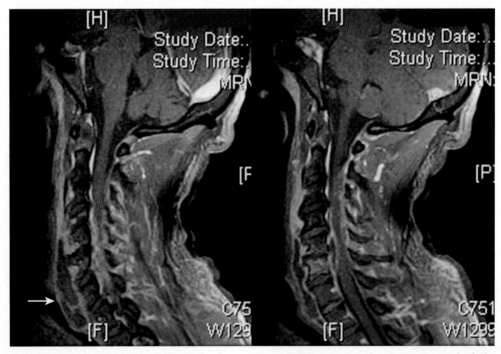

Figure 20-5 Preoperative sagittal contrast-enhanced T1-weighted magnetic resonance imaging showing a prevertebral abscess *(arrow)* and an epidural abscess causing spinal cord compression from C3 to C7 with diskitis at C5-6. *(From Yanni DS, LaBagnara M, Saravanan R, et al: Transcervical drainage of epidural and retropharyngeal abscess,* J Clin Neurosci *17[5]:636–638, 2010.)*

of the cervical spine. The physical examination at this point may reveal posterior pharyngeal swelling. A low-grade fever or night sweats may be present. Theoretically, if the patient has received steroids, these constitutional symptoms may be attenuated, or their onset may be delayed. As the abscess increases in size, the patient appears acutely ill with fever, rigors, and chills. Drooling may be present as the patient finds it increasingly difficult to swallow. Nuchal rigidity and respiratory stridor may also be evident. Spread to the mediastinum and central nervous system is associated with a high mortality rate in spite of aggressive medical and surgical treatment.

TESTING

Lateral radiography of the neck reveals widening of the retropharyngeal soft tissues in more than 80% of patients suffering from retropharyngeal abscess; clearly defined soft tissue masses with air-fluid levels suggestive of abscess are seen in less than 10% of patients (Fig. 20-3). In this era of readily available magnetic resonance imaging (MRI) and high-speed computed tomography (CT) scanning, it may be more prudent to obtain this noninvasive testing first, given the highly specific diagnostic information obtained (Figs. 20-4 and 20-5). Both MRI and CT are highly

TABLE 20-1

Differential Diagnosis of Retropharyngeal Abscess

- Angioedema
- Caustic ingestions
- Cervical epidural abscess
- Cervical subdural abscess
- Epiglottitis
- Esophagitis
- Foreign body of esophagus
- Foreign body of pharynx
- Foreign body of trachea
- Kawasaki's disease
- Mediastinitis
- Meningitis
- Mononucleosis
- Odontogenic infections
- Pediatric fever
- Peritonsillar abscess
- Pharyngitis
- Severe thrush
- Sinusitis

TABLE 20-2

Algorithm for Spinal Cord Compression Resulting From Retropharyngeal Abscess

- Immediately obtain blood and urine cultures.
- Immediately start high-dose antibiotics that cover *Staphylococcus aureus*.
- Immediately obtain the most readily available spinal imaging technique that can confirm the presence of spinal cord compression, such as abscess, tumor, and others.
  - Computed tomography
  - Magnetic resonance imaging
  - Myelography
- Simultaneously obtain emergency consultation from a spinal surgeon.
- Continuously and carefully monitor the patient's neurologic status.
- If any of the above is unavailable, arrange emergency transfer of the patient to a tertiary care center by the most rapidly available transportation.
- Repeat imaging and obtain a repeat surgical consultation if any deterioration in the patient's neurologic status occurs.

accurate in the diagnosis of retropharyngeal abscess and should be obtained on an urgent basis in all patients suspected of suffering from this condition. Ultrasonography may also be useful in identifying retropharyngeal abscess.

All patients suspected of suffering from retropharyngeal abscess should undergo laboratory testing consisting of complete blood cell count, sedimentation rate, and automated blood chemistries. Studies suggest that C-reactive protein testing may also be beneficial because patients with markedly elevated levels have higher morbidity and mortality rates. Blood and urine cultures should be immediately obtained in all patients thought to be suffering from retropharyngeal abscess to allow immediate implementation of antibiotic therapy while the workup is in progress. Gram stains and cultures of the abscess material should also be obtained, but antibiotic treatment should not be delayed while waiting for this information.

DIFFERENTIAL DIAGNOSIS

The diagnosis of retropharyngeal abscess should be strongly considered in any patient with sore throat, fever, neck pain, painful and difficult swallowing, and posterior pharyngeal swelling, especially if the patient has a history of trauma to the retropharyngeal space. Diseases commonly mistaken for retropharyngeal abscess are listed in Table 20-1. Constitutional symptoms associated with serious infection may be attenuated in patients who have been receiving steroids or who are immunocompromised (e.g., acquired immunodeficiency syndrome, malignant disease).

TREATMENT

The rapid initiation of treatment of retropharyngeal abscess is mandatory if the patient is to avoid significant morbidity and mortality. The treatment of retropharyngeal abscess is aimed at two goals: (1) treatment of the infection with antibiotics and (2) drainage of the abscess to relieve compression on adjacent structures including the airway. Because many retropharyngeal abscesses are caused by *Staphylococcus aureus,* the initial antibiotic

regimen should include vancomycin to treat staphylococcal infection. Gram-negative and anaerobic antibiotic coverage should also be started empirically immediately after blood and urine culture samples are taken. Antibiotic therapy can be tailored to the culture and sensitivity reports as they become available. As mentioned, antibiotic therapy should not be delayed while waiting for definitive diagnosis if retropharyngeal abscess is being considered as part of the differential diagnosis.

Antibiotics alone are rarely successful in treatment of retropharyngeal abscess unless the diagnosis is made very early in the course of the disease; surgical drainage of the abscess is required to effect full recovery. Careful attention to airway management is mandatory in patients suspected of suffering from retropharyngeal abscess, and early endotracheal intubation in a controlled setting is preferred to waiting until respiratory compromise is already present.

Serial CT or MRI scans are useful in following the resolution of retropharyngeal abscess. These imaging tests should be repeated immediately at the first sign of negative change in the patient's clinical status.

COMPLICATIONS AND PITFALLS

Failure to diagnose and treat retropharyngeal abscess rapidly and accurately can result only in disaster for the clinician and patient alike. The insidious onset of airway compromise associated with retropharyngeal abscess can lull the clinician into a sense of false security, and failure to recognize the spread of infection into the central nervous system can result in permanent neurologic damage. If retropharyngeal abscess is suspected, the algorithm listed in Table 20-2 should be followed.

Clinical Pearls

Delay in diagnosis puts the patient and clinician at tremendous risk for a poor outcome. The clinician should assume that all patients who present with sore throat, fever, neck pain, painful and difficult swallowing, and posterior pharyngeal swelling are suffering from retropharyngeal abscess until proved otherwise and should treat these patients accordingly. Overreliance on a single negative or equivocal imaging test result is a mistake. Serial CT or MRI testing is indicated should any deterioration in the patient's clinical status occur.

SUGGESTED READINGS

Abu Abeeleh M, Al Smady M, Qasem H, et al: Descending necrotising mediastinitis: a fatal disease to keep in mind, *Heart Lung Circ* 19(4):254–256, 2010.

Beningfield A, Nehus E, Chen AY, et al: Pseudoaneurysm of the internal carotid artery after retropharyngeal abscess, *Otolaryngol Head Neck Surg* 134(2): 338–339, 2006.

Brook I: Microbiology and management of peritonsillar, retropharyngeal, and parapharyngeal abscesses, *J Oral Maxillofac Surg* 62(12):1545–1550, 2004.

Chern S-H, Wei C-P, Hsieh R-L, et al: Methicillin-resistant Staphylococcus aureus retropharyngeal abscess complicated by a cervical spinal subdural empyema, *J Clin Neurosci* 16(1):144–146, 2009.

Wever K, Armstrong A: Retropharyngeal and mediastinal abscesses: postanesthetic complication of gynecologic surgery, *Obstet Gynecol* 94(5):857, 1999.

Yanni DS, LaBagnara M, Saravanan R, et al: Transcervical drainage of epidural and retropharyngeal abscess, *J Clin Neurosci* 17(5):636–638, 2010.

Chapter 21

CERVICOTHORACIC INTERSPINOUS BURSITIS

ICD-9 CODE **727.3**

ICD-10 CODE **M71.50**

THE CLINICAL SYNDROME

The interspinous ligaments of the lower cervical and upper thoracic spine and their associated muscles are susceptible to the development of acute and chronic pain symptoms following overuse. Bursitis is thought to be responsible for this pain. Frequently, the patient presents with midline pain after prolonged activity requiring hyperextension of the neck, such as painting a ceiling, or following prolonged use of a computer monitor with too high a focal point.

SIGNS AND SYMPTOMS

The pain is localized to the interspinous region between C7 and T1 and does not radiate. It is constant, dull, and aching. The patient may attempt to relieve the constant ache by assuming a posture of dorsal kyphosis with a thrusting forward of the neck (Fig. 21-1). In contrast to the pain of cervical strain, the pain of cervicothoracic interspinous bursitis often improves with activity and worsens with rest. On physical examination, tenderness is elicited on deep palpation of the C7-T1 region, often with reflex spasm of the associated paraspinous musculature. Decreased range of motion is invariably present, and pain increases with extension of the lower cervical and upper thoracic spine.

TESTING

No specific test exists for cervicothoracic bursitis, although magnetic resonance imaging (MRI) may reveal inflammation of interspinous bursae (Fig. 21-2). Testing is aimed primarily at identifying an occult pathologic process or other diseases that may mimic cervicothoracic bursitis (see "Differential Diagnosis"). Plain radiographs can delineate any bony abnormality of the cervical spine, including arthritis, fracture, congenital abnormality (e.g., Arnold-Chiari malformation), and tumor. All patients with the recent onset of cervicothoracic bursitis should undergo MRI of the cervical spine and, if significant occipital or headache symptoms are present, of the brain (Fig. 21-3). Screening laboratory tests consisting of a complete blood count, erythrocyte sedimentation rate, antinuclear antibody testing, and automated blood chemistry should be performed to rule out occult inflammatory arthritis, infection, and tumor.

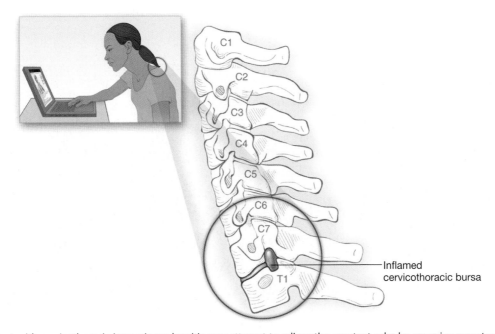

Figure 21-1 A patient with cervicothoracic interspinous bursitis may attempt to relieve the constant ache by assuming a posture of dorsal kyphosis with a thrusting forward of the neck.

DIFFERENTIAL DIAGNOSIS

Cervicothoracic bursitis is a clinical diagnosis of exclusion supported by a combination of clinical history, physical examination, radiography, and MRI. Pain syndromes that may mimic cervicothoracic bursitis include cervical strain, cervical fibromyositis, inflammatory arthritis, and disorders of the cervical spinal cord, roots, plexus, and nerves. Congenital abnormalities such as

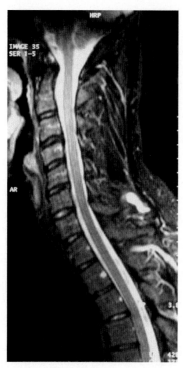

Figure 21-2 Magnetic resonance imaging (T2) of an interspinous bursa measuring 2 × 2 × 2.5 cm between C6 and C7. *(From Perka C, Schneider SV, Buttgereit F, Matziolis G: Development of cervical interspinous bursitis after prolonged sports trauma: a case report,* Joint Bone Spine *73[1]:118–120, 2006.)*

Arnold-Chiari malformation and Klippel-Feil syndrome may also manifest similarly to cervicothoracic bursitis.

TREATMENT

Cervicothoracic bursitis is best treated with a multimodality approach. Physical therapy consisting of the correction of functional abnormalities (e.g., poor posture, improper chair or computer height), heat modalities, and deep sedative massage, combined with nonsteroidal antiinflammatory drugs (NSAIDs) and skeletal muscle relaxants, is a reasonable starting point. If these treatments fail to provide rapid relief, injection of local anesthetic and steroid into the area between the interspinous ligament and the ligamentum flavum is a reasonable next step. For symptomatic relief, cervical epidural block, blockade of the medial branch of the dorsal ramus, or intra-articular injection of the facet joint with local anesthetic and steroid may also be considered. Antimyotonic agents such as tizanidine may be used if symptoms persist. Underlying sleep disturbance and depression are best treated with a tricyclic antidepressant such as nortriptyline, which can be started at a single bedtime dose of 25 mg.

COMPLICATIONS AND PITFALLS

The proximity to the spinal cord and exiting nerve roots makes it imperative that injections be performed only by those familiar with the regional anatomy and experienced in interventional pain management techniques. The proximity to the vertebral artery, combined with the vascular nature of this region, renders the potential for intravascular injection high, and the injection of even a small amount of local anesthetic into the vertebral artery can result in seizures. Given the proximity of the brain and brainstem, ataxia resulting from vascular uptake of local anesthetic is not uncommon after injection in this region. Many patients also complain of a transient increase in headache and cervicalgia after injection of the cervical facet joints.

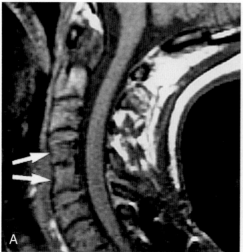
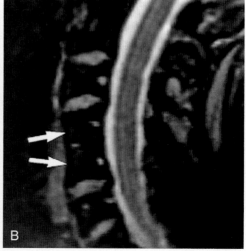

Figure 21-3 Klippel-Feil anomaly. T1-weighted **(A)** and T2-weighted **(B)** sagittal magnetic resonance imaging of the cervical spine that demonstrates lack of segmentation of the C4 and C5 vertebrae *(arrows). (From Edelman RR, Hesselink JR, Zlatkin MB, Crues JV, editors:* Clinical magnetic resonance imaging, *ed 3, Philadelphia, 2006, Saunders, p 2306.)*

Clinical Pearls

Correction of the functional abnormalities responsible for the development of cervicothoracic bursitis is mandatory if long-lasting relief is to be achieved. Physical modalities, including local heat, gentle stretching exercises, and deep sedative massage, are beneficial and may be started concurrently with a trial of NSAIDs. Injection of local anesthetic and steroid is extremely effective in the treatment of cervicothoracic bursitis pain that fails to respond to more conservative measures. Vigorous exercise should be avoided, because it will exacerbate the patient's symptoms.

SUGGESTED READINGS

Linetsky FS, Miguel R, Torres F: Treatment of cervicothoracic pain and cervicogenic headaches with regenerative injection therapy, *Curr Pain Headache Rep* 8(1):41–48, 2004.

Waldman SD: Cervicothoracic interspinous bursitis. In *Pain review,* Philadelphia, 2009, Saunders, pp 238–239.

Waldman SD: Injection technique for cervicothoracic bursitis. In *Atlas of pain management injection techniques,* ed 2, Philadelphia, 2009, Saunders, pp 52–56.

Wasserman AR, Melville LD, Birkhahn RH: Septic bursitis: a case report and primer for the emergency clinician, *J Emerg Med* 37(3):269–272, 2009.

Yung E, Asavasopon S, Joseph J, et al: Screening for head, neck, and shoulder pathology in patients with upper extremity signs and symptoms, *J Hand Ther* 23(2):173–186, 2010.

Chapter **22**

BRACHIAL PLEXOPATHY

ICD-9 CODE `353.0`

ICD-10 CODE `G54.0`

THE CLINICAL SYNDROME

Brachial plexopathy is a constellation of symptoms consisting of neurogenic pain and associated weakness that radiates from the shoulder into the supraclavicular region and upper extremity (Fig. 22-1). Brachial plexopathy has many causes, but some of the more common ones include compression of the plexus by cervical ribs or abnormal muscles (e.g., thoracic outlet syndrome), invasion of the plexus by tumor (e.g., Pancoast's tumor syndrome), direct trauma to the plexus (e.g., stretch injuries and avulsions), inflammatory causes (e.g., Parsonage-Turner syndrome, herpes zoster), and postradiation plexopathy (Fig. 22-2).

SIGNS AND SYMPTOMS

Patients suffering from brachial plexopathy complain of pain radiating to the supraclavicular region and upper extremity. The pain is neuritic and may take on a deep, boring quality as the plexus is invaded by tumor. Movement of the neck and shoulder exacerbates the pain, so patients often try to avoid such movement. Frozen shoulder often results and may confuse the diagnosis. If thoracic outlet syndrome is suspected, the Adson test may be performed

(Fig. 22-3). The test result is positive if the radial pulse disappears with the neck extended and the head turned toward the affected side. Because the Adson test is nonspecific, treatment decisions should not be based on this finding alone (see "Testing"). If the patient presents with severe pain that is followed shortly by profound weakness, brachial plexitis should be considered; this can be confirmed with electromyography (EMG).

TESTING

All patients presenting with brachial plexopathy, especially those without a clear history of antecedent trauma, must undergo magnetic resonance imaging (MRI) of the cervical spine and the brachial plexus. Computed tomography scanning is a reasonable alternative if MRI is contraindicated. EMG and nerve conduction velocity testing are extremely sensitive, and a skilled electromyographer can delineate which portion of the plexus is abnormal. If an inflammatory basis for the plexopathy is suspected, serial EMG is indicated, and MRI of the shoulder muscles often reveals muscle edema and denervation-induced atrophy (Fig. 22-4). If Pancoast's tumor or some other tumor of the brachial plexus is suspected, chest radiographs with apical lordotic views may be helpful. If the diagnosis is in question, screening laboratory tests consisting of a complete blood count, erythrocyte sedimentation rate, antinuclear antibody testing, and automated blood chemistry should be performed to rule out other causes of the patient's pain.

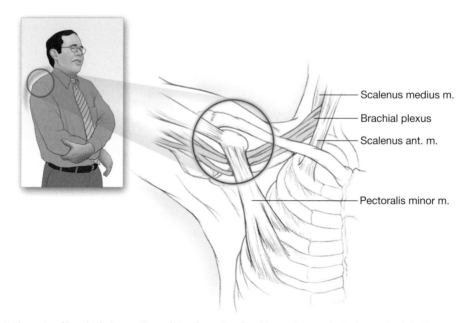

Figure 22-1 The pain of brachial plexopathy radiates from the shoulder and supraclavicular region into the upper extremity.

DIFFERENTIAL DIAGNOSIS

Diseases of the cervical spinal cord, bony cervical spine, and disk can mimic brachial plexopathy. Appropriate testing, including MRI and EMG, can help sort out the myriad possibilities, but the clinician should be aware that more than one pathologic process may be contributing to the patient's symptoms. Syringomyelia, tumor of the cervical spinal cord, and tumor of the cervical nerve root as it exits the spinal cord (e.g., schwannoma) can have an insidious onset and be quite difficult to diagnosis. Pancoast's tumor should be high on the list of diagnostic possibilities in all patients presenting with brachial plexopathy in the absence of clear antecedent trauma, especially if they have a history of tobacco use. Lateral herniated cervical disk, metastatic tumor, or cervical spondylosis resulting in significant nerve root compression may also manifest as brachial plexopathy. Rarely, infection involving the apex of the lung may compress and irritate the plexus.

TREATMENT

Drug Therapy

Gabapentin

Gabapentin is first-line treatment for the neuritic pain of brachial plexopathy. The initial dose is 300 mg gabapentin at bedtime for 2 nights, and the patient should be cautioned about potential side effects, including dizziness, sedation, confusion, and rash. The drug is then increased in 300-mg increments given in equally divided doses over 2 days, as side effects allow, until pain relief is obtained or a total dose of 2400 mg/day is reached. At this point, if the patient has experienced partial pain relief, blood values are measured, and the drug is carefully titrated upward using 100-mg tablets. Rarely is a dose greater than 3600 mg/day required.

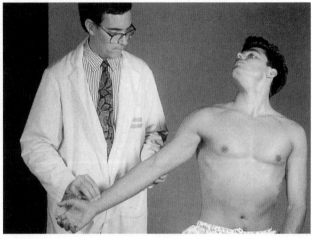

Figure 22-3 The Adson test. The patient inhales deeply, extends the neck fully, and turns the head to the affected side. This maneuver tests for compression in the scalene triangle; the result is positive if the radial pulse diminishes and the patient's symptoms are reproduced. *(From Klippel JH, Dieppe PA: Rheumatology, ed 2, London, 1998, Mosby.)*

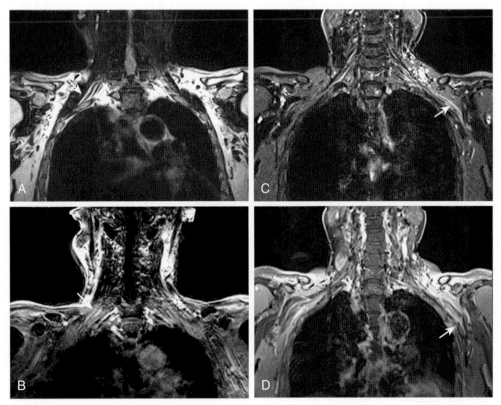

Figure 22-2 Coronal magnetic resonance imaging (MRI) of the brachial plexus. Case 1. MRI obtained 10 days after the onset of motor symptoms shows mild swelling of the brachial plexus with T2 hyperintensity **(A)** and corresponding contrast enhancement **(B),** marked in the upper and middle trunks *(arrows)*. Case 2. MRI obtained 8 weeks after the onset of motor weakness. T2-weighted short tau inversion recovery coronal **(C)** and gadolinium-enhanced turbo spin-echo coronal **(D)** images demonstrate increased signal and intense enhancement in the left brachial plexus at the cord level, marked in the medial cord *(arrows)*. *(From Choi J-Y, Kang CH, Kim B-J, et al: Brachial plexopathy following herpes zoster infection: two cases with MRI findings,* J Neurol Sci 285[1–2]:224–226, 2009.)

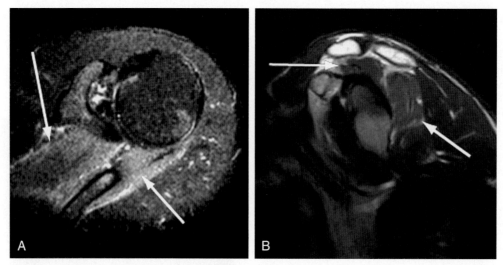

Figure 22-4 Parsonage-Turner syndrome. Axial short tau inversion recovery **(A)** and sagittal oblique T2-weighted **(B)** magnetic resonance images. Increased signal intensity consistent with interstitial muscle edema associated with denervation is seen in the supraspinatus and infraspinatus muscles *(arrows). (From Edelman RR, Hesselink JR, Zlatkin MB, Crues JV, editors:* Clinical magnetic resonance imaging, *ed 3, Philadelphia, 2006, Saunders, p 3272.)*

Pregabalin

Pregabalin represents a reasonable alternative to gabapentin and is better tolerated in some patients. Pregabalin is started at 50 mg three times a day and may be titrated upward to 100 mg three times a day as side effects allow. Because pregabalin is excreted primarily by the kidneys, the dosage should be decreased in patients with compromised renal function.

Carbamazepine

Carbamazepine is useful in patients who do not obtain pain relief with gabapentin. Despite the safety and efficacy of carbamazepine, confusion and anxiety have surrounded its use. The drug is sometimes discontinued owing to laboratory abnormalities erroneously attributed to it. Therefore, baseline laboratory values consisting of a complete blood count, urinalysis, and automated chemistry profile should be obtained before starting the drug.

Carbamazepine should be initiated slowly if the pain is not out of control at a starting dose of 100 to 200 mg at bedtime for 2 nights. The patient should be cautioned about side effects, including dizziness, sedation, confusion, and rash. The drug is increased in 100- to 200-mg increments given in equally divided doses over 2 days, as side effects allow, until pain relief is obtained or a total dose of 1200 mg/day is reached. Careful monitoring of laboratory parameters is mandatory to avoid the rare possibility of a life-threatening blood dyscrasia, and at the first sign of blood count abnormality or rash, the drug should be discontinued. Failure to monitor patients started on carbamazepine can be disastrous, because aplastic anemia can occur. When pain relief is obtained, the patient should be kept at that dosage of carbamazepine for at least 6 months before tapering of the medication is considered. The patient should be instructed that under no circumstances should the drug dosage be changed or the drug refilled or discontinued without the physician's knowledge.

Baclofen

Baclofen may be of value in some patients who fail to obtain relief from gabapentin or carbamazepine. Baseline laboratory tests should be obtained before starting baclofen, and the patient should

be cautioned about potential adverse effects, which are the same as those associated with carbamazepine and gabapentin. Baclofen is started with a 10-mg dose at bedtime for 2 nights; the dosage is then increased in 10-mg increments given in equally divided doses over 7 days, as side effects allow, until pain relief is obtained or a total dose of 80 mg/day is reached. This drug has significant hepatic and central nervous system side effects, including weakness and sedation. As with carbamazepine, careful monitoring of laboratory values is indicated.

When treating individuals with any of these drugs, the physician should make sure that the patient knows that premature tapering or discontinuation of the medication may lead to the recurrence of pain, which will be more difficult to control.

Invasive Therapy
Brachial Plexus Block

Brachial plexus block with local anesthetic and steroid is an excellent adjunct to drug treatment. This technique rapidly relieves pain while medications are being titrated to effective levels. The initial block is carried out with preservative-free bupivacaine combined with methylprednisolone. Subsequent daily nerve blocks are performed in a similar manner, by substituting a lower dose of methylprednisolone. This approach can also be used to control breakthrough pain.

Radiofrequency Destruction of the Brachial Plexus

The brachial plexus can be destroyed by creating a radiofrequency lesion under biplanar fluoroscopic guidance. This procedure is reserved for patients who have failed to respond to all aforementioned treatments and whose pain is secondary to tumor or avulsion of the brachial plexus.

Dorsal Root Entry Zone Lesioning

Dorsal root entry zone lesioning is the neurosurgical procedure of choice for intractable brachial plexopathy in patients who have failed to respond to all aforementioned treatments and whose pain is secondary to tumor or avulsion of the brachial plexus. This is a major neurosurgical procedure and carries significant risks.

Physical Modalities

Physical and occupational therapy to maintain function and palliate pain is a crucial part of the treatment plan for patients suffering from brachial plexopathy. Shoulder abnormalities, including subluxation and adhesive capsulitis, must be treated aggressively. Occupational therapy to assist in activities of daily living is important to avoid further deterioration of function.

COMPLICATIONS AND PITFALLS

The pain of brachial plexopathy is difficult to treat. It responds poorly to opioid analgesics and may respond poorly to the medications discussed. The uncontrolled pain of brachial plexopathy can lead to suicide, and strong consideration should be given to hospitalizing such patients. Correct diagnosis of the underlying cause is crucial to the successful treatment of the pain and dysfunction associated with brachial plexopathy, because stretch injuries and contusions of the plexus may respond with time, but plexopathy secondary to tumor or avulsion of the cervical roots requires aggressive treatment.

Clinical Pearls

Brachial plexus block with local anesthetic and steroid represents an excellent stopgap measure for patients suffering from the uncontrolled pain of brachial plexopathy while waiting for drug treatments to take effect. Correct diagnosis is paramount to allow the clinician to design a logical treatment plan.

SUGGESTED READINGS

Chen AM, Hall W, Guiou M, et al: Brachial plexopathy after radiation therapy for head-and-neck cancer, *Int J Radiat Oncol Biol Phys* 75(3 Suppl 1):S31–S32, 2009.

Choi J-Y, Kang CH, Kim B-J, et al: Brachial plexopathy following herpes zoster infection: two cases with MRI findings, *J Neurol Sci* 285(1–2):224–226, 2009.

Mullins GM, O'Sullivan SS, Neligan A, et al: Non-traumatic brachial plexopathies, clinical, radiological and neurophysiological findings from a tertiary centre, *Clin Neurol Neurosurg* 109(8):661–666, 2007.

Waldman SD: Brachial plexopathy. In *Pain review*, Philadelphia, 2009, Saunders, pp 260–261.

Waldman SD: Brachial plexus block: interscalene approach. In *Atlas of interventional pain management*, ed 3, Philadelphia, 2009, Saunders, pp 195–198.

Chapter 23

PANCOAST'S TUMOR SYNDROME

ICD-9 CODE **162.3**

ICD-10 CODE **C34.10**

THE CLINICAL SYNDROME

Pancoast's tumor syndrome is the result of local growth of tumor from the apex of the lung directly into the brachial plexus. Such tumors usually involve the first and second thoracic nerves, as well as the eighth cervical nerve, and produce a classic clinical syndrome consisting of severe arm pain and, in some patients, Horner's syndrome (Fig. 23-1). Destruction of the first and second ribs is also common. Diagnosis is usually delayed, and patients are often erroneously treated for cervical radiculopathy or primary shoulder disease until the diagnosis becomes clear.

SIGNS AND SYMPTOMS

Patients suffering from Pancoast's tumor syndrome complain of pain radiating to the supraclavicular region and upper extremity (Fig. 23-2). Initially, the lower portion of the brachial plexus is involved because the tumor growth is from below, causing pain in the upper thoracic and lower cervical dermatomes. The pain is neuritic and may take on a deep, boring quality as the tumor invades the brachial plexus. Movement of the neck and shoulder exacerbates the pain, so patients often try to avoid such movement. Frozen shoulder often results and may confuse the diagnosis. As the disease progresses, Horner's syndrome may occur.

TESTING

All patients presenting with brachial plexopathy, especially those without a clear history of antecedent trauma, must undergo magnetic resonance imaging (MRI) of the cervical spine and the brachial plexus (Figs. 23-3 and 23-4). Computed tomography (CT) is a reasonable alternative if MRI is contraindicated. Electromyography (EMG) and nerve conduction velocity testing are extremely sensitive, and a skilled electromyographer can determine which portion of the plexus is abnormal. All patients with a significant smoking history and suspected Pancoast's tumor or other tumor of the brachial plexus should undergo chest radiography with apical lordotic views or CT scanning through the apex of the lung. If the diagnosis is in question, screening laboratory tests consisting of a complete blood count, erythrocyte sedimentation rate, antinuclear antibody testing, and automated blood chemistry should be performed to rule out other causes of the patient's pain.

DIFFERENTIAL DIAGNOSIS

Diseases of the cervical spinal cord, bony cervical spine, and disk can mimic the brachial plexopathy associated with Pancoast's tumor syndrome. Appropriate testing, including MRI and EMG, can help sort out the myriad possibilities, but the clinician should be aware that more than one pathologic process may be contributing to the patient's symptoms. Syringomyelia, tumor of the cervical spinal cord, and tumor of the cervical nerve root as it exits the spinal cord (e.g., schwannoma) can have an insidious onset and be quite difficult to diagnose. Pancoast's tumor should be high on the list of diagnostic possibilities in all patients presenting with brachial plexopathy in the absence of clear antecedent trauma, especially if they have a history of tobacco use. Lateral herniated cervical disk, metastatic tumor, or cervical spondylosis that results in significant nerve root compression may also manifest as brachial plexopathy. Rarely, infection involving the apex of the lung may compress and irritate the plexus.

TREATMENT

The primary treatment of Pancoast's tumor syndrome is aimed at the tumor itself. Based on the cell type and extent of involvement, chemotherapy and radiation therapy may be indicated. Primary surgical treatment of tumors involving the brachial plexus is difficult, and the results are disappointing.

Drug Therapy
Opioid Analgesics

Opioid analgesics are the mainstay of treatment for the pain associated with Pancoast's tumor syndrome. Although neuropathic pain generally responds poorly to opioid analgesics, given the severity of the pain and the lack of other options, a trial of opioid analgesics is warranted. Administration of a short-acting, potent opioid such as oxycodone is a reasonable starting point. Immediate-release morphine or methadone can also be considered. These drugs can be used in combination with nonsteroidal antiinflammatory drugs and the adjuvant analgesics described here.

Gabapentin

Gabapentin is used to treat the neuritic pain of Pancoast's tumor syndrome. The initial dose is 300 mg gabapentin at bedtime for 2 nights, and the patient should be cautioned about potential side effects, including dizziness, sedation, confusion, and rash. The drug is then increased in 300-mg increments given in equally divided doses over 2 days, as side effects allow, until pain relief is obtained or a total dose of 2400 mg/day is reached. At this point, if the patient has experienced partial pain relief, blood values are

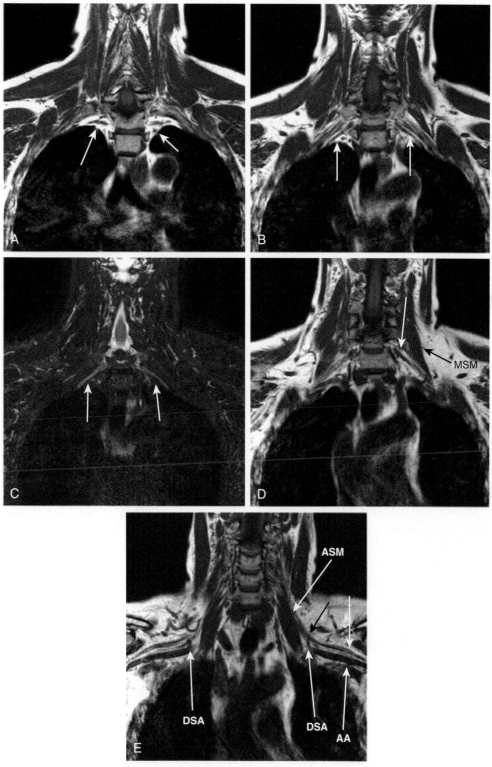

Figure 23-1 Magnetic resonance imaging of normal coronal anatomy. **A,** Most posterior image with the horizontal course of the T1 nerve root *(long arrow),* very close to the lung apex. The *short arrow* points to the stellate ganglion. **A,** Image just anterior to **A** with the C8 nerve roots *(arrows).* **C,** T2-weighted short tau inversion recovery image at the same level as **B** shows the slightly increased signal intensity of the normal C8 nerve roots *(arrows).* **D,** *Arrow* points to the C7 nerve root. MSM, middle scalene muscle. **E,** The cords *(white arrow)* are seen as linear structures above the axillary artery (AA). The dorsal scapular artery (DSA) courses between the trunks of the brachial plexus; the *black arrow* points to the superior trunk. ASM, anterior scalene muscle. *(From Van Es HW, Bollen TL, van Heesewijk HP: MRI of the brachial plexus: a pictorial review,* Eur J Radiol *74[2]:391–402, 2010.)*

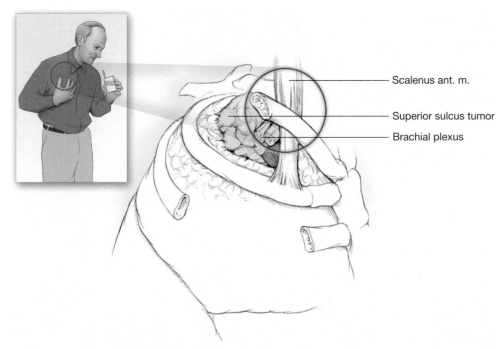

Scalenus ant. m.

Superior sulcus tumor

Brachial plexus

Figure 23-2 Pancoast's tumor should be suspected in patients suffering from shoulder and upper extremity pain who have a history of smoking.

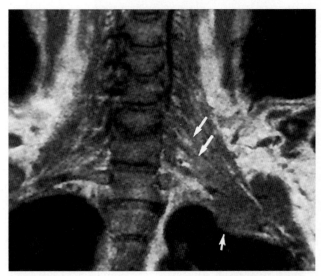

Figure 23-3 Pancoast's tumor (adenocarcinoma) with infiltration of the brachial plexus. A 65-year-old man complained of severe pain in the shoulder radiating to the elbow, the medial side of the forearm, and the fourth and fifth fingers in an ulnar nerve distribution. Screening coronal T1-weighted magnetic resonance imaging shows the brachial plexus from the region of the roots *(long arrows)* to the region of the trunks and divisions, where one sees tumor invasion *(short arrow)* and loss of fat planes on the left. *(From Stark DD, Bradley WG Jr, editors: Magnetic resonance imaging, ed 3, St Louis, 1999, Mosby, p 2399.)*

measured, and the drug is carefully titrated upward using 100-mg tablets. Rarely is a dose greater than 3600 mg/day required.

Pregabalin

Pregabalin represents a reasonable alternative to gabapentin and is better tolerated in some patients. Pregabalin is started at 50 mg three times a day and may be titrated upward to 100 mg three times a day as side effects allow. Because pregabalin is excreted primarily by the kidneys, the dosage should be decreased in patients with compromised renal function.

Carbamazepine

Carbamazepine is useful in patients who do not obtain pain relief with gabapentin. Despite the safety and efficacy of carbamazepine, confusion and anxiety have surrounded its use. The drug is sometimes discontinued owing to laboratory abnormalities erroneously attributed to it. Therefore, baseline laboratory values consisting of a complete blood count, urinalysis, and automated chemistry profile should be obtained before starting the drug.

Carbamazepine should be initiated slowly if the pain is not out of control at a starting dose of 100 to 200 mg at bedtime for 2 nights. The patient should be cautioned about side effects, including dizziness, sedation, confusion, and rash. The drug is increased in 100- to 200-mg increments given in equally divided doses over 2 days, as side effects allow, until pain relief is obtained or a total dose of 1200 mg/day is reached. Careful monitoring of laboratory parameters is mandatory to avoid the rare possibility of a life-threatening blood dyscrasia, and at the first sign of blood count abnormality or rash, the drug should be discontinued. Failure to monitor patients started on carbamazepine can be disastrous, because aplastic anemia can occur. When pain relief is obtained, the patient should be kept at that dosage of carbamazepine for at least 6 months before tapering of the medication is considered. The patient should be instructed that under no circumstances should the drug dosage be changed or the drug refilled or discontinued without the physician's knowledge.

Baclofen

Baclofen may be of value in some patients who fail to obtain relief from the previously mentioned medications. Baseline laboratory tests should be obtained before starting baclofen, and the patient should be cautioned about potential adverse effects, which are the same as those associated with carbamazepine

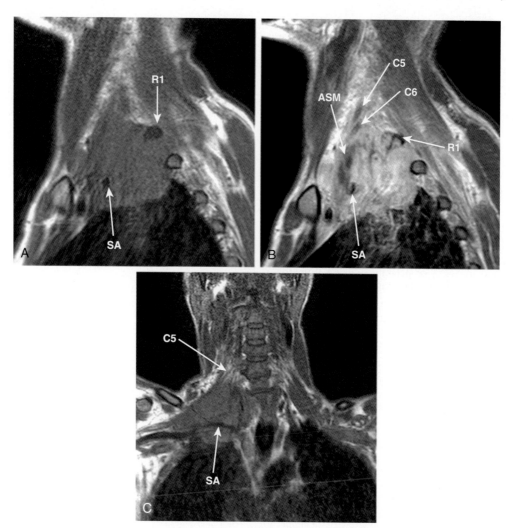

Figure 23-4 Magnetic resonance imaging of an inoperable superior sulcus tumor. **A** and **B**, Sagittal T1-weighted image without **(A)** and with **(B)** intravenous gadolinium show the extension of the non–small cell lung tumor into the interscalene triangle. With intravenous gadolinium, the nonenhancing nerve roots can be discerned from the enhancing tumor, and tumor is visible up to the C5 nerve root. The subclavian artery (SA) is encased, the tumor surrounds the anterior scalene muscle (ASM), and involvement of the first rib (R1) is evident. **C,** Coronal T1-weighted image demonstrates the involvement of the C5 nerve root. *(From Van Es HW, Bollen TL, van Heesewijk HP: MRI of the brachial plexus: a pictorial review,* Eur J Radiol *74[2]:391–402, 2010.)*

and gabapentin. Baclofen is started with a 10-mg dose at bedtime for 2 nights; the drug is then increased in 10-mg increments given in equally divided doses over 7 days, as side effects allow, until pain relief is obtained or a total dose of 80 mg/day is reached. This drug has significant hepatic and central nervous system side effects, including weakness and sedation. As with carbamazepine, careful monitoring of laboratory values is indicated.

Invasive Therapy

Brachial Plexus Block

Brachial plexus block with local anesthetic and steroid is an excellent adjunct to drug treatment of Pancoast's tumor syndrome. This technique rapidly relieves pain while medications are being titrated to effective levels. The initial block is carried out with preservative-free bupivacaine combined with methylprednisolone. Subsequent daily nerve blocks are performed in a similar manner, by substituting a lower dose of methylprednisolone. This approach can also be used to control breakthrough pain.

Radiofrequency Destruction of the Brachial Plexus

The brachial plexus can be destroyed by creating a radiofrequency lesion under biplanar fluoroscopic guidance. This procedure is reserved for patients for whom all aforementioned treatments have failed.

Dorsal Root Entry Zone Lesioning

Dorsal root entry zone lesioning is the neurosurgical procedure of choice for intractable brachial plexopathy associated with Pancoast's tumor in patients who have failed to respond to all aforementioned treatment options. This is a major neurosurgical procedure and carries significant risks.

Other Neurosurgical Options

Cordotomy, deep brain stimulation, and thalamotomy have all been tried, with varying degrees of success.

Physical Modalities

Physical and occupational therapy to maintain function and palliate pain is a crucial part of the treatment plan for patients suffering from Pancoast's tumor syndrome. Shoulder abnormalities, including subluxation and adhesive capsulitis, must be aggressively treated. Occupational therapy to assist in activities of daily living is important to avoid further deterioration of function.

COMPLICATIONS AND PITFALLS

The pain of Pancoast's tumor syndrome is difficult to treat. It may respond poorly to any of or all the recommended medications. The uncontrolled pain of Pancoast's tumor syndrome can lead to suicide, and strong consideration should be given to hospitalizing such patients. Correct diagnosis of the underlying cause is crucial, because the pain and dysfunction associated with brachial plexopathy secondary to Pancoast's tumor require aggressive treatment.

Clinical Pearls

Brachial plexus block with local anesthetic and steroid is an excellent stopgap measure for patients suffering from the uncontrolled pain of brachial plexopathy while waiting for drug treatments to take effect. Correct diagnosis is paramount to allow the clinician to design a logical treatment plan.

SUGGESTED READINGS

Davis GA, Knight SR: Pancoast tumors, *Neurosurg Clin N Am* 23(4):545–557, 2008.

Rusch VW: Management of Pancoast tumours, *Lancet Oncol* 7(12):997–1005, 2006.

Tamura M, Hoda MA, Klepetko W: Current treatment paradigms of superior sulcus tumours, *Eur J Cardiothorac Surg* 36(4):747–753, 2009.

Van Es HW, Bollen TL, van Heesewijk HP: MRI of the brachial plexus: a pictorial review, *Eur J Radiol* 74(2):391–402, 2010.

Waldman SD: Brachial plexopathy. In *Pain review,* Philadelphia, 2009, Saunders, pp 260–261.

Waldman SD: Brachial plexus block: interscalene approach. In *Atlas of interventional pain management,* ed 3, Philadelphia, 2009, Saunders, pp 195–198.

Chapter 24

THORACIC OUTLET SYNDROME

ICD-9 CODE `353.0`

ICD-10 CODE `G54.0`

THE CLINICAL SYNDROME

Thoracic outlet syndrome consists of a constellation of signs and symptoms, including paresthesias and aching pain of the neck, shoulder, and arm. The cause is thought to be compression of the brachial plexus and subclavian artery and vein as they exit the space between the shoulder girdle and the first rib (Fig. 24-1) or compression from congenitally abnormal structures such as cervical ribs. One or all the structures may be compressed, thus giving the syndrome a varied clinical expression. Thoracic outlet syndrome is seen most commonly in women between 25 and 50 years of age. It has been the subject of significant debate, and the diagnosis and treatment of thoracic outlet syndrome remain controversial.

SIGNS AND SYMPTOMS

Although the symptoms of thoracic outlet syndrome vary, compression of neural structures accounts for most of them. Paresthesias of the upper extremity radiating into the distribution of the ulnar nerve may be misdiagnosed as tardy ulnar palsy. Aching and incoordination of the affected extremity are also common findings. If vascular compression exists, edema or discoloration of the arm

may be noted; in rare instances, venous or arterial thrombosis may occur. Rarely, the symptoms of thoracic outlet syndrome are caused by arterial aneurysm, and auscultation of the supraclavicular region reveals a bruit.

The symptoms of thoracic outlet syndrome may be elicited by various maneuvers, including the Adson test and the elevated arm stress test. The Adson test is carried out by palpating the radial pulse on the affected side with the patient's neck extended and the head turned toward the affected side. A diminished pulse suggests thoracic outlet syndrome. The elevated arm stress test is performed by having the patient hold his or her arms over the head and open and close the hands. Normally, patients without thoracic outlet syndrome can perform this maneuver for approximately 3 minutes, whereas those suffering from thoracic outlet syndrome experience the onset of symptoms within 30 seconds.

TESTING

Plain radiographs of the cervical spine should be obtained in all patients suspected of having thoracic outlet syndrome. These films should be carefully reviewed for congenital abnormalities such as cervical ribs or overly elongated transverse processes. Patients should also undergo chest radiography with apical lordotic views to rule out Pancoast's tumor. Magnetic resonance imaging (MRI) of the cervical spine is indicated to identify lesions of the cervical spinal cord and exiting nerve roots, as well as cervical ribs (Fig. 24-2). If the diagnosis is still in doubt, MRI of the brachial

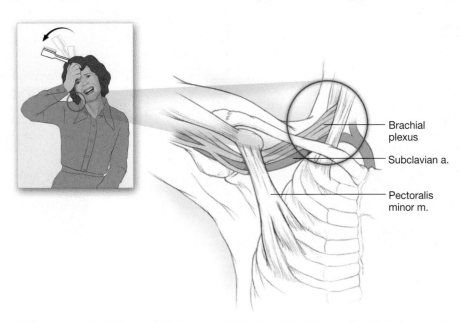

- Brachial plexus
- Subclavian a.
- Pectoralis minor m.

Figure 24-1 Compression of the brachial plexus results in pain and weakness in the affected upper extremity.

plexus is indicated to search for an occult pathologic process, including primary tumors of the plexus. Screening laboratory tests consisting of a complete blood count, erythrocyte sedimentation rate, antinuclear antibody testing, and automated blood chemistry may be performed to exclude other causes of the patient's pain.

DIFFERENTIAL DIAGNOSIS

Diseases of the cervical spinal cord, bony cervical spine, and disk can mimic thoracic outlet syndrome. Appropriate testing, including MRI and electromyography, can help sort out the myriad possibilities, but the clinician should be aware that more than one pathologic process may be contributing to the patient's symptoms. Syringomyelia, tumor of the cervical spinal cord, and tumor of the cervical nerve root as it exits the spinal cord (e.g., schwannoma) can have an insidious onset and may be quite difficult to diagnose. Pancoast's tumor should be high on the list of diagnostic possibilities in the absence of clear antecedent trauma, especially if the patient has a history of tobacco use. Lateral herniated cervical disk, metastatic tumor, or cervical spondylosis that results

in significant nerve root compression should also be considered. Rarely, infection involving the apex of the lung may compress and irritate the plexus.

TREATMENT

Physical Modalities

The primary treatment for patients suffering from thoracic outlet syndrome is the rational use of physical therapy to maintain function and palliate pain. Shoulder abnormalities, including subluxation and adhesive capsulitis, must be aggressively treated. Occupational therapy to assist in activities of daily living is important to avoid further deterioration of function.

Drug Therapy

Gabapentin

Gabapentin is first-line pharmacologic treatment for the neuritic pain of thoracic outlet syndrome. The initial dose is 300 mg gabapentin at bedtime for 2 nights, and the patient should be cautioned

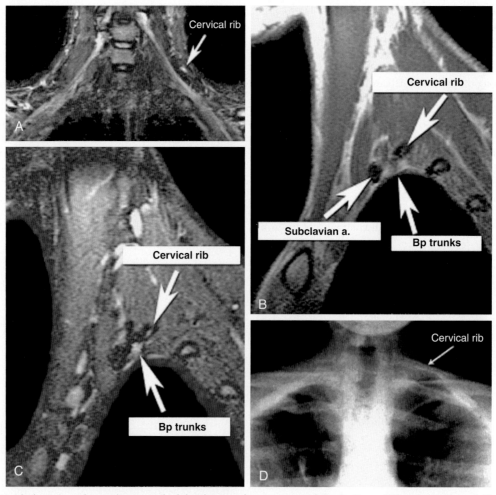

Figure 24-2 Patient with thoracic outlet syndrome on the left side secondary to a cervical rib. **A,** Coronal T2-weighted magnetic resonance imaging (MRI) shows the subtle deviation of the brachial plexus as it crosses the area of the cervical rib. **B** and **C,** Sagittal T1- and T2-weighted MRI at the level of the interscalene triangle shows the close proximity of the cervical rib to the lower trunk of the brachial plexus (Bp). **D,** Plain chest film shows the left cervical rib. The patient underwent surgical removal of the cervical rib, with resulting relief of symptoms. *(From Edelman RR, Hesselink JR, Zlatkin MB, Crues JV, eds:* Clinical magnetic resonance imaging, *ed 3, Philadelphia, 2006, Saunders, p 2382.)*

about potential side effects, including dizziness, sedation, confusion, and rash. The drug is then increased in 300-mg increments given in equally divided doses over 2 days, as side effects allow, until pain relief is obtained or a total dosage of 2400 mg/day is reached. At this point, if the patient has experienced partial pain relief, blood values are measured, and the drug is carefully titrated upward using 100-mg tablets. Rarely is a dosage greater than 3600 mg/day required.

Carbamazepine

Carbamazepine is useful in patients who do not obtain pain relief with gabapentin. Despite the safety and efficacy of carbamazepine, confusion and anxiety have surrounded its use. The drug is sometimes discontinued owing to laboratory abnormalities erroneously attributed to it. Therefore, baseline laboratory values consisting of a complete blood count, urinalysis, and automated chemistry profile should be obtained before starting the drug.

Carbamazepine should be initiated slowly if the pain is not out of control at a starting dose of 100 to 240 mg at bedtime for 2 nights. The patient should be cautioned about side effects, including dizziness, sedation, confusion, and rash. The drug is increased in 100- to 240-mg increments given in equally divided doses over 2 days, as side effects allow, until pain relief is obtained or a total dosage of 1240 mg/day is reached. Careful monitoring of laboratory parameters is mandatory to avoid the rare possibility of a life-threatening blood dyscrasia, and at the first sign of blood count abnormality or rash, the drug should be discontinued. Failure to monitor patients started on carbamazepine can be disastrous, because aplastic anemia can occur. When pain relief is obtained, the patient should be kept at that dosage of carbamazepine for at least 6 months before considering tapering of the medication. The patient should be instructed that under no circumstances should the drug dosage be changed or the drug refilled or discontinued without the physician's knowledge.

Pregabalin

Pregabalin represents a reasonable alternative to gabapentin and is better tolerated in some patients. Pregabalin is started at 50 mg three times a day and may be titrated upward to 100 mg three times a day as side effects allow. Because pregabalin is excreted primarily by the kidneys, the dosage should be decreased in patients with compromised renal function.

Baclofen

Baclofen may be of value in some patients who fail to obtain relief with gabapentin and carbamazepine. Baseline laboratory tests should be obtained before starting baclofen, and the patient should be cautioned about potential adverse effects, which are the same as those associated with carbamazepine and gabapentin. Baclofen is started with a 10-mg dose at bedtime for 2 nights; the drug is then increased in 10-mg increments given in equally divided doses over 7 days, as side effects allow, until pain relief is obtained or a total dosage of 80 mg/day is reached. This drug has significant hepatic and central nervous system side effects, including weakness and sedation. As with carbamazepine, careful monitoring of laboratory values is indicated.

When treating individuals with any of these drugs, the physician should make sure that the patient knows that premature tapering or discontinuation of the medication may lead to the recurrence of pain, which will be more difficult to control.

Invasive Therapy

Brachial Plexus Block

Brachial plexus block with local anesthetic and steroid is an excellent adjunct to drug treatment of thoracic outlet syndrome. This technique rapidly relieves pain while medications are being titrated to effective levels. The initial block is carried out with preservative-free bupivacaine combined with methylprednisolone. Subsequent daily nerve blocks are carried out in a similar manner, by substituting a lower dose of methylprednisolone. This approach can also be used to control breakthrough pain.

Surgery

In the absence of demonstrable disease (e.g., a cervical rib), the outcome of surgical treatment for thoracic outlet syndrome is dismal, regardless of the technique chosen. In patients with a clear cause of their symptoms who have failed to achieve relief from more conservative therapies, however, the judicious use of surgical treatment may be a reasonable last step.

COMPLICATIONS AND PITFALLS

The pain and dysfunction of thoracic outlet syndrome are difficult to treat. Physical therapy should be the primary modality in any well thought out treatment plan. In general, the pain of thoracic outlet syndrome responds poorly to opioid analgesics, and these drugs should be avoided. The careful use of adjuvant analgesics may help palliate the pain and allow the patient to participate in physical therapy. Correct diagnosis is crucial, because stretch injuries and contusions of the plexus may respond with time, but plexopathy secondary to tumor or avulsion of the cervical roots requires aggressive treatment.

Clinical Pearls

Brachial plexus block with local anesthetic and steroid represents an excellent stopgap measure to palliate the pain associated with thoracic outlet syndrome while waiting for drug treatments to take effect. Correct diagnosis is paramount to allow the clinician to design a logical treatment plan.

SUGGESTED READINGS

Abdul-Jabar H, Rashid A, Lam F: Thoracic outlet syndrome, *Orthop Trauma* 23(1):69–73, 2009.

Campbell WW, Landau ME: Controversial entrapment neuropathies, *Neurosurg Clin N Am* 19(4):597–608, 2008.

Lee J, Laker S, Fredericson M: Thoracic outlet syndrome, *PM R* 2(1):64–70, 2010.

Watson LA, Pizzari T, Balster S: Thoracic outlet syndrome. Part 1. Clinical manifestations, differentiation and treatment pathways, *Man Ther* 14(6):586–595, 2009.

White PW, Fox CJ, Feuerstein IM: Cervical rib causing arterial thoracic outlet syndrome, *J Am Coll Surg* 209(1):148–149, 2009.

Chapter 25

ARTHRITIS PAIN OF THE SHOULDER

ICD-9 CODE 715.91

ICD-10 CODE M19.90

THE CLINICAL SYNDROME

The shoulder joint is susceptible to the development of arthritis from various conditions that cause damage to the joint cartilage. Osteoarthritis is the most common cause of shoulder pain and functional disability (Fig. 25-1). It may occur after seemingly minor trauma or may be the result of repeated microtrauma. Pain around the shoulder and upper arm that is worse with activity is present in most patients suffering from osteoarthritis of the shoulder. Difficulty sleeping is also common, as is progressive loss of motion.

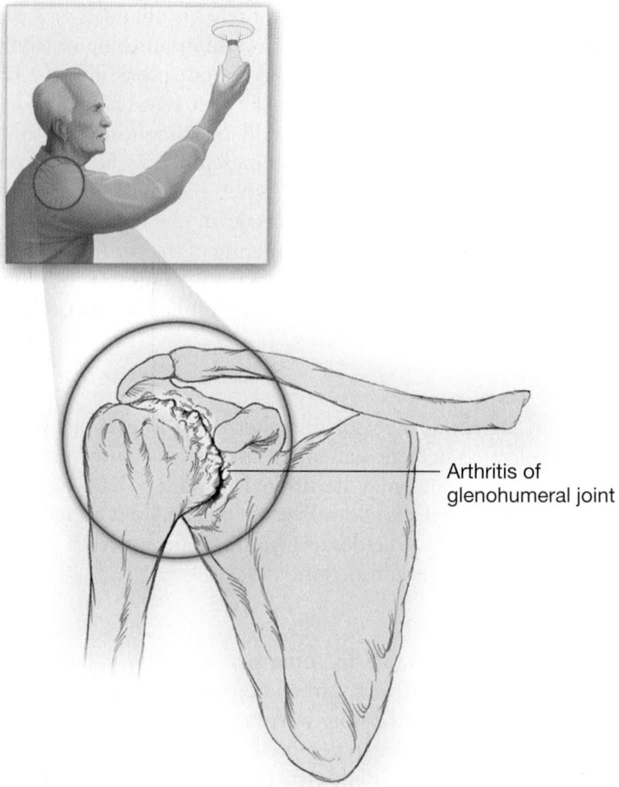

SIGNS AND SYMPTOMS

Most patients presenting with shoulder pain secondary to osteoarthritis, rotator cuff arthropathy, or posttraumatic arthritis complain of pain that is localized around the shoulder and upper arm. Activity makes the pain worse, whereas rest and heat provide some relief. The pain is constant and is characterized as aching; it may interfere with sleep. Some patients complain of a grating or popping sensation with use of the joint, and crepitus may be present on physical examination.

In addition to pain, patients suffering from arthritis of the shoulder joint often experience a gradual reduction in functional ability because of decreasing shoulder range of motion. This change makes simple everyday tasks such as combing one's hair, fastening a brassiere, or reaching overhead quite difficult. With continued disuse, muscle wasting may occur, and a frozen shoulder may develop.

TESTING

Plain radiographs are indicated in all patients who present with shoulder pain (Fig. 25-2). Based on the patient's clinical presentation, additional testing may be indicated, including

Arthritis of glenohumeral joint

Figure 25-1 Range of motion of the shoulder can precipitate the pain of osteoarthritis.

a complete blood count, erythrocyte sedimentation rate, and antinuclear antibody testing. Magnetic resonance imaging of the shoulder is indicated if a rotator cuff tear is suspected. Radionuclide bone scanning is indicated if metastatic disease or primary tumor involving the shoulder is a possibility.

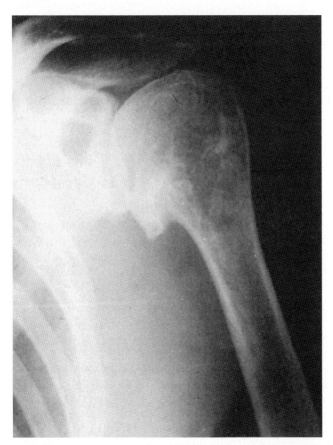

Figure 25-2 Osteoarthritis of the shoulder. The radiograph shows all the characteristic features of a hypertrophic form of osteoarthritis of the glenohumeral joint, with joint space narrowing, subchondral sclerosis, large cysts in the glenoid, and massive inferior osteophytosis. *(From Klippel JH, Dieppe PA:* Rheumatology, *ed 2, London, 1998, Mosby.)*

DIFFERENTIAL DIAGNOSIS

Osteoarthritis of the joint is the most common form of arthritis that results in shoulder pain; however, rheumatoid arthritis, posttraumatic arthritis, and rotator cuff arthropathy are also common causes of shoulder pain. Less common causes of arthritis-induced shoulder pain include collagen vascular diseases, infection, villonodular synovitis, and Lyme disease. Acute infectious arthritis is usually accompanied by significant systemic symptoms, including fever and malaise, and should be easily recognized; it is diagnosed with culture and treated with antibiotics rather than injection therapy. Collagen vascular diseases generally manifest as a polyarthropathy rather than a monarthropathy limited to the shoulder joint; however, shoulder pain secondary to collagen vascular disease responds exceedingly well to the intraarticular injection technique described here.

TREATMENT

Initial treatment of the pain and functional disability associated with osteoarthritis of the shoulder includes a combination of nonsteroidal antiinflammatory drugs (NSAIDs) or cyclooxygenase-2 (COX-2) inhibitors and physical therapy. Local application of heat and cold may also be beneficial. For patients who do not respond to these treatment modalities, intraarticular injection of local anesthetic and steroid is a reasonable next step.

Intraarticular injection of the shoulder is performed by placing the patient in the supine position and preparing the skin overlying the shoulder, subacromial region, and joint space with antiseptic solution. Using strict aseptic technique, the practitioner attaches a sterile syringe containing 2 mL of 0.25% preservative-free bupivacaine and 40 mg methylprednisolone to a 1½-inch, 25-gauge needle. The midpoint of the acromion is identified, and at a point approximately 1 inch below the midpoint, the shoulder joint space is identified. The needle is carefully advanced through the skin and subcutaneous tissues, through the joint capsule, and into the joint. If bone is encountered, the needle is withdrawn into the subcutaneous tissues and is redirected superiorly and slightly more medially. After the joint space is entered, the contents of the syringe are gently injected. Little resistance to injection is felt; if resistance is encountered, the needle is probably in a ligament or tendon and should be advanced slightly into the joint space until the injection can proceed without significant resistance. The needle is then removed, and a sterile pressure dressing and ice pack are applied to the injection site.

Physical modalities, including local heat and gentle range-of-motion exercises, should be introduced several days after the patient undergoes injection for shoulder pain. Vigorous exercises should be avoided, because they will exacerbate the patient's symptoms.

COMPLICATIONS AND PITFALLS

This injection technique is safe if careful attention is paid to the clinically relevant anatomy. Sterile technique must be used to avoid infection, along with universal precautions to minimize any risk to the operator. The incidence of ecchymosis and hematoma formation can be decreased if pressure is applied to the injection site immediately after injection. The major complication of intraarticular injection of the shoulder is infection, although it should be exceedingly rare if strict aseptic technique is followed. Approximately 25% of patients complain of a transient increase in pain after intraarticular injection of the shoulder joint, and they should be warned of this possibility.

Clinical Pearls

Osteoarthritis of the shoulder is a common complaint encountered in clinical practice. It must be distinguished from other causes of shoulder pain, including rotator cuff tears. Intraarticular injection is extremely effective in the treatment of pain secondary to arthritis of the shoulder joint. Coexistent bursitis and tendinitis may contribute to shoulder pain and necessitate additional treatment with more localized injection of local anesthetic and methylprednisolone. Simple analgesics and NSAIDs or COX-2 inhibitors can be used concurrently with this injection technique.

SUGGESTED READINGS

Andrews JR: Diagnosis and treatment of chronic painful shoulder: review of nonsurgical interventions, *Arthroscopy* 21(3):333–347, 2005.
Dalton SE: Clinical examination of the painful shoulder, *Baillieres Clin Rheumatol* 3(3):453–474, 1989.
Davies AM: Imaging the painful shoulder, *Curr Orthop* 6(1):32–38, 1992.
Monach PA: Shoulder pain. In Mushlin SB, Greene HL II, editors: *Decision making in medicine,* ed 3, Philadelphia, 2010, Mosby, pp 522–523.
Reutter TRC: Shoulder pain. In Ramamurthy S, Alanmanou E, Rogers JN, editors: *Decision making in pain management,* ed 2, St Louis, 2006, Mosby, pp 160–162.

Chapter 26

ACROMIOCLAVICULAR JOINT PAIN

ICD-9 CODE **719.41**

ICD-10 CODE **M25.519**

THE CLINICAL SYNDROME

The acromioclavicular joint is vulnerable to injury from both acute trauma and repeated microtrauma. Acute injuries are frequently the result of falling directly onto the shoulder when playing sports or riding a bicycle. Repeated strain from throwing or working with the arm raised across the body may also result in trauma to the joint. After trauma, the joint may become acutely inflamed, and if the condition becomes chronic, arthritis of the acromioclavicular joint may develop. Cysts of the acromioclavicular joint can become quite large and contribute to functional disability and pain (Fig. 26-1). Rarely, infection of the acromioclavicular joint may occur.

SIGNS AND SYMPTOMS

Patients suffering from acromioclavicular joint dysfunction frequently complain of pain when reaching across the chest (Fig. 26-2). Often, patients are unable to sleep on the affected shoulder and may complain of a grinding sensation in the joint, especially on first awakening. Physical examination may reveal enlargement or swelling of the joint, with tenderness to palpation. Downward traction or passive adduction of the affected shoulder may cause increased pain. If the ligaments of the acromioclavicular joint are disrupted, these maneuvers may reveal joint instability.

TESTING

Plain radiographs of the joint may reveal narrowing or sclerosis, consistent with osteoarthritis or actual separation or dislocation of the joint (Fig. 26-3). Magnetic resonance imaging (MRI) is indicated if disruption of the ligaments is suspected and to clarify the extent of ligamentous injury or to help rule out infection (Fig. 26-4). Ultrasound evaluation of the joint is also useful if a cyst is suspected. The injection technique described later serves as both a diagnostic and a therapeutic maneuver. If polyarthritis is present, screening laboratory tests consisting of a complete blood count, erythrocyte sedimentation rate, and antinuclear antibody testing should be performed.

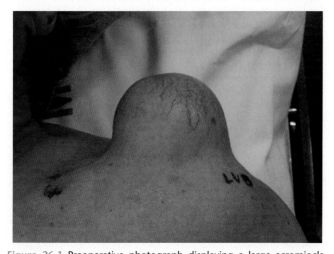

Figure 26-1 Preoperative photograph displaying a large acromioclavicular joint cyst with telangiectatic vessels. *(From Nowak DD, Covey AS, Grant RT, Bigliani LU: Massive acromioclavicular joint cyst,* J Shoulder Elbow Surg *18[5]:e12–e14, 2009.)*

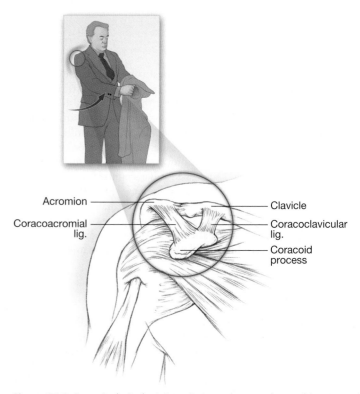

Figure 26-2 Acromioclavicular joint pain is made worse by reaching across the chest.

DIFFERENTIAL DIAGNOSIS

Osteoarthritis of the acromioclavicular joint is a frequent cause of shoulder pain, and it is usually the result of trauma. However, rheumatoid arthritis and rotator cuff arthropathy are also common causes of shoulder pain that may mimic acromioclavicular joint pain and confuse the diagnosis. Less common causes of arthritis-induced shoulder pain include the collagen vascular diseases, infection, and Lyme disease. Acute infectious arthritis is usually accompanied by significant systemic symptoms, including fever and malaise, and should be easily recognized; it is treated with culture, antibiotics, and surgical drainage, rather than injection therapy. Collagen

vascular diseases generally manifest as polyarthropathy rather than monarthropathy limited to the shoulder joint; however, shoulder pain secondary to collagen vascular disease responds exceedingly well to the intraarticular injection technique described here.

TREATMENT

Initial treatment of the pain and functional disability associated with acromioclavicular joint pain includes a combination of nonsteroidal antiinflammatory drugs (NSAIDs) or cyclooxygenase-2 (COX-2) inhibitors and physical therapy. Local application of heat and cold may also be beneficial. For patients who do not respond to these treatment modalities, intraarticular injection of local anesthetic and steroid is a reasonable next step.

Intraarticular injection of the acromioclavicular joint is performed by placing the patient in the supine position and preparing the skin overlying the superior shoulder and distal clavicle with antiseptic solution. A sterile syringe containing 1 mL of 0.25% preservative-free bupivacaine and 40 mg methylprednisolone is attached to a 1½-inch, 25-gauge needle using strict aseptic technique. The top of the acromion is identified, and at a point approximately 1 inch medially, the acromioclavicular joint space is identified. The needle is carefully advanced through the skin and subcutaneous tissues, through the joint capsule, and into the joint (Fig. 26-5). If bone is encountered, the needle is withdrawn into the subcutaneous tissues and is redirected slightly more medially. After the joint space is entered, the contents of the syringe are gently injected. Some resistance to injection should be felt, because the joint space is small and the joint capsule is dense. If significant resistance is encountered, however, the needle is probably in a ligament and should be advanced slightly into the joint space until the injection can proceed with only limited resistance. If no resistance is encountered on injection, the joint space is probably

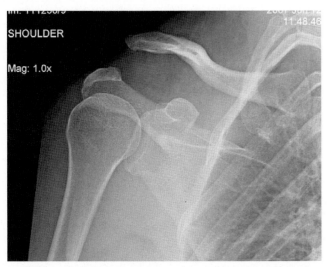

Figure 26-3 Type V superior dislocation of the acromioclavicular joint. *(From MacDonald PB, Lapointe P: Acromioclavicular and sternoclavicular joint injuries,* Orthop Clin North Am *39[4]:535–545, 2008.)*

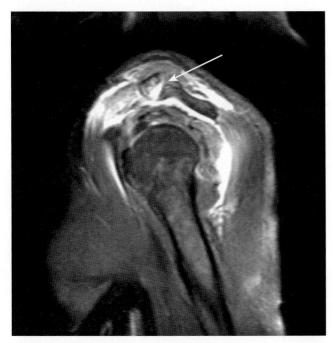

Figure 26-4 T2-weighted sagittal magnetic resonance image of the shoulder demonstrates inflammation and distention of the acromioclavicular joint space *(arrow). (From Hammel JM, Kwon N: Septic arthritis of the acromioclavicular joint,* J Emerg Med *29[4]:425–427, 2005.)*

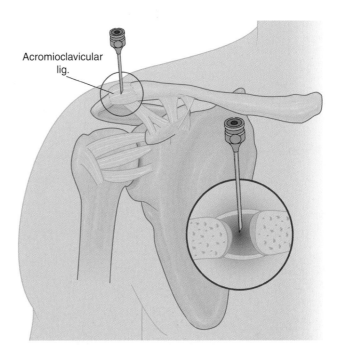

Figure 26-5 Proper needle placement for acromioclavicular joint injection. *(From Waldman SD:* Atlas of pain management injection techniques, *Philadelphia, 2000, Saunders, p 41.)*

not intact, and MRI is recommended. After injection, the needle is removed, and a sterile pressure dressing and ice pack are applied to the injection site.

Physical modalities, including local heat and gentle range-of-motion exercises, should be introduced several days after the patient undergoes injection for shoulder pain. Vigorous exercises should be avoided, because they will exacerbate the patient's symptoms.

COMPLICATIONS AND PITFALLS

This injection technique is safe if careful attention is paid to the clinically relevant anatomy. Sterile technique must be used to avoid infection, along with universal precautions to minimize any risk to the operator. The incidence of ecchymosis and hematoma formation can be decreased if pressure is applied to the injection site immediately after injection. The major complication of intraarticular injection of the acromioclavicular joint is infection, although it should be exceedingly rare if strict aseptic technique is followed. Approximately 25% of patients complain of a transient increase in pain after intraarticular injection of the acromioclavicular joint, and patients should be warned of this possibility.

Clinical Pearls

Intraarticular injection is extremely effective in the treatment of pain secondary to arthritis of the acromioclavicular joint. Coexistent bursitis and tendinitis may contribute to shoulder pain and necessitate additional treatment with more localized injection of local anesthetic and methylprednisolone. Simple analgesics and NSAIDs or COX-2 inhibitors can be used concurrently with this injection technique.

SUGGESTED READINGS

Ballesta Moratalla M, Fernández Gabarda R: Acromioclavicular joint ganglion, *Eur J Radiol Extra* 63(1):21–23, 2007.

Hammel JM, Kwon N: Septic arthritis of the acromioclavicular joint, *J Emerg Med* 29(4):425–427, 2005.

Hossain S, Jacobs LG, Hashmi R: The long-term effectiveness of steroid injections in primary acromioclavicular joint arthritis: a five-year prospective study, *J Shoulder Elbow Surg* 17(4):535–538, 2008.

Kippe MA, Wiater JM: Functional anatomy of the shoulder. In Placzek JD, Boyce DA, editors: *Orthopaedic physical therapy secrets,* ed 2, St Louis, 2006, Mosby, pp 321–330.

Chapter 27

SUBDELTOID BURSITIS

ICD-9 CODE `726.10`

ICD-10 CODE `M75.50`

THE CLINICAL SYNDROME

The subdeltoid bursa lies primarily under the acromion and extends laterally between the deltoid muscle and the joint capsule under the deltoid muscle (Fig. 27-1). It may exist as a single bursal sac or, in some patients, as a multisegmented series of loculated sacs. The subdeltoid bursa is vulnerable to injury from both acute trauma and repeated microtrauma. Acute injuries frequently take the form of direct trauma to the shoulder when playing sports or falling off a bicycle. Repeated strain from throwing, bowling, carrying a heavy briefcase, working with the arm raised across the body, rotator cuff injuries, or repetitive motion associated with assembly-line work may result in inflammation of the subdeltoid bursa. If the inflammation becomes chronic, calcification of the bursa may occur.

Patients suffering from subdeltoid bursitis frequently complain of pain with any movement of the shoulder, but especially with abduction (Fig. 27-2). The pain is localized to the subdeltoid area, with referred pain often noted at the insertion of the deltoid at the deltoid tuberosity on the upper third of the humerus. Patients are often unable to sleep on the affected shoulder and may complain of a sharp, catching sensation when abducting the shoulder, especially on first awakening.

SIGNS AND SYMPTOMS

Physical examination may reveal point tenderness over the acromion; occasionally, swelling of the bursa gives the affected deltoid muscle an edematous feel. Passive elevation and medial rotation of the affected shoulder reproduce the pain, as do resisted abduction and lateral rotation. Sudden release of resistance during this maneuver markedly increases the pain. Rotator cuff tear may mimic or coexist with subdeltoid bursitis and may confuse the diagnosis (see "Differential Diagnosis").

TESTING

Plain radiographs of the shoulder may reveal calcification of the bursa and associated structures, consistent with chronic inflammation. Magnetic resonance imaging is indicated if tendinitis, partial disruption of the ligaments, or rotator cuff tear is being considered (Fig. 27-3). Based on the patient's clinical presentation, additional testing may be indicated, including a complete blood count, erythrocyte sedimentation rate, and antinuclear antibody testing. Radionuclide bone scanning is indicated if metastatic disease or primary tumor involving the shoulder is a possibility. The injection technique described later serves as both a diagnostic and a therapeutic maneuver.

DIFFERENTIAL DIAGNOSIS

Subdeltoid bursitis is one of the most common causes of shoulder joint pain. Osteoarthritis, rheumatoid arthritis, posttraumatic arthritis, and rotator cuff arthropathy are also common causes of shoulder pain that may coexist with subdeltoid bursitis. Less common causes of arthritis-induced shoulder pain include collagen vascular diseases, infection, villonodular synovitis, and Lyme disease. Acute infectious arthritis is usually accompanied by significant systemic symptoms, including fever and malaise, and should be easily recognized; it is treated with culture and antibiotics, rather than with injection therapy. Collagen vascular diseases generally manifest as polyarthropathy rather than monarthropathy limited to the shoulder joint; however, shoulder pain secondary to collagen vascular disease responds exceedingly well to the injection technique described here.

TREATMENT

Initial treatment of the pain and functional disability associated with subdeltoid bursitis includes a combination of nonsteroidal antiinflammatory drugs (NSAIDs) or cyclooxygenase-2 inhibitors and physical therapy. Local application of heat and cold may also be beneficial. For patients who do not respond to these treatment modalities, injection of local anesthetic and steroid into the subdeltoid bursa is a reasonable next step.

Injection into the subdeltoid bursa is performed by placing the patient in the supine position and preparing the skin overlying the superior shoulder, acromion, and distal clavicle with antiseptic solution. A sterile syringe containing 4 mL of 0.25% preservative-free bupivacaine and 40 mg methylprednisolone is attached to a 1½-inch, 25-gauge needle using strict aseptic technique. The lateral edge of the acromion is identified, and at the midpoint of the lateral edge, the injection site is identified. At this point, the needle is carefully advanced with a slightly cephalad trajectory through the skin and subcutaneous tissues beneath the acromion capsule and into the bursa (Fig. 27-4). If bone is encountered, the needle is withdrawn into the subcutaneous tissues and is redirected slightly more inferiorly. After the bursa is entered, the contents of the syringe are gently injected while the needle is slowly withdrawn. Resistance to injection should be minimal unless calcification of the bursal sac is present, in which

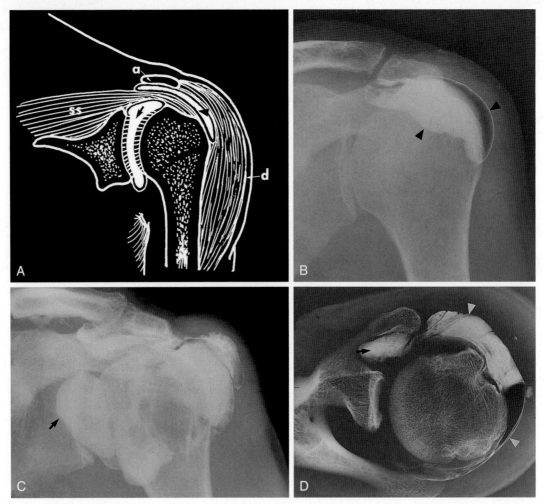

Figure 27-1 Normal anatomy of the subacromial (subdeltoid) bursa. **A,** Diagram of a coronal section of the shoulder shows the glenohumeral joint *(arrow)* and subacromial (subdeltoid) bursa *(arrowhead),* separated by a portion of the rotator cuff (i.e., supraspinatus tendon). The supraspinatus (ss) and deltoid (d) muscles and the acromion (a) are indicated. **B,** Subdeltoid-subacromial bursogram, accomplished with the injection of both radiopaque contrast material and air, shows the bursa *(arrowheads)* sitting like a cap on the humeral head and greater tuberosity of the humerus. Note that the joint is not opacified, indicative of an intact rotator cuff. **C,** In a different cadaver, a subacromial-subdeltoid bursogram shows much more extensive structure as a result of opacification of the subacromial, subdeltoid, and subcoracoid *(arrow)* portions of the bursa. **D,** Radiograph of a transverse section of the specimen illustrated in **C** shows both the subdeltoid *(arrowheads)* and subcoracoid *(arrow)* portions of the bursa. The glenohumeral joint is not opacified. *(From Resnick D:* Diagnosis of bone and joint disorders, *ed 4, Philadelphia, 2002, Saunders, p 3072.)*

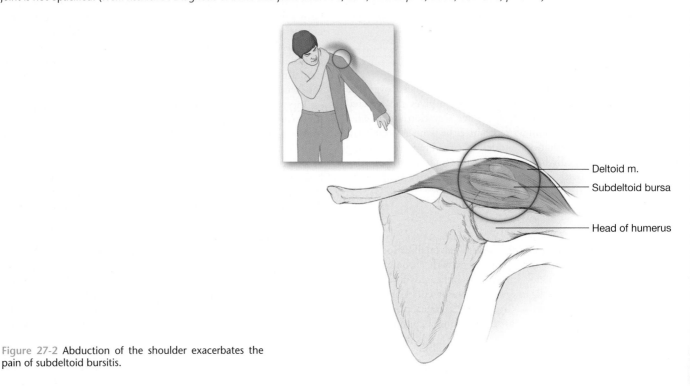

Deltoid m.
Subdeltoid bursa
Head of humerus

Figure 27-2 Abduction of the shoulder exacerbates the pain of subdeltoid bursitis.

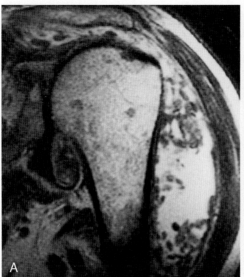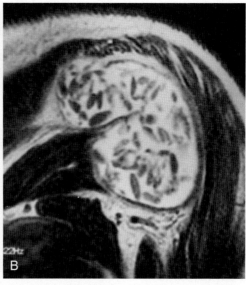

Figure 27-3 Subacromial-subdeltoid bursitis. **A** and **B,** Oblique, coronal, fast spin-echo (TR 300, TE 99) magnetic resonance images (**B** is posterior to **A**) show massive distention of the bursa with fluid of high signal intensity, and synovial proliferative tissue and rice bodies of low signal intensity, in a patient with probable rheumatoid arthritis. The rotator cuff is torn and retracted, and the glenohumeral joint is also involved. *(From Resnick D: Diagnosis of bone and joint disorders, ed 4, Philadelphia, 2002, Saunders, p 4256.)*

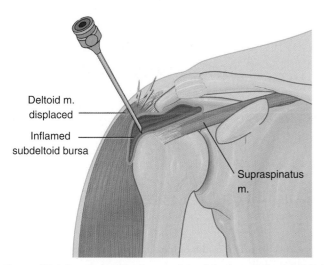

Deltoid m. displaced

Inflamed subdeltoid bursa

Supraspinatus m.

Figure 27-4 Proper needle placement for injection of the subdeltoid bursa. *(From Waldman SD: Atlas of pain management injection techniques, Philadelphia, 2000, Saunders.)*

case resistance to needle advancement is associated with a gritty feel. Significant calcific bursitis may ultimately require surgical excision to achieve complete relief of symptoms. After injection, the needle is removed, and a sterile pressure dressing and ice pack are applied to the injection site.

Physical modalities, including local heat and gentle range-of-motion exercises, should be introduced several days after the patient undergoes injection for shoulder pain. Vigorous exercises should be avoided, because they will exacerbate the patient's symptoms.

COMPLICATIONS AND PITFALLS

This injection technique is safe if careful attention is paid to the clinically relevant anatomy. Sterile technique must be used to avoid infection, along with universal precautions to minimize any risk to the operator. The incidence of ecchymosis and hematoma formation can be decreased if pressure is applied to the injection site immediately after injection. The major complication of injection of the subdeltoid bursa is infection, although it should be exceedingly rare if strict aseptic technique is followed. Approximately 25% of patients complain of a transient increase in pain after injection of the subdeltoid bursa, and patients should be warned of this possibility.

Clinical Pearls

This injection technique is extremely effective in the treatment of pain secondary to subdeltoid bursitis. Coexistent arthritis and tendinitis may contribute to shoulder pain, necessitating additional treatment with more localized injection of local anesthetic and methylprednisolone. Simple analgesics and NSAIDs can be used concurrently with this injection technique.

SUGGESTED READINGS

Andrews JR: Diagnosis and treatment of chronic painful shoulder: review of nonsurgical interventions, *Arthroscopy* 21(3):333–347, 2005.
Cowderoy GA, Lisle DA, O'Connell PT: Overuse and impingement syndromes of the shoulder in the athlete, *Magn Reson Imaging Clin N Am* 17(4):577–593, 2009.
Monach PA: Shoulder pain. In Mushlin SB, Greene HL II, editors: *Decision making in medicine,* ed 3, Philadelphia, 2010, Mosby, pp 522–523.
Waldman SD: Injection technique for subdeltoid bursitis pain. In *Pain review,* Philadelphia, 2009, Saunders, p 456.
Waldman SD: The subdeltoid bursa. In *Pain review,* Philadelphia, 2009, Saunders, p 83.

Chapter **28**

BICIPITAL TENDINITIS

ICD-9 CODE **726.12**

ICD-10 CODE **M75.20**

THE CLINICAL SYNDROME

The tendons of the long and short heads of the biceps are particularly prone to the development of tendinitis. Bicipital tendinitis is usually caused at least partially by impingement on the tendons of the biceps at the coracoacromial arch. The onset of bicipital tendinitis is generally acute, occurring after overuse or misuse of the shoulder joint, such as trying to start a recalcitrant lawn mower, practicing an overhead tennis serve, or performing an overaggressive follow-through when driving golf balls. The biceps muscle and tendons are susceptible to trauma and to wear and tear. If the damage is severe enough, the tendon of the long head of the biceps can rupture, leaving the patient with a telltale "Popeye" biceps (named after the cartoon character). This deformity can be accentuated by having the patient perform Ludington's maneuver: placing his or her hands behind the head and flexing the biceps muscle (see Chapter 31).

SIGNS AND SYMPTOMS

The pain of bicipital tendinitis is constant and severe and is localized in the anterior shoulder over the bicipital groove (Fig. 28-1). A catching sensation may accompany the pain. Significant sleep disturbance is often reported. The patient may attempt to splint the inflamed tendons by internal rotation of the humerus, which moves the biceps tendon from beneath the coracoacromial arch. Patients with bicipital tendinitis have a positive Yergason's test result—that is, production of pain on active supination of the forearm against resistance with the elbow flexed at a right angle (Fig. 28-2). Bursitis often accompanies bicipital tendinitis.

In addition to pain, patients suffering from bicipital tendinitis often experience a gradual reduction in functional ability because of decreasing shoulder range of motion that makes simple everyday tasks such as combing one's hair, fastening a brassiere, and reaching overhead quite difficult. With continued disuse, muscle wasting may occur, and a frozen shoulder may develop.

TESTING

Plain radiographs are indicated for all patients who present with shoulder pain. Based on the patient's clinical presentation, additional testing may be indicated, including a complete blood count, erythrocyte sedimentation rate, and antinuclear antibody testing. Magnetic resonance imaging of the shoulder is indicated if

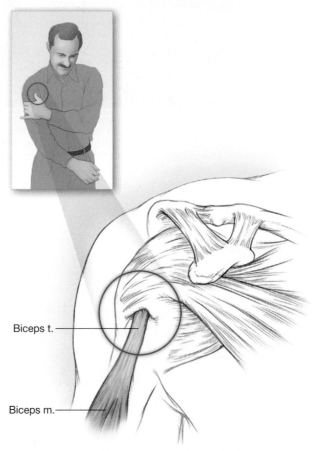

Biceps t.

Biceps m.

Figure 28-1 Palpation of the bicipital groove exacerbates the pain of bicipital tendinitis.

rotator cuff tear is suspected (Fig. 28-3). The injection technique described later serves as both a diagnostic and a therapeutic maneuver.

DIFFERENTIAL DIAGNOSIS

Bicipital tendinitis is usually a straightforward clinical diagnosis. However, coexisting bursitis or tendinitis of the shoulder from overuse or misuse may confuse the diagnosis. Occasionally, partial rotator cuff tear can be mistaken for bicipital tendinitis. In some clinical situations, consideration should be given to primary or secondary tumors involving the shoulder, superior sulcus of the lung, or proximal humerus. The pain of acute herpes zoster, which occurs before eruption of a vesicular rash, can also mimic bicipital tendinitis.

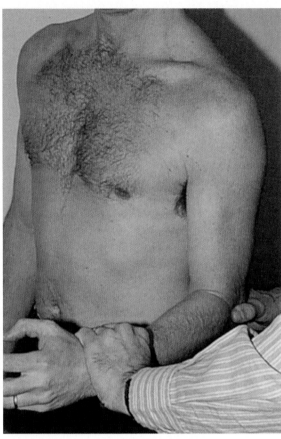

Figure 28-2 Yergason's test for bicipital tendinitis. *(From Klippel JH, Dieppe PA:* Rheumatology, *ed 2, London, 1998, Mosby.)*

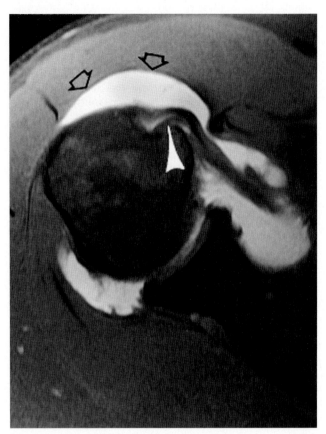

Figure 28-3 "Perched" biceps tendon. Fat-suppressed, T1-weighted, axial magnetic resonance arthrogram reveals a flattened biceps tendon *(large arrowhead)* draped over the lesser tuberosity in the presence of a normally configured bicipital groove. The presence of contrast material in the subacromial-subdeltoid bursa *(open arrowheads)* indicates a coexisting full-thickness tear of the rotator cuff. *(From Edelman RR, Hesselink JR, Zlatkin MB, Crues JV, editors:* Clinical magnetic resonance imaging, *ed 3, Philadelphia, 2005, Saunders, p 3161.)*

TREATMENT

Initial treatment of the pain and functional disability associated with bicipital tendinitis includes a combination of nonsteroidal antiinflammatory drugs (NSAIDs) or cyclooxygenase-2 (COX-2) inhibitors and physical therapy. Local application of heat and cold may also be beneficial. For patients who do not respond to these treatment modalities, injection with local anesthetic and steroid is a reasonable next step.

Injection for bicipital tendinitis is carried out by placing the patient in the supine position with the arm externally rotated approximately 45 degrees. The coracoid process is identified anteriorly. Just lateral to the coracoid process is the lesser tuberosity, which can be more easily palpated as the arm is passively rotated. The point overlying the tuberosity is marked with a sterile marker. The skin overlying the anterior shoulder is prepared with antiseptic solution. A sterile syringe containing 1 mL of 0.25% preservative-free bupivacaine and 40 mg methylprednisolone is attached to a 1½-inch, 25-gauge needle using strict aseptic technique. The previously marked point is palpated, and the insertion of the biceps tendon is reidentified with the gloved finger. The needle is carefully advanced at this point through the skin, subcutaneous tissues, and underlying tendon until it impinges on bone. The needle is then withdrawn 1 to 2 mm out of the periosteum of the humerus, and the contents of the syringe are gently injected. The clinician should feel slight resistance to injection. If no resistance is encountered, either the needle tip is in the joint space itself or the tendon is ruptured. If resistance is significant, the needle tip is probably in the substance of a ligament or tendon and should be advanced or withdrawn

slightly until the injection can proceed without significant resistance. The needle is then removed, and a sterile pressure dressing and ice pack are applied to the injection site.

Physical modalities, including local heat and gentle range-of-motion exercises, should be introduced several days after the patient undergoes injection. Vigorous exercises should be avoided, because they will exacerbate the patient's symptoms.

COMPLICATIONS AND PITFALLS

This injection technique is safe if careful attention is paid to the clinically relevant anatomy. Sterile technique must be used to avoid infection, along with universal precautions to minimize any risk to the operator. The incidence of ecchymosis and hematoma formation can be decreased if pressure is applied to the injection site immediately after injection. The major complication of this injection technique is infection, although it should be exceedingly rare if strict aseptic technique is followed. Trauma to the biceps tendon from the injection itself is also a possibility. Tendons that are highly inflamed or previously damaged are subject to rupture if they are injected directly. This complication can often be avoided if the clinician uses a gentle technique and stops injecting immediately if significant resistance is encountered. Approximately 25% of patients complain of a transient increase in pain after injection, and patients should be warned of this possibility.

Clinical Pearls

The musculotendinous unit of the shoulder joint is susceptible to the development of tendinitis for several reasons. First, the joint is subjected to many different repetitive motions. Second, the space in which the musculotendinous unit functions is restricted by the coracoacromial arch, a configuration that makes impingement likely with extreme movements of the joint. Third, the blood supply to the musculotendinous unit is poor, and this complicates the healing of microtrauma. All these factors can contribute to tendinitis. If the inflammation continues, calcium deposition around the tendon may occur and make subsequent treatment more difficult.

The injection technique described is extremely effective in the treatment of pain secondary to bicipital tendinitis. Coexistent bursitis and arthritis may contribute to shoulder pain, thus necessitating additional treatment with more localized injection of local anesthetic and methylprednisolone. Simple analgesics and NSAIDs or COX-2 inhibitors can be used concurrently with this injection technique.

SUGGESTED READINGS

Karistinos A, Paulos LE: Anatomy and function of the tendon of the long head of the biceps muscle, *Oper Tech Sports Med* 15(1):2–6, 2007.

Schultz JS: Clinical evaluation of the shoulder, *Phys Med Rehabil Clin N Am* 15(2):351–371, 2004.

Waldman SD: Bicipital tendinitis. In *Atlas of pain management injection techniques,* ed 2, Philadelphia, 2007, Saunders, pp 91–96.

Waldman SD: The biceps tendon. In *Pain review,* Philadelphia, 2009, Saunders, pp 84–85.

Weiland DE, Rodosky MW: Biceps tendon disorders. In *Clinical sports medicine,* New York, 2006, McGraw-Hill, pp 235–241.

Chapter 29

AVASCULAR NECROSIS OF THE GLENOHUMERAL JOINT

ICD-9 CODE **733.41**

ICD-10 CODE **M87.029**

THE CLINICAL SYNDROME

Avascular necrosis of the glenohumeral joint is an often missed diagnosis. Like the scaphoid, the glenohumeral joint is extremely susceptible to this disease because of the tenuous blood supply of the articular cartilage, which is only 1.0 to 1.2 mm thick at the center of the humeral head. This blood supply is easily disrupted, often leaving the proximal portion of the bone without nutrition leading to osteonecrosis (Fig. 29-1). Avascular necrosis of the glenohumeral joint is a disease of the fourth and fifth decades, except when it is secondary to collagen vascular disease. Avascular necrosis of the glenohumeral joint is more common in men. The disease is bilateral in 50% to 55% of cases.

Factors predisposing to avascular necrosis of the glenohumeral joint are listed in Table 29-1. They include trauma to the joint, corticosteroid use, Cushing's disease, alcohol abuse, connective tissue diseases especially systemic lupus erythematosus, osteomyelitis, human immunodeficiency virus infection, organ transplantation, hemoglobinopathies including sickle cell disease, hyperlipidemia, gout, renal failure, pregnancy, and radiation therapy involving the femoral head.

The patient with avascular necrosis of the glenohumeral joint complains of pain over the affected glenohumeral joint or glenohumeral joints that may radiate into the proximal upper extremity and shoulder. The pain is deep and aching, and patients often complain of a catching sensation with range of motion of the affect glenohumeral joint or glenohumeral joints. Range of motion decreases as the disease progresses.

SIGNS AND SYMPTOMS

Physical examination of patients suffering from avascular necrosis of the glenohumeral joint reveals pain to deep palpation of the glenohumeral joint. The pain can be worsened by passive and active range of motion. A click or crepitus may also be appreciated by the examiner during range of motion of the glenohumeral joint. Range of motion is invariably decreased.

TESTING

Plain radiographs are indicated in all patients who present with avascular necrosis of the glenohumeral joint, to rule out underlying occult bony disease and to identify sclerosis and fragmentation of

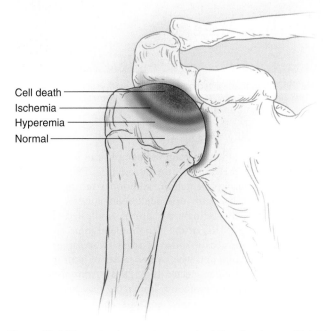

Cell death
Ischemia
Hyperemia
Normal

Figure 29-1 The pain of avascular necrosis of the glenohumeral joint is worsened by passive and active range of motion.

TABLE 29-1
Predisposing Factors for Avascular Necrosis of the Glenohumeral Joint

- Trauma to the glenohumeral joint
- Steroids
- Cushing's disease
- Alcohol abuse
- Connective tissue diseases especially systemic lupus erythematosus
- Osteomyelitis
- Human immunodeficiency virus infection
- Organ transplantation,
- Hemoglobinopathies including sickle cell disease
- Hyperlipidemia
- Gout
- Renal failure
- Pregnancy
- Radiation therapy

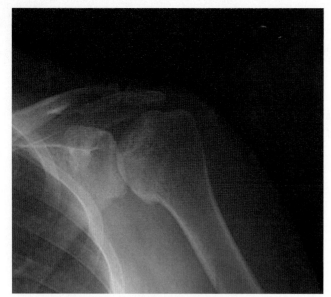

Figure 29-2 Preoperative radiographs from a 60-year-old patient with avascular necrosis. *(From Hollis R, Yamaguchi K: Avascular necrosis of the shoulder, Semin Arthroplasty 19[1]:19–22, 2008.)*

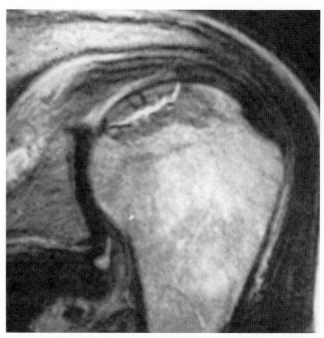

Figure 29-3 Osteonecrosis: humeral head. A coronal oblique T2-weighted (TR/TE, 3600/96) fast spin-echo magnetic resonance image shows the classic features of osteonecrosis, including a crescent sign. *(Courtesy of S. Eilenberg, M.D., San Diego. From Resnick D, Kang HS, Pretterklieber ML, editors: Internal derangement of joints, ed 2, Philadelphia, 2007, Saunders, p 404.)*

the humoral head, although plain radiographs can be notoriously unreliable early in the course of the disease (Fig. 29-2). Based on the patient's clinical presentation, additional testing including complete blood cell count, uric acid, sedimentation rate, and antinuclear antibody testing may also be indicated. Magnetic resonance imaging (MRI) of the glenohumeral joint is indicated in all patients suspected of suffering from avascular necrosis of the glenohumeral joint and when other causes of joint instability, infection, or tumor are suspected (Fig. 29-3). Administration of gadolinium followed by postcontrast imaging may help delineate the adequacy of blood supply; contrast enhancement of the glenohumeral joint is a good prognostic sign. Electromyography is indicated if coexistent cervical radiculopathy or brachial plexopathy is suspected. A very gentle intraarticular injection of the glenohumeral joint with small volumes of local anesthetic provides immediate improvement of the pain and helps demonstrate that the nidus of the patient's pain is in fact the glenohumeral joint. Ultimately, total joint replacement will be required in most patients suffering from avascular necrosis of the glenohumeral joint, although newer joint preservation techniques are becoming more popular in younger, more active patients, given the short life expectancy of total shoulder prostheses.

DIFFERENTIAL DIAGNOSIS

Coexistent arthritis and gout of the glenohumeral joint, bursitis, and tendinitis may also coexist with avascular necrosis of the glenohumeral joints and exacerbate the pain and disability of the patient. Tears of the labrum, ligament tears, bone cysts, bone contusions, and fractures may also mimic the pain of avascular necrosis of the glenohumeral joint, as can occult metastatic disease.

TREATMENT

Initial treatment of the pain and functional disability associated with avascular necrosis of the glenohumeral joint should include a combination of the nonsteroidal antiinflammatory drugs (NSAIDs) or cyclooxygenase-2 (COX-2) inhibitors and decreased weight bearing of the affected glenohumeral joint. The local application of heat and cold may also be beneficial. For patients who do not respond to these treatment modalities, an injection of a local anesthetic into the glenohumeral joint may be a reasonable next step to provide palliation of acute pain. Vigorous exercises should be avoided because they will exacerbate the patient's symptoms. Ultimately, surgical repair in the form of total joint arthroplasty is the treatment of choice.

COMPLICATIONS AND PITFALLS

Failure to treat significant avascular necrosis of the glenohumeral joint surgically usually results in continued pain and disability and, in most patients, leads to ongoing damage to the glenohumeral joint (see Fig. 29-2). Injection of the joint with local anesthetic is a relatively safe technique if the clinician is attentive to detail, uses small amounts of local anesthetic, and avoids high injection pressures that may further damage the joint. Another complication of this injection technique is infection. This complication should be exceedingly rare if strict aseptic technique is followed. Approximately 25% of patients complain of a transient increase in pain after this injection technique, and patients should be warned of this possibility.

Clinical Pearls

Avascular necrosis of the glenohumeral joint is a diagnosis that is often missed, leading to much unnecessary pain and disability. The clinician should include avascular necrosis of the glenohumeral joint in his or her differential diagnosis for all patients complaining of shoulder joint pain, especially if any of the predisposing factors listed in Table 29-1 are present. Coexistent arthritis, tendinitis, and gout may also contribute to the pain and may require additional treatment. The use of physical modalities, including local heat and cold, as well as decreased weight bearing, may provide symptomatic relief. Vigorous exercises should be avoided because they will exacerbate the patient's symptoms and may cause further damage to the wrist. Simple analgesics and NSAIDs may be used concurrently with this injection technique.

SUGGESTED READINGS

Elser F, Braun S, Dewing CB, et al: Glenohumeral joint preservation: current options for managing articular cartilage lesions in young, active patients, *Arthroscopy* 26(5):685–696, 2010.

Hasan SS, Anthony A, Romeo AA: Nontraumatic osteonecrosis of the humeral head, *J Shoulder Elbow Surg* 11(3):281–298, 2002.

Hollis R, Yamaguchi K: Avascular necrosis of the shoulder, *Semin Arthroplasty* 19(1):19–22, 2008.

Savini CJ, James CW: HIV infection and avascular necrosis, *J Assoc Nurses AIDS Care* 12(5):83–85, 2001.

Chapter **30**

ADHESIVE CAPSULITIS

ICD-9 CODE **726.0**

ICD-10 CODE **M75.00**

THE CLINICAL SYNDROME

The shoulder joint is susceptible to the development of various conditions that cause damage or inflammation to the joint cartilage, ligaments, tendons, and soft tissues. Although most of these conditions can cause pain and functional disability, a favorable outcome is expected when they are properly managed. In some patients, however, increasing pain and inflammation lead to the development of edema and stiffness of the soft and connective tissues of the shoulder and result in the formation of fibrous adhesions that severely restrict the range of motion of the joint. If this condition is untreated, significant pain and functional disability can result.

Diseases that predispose the patient to the development of adhesive capsulitis can be divided into two general categories: (1) those within the shoulder and proximal upper extremity (e.g., rotator cuff tendinopathy, subdeltoid bursitis, and biceps tendon tendinopathy) and (2) diseases outside the shoulder region (e.g., stroke, diabetes, myocardial infarction, and reflex sympathetic dystrophy).

Regardless of the underlying cause of adhesive capsulitis, failure of prompt diagnosis and treatment of this condition uniformly results in a poor clinical outcome.

SIGNS AND SYMPTOMS

Most patients presenting with shoulder pain secondary to adhesive capsulitis complain of pain that is localized around the shoulder and upper arm. Activity makes the pain worse, whereas rest and heat provide some relief. The pain is constant and is characterized as aching; it may interfere with sleep. Some patients complain of a grating or popping sensation with use of the joint, and crepitus may be present on physical examination.

In addition to pain, patients suffering from adhesive capsulitis of the shoulder joint often experience a gradual reduction in functional ability because of decreasing shoulder range of motion that makes simple everyday tasks, such as combing one's hair, fastening a brassiere, or reaching overhead, quite difficult (Fig. 30-1). With

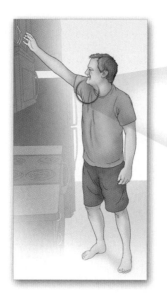

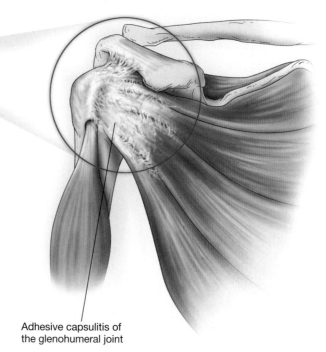

Adhesive capsulitis of
the glenohumeral joint

Figure 30-1 Patients suffering from adhesive capsulitis of the shoulder joint often experience a gradual reduction in functional ability because of decreasing shoulder range of motion that makes simple everyday tasks quite difficult.

continued disuse, muscle wasting may occur, and a frozen shoulder may develop. Sleep disturbance is quite common in patients suffering from adhesive capsulitis and may further exacerbate the patient's pain.

TESTING

Plain radiographs are indicated in all patients who are suspected of suffering from adhesive capsulitis, to rule out other causes of shoulder pain. Based on the patient's clinical presentation, additional testing may be indicated, including a complete blood count, erythrocyte sedimentation rate, and antinuclear antibody testing. Magnetic resonance imaging of the shoulder is indicated to identify treatable shoulder abnormalities (e.g., rotator cuff tears), as well as define the extent of adhesive capsulitis (Figs. 30-2 and 30-3). Radionuclide bone scanning is indicated if metastatic disease or primary tumor involving the shoulder is a possibility. Diseases outside the shoulder region may cause shoulder pain (e.g., pericarditis and reflex sympathetic dystrophy), and specific testing to rule these disorders out is mandatory if successful diagnosis and treatment are to be expected.

DIFFERENTIAL DIAGNOSIS

Osteoarthritis of the joint is the most common form of arthritis that results in shoulder pain; however, rheumatoid arthritis, post-traumatic arthritis, and rotator cuff arthropathy are also common causes of shoulder pain. Less common causes of arthritis-induced shoulder pain include collagen vascular diseases, infection, villonodular synovitis, and Lyme disease. Acute infectious arthritis is usually accompanied by significant systemic symptoms, including fever and malaise and should be easily recognized; it is diagnosed with culture and treated with antibiotics, rather than with injection therapy. Collagen vascular diseases generally manifest as polyarthropathy rather than as monarthropathy limited to the shoulder joint; however, shoulder pain secondary to collagen vascular disease responds exceedingly well to the intraarticular injection technique described here.

TREATMENT

Initial treatment of the pain and functional disability associated with adhesive capsulitis of the shoulder includes a combination of nonsteroidal antiinflammatory drugs (NSAIDs) or cyclooxygenase-2 (COX-2) inhibitors and physical therapy. Local application of heat and cold may also be beneficial. For patients who do not respond to these treatment modalities, intraarticular injection of local anesthetic and steroid is a reasonable next step (Fig. 30-4).

Intraarticular injection of the shoulder is performed by placing the patient in the supine position and preparing the skin overlying the shoulder, subacromial region, and joint space with antiseptic solution. A sterile syringe containing 2 mL of 0.30% preservative-free bupivacaine and 40 mg methylprednisolone is attached to a 1½-inch, 30-gauge needle using strict aseptic technique. The midpoint of the acromion is identified, and at a point approximately 1 inch below the midpoint, the shoulder joint space is identified. The needle is carefully advanced through the skin and subcutaneous tissues, through the joint capsule, and into the joint. If bone

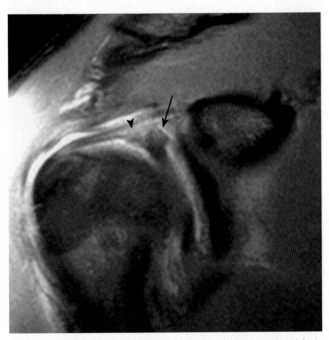

Figure 30-2 Superior labral tear from anterior to posterior (SLAP) lesion demonstrated on magnetic resonance imaging of the shoulder. Coronal oblique fat-suppressed T1-weighted fast spin-echo direct magnetic resonance arthrogram image demonstrating a detached tear of the superior glenoid labrum *(arrow)* extending into the long head of biceps tendon *(arrowhead)*. (From Lee JC, Guy S, Connell D, et al: MRI of the rotator interval of the shoulder, Clin Radiol *62[5]:416–423, 2007.)*

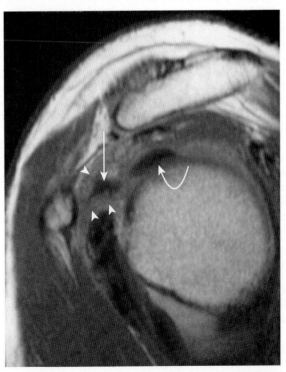

Figure 30-3 Adhesive capsulitis demonstrated on magnetic resonance imaging (MRI). Sagittal oblique T1-weighted fast spin-echo magnetic resonance imaging demonstrating enhancing soft tissue *(arrowheads)* surrounding the coracohumeral ligament *(straight arrow)* and extending toward the intraarticular portion of the long head of the biceps tendon *(curved arrow)*. (From Lee JC, Guy S, Connell D, et al: MRI of the rotator interval of the shoulder, Clin Radiol *62[5]:416–423, 2007.)*

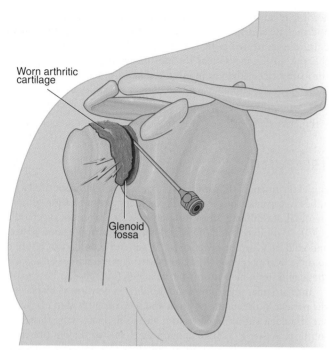

Figure 30-4 Injection technique for adhesive capsulitis of the shoulder. *(From Waldman SD: Atlas of pain management injection techniques, ed 2, Philadelphia, 2007, Saunders, p 58.)*

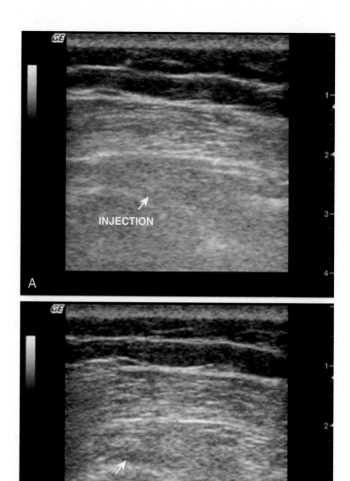

Figure 30-5 Ultrasound study showing **(A)** the needle tip in the articular capsule and **(B)** the capsular distention. *(From Lee H-J, Lim K-B, Kim D-Y, Lee K-T: Randomized controlled trial for efficacy of intraarticular injection for adhesive capsulitis: ultrasonography-guided versus blind technique, Arch Phys Med Rehabil 90[12]:1997–2002, 2009.)*

is encountered, the needle is withdrawn into the subcutaneous tissues and is redirected superiorly and slightly more medially. After the joint space is entered, the contents of the syringe are gently injected. Little resistance to injection should be felt; if resistance is encountered, the needle is probably in a ligament or tendon and should be advanced slightly into the joint space until the injection can proceed without significant resistance. The needle is then removed, and a sterile pressure dressing and ice pack are applied to the injection site. Studies suggest that the use of ultrasound guidance may improve the accuracy of needle placement for those less familiar with this technique (Fig. 30-5).

Physical modalities, including local heat and gentle range-of-motion exercises, should be introduced several days after the patient undergoes injection for shoulder pain. Vigorous exercises should be avoided, because they will exacerbate the patient's symptoms. Treatment of any underlying reflex sympathetic dystrophy of the affected extremity with stellate ganglion blocks should be introduced early in course of the disease.

COMPLICATIONS AND PITFALLS

This injection technique is safe if careful attention is paid to the clinically relevant anatomy. Sterile technique must be used to avoid infection, along with universal precautions to minimize any risk to the operator. The incidence of ecchymosis and hematoma formation can be decreased if pressure is applied to the injection site immediately after injection. The major complication of intraarticular injection of the shoulder is infection, although it should be exceedingly rare if strict aseptic technique is followed. Approximately 30% of patients complain of a transient increase in pain after intraarticular injection of the shoulder joint, and patients should be warned of this possibility.

Clinical Pearls

Adhesive capsulitis of the shoulder is a common complaint encountered in clinical practice. It must be distinguished from other causes of shoulder pain, including rotator cuff tears. Diseases outside the shoulder region may be responsible for the development of adhesive capsulitis and must be diagnosed and treated if a successful clinical outcome is to be expected. Intraarticular injection is extremely effective in the treatment of pain secondary to arthritis of the shoulder joint. Coexistent bursitis and tendinitis may contribute to shoulder pain and necessitate additional treatment with more localized injection of local anesthetic and methylprednisolone. Simple analgesics and NSAIDs or COX-2 inhibitors can be used concurrently with this injection technique.

SUGGESTED READINGS

Cain EL, Kocaj SM, Wilk KE: Adhesive capsulitis of the shoulder. In Andrews JR, Wilk KE, Reinold MM, editors: *The athlete's shoulder,* ed 2, Philadelphia, 2009, Churchill Livingstone, pp 293–301.

Dalton SE: Clinical examination of the painful shoulder, *Baillieres Clin Rheumatol* 3(3):453–474, 1989.

Davies AM: Imaging the painful shoulder, *Curr Orthop* 6(1):32–38, 1992.

Lee H-J, Lim K-B, Kim D-Y, et al: Randomized controlled trial for efficacy of intraarticular injection for adhesive capsulitis: ultrasonography-guided versus blind technique, *Arch Phys Med Rehabil* 90(12):1997–2002, 2009.

Monach PA: Shoulder pain. In Mushlin SB Greene HL, II, editors: *Decision making in medicine,* ed 3, Philadelphia, 2010, Mosby, pp 522–523.

Reutter TRC: Shoulder pain. In Ramamurthy S, Alanmanou E, Rogers JN, editors: *Decision making in pain management,* ed 2, St Louis, 2006, Mosby, pp 160–162.

Chapter 31

BICEPS TENDON TEAR

ICD-9 CODE 727.62

ICD-10 CODE M66.829

The Clinical Syndrome

The tendons of the long and short heads of the biceps are particularly prone to the development of tendinitis. Biceps tendon tear is usually caused at least partially by impingement on the tendons of the biceps at the coracoacromial arch. The onset of pain and functional disability associated biceps tendon tear is generally acute, occurring after overuse or misuse of the shoulder joint, such as trying to start a recalcitrant lawn mower, practicing an overhead tennis serve, or performing an overaggressive follow-through when driving golf balls (Fig. 31-1). More common in men, proximal rupture of the tendon of the long head of the biceps tendon accounts for more than 97% of biceps tendon ruptures; ruptures of the distal portion of the biceps tendon occur less than 3% of the time. Rupture of the long head of the biceps tendon generally occurs in the fourth to sixth decades, but it can occur in younger age groups involved in high-risk activities such as snowboarding.

The biceps muscle and tendons are intimately involved in shoulder and upper extremity function and are susceptible to trauma and to wear and tear. If the damage is severe enough, the tendon of the long head of the biceps can rupture, leaving the patient with a telltale "Popeye" biceps (named after the cartoon character). This deformity can be accentuated by having the patient perform Ludington's maneuver: placing his or her hands behind the head and flexing the biceps muscle (Fig. 31-2).

Signs and Symptoms

In most patients, the pain of biceps tendon tear occurs acutely and is accompanied by a pop or snapping sound. The pain is constant and severe and is localized in the anterior shoulder over the bicipital groove. Ecchymosis may be present if the trauma is acute and severe. Significant sleep disturbance is often reported. Patients with a partial tendon tear and significant tendinitis may attempt to splint the affected shoulder by internal rotation of the humerus,

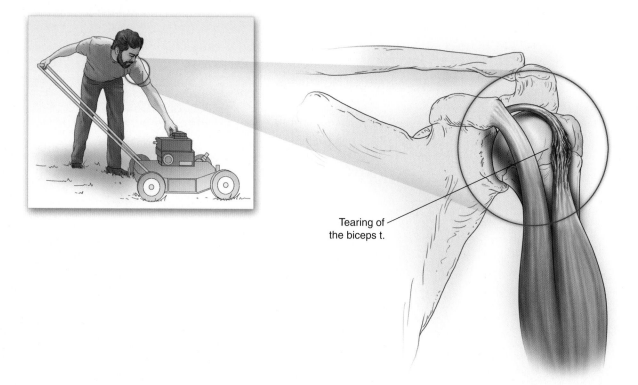

Tearing of
the biceps t.

Figure 31-1 The onset of pain and functional disability associated with biceps tendon tear is generally acute, occurring after overuse or misuse of the shoulder joint, such as trying to start a recalcitrant lawn mower.

which moves the biceps tendon from beneath the coracoacromial arch. Patients with biceps tendon tear have a positive Ludington's test result, as described earlier. Bursitis and tendinitis often accompany biceps tendon tear. Occasionally, patients with acute tear of the long tendon of the biceps may experience only vague discomfort and seek medical attention only because of the cosmetic abnormality of retracted biceps tendon and muscle. Occasionally, without treatment, frozen shoulder may develop.

TESTING

Plain radiographs are indicated for all patients who present with shoulder pain. Based on the patient's clinical presentation, additional testing may be indicated, including a complete blood count, erythrocyte sedimentation rate, and antinuclear antibody testing. Magnetic resonance imaging of the shoulder is indicated if tendinopathy or tear of the biceps tendon is suspected (Figs. 31-3 and 31-4). The injection technique described later serves as both a diagnostic and a therapeutic maneuver.

DIFFERENTIAL DIAGNOSIS

Biceps tendon tear is usually a straightforward clinical diagnosis. However, coexisting bursitis or tendinitis of the shoulder from overuse or misuse may confuse the diagnosis. Occasionally, partial rotator cuff tear can be mistaken for biceps tendon tear. In some clinical situations, consideration should be given to primary or secondary tumors involving the shoulder, superior sulcus of the lung, or proximal humerus. The pain of acute herpes zoster, which occurs before eruption of a vesicular rash, can also mimic biceps tendon tear.

TREATMENT

Initial treatment of the pain and functional disability associated with biceps tendon tear includes a combination of nonsteroidal antiinflammatory drugs (NSAIDs) or cyclooxygenase-2 (COX-2)

inhibitors and physical therapy. Local application of heat and cold may also be beneficial. For patients who do not respond to these treatment modalities and who appear to have significant local pain in the region of the bicipital groove, injection with local anesthetic and steroid is a reasonable next step.

Injection for biceps tendon tear is carried out by placing the patient in the supine position with the arm externally rotated approximately 45 degrees. The coracoid process is identified anteriorly. Just lateral to the coracoid process is the lesser tuberosity, which can be more easily palpated as the arm is passively rotated. The point overlying the tuberosity is marked with a sterile marker. The skin overlying the anterior shoulder is prepared with antiseptic solution. A sterile syringe containing 1 mL of 0.25% preservative-free bupivacaine and 40 mg methylprednisolone is attached to a 1½-inch, 25-gauge needle using strict aseptic technique. The previously marked point is palpated, and the insertion of the biceps tendon is reidentified with the gloved finger. The needle is carefully advanced at this point through the skin, subcutaneous tissues, and underlying tendon until it impinges on bone. The needle is then withdrawn 1 to 2 mm out of the periosteum of the humerus, and the contents of the syringe are gently injected. Slight resistance to injection should be felt. If no resistance is encountered, either the needle tip is in the joint space itself or the tendon is ruptured. If resistance is significant, the needle tip is probably in the substance of a ligament or tendon and should be advanced or withdrawn slightly until the injection can proceed without significant resistance. The needle is then removed, and a sterile pressure dressing and ice pack are applied to the injection site.

Physical modalities, including local heat and gentle range-of-motion exercises, should be introduced several days after the patient undergoes injection. Vigorous exercises should be avoided, because they will exacerbate the patient's symptoms. Occasionally, surgical repair of the tendon is undertaken if the patient is experiencing significant functional disability or is unhappy with the cosmetic defect resulting from the retracted tendon and muscle.

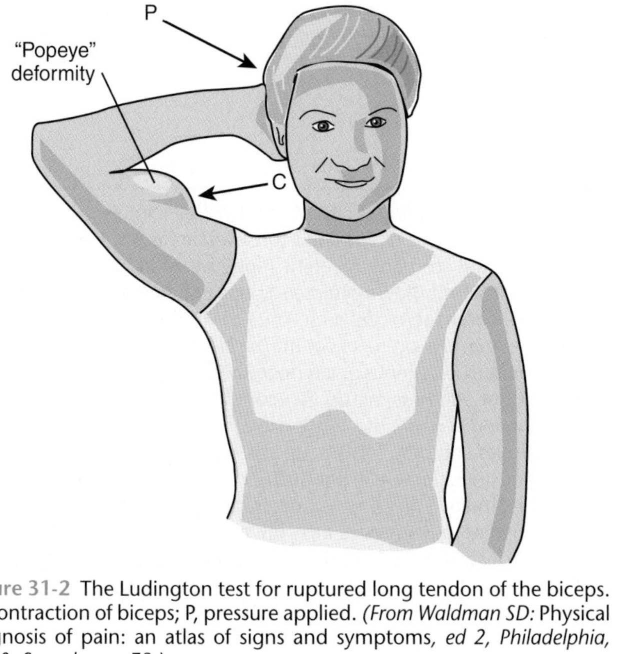

Figure 31-2 The Ludington test for ruptured long tendon of the biceps. C, contraction of biceps; P, pressure applied. *(From Waldman SD: Physical diagnosis of pain: an atlas of signs and symptoms, ed 2, Philadelphia, 2010, Saunders, p 78.)*

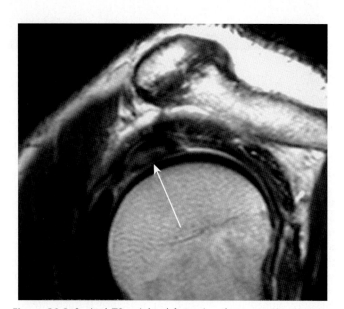

Figure 31-3 Sagittal T2-weighted fast spin-echo magnetic resonance image demonstrates a swollen, hyperintense, but intact long head of biceps tendon within the rotator interval, indicative of biceps tendinopathy *(arrow)*.

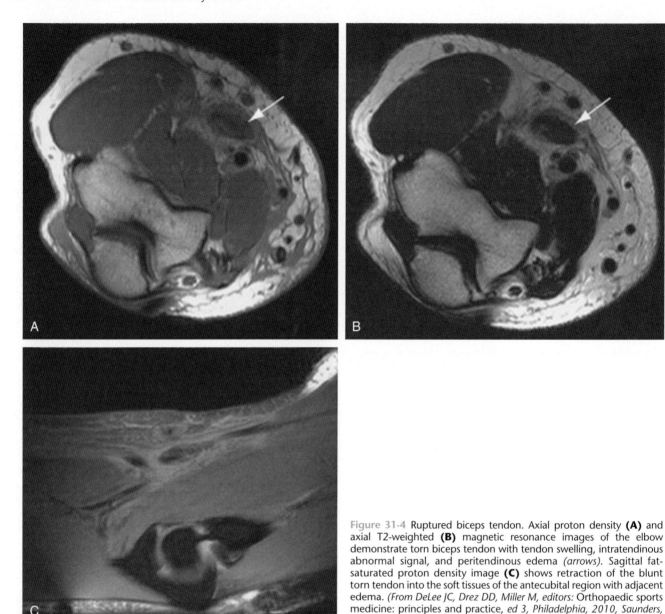

Figure 31-4 Ruptured biceps tendon. Axial proton density **(A)** and axial T2-weighted **(B)** magnetic resonance images of the elbow demonstrate torn biceps tendon with tendon swelling, intratendinous abnormal signal, and peritendinous edema *(arrows)*. Sagittal fat-saturated proton density image **(C)** shows retraction of the blunt torn tendon into the soft tissues of the antecubital region with adjacent edema. *(From DeLee JC, Drez DD, Miller M, editors: Orthopaedic sports medicine: principles and practice, ed 3, Philadelphia, 2010, Saunders, p 570.)*

COMPLICATIONS AND PITFALLS

This injection technique is safe if careful attention is paid to the clinically relevant anatomy. Sterile technique must be used to avoid infection, along with universal precautions to minimize any risk to the operator. The incidence of ecchymosis and hematoma formation can be decreased if pressure is applied to the injection site immediately after injection. The major complication of this injection technique is infection, although it should be exceedingly rare if strict aseptic technique is followed. Trauma to the biceps tendon from the injection itself is also a possibility. Tendons that are highly inflamed or previously damaged are subject to rupture if they are injected directly. This complication can often be avoided if the clinician uses a gentle technique and stops injecting immediately if significant resistance is encountered. Approximately 25% of patients complain of a transient increase in pain after injection, and patients should be warned of this possibility.

Clinical Pearls

The musculotendinous unit of the shoulder joint is susceptible to the development of tendinitis for several reasons. First, the joint is subjected to many different repetitive motions. Second, the space in which the musculotendinous unit functions is restricted by the coracoacromial arch, thus making impingement likely with extreme movements of the joint. Third, the blood supply to the musculotendinous unit is poor, so the healing of microtrauma is difficult. All these factors can contribute to tendinitis. Calcium deposition around the tendon may occur if the inflammation continues and may complicate subsequent treatment.

The injection technique described is extremely effective in the treatment of pain secondary to biceps tendon tear. Coexistent bursitis and arthritis may contribute to shoulder pain, necessitating additional treatment with more localized injection of local anesthetic and methylprednisolone. Simple analgesics and NSAIDs or COX-2 inhibitors can be used concurrently with this injection technique.

SUGGESTED READINGS

Karistinos A, Paulos LE: Anatomy and function of the tendon of the long head of the biceps muscle, *Oper Tech Sports Med* 15(1):2–6, 2007.

Lee JC, Guy S, Connell D, et al: MRI of the rotator interval of the shoulder, *Clin Radiol* 62(5):416–423, 2007.

Schultz JS: Clinical evaluation of the shoulder, *Phys Med Rehabil Clin N Am* 15(2):351–371, 2004.

Waldman SD: Bicipital tendinitis. In *Atlas of pain management injection techniques,* ed 2, Philadelphia, 2007, Saunders, pp 91–96.

Waldman SD: The biceps tendon. In *Pain review,* Philadelphia, 2009, Saunders, pp 84–85.

Weiland DE, Rodosky MW: Biceps tendon disorders. In *Clinical sports medicine,* New York, 2006, McGraw-Hill, pp 235–241.

Chapter 32

SUPRASPINATUS SYNDROME

ICD-9 CODE 729.1

ICD-10 CODE M79.7

THE CLINICAL SYNDROME

The supraspinatus muscle is susceptible to the development of myofascial pain syndrome. Flexion-extension and lateral motion stretch injuries to the neck, shoulder, and upper back or repeated microtrauma secondary to activities that require working overhead or repeatedly reaching across one's body, such as painting ceilings, assembly-line work, or even watching television while reclining on a couch, may result in the development of myofascial pain in the supraspinatus muscle.

Myofascial pain syndrome is a chronic pain syndrome that affects a focal or regional portion of the body. The sine qua non of myofascial pain syndrome is the finding of myofascial trigger points on physical examination. Although these trigger points are generally localized to the part of the body affected, the pain is often referred to other areas. This referred pain may be misdiagnosed or attributed to other organ systems, thus leading to extensive evaluation and ineffective treatment. Patients with myofascial pain syndrome involving the supraspinatus muscle often have referred pain in the shoulder that radiates down into the upper extremity.

The trigger point is pathognomonic of myofascial pain syndrome and is characterized by a local point of exquisite tenderness in the affected muscle. Mechanical stimulation of the trigger point by palpation or stretching produces not only intense local pain but referred pain as well. In addition, one often sees an involuntary withdrawal of the stimulated muscle, called a jump sign, which is characteristic of myofascial pain syndrome. In patients with supraspinatus syndrome, the trigger point overlies the superior border of the scapula (Fig. 32-1).

Taut bands of muscle fibers are often identified when myofascial trigger points are palpated. In spite of this consistent physical finding, the pathophysiology of the myofascial trigger point remains elusive, but trigger points are thought to result from microtrauma to the affected muscle. This trauma may occur from a single injury, repetitive microtrauma, or chronic deconditioning of the agonist and antagonist muscle unit.

In addition to muscle trauma, various other factors seem to predispose patients to the development of myofascial pain syndrome. For instance, a weekend athlete who subjects his or her body to unaccustomed physical activity may develop myofascial pain syndrome. Poor posture while sitting at a computer or while watching television has also been implicated as a predisposing factor. Previous injuries may result in abnormal muscle function and lead to the development of myofascial pain syndrome. All

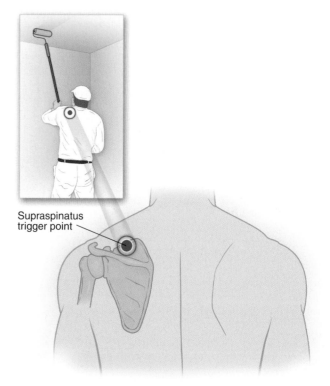

Supraspinatus trigger point

Figure 32-1 In patients with supraspinatus syndrome, the trigger point overlies the superior border of the scapula.

these factors may be intensified if the patient also suffers from poor nutritional status or coexisting psychological or behavioral abnormalities, including chronic stress and depression. The supraspinatus muscle seems to be particularly susceptible to stress-induced myofascial pain syndrome.

Stiffness and fatigue often coexist with pain, and they increase the functional disability associated with this disease and complicate its treatment. Myofascial pain syndrome may occur as a primary disease state or in conjunction with other painful conditions, including radiculopathy and chronic regional pain syndromes. Psychological or behavioral abnormalities, including depression, frequently coexist with the muscle abnormalities, and management of these psychological disorders is an integral part of any successful treatment plan.

SIGNS AND SYMPTOMS

The sine qua non of supraspinatus syndrome is the identification of a myofascial trigger point—a local point of exquisite tenderness—overlying the superior border of the scapula. Mechanical stimulation of the trigger point by palpation or stretching produces intense

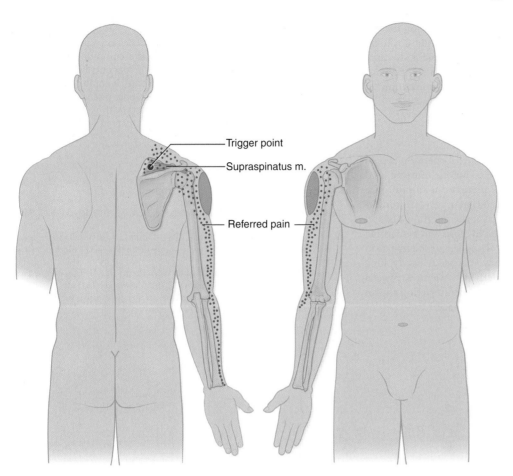

Figure 32-2 Pain on range of motion and pain referred to the shoulder and upper extremities in a nondermatomal pattern are characteristic of supraspinatus syndrome. *(From Waldman SD: Atlas of pain management injection techniques, ed 2, Philadelphia, 2007, Saunders.)*

local pain as well as referred pain, and the jump sign may be present. Other findings characteristic of supraspinatus syndrome are pain on range of motion of the affected scapula and shoulder and pain referred to the shoulder and upper extremities in a nondermatomal pattern (Fig. 32-2).

TESTING

Biopsies of clinically identified trigger points have not revealed consistently abnormal histologic features. The muscle hosting the trigger points has been described either as "moth-eaten" or as containing "waxy degeneration." Increased plasma myoglobin has been reported in some patients with supraspinatus syndrome, but this finding has not been corroborated by other investigators. Electrodiagnostic testing of patients suffering from supraspinatus syndrome has revealed an increase in muscle tension in some patients, but again, this finding has not been reproducible. Because of the lack of objective testing, the clinician must use electrodiagnostic and radiographic means to rule out other disease processes that may mimic supraspinatus syndrome (see "Differential Diagnosis").

DIFFERENTIAL DIAGNOSIS

The diagnosis of supraspinatus syndrome is made on the basis of clinical findings rather than specific laboratory, electrodiagnostic, or radiographic testing. For this reason, a targeted history and physical examination, with a systematic search for trigger points and identification of a positive jump sign, must be carried out in every patient suspected of having supraspinatus syndrome. The

clinician must rule out other coexisting disease processes that may mimic supraspinatus syndrome, including primary inflammatory muscle disease, multiple sclerosis, and collagen vascular disease. Electrodiagnostic and radiographic testing can help identify coexisting disorders such as shoulder bursitis, tendinitis, and rotator cuff tears. The clinician must also identify coexisting psychological and behavioral abnormalities that may mask or exacerbate the symptoms associated with supraspinatus syndrome.

TREATMENT

Treatment is focused on blocking the myofascial trigger and achieving prolonged relaxation of the affected muscle. It is hoped that interrupting the pain cycle in this way will allow the patient to obtain long-term pain relief. Because the mechanism of action of the treatment modalities used is poorly understood, an element of trial and error is involved in developing a treatment plan.

Conservative therapy consisting of trigger point injection with local anesthetic or saline solution is the initial treatment of supraspinatus syndrome. The use of pregabalin is a reasonable next step in patients who do not respond to trigger point injections. Starting at a bedtime dose of 50 to 100 mg, this drug can be titrated upward to a dose of 100 mg three times a day as side effects allow. The dosage should be decreased in patients with impaired renal function. Adjunct therapies, including physical therapy, therapeutic heat and cold, transcutaneous nerve stimulation, and electrical stimulation, can be used on a case-by-case basis. For patients who do not respond to these traditional measures, consideration should be given to the use of botulinum toxin type A; although not currently approved by the Food and Drug Administration for this indication, the injection of minute quantities of botulinum toxin type A directly into trigger points has been successful. Because underlying depression and anxiety are present in many patients suffering from supraspinatus syndrome, the administration of antidepressants is an integral part of most treatment plans.

COMPLICATIONS AND PITFALLS

Trigger point injection is extremely safe if careful attention is paid to the clinically relevant anatomy. Sterile technique must be used to avoid infection, along with universal precautions to minimize any risk to the operator. Most complications of trigger point injection are related to needle-induced trauma at the injection site and in underlying tissues. The incidence of ecchymosis and hematoma formation can be decreased if pressure is applied to the injection site immediately after injection. The avoidance of overly long needles can decrease the trauma to underlying structures. Special care must be taken to avoid pneumothorax when injecting trigger points in proximity to the underlying pleural space.

Clinical Pearls

Although supraspinatus syndrome is a common disorder, it is often misdiagnosed. Therefore, in patients suspected of suffering from supraspinatus syndrome, a careful evaluation is mandatory to identify any underlying disease processes. Supraspinatus syndrome often coexists with various somatic and psychological disorders.

SUGGESTED READINGS

Bradley LA: Pathophysiology of fibromyalgia, *Am J Med* 122(12 Suppl 1):S22–S30, 2009.

Ge H-Y, Nie H, Madeleine P, et al: Contribution of the local and referred pain from active myofascial trigger points in fibromyalgia syndrome, *Pain* 147(1–3):233–240, 2009.

Monach PA: Shoulder pain. In Mushlin SB, Greene HL, II, editors: *Decision making in medicine,* ed 3, Philadelphia, 2010, Mosby, pp 522–523.

Waldman SD: Supraspinatus syndrome. In *Atlas of pain management injection techniques,* ed 2, Philadelphia, 2007, Saunders, pp 68–70.

Chapter **33**

ROTATOR CUFF TEAR

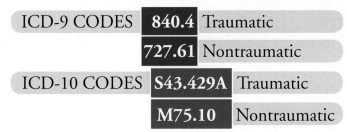

ICD-9 CODES	**840.4**	Traumatic
	727.61	Nontraumatic
ICD-10 CODES	**S43.429A**	Traumatic
	M75.10	Nontraumatic

THE CLINICAL SYNDROME

Rotator cuff tears are a common cause of shoulder pain and dysfunction. A rotator cuff tear frequently occurs after seemingly minor trauma to the musculotendinous unit of the shoulder. However, in most cases, the pathologic process responsible for the tear has been a long time in the making and is the result of ongoing tendinitis. The rotator cuff is made up of the subscapularis, supraspinatus, infraspinatus, and teres minor muscles and the associated tendons (Fig. 33-1). The function of the rotator cuff is to rotate the arm and help provide shoulder joint stability along with the other muscles, tendons, and ligaments of the shoulder.

The supraspinatus and infraspinatus muscle tendons are particularly susceptible to the development of tendinitis, for several reasons. First, the joint is subjected to many different repetitive motions. Second, the space in which the musculotendinous unit functions is restricted by the coracoacromial arch, thus making impingement likely with extreme movements of the joint. Third, the blood supply to the musculotendinous unit is poor, and this makes healing of microtrauma difficult. All these factors can contribute to tendinitis of one or more tendons of the shoulder joint. Calcium deposition around the tendon may occur if the inflammation continues and complicates subsequent treatment. Bursitis often accompanies rotator cuff tears and may require specific treatment.

In addition to pain, patients suffering from rotator cuff tear often experience a gradual reduction in functional ability because of decreasing shoulder range of motion that makes simple everyday tasks such as combing one's hair, fastening a brassiere, or reaching overhead quite difficult. With continued disuse, muscle wasting may occur, and a frozen shoulder may develop.

SIGNS AND SYMPTOMS

Patients presenting with rotator cuff tear frequently complain that they cannot raise the affected arm above the level of the shoulder without using the other arm to lift it (Fig. 33-2). On physical examination, weakness on external rotation is noted if the infraspinatus is involved, and weakness on abduction above the level of the shoulder is evident if the supraspinatus is involved. Tenderness to palpation in the subacromial region is often present. Patients with partial rotator cuff tears lose the ability to reach overhead smoothly. Patients with complete tears exhibit anterior migration of the humeral head, as well as a complete inability to reach above the level of the shoulder. A positive drop arm test—the inability to hold the arm abducted at the level of the shoulder after the supported arm is released—is often seen with complete tears of the rotator cuff (Fig. 33-3). The result of Moseley's test for rotator cuff tear is also positive; this test is performed by having the patient actively abduct the arm to 80 degrees and then adding gentle resistance, which forces the arm to drop if complete rotator cuff tear is present. Passive range of motion of the shoulder is normal, but active range of motion is limited.

The pain of rotator cuff tear is constant and severe and is made worse with abduction and external rotation of the shoulder. Significant sleep disturbance is often reported. Patients may attempt to splint the inflamed subscapularis tendon by limiting medial rotation of the humerus.

TESTING

Plain radiographs are indicated in all patients who present with shoulder pain. Based on the patient's clinical presentation, additional testing may be indicated, including a complete blood count, erythrocyte sedimentation rate, and antinuclear antibody testing. Magnetic resonance imaging (MRI) of the shoulder is indicated if rotator cuff tear is suspected (Fig. 33-4).

DIFFERENTIAL DIAGNOSIS

Because rotator cuff tears may occur after seemingly minor trauma, the diagnosis is often delayed. The tear may be either partial or complete, further confusing the diagnosis, although a careful physical examination can distinguish between the two. Tendinitis of the musculotendinous unit of the shoulder frequently coexists with bursitis of the associated bursae of the shoulder joint and creates additional pain and functional disability. This pain can cause the patient to splint the shoulder group, with resulting abnormal movement of the shoulder that puts additional stress on the rotator cuff and can lead to further trauma. With rotator cuff tears, passive range of motion is normal, but active range of motion is limited; with frozen shoulder, both passive range of motion and active range of motion are limited. Rotator cuff tear rarely occurs before age 40 years, except in cases of severe acute trauma to the shoulder.

TREATMENT

Initial treatment of the pain and functional disability associated with rotator cuff tear includes a combination of nonsteroidal anti-inflammatory drugs (NSAIDs) or cyclooxygenase-2 inhibitors

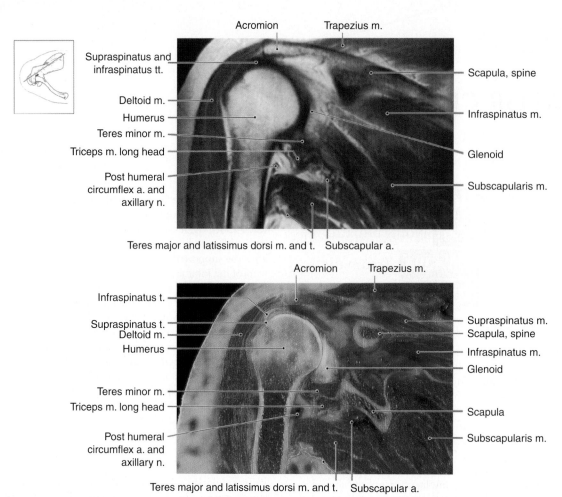

Figure 33-1 Muscles and tendons of the rotator cuff. *(From Kang HS, Ahn JM, Resnick D: MRI of the extremities: an anatomic atlas, ed 2, Philadelphia, 2002, Saunders, p 5.)*

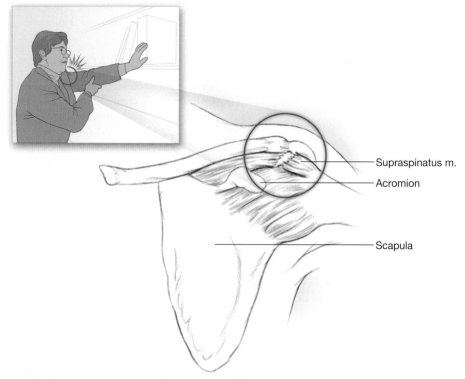

Figure 33-2 Inability to elevate the arm above the level of the shoulder is the hallmark of rotator cuff dysfunction.

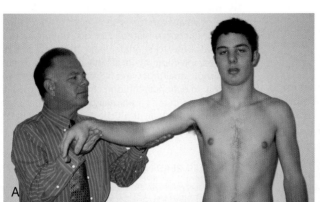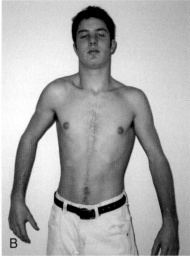

Figure 33-3 **A,** The drop arm test for complete rotator cuff tear. **B,** A patient with a complete rotator cuff tear is unable to hold the arm in the abducted position, and it falls to the patient's side. The patient often shrugs or hitches the shoulder forward to use the intact muscles of the rotator cuff and the deltoid to keep the arm in the abducted position. *(From Waldman SD:* Physical diagnosis of pain: an atlas of signs and symptoms, *Philadelphia, 2006, Saunders, pp 91–92.)*

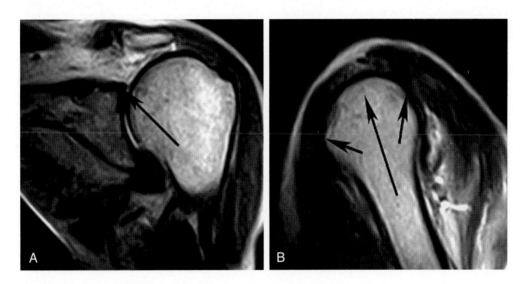

Figure 33-4 Massive tear of the rotator cuff. **A,** Coronal oblique T2-weighted magnetic resonance imaging (MRI). The supraspinatus tendon is retracted to the medial glenoid margin *(arrow).* Severe atrophy is evident. **B,** Sagittal oblique T2-weighted MRI. Note the "bald" humeral head. The tear extends from the subscapularis to the infraspinatus tendon *(arrows). (From Edelman RR, Hesselink JR, Zlatkin MB, Crues JV, editors:* Clinical magnetic resonance imaging, *ed 3, Philadelphia, 2006, Saunders, p 3225.)*

and physical therapy. Local application of heat and cold may also be beneficial. For patients who do not respond to these treatment modalities, the injection technique described here is a reasonable next step before surgical intervention.

Injection for rotator cuff tear is carried out by placing the patient in the supine position and preparing the skin overlying the superior shoulder, acromion, and distal clavicle with antiseptic solution. A sterile syringe containing 4 mL of 0.25% preservative-free bupivacaine and 40 mg methylprednisolone is attached to a 1½-inch, 25-gauge needle using strict aseptic technique. The lateral edge of the acromion is identified, and at the midpoint of the lateral edge, the injection site is identified. With a slightly cephalad trajectory, the needle is carefully advanced through the skin, subcutaneous tissues, and deltoid muscle

beneath the acromion process. If bone is encountered, the needle is withdrawn into the subcutaneous tissues and is redirected slightly more inferiorly. After the needle is in place, the contents of the syringe are gently injected. Resistance to injection should be minimal unless calcification of the subacromial bursal sac is present. This calcification can be recognized as resistance to needle advancement, with an associated gritty feel. Significant calcific bursitis may ultimately require surgical excision to obtain complete relief of symptoms. After injection the needle is removed, and a sterile pressure dressing and ice pack are applied to the injection site.

Physical modalities, including local heat and gentle range-of-motion exercises, should be introduced several days after the patient undergoes injection. Vigorous exercises should be avoided, because they will exacerbate the patient's symptoms and may lead to complete tendon rupture.

COMPLICATIONS AND PITFALLS

One major complication is failure to identify a partial rotator cuff tear correctly and to treat it before it becomes complete. This usually occurs because MRI of the shoulder is not performed and the diagnosis is made on clinical grounds alone.

The injection technique described is safe if careful attention is paid to the clinically relevant anatomy. Sterile technique must be used to avoid infection, along with universal precautions to minimize any risk to the operator. The incidence of ecchymosis and hematoma formation can be decreased if pressure is applied to the injection site immediately after injection. The major complication of the injection technique is infection, although it should be exceedingly rare if strict aseptic technique is followed. Trauma to the rotator cuff from the injection itself is also a possibility. Tendons that are highly inflamed or previously damaged are subject to rupture if they are injected directly, which could convert a partial tear into a complete one. This complication can be avoided if the clinician uses gentle technique and stops injecting immediately if significant resistance is encountered. Approximately 25% of patients complain of a transient increase in pain after injection, and patients should be warned of this possibility.

Clinical Pearls

Injection is extremely effective in the treatment of pain secondary to rotator cuff tear. This technique is not a substitute for surgery, but it can be used to palliate the pain of partial tears or when surgery for complete tears is not being contemplated. Coexistent bursitis and arthritis may contribute to shoulder pain, thus necessitating more localized injection of local anesthetic and methylprednisolone. Simple analgesics and NSAIDs can be used concurrently with this injection technique. Partial tears may be amenable to arthroscopic or minimal-incision surgery, and the clinician should not wait until the tear is complete before obtaining orthopedic consultation.

SUGGESTED READINGS

Baring T, Emery R, Reilly P: Management of rotator cuff disease: specific treatment for specific disorders, *Best Pract Res Clin Rheumatol* 21(2):279–294, 2007.

Beaudreuil J, Dhénain M, Coudane H, et al: Clinical practice guidelines for the surgical management of rotator cuff tears in adults, *Orthop Traumatol Surg Res* 96(2):175–179, 2010.

Henshaw DR, Craig EV: Disorders of the rotator cuff. In Waldman SD, editor: *Pain management,* Philadelphia, 2006, Saunders.

Lin JC, Weintraub N, Aragaki DR: Nonsurgical treatment for rotator cuff injury in the elderly, *J Am Med Dir Assoc* 9(9):626–632, 2008.

Waldman SD: Function anatomy of the rotator cuff. In *Pain review,* Philadelphia, 2009, Saunders, pp 85–86.

Chapter **34**

DELTOID SYNDROME

ICD-9 CODE **729.1**

ICD-10 CODE **M79.7**

THE CLINICAL SYNDROME

The deltoid muscle is susceptible to the development of myofascial pain syndrome. Flexion-extension and lateral motion stretch injuries or impact injuries to the deltoid muscle during football or repeated microtrauma secondary to jobs that require prolonged lifting may result in the development of myofascial pain in the deltoid muscle (Fig. 34-1).

Myofascial pain syndrome is a chronic pain syndrome that affects a focal or regional portion of the body. The sine qua non of myofascial pain syndrome is the finding of myofascial trigger points on physical examination. Although these trigger points are generally localized to the part of the body affected, the pain is often referred to other areas. This referred pain may be misdiagnosed or attributed to other organ systems, thus leading to extensive evaluation and ineffective treatment. Patients with myofascial pain syndrome involving the deltoid muscle often have referred pain in the shoulder that radiates down into the upper extremity.

The trigger point is pathognomonic of myofascial pain syndrome and is characterized by a local point of exquisite tenderness in the affected muscle. Mechanical stimulation of the trigger point by palpation or stretching produces not only intense local pain but also referred pain. In addition, one often sees an involuntary withdrawal of the stimulated muscle, called a jump sign, characteristic of myofascial pain syndrome. Patients with deltoid syndrome exhibit trigger points in both the anterior and posterior fibers of the muscle (Fig. 34-2).

Taunt bands of muscle fibers are often identified when myofascial trigger points are palpated. In spite of this consistent physical finding, the pathophysiology of the myofascial trigger point remains elusive, although trigger points are believed to result from microtrauma to the affected muscle. This trauma may occur from

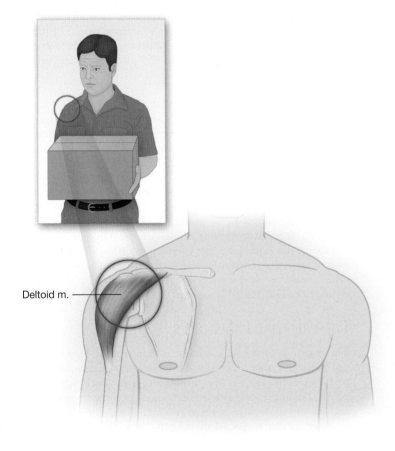

Deltoid m.

Figure 34-1 Jobs that require prolonged lifting may lead to the development of myofascial pain in the deltoid muscle.

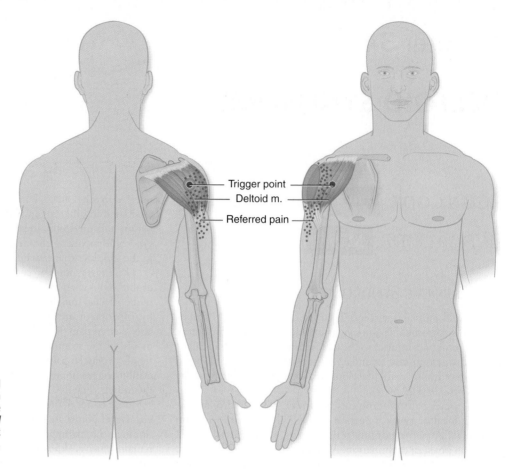

Figure 34-2 Patients with deltoid syndrome have trigger points in both the anterior and posterior fibers of the muscle. *(From Waldman SD: Deltoid syndrome. In* Atlas of pain management injection techniques, *ed 2, Philadelphia, 2007, Saunders, p 83.)*

a single injury, repetitive microtrauma, or chronic deconditioning of the agonist and antagonist muscle unit.

In addition to muscle trauma, various other factors seem to predispose patients to develop myofascial pain syndrome. For instance, a weekend athlete who subjects his or her body to unaccustomed physical activity may develop myofascial pain syndrome. Poor posture while sitting at a computer or while watching television has also been implicated as a predisposing factor. Previous injuries may result in abnormal muscle function and lead to the development of myofascial pain syndrome. All these factors may be intensified if the patient also suffers from poor nutritional status or coexisting psychological or behavioral abnormalities, including chronic stress and depression. The deltoid muscle seems to be particularly susceptible to stress-induced myofascial pain syndrome.

Stiffness and fatigue often coexist with pain, and they increase the functional disability associated with this disease and complicate its treatment. Myofascial pain syndrome may occur as a primary disease state or in conjunction with other painful conditions, including radiculopathy and chronic regional pain syndromes. Psychological or behavioral abnormalities, including depression, frequently coexist with the muscle abnormalities, and management of these psychological disorders is an integral part of any successful treatment plan.

SIGNS AND SYMPTOMS

The sine qua non of deltoid syndrome is the identification of a myofascial trigger point—a local point of exquisite tenderness—overlying the superior border of the scapula. Mechanical stimulation of the trigger point by palpation or stretching produces not only intense local pain but also referred pain. The jump sign is also characteristic of deltoid syndrome, as is pain over the deltoid muscle that is referred into the proximal lateral upper extremity (see Fig. 34-2).

TESTING

Biopsies of clinically identified trigger points have not revealed consistently abnormal histologic features. The muscle hosting the trigger points has been described either as "moth-eaten" or as containing "waxy degeneration." Increased plasma myoglobin has been reported in some patients with deltoid syndrome, but this finding has not been corroborated by other investigators. Electrodiagnostic testing of patients suffering from deltoid syndrome has revealed an increase in muscle tension in some patients, but again, this finding has not been reproducible. Because of the lack of objective diagnostic testing, the clinician must rule out other coexisting disease processes that may mimic deltoid syndrome (see "Differential Diagnosis").

DIFFERENTIAL DIAGNOSIS

The diagnosis of deltoid syndrome is made on the basis of clinical findings rather than specific laboratory, electrodiagnostic, or radiographic testing. For this reason, a targeted history and physical examination, with a systematic search for trigger points and identification of a positive jump sign, must be carried out in every patient suspected of suffering from deltoid syndrome. The clinician must rule out other coexisting disease processes that

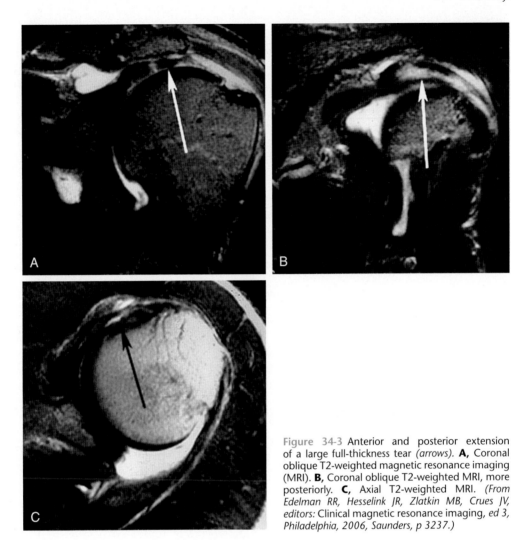

Figure 34-3 Anterior and posterior extension of a large full-thickness tear *(arrows)*. **A,** Coronal oblique T2-weighted magnetic resonance imaging (MRI). **B,** Coronal oblique T2-weighted MRI, more posteriorly. **C,** Axial T2-weighted MRI. *(From Edelman RR, Hesselink JR, Zlatkin MB, Crues JV, editors: Clinical magnetic resonance imaging, ed 3, Philadelphia, 2006, Saunders, p 3237.)*

may mimic deltoid syndrome, including primary inflammatory muscle disease, multiple sclerosis, and collagen vascular disease. Electrodiagnostic and radiographic testing can help identify coexisting disorders such as bursitis, tendinitis, and rotator cuff tears (Fig. 34-3). The clinician must also identify coexisting psychological and behavioral abnormalities that may mask or exacerbate the symptoms associated with deltoid syndrome.

TREATMENT

Treatment is focused on blocking the myofascial trigger and achieving prolonged relaxation of the affected muscle. It is hoped that interrupting the pain cycle in this way will allow the patient to obtain long-term pain relief. Because the mechanism of action of the treatment modalities used is poorly understood, an element of trial and error is involved in developing a treatment plan.

Conservative therapy consisting of trigger point injections with local anesthetic or saline solution is the initial treatment of deltoid syndrome. The use of pregabalin is a reasonable next step in patients who do not respond to trigger point injections. Starting at a bedtime dose of 50 to 100 mg, this drug can be titrated upward to a dose of 100 mg three times a day as side effects allow. The dosage should be decreased in patients with impaired renal function. Adjunct therapies, including physical therapy, therapeutic heat and cold, transcutaneous nerve stimulation, and electrical stimulation, can be used on a case-by-case basis. For patients who do not respond to these traditional measures, consideration should be given to the use of botulinum toxin type A; although not currently approved by the Food and Drug Administration for this indication, the injection of minute quantities of botulinum toxin type A directly into trigger points has been successful. Because underlying depression and anxiety are present in many patients suffering from deltoid syndrome, the administration of antidepressants is an integral part of most treatment plans.

COMPLICATIONS AND PITFALLS

Trigger point injections are extremely safe if careful attention is paid to the clinically relevant anatomy. Sterile technique must be used to avoid infection, along with universal precautions to minimize any risk to the operator. Most complications of trigger point injection are related to needle-induced trauma at the injection site and in underlying tissues. The incidence of ecchymosis and hematoma formation can be decreased if pressure is applied to the injection site immediately after injection. The avoidance of overly long needles can decrease the incidence of trauma to underlying structures. Special care must be taken to avoid pneumothorax when injecting trigger points in proximity to the underlying pleural space.

Clinical Pearls

Although deltoid syndrome is a common disorder, it is often misdiagnosed. Therefore, in patients suspected of suffering from deltoid syndrome, a careful evaluation to identify underlying disease processes is mandatory. Deltoid syndrome often coexists with various somatic and psychological disorders.

SUGGESTED READINGS

Bradley LA: Pathophysiology of fibromyalgia, *Am J Med* 122(12 Suppl 1):S22–S30, 2009.

Ge H-Y, Nie H, Madeleine P, et al: Contribution of the local and referred pain from active myofascial trigger points in fibromyalgia syndrome, *Pain* 147(1–3): 233–240, 2009.

Monach PA: Shoulder pain. In Mushlin SB, Greene HL II, editors: *Decision making in medicine,* ed 3, Philadelphia, 2010, Mosby, pp 522–523.

Schultz JS: Clinical evaluation of the shoulder, *Phys Med Rehabil Clin N Am* 15(2):351–371, 2004.

Waldman SD: Deltoid syndrome. In *Atlas of pain management injection techniques,* ed 2, Philadelphia, 2007, Saunders, pp 82–84.

Chapter **35**

TERES MAJOR SYNDROME

ICD-9 CODE **729.1**

ICD-10 CODE **M79.7**

THE CLINICAL SYNDROME

The teres major muscle is susceptible to the development of myofascial pain syndrome. Stretch or impact injuries to the teres major muscle sustained while playing sports or in motor vehicle accidents, as well as falls onto the lateral scapula, have been implicated in the evolution of teres major syndrome. In addition, repeated microtrauma secondary to reaching up and behind, such as when retrieving a briefcase from the backseat of a car, overhead throwing, and other sports injuries may result in the development of myofascial pain in the teres major muscle (Figs. 35-1 and 35-2).

Myofascial pain syndrome is a chronic pain syndrome that affects a focal or regional portion of the body. The sine qua non of myofascial pain syndrome is the finding of myofascial trigger points on physical examination. Although these trigger points are generally localized to the part of the body affected, the pain is often referred to other areas. This referred pain may be misdiagnosed or attributed to other organ systems, thus leading to extensive evaluation and ineffective treatment. Patients with myofascial pain syndrome involving the teres major muscle often have referred pain in the shoulder that radiates down into the upper extremity.

The trigger point is pathognomonic of myofascial pain syndrome and is characterized by a local point of exquisite tenderness. Mechanical stimulation of the trigger point by palpation or stretching produces not only intense local pain but also referred pain. In addition, involuntary withdrawal of the stimulated muscle, called a jump sign, is often seen and is characteristic of

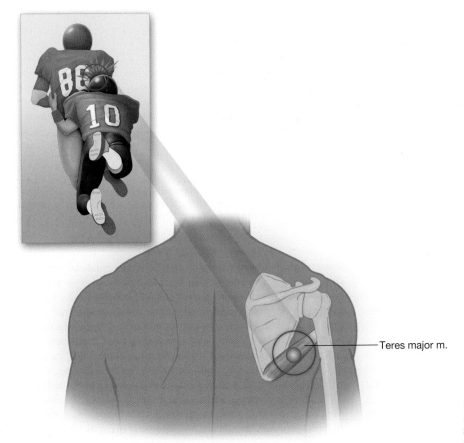

Teres major m.

Figure 35-1 Repeated microtrauma secondary to reaching up and behind, as well as playing sports such as football, may result in the development of myofascial pain in the teres major muscle.

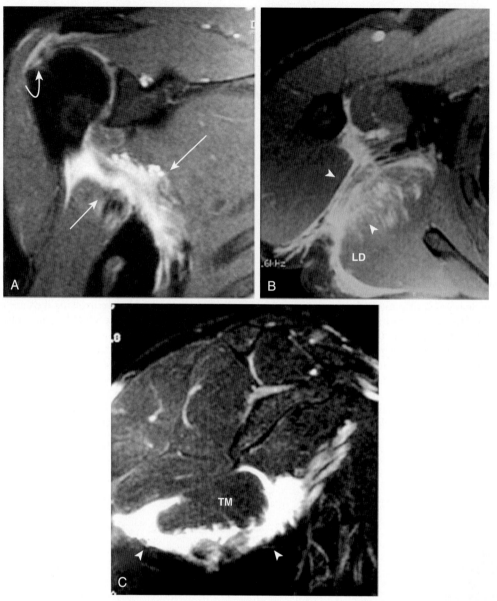

Figure 35-2 Teres major injury in a professional baseball player: magnetic resonance imaging (MRI). Coronal oblique **(A)** and axial T1-weighted spin-echo fat-suppressed **(B)** images of the right shoulder acquired using a 1.5-Tesla magnet after the administration of intravenous contrast from patient 1 demonstrate enhancing fluid *(straight arrows* and *arrowheads)* tracking caudally and posteriorly from the inferior aspect of the glenohumeral joint and indicating an acute, traumatic soft tissue injury of the teres major muscle, consistent with a grade II strain. Also visible is enhancement at the distal supraspinatus footprint *(curved arrow)* that is typical of degenerative tendinosis associated with overhand throwing. LD, latissimus dorsi muscle. **C,** Sagittal oblique T2-weighted fast spin-echo fat-suppressed image shows hyperintense fluid signal outlining the teres major proximal myotendinous junction (TM), as well as intramuscular "feathery" edema *(arrowheads)* typical of an acute myotendinous strain. *(From Leland M, Ciccotti MG, Cohen SB, et al: Teres major injuries in two professional baseball pitchers,* J Shoulder Elbow Surg 18[6]:e1–e5, 2009.)

myofascial pain syndrome. Patients with teres major syndrome exhibit trigger points lateral to the scapula in the teres major muscle (Fig. 35-3).

Taut bands of muscle fibers are often identified when myofascial trigger points are palpated. In spite of this consistent physical finding, the pathophysiology of the myofascial trigger point remains elusive, but trigger points are thought to result from microtrauma to the affected muscle. This trauma may occur from a single injury, repetitive microtrauma, or chronic deconditioning of the agonist and antagonist muscle unit.

In addition to muscle trauma, various other factors seem to predispose patients to the development of myofascial pain syndrome. For instance, a weekend athlete who subjects his or her body to unaccustomed physical activity may develop myofascial pain syndrome. Poor posture while sitting at a computer or while watching television has also been implicated as a predisposing factor. Previous injuries may result in abnormal muscle function and lead to the development of myofascial pain syndrome. All these factors may be intensified if the patient also suffers from poor nutritional status or coexisting psychological or behavioral abnormalities, including chronic stress and depression. The teres major muscle seems to be particularly susceptible to stress-induced myofascial pain syndrome.

Stiffness and fatigue often coexist with pain, and they increase the functional disability associated with this disease and complicate its treatment. Myofascial pain syndrome may occur as a primary disease state or in conjunction with other painful conditions, including

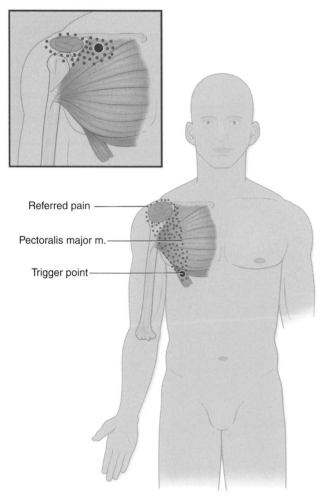

Referred pain

Pectoralis major m.

Trigger point

Figure 35-3 Patients with teres major syndrome have a trigger point lateral to the scapula in the teres major muscle. *(From Waldman SD: Atlas of pain management injection techniques, ed 2, Philadelphia, 2007, Saunders, 2007, p 86.)*

radiculopathy and chronic regional pain syndromes. Psychological or behavioral abnormalities, including depression, frequently coexist with the muscle abnormalities, and management of these psychological disorders is an integral part of any successful treatment plan.

SIGNS AND SYMPTOMS

The trigger point is the pathologic lesion of teres major syndrome and is characterized by a local point of exquisite tenderness in the axillary or posterior portion of the muscle. Mechanical stimulation of the trigger point by palpation or stretching produces both intense local pain and referred pain. In addition, the jump sign is characteristic of teres major syndrome, as is pain over the teres major muscle that is referred to the proximal portion of the posterolateral upper extremity (see Fig. 34-2).

TESTING

Biopsies of clinically identified trigger points have not revealed consistently abnormal histologic features. The muscle hosting the trigger points has been described either as "moth-eaten" or as containing "waxy degeneration." Increased plasma myoglobin has been reported in some patients with teres major syndrome, but this finding has not been corroborated by other investigators.

Electrodiagnostic testing of patients suffering from teres major syndrome has revealed an increase in muscle tension in some patients, but again, this finding has not been reproducible. Because of the lack of objective diagnostic testing, the clinician must rule out other coexisting disease processes that may mimic teres major syndrome (see "Differential Diagnosis").

DIFFERENTIAL DIAGNOSIS

The diagnosis of teres major syndrome is made on the basis of clinical findings rather than specific laboratory, electrodiagnostic, or radiographic testing. For this reason, a targeted history and physical examination, with a systematic search for trigger points and identification of a positive jump sign, must be carried out in every patient suspected of suffering from teres major syndrome. The clinician must rule out other coexisting disease processes that may mimic teres major syndrome, including primary inflammatory muscle disease, multiple sclerosis, and collagen vascular disease. Electrodiagnostic and radiographic testing can help identify coexisting disorders such as shoulder bursitis, tendinitis, and rotator cuff tears. The clinician must also identify coexisting psychological and behavioral abnormalities that may mask or exacerbate the symptoms associated with teres major syndrome.

TREATMENT

Treatment is focused on blocking the myofascial trigger and achieving prolonged relaxation of the affected muscle. Because the mechanism of action is poorly understood, an element of trial and error is often required when developing a treatment plan. Conservative therapy consisting of trigger point injections with local anesthetic or saline solution is the starting point. Because underlying depression and anxiety are present in many patients suffering from fibromyalgia, the administration of antidepressants is an integral part of most treatment plans. Pregabalin and gabapentin have also been shown to provide some palliation of the symptoms associated with fibromyalgia.

In addition, several adjuvant methods are available for the treatment of fibromyalgia of the cervical spine. The therapeutic use of heat and cold is often combined with trigger point injections and antidepressants to achieve pain relief. Some patients experience decreased pain with the application of transcutaneous nerve stimulation or electrical stimulation to fatigue the affected muscles. Exercise may also provide some palliation of symptoms and improve the fatigue associated with this disease. Although not currently approved by the Food and Drug Administration for this indication, the injection of minute quantities of botulinum toxin type A directly into trigger points has been used with success in patients who have not responded to traditional treatment modalities.

COMPLICATIONS AND PITFALLS

Trigger point injections are extremely safe if careful attention is paid to the clinically relevant anatomy. Sterile technique must be used to avoid infection, along with universal precautions to minimize any risk to the operator. Most complications of trigger point injection are related to needle-induced trauma at the injection site and in underlying tissues. The incidence of ecchymosis and hematoma formation can be decreased if pressure is applied to the injection site immediately after injection. The avoidance of overly long needles can decrease the incidence of trauma to underlying structures. Special care must be taken to avoid pneumothorax when injecting trigger points in proximity to the underlying pleural space.

Clinical Pearls

> Although teres major syndrome is a common disorder, it is often misdiagnosed. Therefore, in patients suspected of suffering from teres major syndrome, a careful evaluation to identify underlying disease processes is mandatory. Teres major syndrome commonly coexists with various somatic and psychological disorders.

SUGGESTED READINGS

Bradley LA: Pathophysiology of fibromyalgia, *Am J Med* 122(12 Suppl 1):S22–S30, 2009.

Ge H-Y, Nie H, Madeleine P, et al: Contribution of the local and referred pain from active myofascial trigger points in fibromyalgia syndrome, *Pain* 147(1–3): 233–240, 2009.

Monach PA: Shoulder pain. In Mushlin SB, Greene HL, II, editors: *Decision making in medicine,* ed 3, Philadelphia, 2010, Mosby, pp 522–523.

Schultz JS: Clinical evaluation of the shoulder, *Phys Med Rehabil Clin N Am* 15(2):351–371, 2004.

Waldman SD: Teres major syndrome. In *Atlas of pain management injection techniques,* ed 2, Philadelphia, 2007, Saunders, pp 88–90.

Chapter **36**

SCAPULOCOSTAL SYNDROME

ICD-9 CODE	**354.8**

ICD-10 CODE	**G56.80**

THE CLINICAL SYNDROME

Scapulocostal syndrome consists of a constellation of symptoms including unilateral pain and associated paresthesias at the medial border of the scapula, referred pain radiating from the deltoid region to the dorsum of the hand, and decreased range of motion of the scapula (Fig. 36-1). Scapulocostal syndrome is commonly referred to as traveling salesman's shoulder, because it is frequently seen in individuals who repeatedly reach backward to retrieve something from the back seat of a car (Fig. 36-2). Scapulocostal syndrome is an overuse syndrome caused by repeated improper use of the muscles of scapular stabilization—the levator scapulae, pectoralis minor, serratus anterior, rhomboids, and, to a lesser extent, infraspinatus and teres minor.

Scapulocostal syndrome is a chronic myofascial pain syndrome, and the sine qua non of myofascial pain syndrome is the finding of myofascial trigger points on physical examination. Although these trigger points are generally localized to the part of the body affected, the pain is often referred to other areas. This referred pain may be misdiagnosed or attributed to other organ systems, thus leading to extensive evaluation and ineffective treatment. Mechanical stimulation of the trigger point by palpation or stretching produces both intense local pain and referred pain. In addition, involuntary withdrawal of the stimulated muscle, called a jump sign, is often seen and is characteristic of myofascial pain syndrome. Almost all patients with scapulocostal syndrome have a prominent infraspinatus trigger point, which is best demonstrated by having the patient place the hand of the affected side over the deltoid of the opposite shoulder (Fig. 36-3). This maneuver laterally rotates the affected scapula and allows palpation and subsequent injection of the infraspinatus trigger point. Other trigger points along the medial border of the scapula may be present and may be amenable to injection therapy.

Taut bands of muscle fibers are often identified when myofascial trigger points are palpated. In spite of this consistent physical finding, the pathophysiology of the myofascial trigger point remains elusive, although trigger points are believed to result from microtrauma to the affected muscle. This trauma may occur from a single injury, repetitive microtrauma, or chronic deconditioning of the agonist and antagonist muscle unit.

In addition to muscle trauma, various other factors seem to predispose patients to develop myofascial pain syndrome. For instance, a weekend athlete who subjects his or her body to

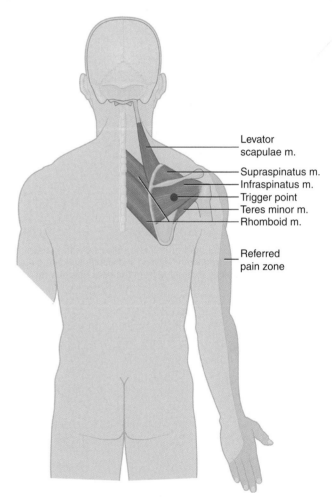

Levator scapulae m.

Supraspinatus m.
Infraspinatus m.
Trigger point
Teres minor m.
Rhomboid m.

Referred pain zone

Figure 36-1 Scapulocostal syndrome involves unilateral pain and associated paresthesias at the medial border of the scapula, referred pain radiating from the deltoid region to the dorsum of the hand, and decreased range of motion of the scapula. *(From Waldman SD: Atlas of pain management injection techniques, ed 2, Philadelphia, 2007, Saunders.)*

unaccustomed physical activity may develop myofascial pain syndrome. Poor posture while sitting at a computer or while watching television has also been implicated as a predisposing factor. Previous injuries may result in abnormal muscle function and lead to the development of myofascial pain syndrome. All these factors may be intensified if the patient also suffers from poor nutritional status or coexisting psychological or behavioral abnormalities, including chronic stress and depression. The muscle groups involved in scapulocostal syndrome seem to be particularly susceptible to stress-induced myofascial pain syndrome.

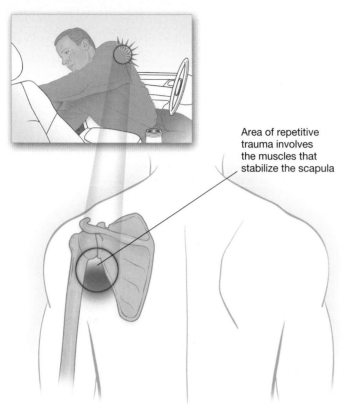

Area of repetitive trauma involves the muscles that stabilize the scapula

Figure 36-2 Scapulocostal syndrome is also called traveling salesman's shoulder because it is frequently seen in individuals who repeatedly reach backward to retrieve something from the back seat of a car.

Stiffness and fatigue often coexist with pain, and they increase the functional disability associated with this disease and complicate its treatment. Myofascial pain syndrome may occur as a primary disease state or in conjunction with other painful conditions, including radiculopathy and chronic regional pain syndromes. Psychological or behavioral abnormalities, including depression, frequently coexist with the muscle abnormalities, and management of these psychological disorders is an integral part of any successful treatment plan.

SIGNS AND SYMPTOMS

The trigger point is the pathologic lesion of scapulocostal syndrome, and it is characterized by a local point of exquisite tenderness in the infraspinatus muscle. As noted earlier, this infraspinatus trigger point can best be demonstrated by having the patient place the hand of the affected side over the deltoid of the opposite shoulder. Other trigger points may be present along the medial border of the scapula.

Mechanical stimulation of the trigger point by palpation or stretching produces intense local pain as well as referred pain. The jump sign is characteristic of scapulocostal syndrome, as is pain over the infraspinatus muscle that radiates from the deltoid region to the dorsum of the hand.

TESTING

Biopsies of clinically identified trigger points have not revealed consistently abnormal histologic features. The muscle hosting the trigger points has been described either as "moth-eaten" or as containing "waxy degeneration." Increased plasma myoglobin

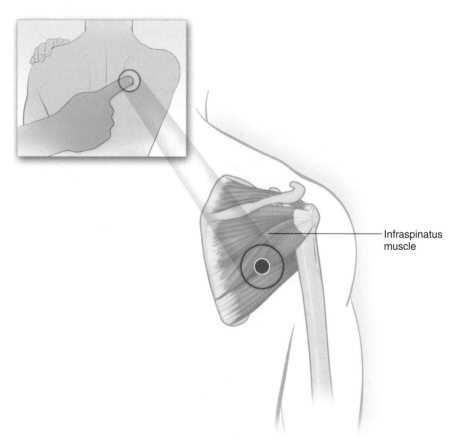

Infraspinatus muscle

Figure 36-3 The infraspinatus trigger point can be demonstrated by having the patient place the hand of the affected side over the deltoid of the opposite shoulder.

has been reported in some patients with scapulocostal syndrome, but this finding has not been corroborated by other investigators. Electrodiagnostic testing of patients suffering from scapulocostal syndrome has revealed an increase in muscle tension in some patients, but again, this finding has not been reproducible. Because of the lack of objective diagnostic testing, the clinician must rule out other coexisting disease processes that may mimic scapulocostal syndrome (see "Differential Diagnosis").

DIFFERENTIAL DIAGNOSIS

The diagnosis of scapulocostal syndrome is made on the basis of clinical findings rather than specific laboratory, electrodiagnostic, or radiographic testing. For this reason, a targeted history and physical examination, with a systematic search for trigger points and identification of a positive jump sign, must be carried out in every patient suspected of suffering from scapulocostal syndrome. The clinician must rule out other coexisting disease processes that may mimic scapulocostal syndrome, including primary inflammatory muscle disease, isolated tears of the infraspinatus musculotendinous unit, multiple sclerosis, and collagen vascular disease (Fig. 36-4). Electrodiagnostic and radiographic testing can help identify coexisting disorders such as shoulder bursitis, tendinitis, and rotator cuff tears. The clinician must also identify coexisting psychological and behavioral abnormalities that may mask or exacerbate the symptoms associated with scapulocostal syndrome.

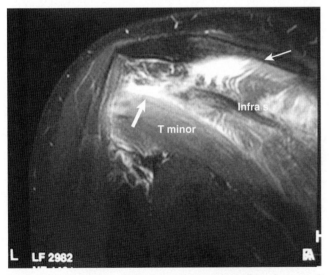

Figure 36-4 Disruption of the infraspinatus musculotendinous unit. Coronal T2-weighted magnetic resonance imaging scan showing high signal at the site of the disruption *(large white arrow)* and an increased pennate angle *(small white arrow)* resulting from muscular retraction of the infraspinatus. Edema is also seen in the infraspinatus muscle belly. Infra s, infraspinatus; T minor, teres minor. *(From Lunn JV, Castellanos-Rosas J, Tavernier T, et al: A novel lesion of the infraspinatus characterized by musculotendinous disruption, edema, and late fatty infiltration, J Shoulder Elbow Surg 17[4]:546–553, 2008.)*

TREATMENT

Treatment is focused on blocking the myofascial trigger and achieving prolonged relaxation of the affected muscle. Because the mechanism of action is poorly understood, an element of trial and error is often required when developing a treatment plan. Conservative therapy consisting of trigger point injections with local anesthetic or saline solution is the starting point. Because underlying depression and anxiety are present in many patients suffering from fibromyalgia, the administration of antidepressants is an integral part of most treatment plans. Pregabalin and gabapentin have also been shown to provide some palliation of the symptoms associated with fibromyalgia.

In addition, several adjuvant methods are available for the treatment of fibromyalgia of the cervical spine. The therapeutic use of heat and cold is often combined with trigger point injections and antidepressants to achieve pain relief. Some patients experience decreased pain with the application of transcutaneous nerve stimulation or electrical stimulation to fatigue the affected muscles. Exercise may also provide some palliation of symptoms and improve the fatigue associated with this disease. Although not currently approved by the Food and Drug Administration for this indication, the injection of minute quantities of botulinum toxin type A directly into trigger points has been used with success in patients who have not responded to traditional treatment modalities.

COMPLICATIONS AND PITFALLS

Trigger point injections are extremely safe if careful attention is paid to the clinically relevant anatomy. Sterile technique must be used to avoid infection, along with universal precautions to minimize any risk to the operator. Most complications of trigger point injection are related to needle-induced trauma at the injection site and in underlying tissues. The incidence of ecchymosis and hematoma formation can be decreased if pressure is applied to the injection site immediately after injection. The avoidance of overly long needles can decrease the incidence of trauma to underlying structures. Special care must be taken to avoid pneumothorax when injecting trigger points in proximity to the underlying pleural space.

Clinical Pearls

Although scapulocostal syndrome is a common disorder, it is often misdiagnosed. Therefore, in patients suspected of suffering from scapulocostal syndrome, a careful evaluation to identify underlying disease processes is mandatory. Scapulocostal syndrome commonly coexists with various somatic and psychological disorders.

SUGGESTED READINGS

Cohen CA: Scapulocostal syndrome: diagnosis and treatment, *South Med J* 73(4):433–477, 1980.
Fourie LJ: The scapulocostal syndrome, *S Afr Med J* 79(12):721–724, 1991.
Ormandy L: Scapulocostal syndrome, *Va Med Q* 121(2):105–108, 1994.
Waldman SD: Scapulocostal syndrome. In *Atlas of pain management injection techniques,* ed 2, Philadelphia, 2007, Saunders, pp 123–128.
Weed ND: When shoulder pain isn't bursitis: the myofascial pain syndrome, *Postgrad Med* 74(3):97–98, 101–102, 104, 1983.

Chapter **37**

ARTHRITIS PAIN OF THE ELBOW

ICD-9 CODE **715.33**

ICD-10 CODE **M19.90**

THE CLINICAL SYNDROME

Elbow pain secondary to degenerative arthritis is frequently encountered in clinical practice. Osteoarthritis is the most common form of arthritis that results in elbow joint pain. Tendinitis and bursitis may coexist with arthritis pain, and they make the correct diagnosis more difficult. The olecranon bursa lies in the posterior aspect of the elbow joint and may become inflamed as a result of direct trauma or overuse of the joint. Bursae susceptible to the development of bursitis also exist between the insertion of the biceps and the head of the radius, as well as in the antecubital and cubital areas.

In addition to pain, patients suffering from arthritis of the elbow joint often experience a gradual reduction in functional ability because of decreasing elbow range of motion that makes simple everyday tasks such as using a computer keyboard, holding a coffee cup, or turning a doorknob quite difficult (Fig. 37-1). With continued disuse, muscle wasting may occur, and adhesive capsulitis with subsequent ankylosis may develop.

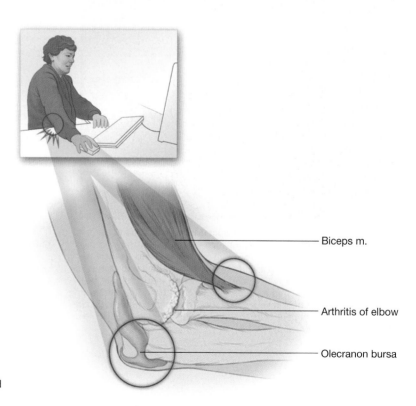

Biceps m.

Arthritis of elbow

Olecranon bursa

Figure 37-1 Arthritis of the elbow can cause pain and functional disability during common everyday tasks.

SIGNS AND SYMPTOMS

Most patients with elbow pain secondary to osteoarthritis or posttraumatic arthritis complain of pain that is localized around the elbow and forearm. Activity makes the pain worse, whereas rest and heat provide some relief. The pain is constant and is characterized as aching; it may interfere with sleep. Some patients also complain of a grating or popping sensation with use of the joint, and crepitus may be present on physical examination.

TESTING

Plain radiographs should be obtained in all patients who present with elbow pain. Based on the patient's clinical presentation, additional testing may be warranted, including a complete blood count, erythrocyte sedimentation rate, and antinuclear antibody testing. Magnetic resonance imaging of the elbow is indicated if joint instability, nerve entrapment, tumor, or other soft tissue abnormalities is suspected (Fig. 37-2).

DIFFERENTIAL DIAGNOSIS

Rheumatoid arthritis, posttraumatic arthritis, and psoriatic arthritis are common causes of elbow pain. Less common causes of arthritis-induced elbow pain include collagen vascular diseases, infection, and Lyme disease. Acute infectious arthritis is usually accompanied by significant systemic symptoms, including fever and malaise, and should be easily recognized; treatment is with culture and antibiotics rather than injection therapy. Collagen vascular diseases generally manifest as polyarthropathy rather than as monarthropathy limited to the elbow joint; however, elbow pain secondary to collagen vascular disease responds exceedingly well to the intraarticular injection technique described later.

TREATMENT

Initial treatment of the pain and functional disability associated with arthritis of the elbow includes a combination of nonsteroidal antiinflammatory drugs (NSAIDs) or cyclooxygenase-2 (COX-2) inhibitors and physical therapy. Local application of heat and cold may also be beneficial. For patients who do not respond to these treatment modalities, intraarticular injection of local anesthetic and steroid is a reasonable next step.

Intraarticular injection of the elbow is carried out with the patient in the supine position, the arm fully adducted at the patient's side, the elbow flexed, and the dorsum of the hand resting on a folded towel. A total of 5 mL local anesthetic and 40 mg methylprednisolone is drawn up in a 12-mL sterile syringe. After sterile preparation of the skin overlying the posterolateral aspect of the joint, the head of the radius is identified. Just superior to the head of the radius is an indentation that represents the space between the radial head and the humerus. Using strict aseptic technique, a 1-inch, 25-gauge needle is inserted just above the superior aspect of the head of the radius through the skin, subcutaneous tissues, and joint capsule and into the joint (Fig. 37-3). If bone is encountered, the needle is withdrawn into the subcutaneous tissues and is redirected superiorly. After the joint space has been entered, the contents of the syringe are gently

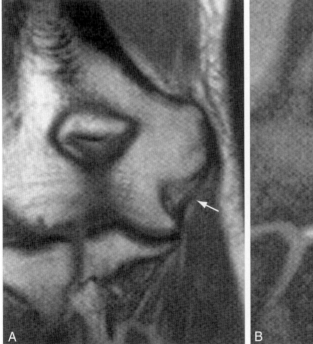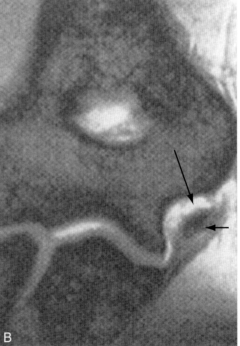

Figure 37-2 Tear of the medial (ulnar) collateral ligament (MCL) of the elbow. **A,** Coronal T1-weighted magnetic resonance imaging (MRI) of a normal elbow demonstrates an intact MCL as a linear, low-signal structure extending from the medial humeral epicondyle to the proximal ulna *(arrow).* **B,** Coronal T2-weighted MRI from a different patient demonstrates disruption of the MCL, with high signal intensity at the expected site of humeral attachment *(long arrow).* The small focus of low signal noted at the proximal end of the ligament may represent an avulsion fragment *(short arrow).* The patient was a professional baseball pitcher; these athletes are prone to MCL tears because of the marked valgus stress when throwing a ball. *(From Grainger RG, Allison DJ, Adam A, Dixon AK:* Grainger & Allison's diagnostic radiology: a textbook of medical imaging, *ed 4, Philadelphia, 2002, Churchill Livingstone.)*

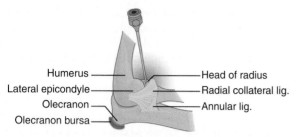

Figure 37-3 Proper needle placement for intraarticular injection of the elbow. *(From Waldman SD: Atlas of pain management injection techniques, Philadelphia, 2000, Saunders.)*

injected. Little resistance to injection should be felt. If resistance is encountered, the needle is probably in a ligament or tendon and should be advanced slightly into the joint space until the injection can proceed without significant resistance. The needle is then removed, and a sterile pressure dressing and ice pack are applied to the injection site.

Physical modalities, including local heat and gentle range-of-motion exercises, should be introduced several days after the patient undergoes injection for elbow pain. Vigorous exercises should be avoided, because they will exacerbate the patient's symptoms.

COMPLICATIONS AND PITFALLS

This injection technique is safe if careful attention is paid to the clinically relevant anatomy. Sterile technique must be used to avoid infection, along with universal precautions to minimize any risk to the operator. The major complication of intraarticular injection of the elbow is infection, although it should be exceedingly rare if strict aseptic technique is followed. The ulnar nerve is especially susceptible to damage at the elbow, and care must be taken to avoid this structure when performing intraarticular injection. Approximately 25% of patients complain of a transient increase in pain after intraarticular injection of the elbow joint, and patients should be warned of this possibility.

Clinical Pearls

Pain and functional disability of the elbow are often the result of degenerative arthritis of the joint. Coexistent bursitis and tendinitis may contribute to elbow pain and may confuse the diagnosis. Simple analgesics and NSAIDs or COX-2 inhibitors can be used concurrently with the intraarticular injection technique.

SUGGESTED READINGS

Chung CB, Kim H-J: Sports injuries of the elbow, *Magn Reson Imaging Clin N Am* 11(2):239–253, 2003.

Hayter CL, Giuffre BM: Overuse and traumatic injuries of the elbow, *Magn Reson Imaging Clin N Am* 17(4):617–638, 2009.

Howard TM, Shaw JL, Phillips J: Physical examination of the elbow. In Seidenberg PH, Beutler A, editors: *The sports medicine resource manual,* Philadelphia, 2008, Saunders, pp 71–78.

Sellards R, Kuebrich C: The elbow: diagnosis and treatment of common injuries, *Prim Care* 32(1):1–16, 2005.

Waldman SD: Intraarticular injection of the elbow. In *Atlas of pain management injection techniques,* ed 2, Philadelphia, 2007, Saunders, pp 129–132.

Chapter 38

TENNIS ELBOW

ICD-9 CODE `726.32`

ICD-10 CODE `M77.10`

THE CLINICAL SYNDROME

Tennis elbow (also known as lateral epicondylitis) is caused by repetitive microtrauma to the extensor tendons of the forearm. The pathophysiology of tennis elbow initially involves microtearing at the origin of the extensor carpi radialis and extensor carpi ulnaris. Secondary inflammation may become chronic as a result of continued overuse or misuse of the extensors of the forearm. Coexistent bursitis, arthritis, or gout may perpetuate the pain and disability of tennis elbow.

The most common nidus of pain from tennis elbow is the bony origin of the extensor tendon of the extensor carpi radialis brevis at the anterior facet of the lateral epicondyle. Less commonly, tennis

elbow pain originates from the origin of the extensor carpi radialis longus at the supracondylar crest; rarely, it originates more distally, at the point where the extensor carpi radialis brevis overlies the radial head. The olecranon bursa lies in the posterior aspect of the elbow joint and may also become inflamed (bursitis) as a result of direct trauma to the joint or its overuse. Other bursae susceptible to the development of bursitis lie between the insertion of the biceps and the head of the radius, as well as in the antecubital and cubital areas.

Tennis elbow occurs in individuals engaged in repetitive activities such as hand grasping (e.g., shaking hands) or high-torque wrist turning (e.g., scooping ice cream) (Fig. 38-1). Tennis players develop tennis elbow by two different mechanisms: (1) increased pressure grip strain as a result of playing with too heavy a racket, and (2) making backhand shots with a leading shoulder and elbow rather than keeping the shoulder and elbow parallel to the net. Other racket sports players are also susceptible to the development of tennis elbow.

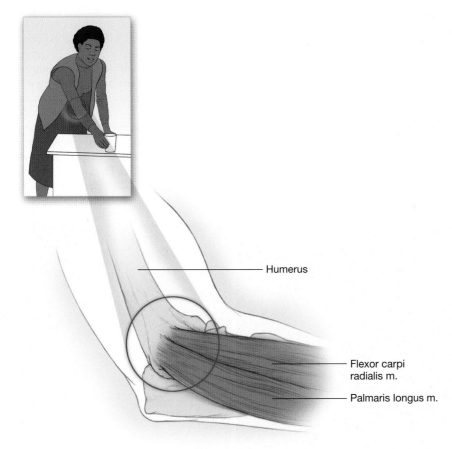

Humerus

Flexor carpi radialis m.

Palmaris longus m.

Figure 38-1 The pain of tennis elbow is localized to the lateral epicondyle.

SIGNS AND SYMPTOMS

The pain of tennis elbow is localized to the region of the lateral epicondyle. This pain is constant and is made worse with active contraction of the wrist. Patients note the inability to hold a coffee cup or use a hammer. Sleep disturbance is common. On physical examination, tenderness is elicited along the extensor tendons at or just below the lateral epicondyle. Many patients with tennis elbow exhibit a bandlike thickening within the affected extensor tendons. Elbow range of motion is normal, but grip strength on the affected side is diminished. Patients with tennis elbow have a positive tennis elbow test result. This test is performed by stabilizing the patient's forearm and then having the patient clench his or her fist and actively extend the wrist. The examiner then attempts to force the wrist into flexion (Fig. 38-2). Sudden severe pain is highly suggestive of tennis elbow.

TESTING

Electromyography can help distinguish cervical radiculopathy and radial tunnel syndrome from tennis elbow. Plain radiographs should be obtained in all patients who present with elbow pain to rule out joint mice and other occult bony disease. Based on the patient's clinical presentation, additional testing may be warranted, including a complete blood count, uric acid level, erythrocyte sedimentation rate, and antinuclear antibody testing. Magnetic resonance imaging of the elbow is indicated if joint instability is suspected or if the symptoms of tennis elbow persist (Fig. 38-3). The injection technique described later serves as both (Fig. 38-4) a diagnostic and a therapeutic maneuver.

DIFFERENTIAL DIAGNOSIS

Radial tunnel syndrome and, occasionally, C6-7 radiculopathy can mimic tennis elbow. Radial tunnel syndrome is caused by entrapment of the radial nerve below the elbow. With radial tunnel syndrome, the maximal tenderness to palpation is distal to the lateral epicondyle over the radial nerve, whereas with tennis elbow, the maximal tenderness to palpation is over the lateral epicondyle.

TREATMENT

Initial treatment of the pain and functional disability associated with tennis elbow includes a combination of nonsteroidal antiinflammatory drugs (NSAIDs) or cyclooxygenase-2 inhibitors and physical therapy. Local application of heat and cold may also be beneficial. Any repetitive activity that may exacerbate the patient's symptoms should be avoided. For patients who do not respond to these treatment modalities, injection of local anesthetic and steroid is a reasonable next step.

Injection for tennis elbow is performed by placing the patient in the supine position with the arm fully adducted at the patient's side, the elbow flexed, and the dorsum of the hand resting on a folded towel to relax the affected tendons. A total of 1 mL local anesthetic and 40 mg methylprednisolone is drawn up in a 5-mL sterile syringe. After sterile preparation of the skin overlying the posterolateral aspect of the joint, the lateral epicondyle is identified. Using strict aseptic technique, a 1-inch, 25-gauge needle is inserted perpendicular to the lateral epicondyle through the skin and into the subcutaneous tissue overlying the affected tendon (see Fig. 38-4). If bone is encountered, the needle is withdrawn into the subcutaneous tissue. The contents of the syringe are then gently injected. Little resistance to injection should be felt. If resistance is encountered, the needle is probably in the tendon and should be withdrawn until the injection can proceed without significant resistance. The needle is then removed, and a sterile pressure dressing and ice pack are applied to the injection site.

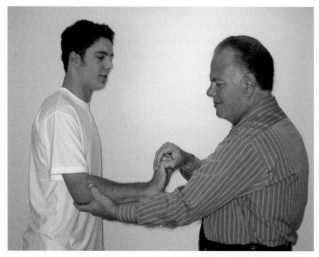

Figure 38-2 Test for tennis elbow. *(From Waldman SD: Physical diagnosis of pain: an atlas of signs and symptoms, Philadelphia, 2006, Saunders, p 138.)*

Figure 38-3 Lateral epicondylitis and tennis elbow. **A,** Coronal inversion recovery magnetic resonance image shows marrow edema in the lateral epicondyle *(arrow)* and subtle edema adjacent to the mildly thickened common extensor tendon *(arrowhead).* **B,** Radiograph shows calcific tendinitis of the common extensor tendon *(arrowheads). (From Manaster BJ, May DA, Disler DG: Musculoskeletal imaging: the requisites, ed 3, Philadelphia, 2007, Mosby, p 128.)*

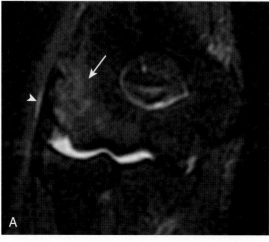

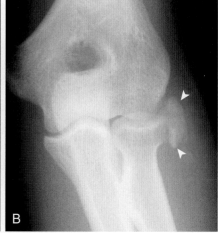

Physical modalities, including local heat and gentle range-of-motion exercises, should be introduced several days after the patient undergoes injection for tennis elbow. A Velcro band placed around the extensor tendons may also help relieve the symptoms. Vigorous exercises should be avoided, because they will exacerbate the patient's symptoms.

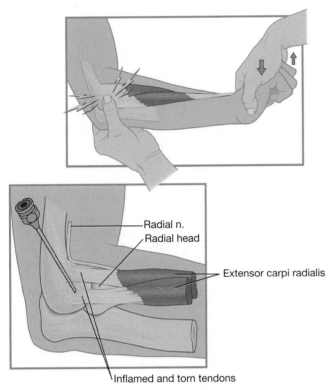

Figure 38-4 Proper needle placement for injection for tennis elbow. *(From Waldman SD: Atlas of pain management injection techniques, Philadelphia, 2000, Saunders.)*

Radial n.
Radial head
Extensor carpi radialis
Inflamed and torn tendons

COMPLICATIONS AND PITFALLS

The major complication associated with tennis elbow is rupture of the inflamed tendon either from repetitive trauma or from injection directly into the tendon. To prevent inflamed and previously damaged tendons from rupturing, the needle position should be confirmed to be outside the tendon before the clinician proceeds with the injection. Another complication of injection is infection, although it should be exceedingly rare if strict aseptic technique is followed. The injection technique is safe if careful attention is paid to the clinically relevant anatomy; in particular, the ulnar nerve is susceptible to damage at the elbow. Approximately 25% of patients complain of a transient increase in pain after injection, and patients should be warned of this possibility.

Clinical Pearls

The injection technique described is extremely effective in the treatment of pain secondary to tennis elbow. Coexistent bursitis and tendinitis may contribute to elbow pain, thus necessitating additional treatment with more localized injection of local anesthetic and methylprednisolone. Simple analgesics and NSAIDs can be used concurrently with the injection technique. Cervical radiculopathy and radial tunnel syndrome may mimic tennis elbow and must be excluded.

SUGGESTED READINGS

Waldman SD, editor: Tennis elbow. In *Pain management*, Philadelphia, 2007, Saunders, pp 633–638.
Waldman SD: Tennis elbow. In *Atlas of pain management injection techniques,* ed 3, Philadelphia, 2009, Saunders, pp 137–144.
Waldman SD: Tennis elbow. In *Pain review,* Philadelphia, 2009, Saunders, pp 266–267.
Whaley AL, Baker CL: Lateral epicondylitis, *Clin Sports Med* 23(4):677–691, 2004.
Wilhelm A: Lateral epicondylitis: review and current concepts, *J Hand Surg* 34(7):1358–1359, 2009.

Chapter **39**

GOLFER'S ELBOW

ICD-9 CODE **726.31**

ICD-10 CODE **M77.00**

THE CLINICAL SYNDROME

Golfer's elbow (also known as medial epicondylitis) is caused by repetitive microtrauma to the flexor tendons of the forearm in a manner analogous to tennis elbow. The pathophysiology of golfer's elbow initially involves microtearing at the origin of the pronator teres, flexor carpi radialis, flexor carpi ulnaris, and palmaris longus (Fig. 39-1). Secondary inflammation may become chronic as a result of continued overuse or misuse of the flexors of the forearm. The most common nidus of pain from golfer's elbow is the bony origin of the flexor tendon of the flexor carpi radialis and the humeral heads of the flexor carpi ulnaris and pronator teres at the medial epicondyle of the humerus. Less commonly, golfer's elbow pain originates from the ulnar head of the flexor carpi ulnaris at the medial aspect of the olecranon process. Coexistent bursitis, arthritis, or gout may perpetuate the pain and disability of golfer's elbow.

Golfer's elbow occurs in individuals engaged in repetitive flexion activities, such as throwing baseballs or footballs, carrying heavy suitcases, and driving golf balls. These activities have in common repetitive flexion of the wrist and strain on the flexor tendons resulting from excessive weight or sudden arrested motion. Many of the activities that cause tennis elbow can also cause golfer's elbow.

SIGNS AND SYMPTOMS

The pain of golfer's elbow is localized to the region of the medial epicondyle (Fig. 39-2). This pain is constant and is made worse with active contraction of the wrist. Patients note the inability to hold a coffee cup or use a hammer. Sleep disturbance is common. On physical examination, tenderness is elicited along the flexor tendons at or just below the medial epicondyle. Many patients with golfer's elbow exhibit a bandlike thickening within the affected flexor tendons. Elbow range of motion is normal, but grip strength on the affected side is diminished. Patients with golfer's elbow have a positive golfer's elbow test result. This test is performed by stabilizing the patient's forearm and then having the patient actively flex the wrist. The examiner then attempts to force the wrist into extension (Fig. 39-3). Sudden severe pain is highly suggestive of golfer's elbow.

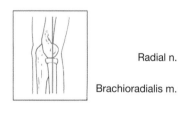

Radial n. ——————————————————— Brachialis m.

Brachioradialis m. ——————————————————

Extensor carpi radialis longus m. —————— Ant. fat pad

Capitulum ——————

Common extensor t. —————— Trochlea
                                    Coronoid

Lat collateral and annular ligs. —————— Pronator teres m.

Radius, head —————— Brachialis m. and t.
Radius, tuberosity —————— Palmaris longus m.
Supinator m., deep portion —————— Flexor carpi radialis m.

Radial n., deep branch —————— Median n.
Supinator m., superficial portion —————— Ulnar a.
                                    Pronator teres t.
Extensor carpi radialis brevis m. —————— ulnar head
                                    Flexor digitorum superficialis m.

Figure 39-1 Origins of the pronator teres, flexor carpi radialis, flexor carpi ulnaris, palmaris longus, and medial epicondyle. *(From Kang HS, Ahn JM, Resnick D: MRI of the extremities: an anatomic atlas, ed 2, Philadelphia, 2002, Saunders, p 89.)*

TESTING

Plain radiographs should be obtained in all patients who present with elbow pain to rule out joint mice and other occult bony disease. Based on the patient's clinical presentation, additional testing may be warranted, including a complete blood count, uric acid level, erythrocyte sedimentation rate, and antinuclear antibody testing. Magnetic resonance imaging of the elbow is indicated if joint instability is suspected or if the symptoms of golfer's elbow persists (Fig. 39-4). Electromyography (EMG) is indicated to diagnosis entrapment neuropathy at the elbow and to distinguish golfer's elbow from cervical radiculopathy. The injection technique described later serves as both a diagnostic and a therapeutic maneuver.

DIFFERENTIAL DIAGNOSIS

Occasionally, C6-7 radiculopathy mimics golfer's elbow; however, patients suffering from cervical radiculopathy usually have neck pain and proximal upper extremity pain in addition to symptoms below the elbow. As noted earlier, EMG can distinguish radiculopathy from golfer's elbow. Bursitis, arthritis, and gout may also mimic golfer's elbow, thus confusing the diagnosis. The olecranon bursa lies in the posterior aspect of the elbow joint and may become inflamed as a result of direct trauma to the joint or its overuse. Other bursae susceptible to the development of bursitis are located between the insertion of the biceps and the head of the radius, as well as in the antecubital and cubital areas.

TREATMENT

Initial treatment of the pain and functional disability associated with golfer's elbow includes a combination of nonsteroidal antiinflammatory drugs (NSAIDs) or cyclooxygenase-2 inhibitors and physical therapy. Local application of heat and cold may also be beneficial. Any repetitive activity that may exacerbate the patient's symptoms should be avoided. For patients who do not respond to these treatment modalities, injection with local anesthetic and steroid is a reasonable next step.

Injection for golfer's elbow is carried out by placing the patient in the supine position with the arm fully adducted at the patient's side, the elbow fully extended, and the dorsum of the hand resting on a folded towel to relax the affected tendons.

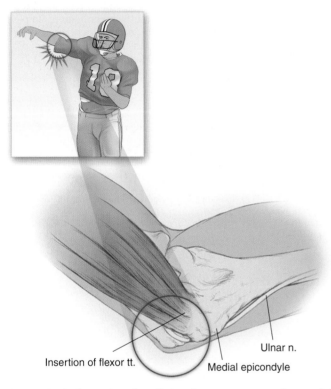

Insertion of flexor tt.

Ulnar n.

Medial epicondyle

Figure 39-2 The pain of golfer's elbow occurs at the medial epicondyle.

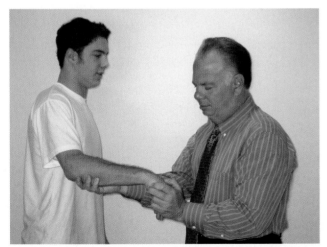

Figure 39-3 Test for golfer's elbow. *(From Waldman SD: Physical diagnosis of pain: an atlas of signs and symptoms, Philadelphia, 2006, Saunders, p 140.)*

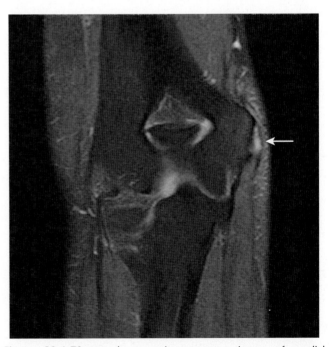

Figure 39-4 T2-coronal magnetic resonance image of medial epicondylitis with a pathologic increase in signal intensity at the origin of the flexor-pronator mass *(arrow)*. *(From Van Hofwegen C, Baker CL III, Baker CL Jr: Epicondylitis in the athlete's elbow, Clin Sports Med 29[4]:577–597, 2010.)*

A total of 1 mL local anesthetic and 40 mg methylprednisolone is drawn up in a 5-mL sterile syringe. After sterile preparation of the skin overlying the medial aspect of the joint, the medial epicondyle is identified. Using strict aseptic technique, a 1-inch, 25-gauge needle is inserted perpendicular to the medial epicondyle through the skin and into the subcutaneous tissue overlying the affected tendon. If bone is encountered, the needle is withdrawn into the subcutaneous tissue. The contents of the syringe are then gently injected. Little resistance to injection should be felt. If significant resistance is encountered, the needle is probably in the tendon and should be withdrawn until the injection can proceed with less resistance. The needle is then removed, and a sterile pressure dressing and ice pack are applied to the injection site.

Physical modalities, including local heat and gentle range-of-motion exercises, should be introduced several days after the patient undergoes injection for elbow pain. A Velcro band placed around the flexor tendons may also help relieve the symptoms. Vigorous exercises should be avoided, because they will exacerbate the patient's symptoms.

COMPLICATIONS AND PITFALLS

The major complications associated with this injection technique are related to trauma to the inflamed and previously damaged tendon, which may rupture if injected directly. Therefore, the needle position should be confirmed to be outside the tendon before the clinician proceeds with the injection. Another complication of the injection technique is infection, although it should be exceedingly rare if strict aseptic technique is followed. Injection is safe if careful attention is paid to the clinically relevant anatomy; in particular, the ulnar nerve is susceptible to damage at the elbow. Approximately 25% of patients complain of a transient increase in pain after intraarticular injection of the elbow joint, and patients should be warned of this possibility.

Clinical Pearls

The injection technique described is extremely effective in the treatment of pain secondary to golfer's elbow. Coexistent bursitis and tendinitis may contribute to elbow pain, thus necessitating additional treatment with more localized injection of local anesthetic and methylprednisolone. Simple analgesics and NSAIDs can be used concurrently with this injection technique. Cervical radiculopathy may mimic golfer's elbow and must be excluded.

SUGGESTED READINGS

Ciccotti MC, Schwartz MA, Ciccotti MG: Diagnosis and treatment of medial epicondylitis of the elbow, *Clin Sports Med* 23(4):693–705, 2004.

Rineer CA, Ruch DS: Elbow tendinopathy and tendon ruptures: epicondylitis, biceps and triceps ruptures, *J Hand Surg* 34(3):566–576, 2009.

Waldman SD: Golfer's elbow. In *Atlas of pain management injection techniques,* ed 3, Philadelphia, 2009, Saunders, pp 148–153.

Waldman SD: Golfer's elbow. In *Pain management,* Philadelphia, 2007, Saunders, pp 637–640.

Waldman SD: Golfer's elbow. In *Pain review,* Philadelphia, 2009, Saunders, pp 267–268.

Chapter **40**

DISTAL BICEPS TENDON TEAR

ICD-9 CODE `841.8`

ICD-10 CODE `S53.499A`

THE CLINICAL SYNDROME

Rupture of the distal tendon of the biceps occurs much less frequently than rupture of the long head of the biceps. Proximal rupture of the tendon of the long head of the biceps tendon accounts for more than 97% of biceps tendon ruptures, whereas ruptures of the distal portion of the biceps tendon occur less than 3% of the time. Occurring most commonly in men in the forth to sixth decades, disruption of the distal biceps tendon is usually the result of an acute traumatic event secondary to a sudden eccentric load on the tendon, such as trying to start a recalcitrant lawn mower, practicing an overhead tennis serve, lifting weights, or performing overaggressive follow-through when driving golf balls (Fig. 40-1). Falls on a flexed and supinated elbow have also been associated with tears and rupture of the distal biceps tendon, as has abuse of anabolic steroids in athletes.

The biceps muscle and proximal and distal tendons are intimately involved in shoulder and elbow function and are susceptible to trauma and to wear and tear. If the damage is severe enough, the distal tendon of the biceps can rupture, leaving the patient with a palpable defect in the antecubital fossa and weakness of upper extremity flexion and supination (Fig. 40-2).

SIGNS AND SYMPTOMS

In most patients, the pain of distal biceps tendon tear occurs acutely, is often quite severe, and is accompanied by a pop or snapping sound. The pain is constant and severe and is localized to the region surrounding the antecubital fossa. Patients with complete distal biceps tendon tear experience weakness of upper extremity flexion and supination. An obvious defect is palpable in the antecubital fossa in patients with complete rupture of the distal biceps tendon.

TESTING

Plain radiographs are indicated for all patients who present with elbow pain. Based on the patient's clinical presentation, additional testing may be indicated, including a complete blood count,

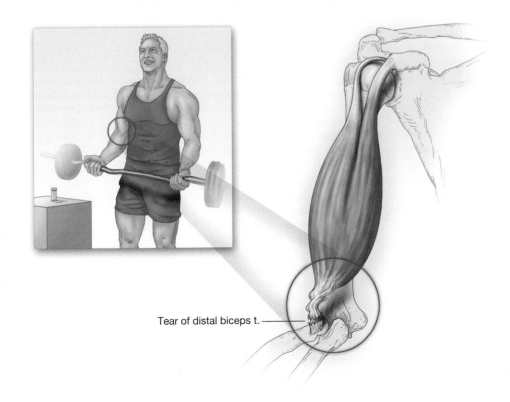

Tear of distal biceps t. —

Figure 40-1 Patients with tears of the distal biceps tendon experience weakness of flexion and supination of the affected extremity.

Right   Left

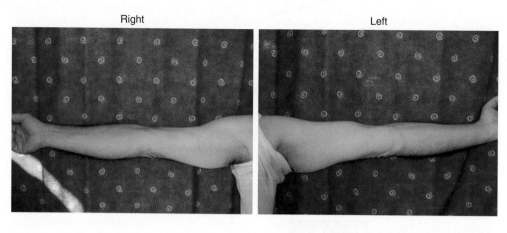

Figure 40-2 A 49-year-old man, 2 years following nonoperative management of a complete avulsion of the right distal biceps tendon. A deficit of distal biceps brachii mass in the right distal arm is clearly seen. *(From Hetsroni I, Pilz-Burstein R, Nyska M, et al: Avulsion of the distal biceps brachii tendon in middle-aged population: is surgical repair advisable? A comparative study of 22 patients treated with either nonoperative management or early anatomical repair, Injury 39[7]:753–760, 2008.)*

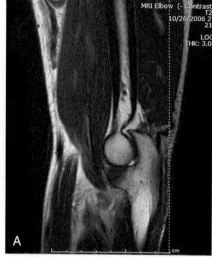 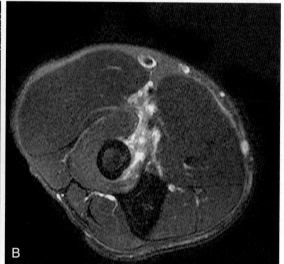

Figure 40-3 T2-weighted magnetic resonance imaging of a distal biceps tendon tear. **A,** Sagittal image with a retracted tendon stump. **B,** Axial image with visible hemorrhage surrounding the insertion site at the bicipital tuberosity of the proximal radius. *(Courtesy of Glenn M. Garcia, MD, Department of Radiology, University of Texas Health Science Center, San Antonio. From DeLee JC, Drez DD, Miller M, editors: Orthopaedic sports medicine: principles and practice, ed 3, Philadelphia, 2010, Saunders, p 1169.)*

erythrocyte sedimentation rate, and antinuclear antibody testing. Magnetic resonance imaging of the elbow is indicated if tendinopathy or if partial tear or complete rupture of the biceps tendon is suspected (Fig. 40-3).

DIFFERENTIAL DIAGNOSIS

Tear of the distal biceps tendon is usually a straightforward clinical diagnosis. However, coexisting bursitis or tendinitis of the elbow from overuse or misuse may confuse the diagnosis. In some clinical situations, consideration should be given to primary or secondary tumors involving the elbow. Nerve entrapments of the elbow and forearm can also complicate the diagnosis.

TREATMENT

Initial treatment of the pain and functional disability associated with distal biceps tendon tear includes a combination of nonsteroidal antiinflammatory drugs (NSAIDs) or cyclooxygenase-2 (COX-2) inhibitors and physical therapy. Local application of heat and cold may also be beneficial. For patients who do not respond to these treatment modalities and who appear to have significant local pain in the region of the distal biceps tendon, careful injection with local anesthetic and steroid is a reasonable next step.

Injection for distal biceps tendon tear is carried out by placing the patient in the sitting position with the elbow flexed to approximately 90 degrees. If intact, the distal biceps tendon is easily identified by palpation at the antecubital fossa. If the tendon is absent, the area of defect is identified. The point overlying the distal tendon or defect is marked with a sterile marker. The skin overlying antecubital fossa is then prepared with antiseptic solution. A sterile syringe containing 1 mL of 0.25% preservative-free bupivacaine and 40 mg methylprednisolone is attached to a 1½-inch, 25-gauge needle using strict aseptic technique. The previously marked point is palpated, and the distal biceps tendon or area of defect is reidentified with the gloved finger. The needle is carefully advanced at this point through the skin and subcutaneous tissues until it impinges on the distal biceps tendon or enters the area of defect. The needle is then withdrawn 1 to 2 mm out of the substance of the tendon, and the contents of the syringe are gently injected. Slight resistance to injection should be felt. If no resistance is encountered, the tendon is ruptured. If resistance is significant, the needle tip is probably in the substance of the tendon and should be advanced or withdrawn slightly until the injection can proceed without significant resistance. The needle is then removed, and a sterile pressure dressing and ice pack are applied to the injection site.

Physical modalities, including local heat and gentle range-of-motion exercises, should be introduced several days after the patient undergoes injection. Vigorous exercises should be avoided, because they will exacerbate the patient's symptoms. Occasionally, surgical repair of the tendon is undertaken if the patient is experiencing significant functional disability or is unhappy with the cosmetic defect caused by the retracted tendon and muscle.

COMPLICATIONS AND PITFALLS

This injection technique is safe if careful attention is paid to the clinically relevant anatomy. Sterile technique must be used to avoid infection, along with universal precautions to minimize any risk to the operator. The incidence of ecchymosis and hematoma formation can be decreased if pressure is applied to the injection site immediately after injection. The major complication of this injection technique is infection, although it should be exceedingly rare if strict aseptic technique is followed. Trauma to the distal biceps tendon from the injection itself is also a possibility. Tendons that are highly inflamed or previously damaged are subject to rupture if they are injected directly. This complication can often be avoided if the clinician uses a gentle technique and stops injecting immediately if significant resistance is encountered. Approximately 25% of patients complain of a transient increase in pain after injection, and patients should be warned of this possibility.

Clinical Pearls

The distal biceps tendon ruptures much less commonly than the proximal long head of the biceps tendon, although the forces that can cause either end of the tendon to rupture are similar. The injection technique described is extremely effective in the treatment of pain secondary to biceps tendon tear. Coexistent bursitis and arthritis may contribute to shoulder pain, thus necessitating additional treatment with more localized injection of local anesthetic and methylprednisolone. Simple analgesics and NSAIDs or COX-2 inhibitors can be used concurrently with this injection technique.

SUGGESTED READINGS

Hayter CL, Giuffre BM: Overuse and traumatic injuries of the elbow, *Magn Reson Imaging Clin N Am* 17(4):617–638, 2009.

Mazzocca AD, Spang JT, Arciero RA: Distal biceps rupture, *Orthop Clin North Am* 39(2):237–249, 2008.

Sarris I, Sotereanos DG: Distal biceps tendon ruptures, *J Am Soc Surg Hand* 2(3):121–128, 2002.

Schneider A, Bennett JM, O'Connor DP, et al: Bilateral ruptures of the distal biceps brachii tendon, *J Shoulder Elbow Surg* 18(5):804–807, 2009.

Waldman SD: The biceps tendon. In *Pain review*, Philadelphia, 2009, Saunders, pp 84–85.

Weiland DE, Rodosky MW: Biceps tendon disorders. In Brukner P, Khan K, editors: *Clinical sports medicine*, ed 3, New York, 2006, McGraw-Hill Medical, pp 235–241.

Chapter 41

THROWER'S ELBOW

ICD-9 CODE `718.82`

ICD-10 CODE `M24.829`

THE CLINICAL SYNDROME

Thrower's elbow is a valgus stress overload syndrome caused by continual microtrauma to the medial and lateral elbow from repetitive throwing motion. The pathophysiology of thrower's elbow initially involves damage secondary to significant valgus stress placed in the medial structures and compression of the lateral structures of the elbow during throwing activities. The medial epicondyle, medial collateral ligaments, and the medial epicondylar apophysis are especially prone to this repetitive stress, and ongoing tissue damage often exceeds the ability of the athlete's body to repair the damage (see Fig. 39-1). When this occurs, the result is acute, localized, medial elbow pain combined with decreased throwing accuracy and throwing distance.

Thrower's elbow is the name given the constellation of symptoms, rather than a single pathologic process, that results from this repetitive microtrauma to the elbow. Contributing to this symptom complex are medial epicondylitis (golfer's elbow), growth abnormalities of the medial epicondyle (medial epicondylar apophysitis), medial epicondylar fragmentation, stress fractures involving the medial epicondylar epiphysis, and avulsion fractures of the medial epicondyle. In addition, the findings of osteochondrosis of the humeral capitellum, osteochondritis dissecans of the humeral capitellum, osteochondritis of the radial head, hypertrophy of the ulna, traction apophysis of the olecranon, triceps tendinitis, and mild instability of the ulnar collateral ligament complex may be observed alone or in combination with the foregoing pathologic processes. Less commonly, nerve entrapment syndromes and subluxation of the ulnar nerve can also occur (Table 41-1).

SIGNS AND SYMPTOMS

The pain of thrower's elbow almost always includes pain localized to the region of the medial epicondyle in a manner analogous to golfer's elbow (Fig. 41-1). The patient may note the inability to hold a coffee cup or use a hammer, and the examiner may notice reduced grip strength. Sleep disturbance is common.

Other symptoms are the result of the other specific pathologic processes at play at the time of the examination. Patients suffering from thrower's elbow may exhibit mild instability of the ulnar collateral ligament complex caused by repetitive stretch injuries, as well as a decreased ability to extend the elbow fully. Active compression across the radiocapitellar joint

TABLE 41-1
Pathology Contributing to Thrower's Elbow
• Medial epicondylitis (golfer's elbow)
• Medial epicondylar apophysitis
• Medial epicondylar fragmentation
• Stress fractures involving the medial epicondylar epiphysis
• Avulsion fractures of the medial epicondyle
• Osteochondrosis of the humeral capitellum
• Osteochondritis dissecans of the humeral capitellum
• Osteochondritis of the radial head
• Hypertrophy of the ulna
• Traction apophysitis of the olecranon
• Triceps tendinitis
• Mild instability of the ulnar collateral ligament complex

from muscular forces may reproduce the patient's pain, as will an active radiocapitellar compression test, which is performed by having the patient pronate and supinate the forearm in full extension (Fig. 41-2).

Physical examination may also reveal localized tenderness along the flexor tendons at or just below the medial epicondyle. If the patient has an acute injury to the elbow, swelling and ecchymosis may be present. Increased valgus angle greater than 11 degrees in male patients and 13 degrees in female patients may also be noted. Flexion contracture may be present and results in a loss of full elbow extension (Fig. 41-3). In some high-performing athletes, these range-of-motion abnormalities represent adaptive changes and are not often the sole cause of the patient's pain symptoms. Palpation of the ulnar collateral ligament may reveal tenderness to palpation or complete disruption (Fig. 41-4A). Valgus instability in the patient suspected of suffering from thrower's elbow can best be assessed by perform the milking maneuver of Veltri, which is done by grasping the thrower's thumb with the arm in the fully cocked position (90 degrees of shoulder abduction and 90 degrees of elbow flexion) and then applying valgus stress by pulling down on the thumb (see Fig. 41-4B). The test result is considered positive if the patient's pain is reproduced.

The point at which the patient notes the onset of pain during the five-step throwing sequence may give the clinician a clue to the pathologic process primarily responsible for the pain; this knowledge can be especially useful when many elbow abnormalities are occurring simultaneously (Fig. 41-5). If the patient's pain occurs primarily during the acceleration phase, the clinician should pay special attention to the ulnar collateral ligament complex because the pain is often the result of elbow instability caused by stretching injuries. If the pain occurs primarily during

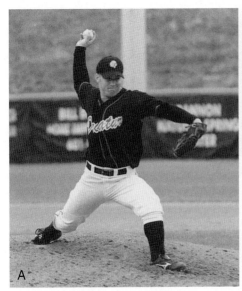
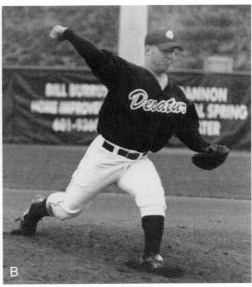

Figure 41-1 Adult male pitcher at the beginning **(A)** and end **(B)** of the late cocking phase of the throwing motion. This phase begins as the foot contacts the ground and ends as the arm reaches maximal external rotation. *(From DeLee JC, Drez DD, Miller M, editors: Orthopaedic sports medicine: principles and practice, ed 3, Philadelphia, 2010, Saunders, p 1215.)*

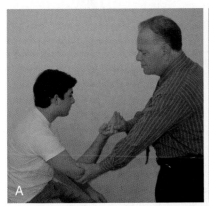
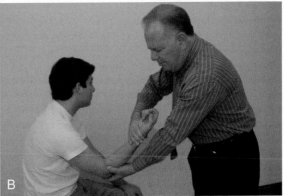

Figure 41-2 The active radiocapitellar compression test is performed by having the patient pronate and supinate the forearm in full extension. **A,** The wrist of the affected extremity is extended and deviated radially. **B,** The radiocapitellar joint is then compressed while the patient's elbow is actively flexed and extended and the forearm is pronated and supinated.

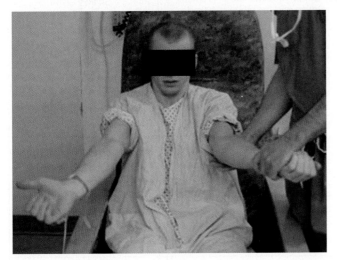

Figure 41-3 The patient is unable to extend his left elbow fully. *(From Erne HC, Zouzias IC, Rosenwasser MP: Medial collateral ligament reconstruction in the baseball pitcher's elbow, Hand Clin 25[3]:339–346, 2009.)*

late deceleration, medial epicondylitis and, less commonly, an ulnar nerve disorder are often the cause. Pain during deceleration should alert the clinician to pay special attention to the posterior elements of the elbow because olecranon and triceps tendon abnormalities and joint mice may be the problem.

TESTING

Plain radiographs should be obtained in all patients who present with elbow pain, to rule out joint mice and other occult bony pathologic processes such as avulsion fractures of the olecranon (Fig. 41-6). Based on the patient's clinical presentation, additional testing may be warranted, including a complete blood count, uric acid level, erythrocyte sedimentation rate, and antinuclear antibody testing. Magnetic resonance imaging of the elbow is indicated if joint instability is suspected or if the symptoms of thrower's elbow persist (Fig. 41-7). Electromyography (EMG) is indicated to diagnosis entrapment neuropathy at the elbow and to rule out cervical radiculopathy. The injection technique described later serves as both a diagnostic and a therapeutic maneuver.

DIFFERENTIAL DIAGNOSIS

Occasionally, cervical radiculopathy mimics thrower's elbow; however, patients suffering from cervical radiculopathy usually have neck pain and proximal upper extremity pain in addition to symptoms below the elbow. As noted earlier, EMG can distinguish radiculopathy from thrower's elbow. Bursitis, arthritis, and gout may also mimic thrower's elbow and confuse the diagnosis. The olecranon bursa lies in the posterior aspect of the elbow joint and may become inflamed as a result

Figure 41-4 A, Palpation of the ulnar collateral ligament. Palpation of the anterior band of the ulnar collateral ligament is performed with the elbow in 70 to 90 degrees of flexion. **B,** The milking maneuver of Veltri is performed by grasping the thrower's thumb with the arm in the fully cocked position and then applying valgus stress by pulling down on the thumb in a manner analogous to milking a cow.

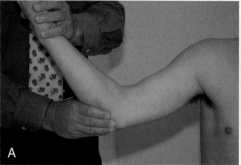 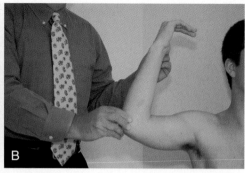

Phase 1: Windup	Begins with the pitcher balancing his or her weight over the rear leg, with the elbow flexed and the forward leg flexed at least 90 degrees.	
Phase 2: Early cocking/stride	Starts with the lead leg beginning to descend toward the plate, and the two arms separate. The elbow moves from extension into flexion of 80 to 100 degrees.	
Phase 3: Late cocking	Begins when the humerus is in extreme abduction and external rotation and the elbow is flexed. The lead foot contacts the ground, the pelvis and trunk rotate, and elbow torque transfers valgus force across the elbow joint. During this phase, medial tension and lateral compression forces are applied to the elbow.	
Phase 4: Acceleration/deceleration	Begins at ball release. Maximal external shoulder rotation occurs to release ball, with trunk rotating and the elbow rapidly extending. Ends when the shoulder has reached full internal rotation with the body decelerating the arm and dissipating the forces in the elbow and shoulder.	
Phase 5: Follow-through	Final phase of the baseball pitch and ends with the pitcher reaching a balanced fielding position with full-trunk rotation and the body weight fully transferred from the rear leg to the forward leg and the elbow flexing into a relaxed position.	

Figure 41-5 The throwing sequence. *(Modified from DeLee JC, Drez DD, Miller M, editors: Orthopaedic sports medicine: principles and practice, ed 3, Philadelphia, 2010, Saunders, p 1232.)*

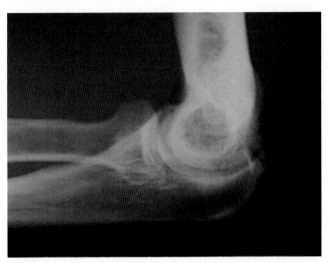

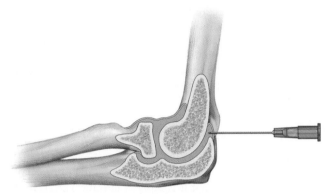

Figure 41-8 Elbow joint injection: posterior approach. A posterior puncture site between the medial and lateral epicondyles just proximal to the olecranon can be used to enter the elbow joint, although this is not recommended because the needle is not seen along its axis and is therefore more difficult to control precisely. *(From Peterson JJ, Fenton DS, Czervionke LF, editors:* Image-guided musculoskeletal interventions, *Philadelphia, 2008, Saunders, p 52.)*

Figure 41-6 Lateral radiograph demonstrating a posteromedial osteophyte involving the olecranon. Such pathologic findings are consistent with valgus extension overload secondary to persistent valgus instability. *(From Dodson CC, Altchek DW: Management of medial collateral ligament tears in the athlete,* Oper Tech Sports Med *14[2]:75–80, 2006.)*

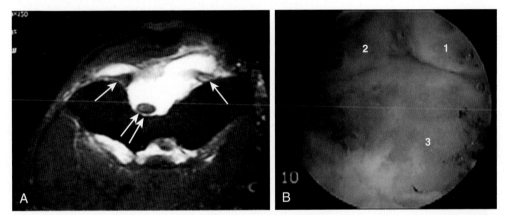

Figure 41-7 The changes that occur in the posterior elbow secondary to overloading. **A,** Axial magnetic resonance imaging of the distal humerus demonstrates an effusion, humeral osteophytes *(single arrows)*, and a loose body in olecranon fossa *(double arrows)*. Up is posterior in this image. **B,** Arthroscopic view of the medial elbow (left is medial, up is distal), demonstrates the tip of olecranon (1), a posteromedial olecranon osteophyte (2), and the olecranon fossa (3). *(From Hsu J, Gould JL, Fonseca-Sabune H, Hausman MH: The emerging role of elbow arthroscopy in chronic use injuries and fracture care,* Hand Clin *25[3]:305–321, 2009.)*

of direct trauma to the joint or its overuse. Other bursae susceptible to the development of bursitis are located between the insertion of the biceps and the head of the radius, as well as in the antecubital and cubital areas.

TREATMENT

Initial treatment of the pain and functional disability associated with thrower's elbow includes a combination of nonsteroidal anti-inflammatory drugs (NSAIDs) or cyclooxygenase-2 inhibitors and physical therapy. Local application of heat and cold may also be beneficial. Any repetitive activity that may exacerbate the patient's symptoms should be avoided. For patients who do not respond to these treatment modalities, injection with local anesthetic and steroid is a reasonable next step.

Injection for thrower's elbow is carried out by placing the patient in the supine position with the arm fully adducted at the

patient's side, the elbow fully extended, and the dorsum of the hand resting on a folded towel to relax the affected tendons. A total of 1 mL local anesthetic and 40 mg methylprednisolone is drawn up in a 5-mL sterile syringe. After sterile preparation of the skin overlying the medial aspect of the joint, the medial epicondyle is identified. Using strict aseptic technique, a 1-inch, 25-gauge needle is inserted perpendicular to the medial epicondyle through the skin and into the subcutaneous tissue overlying the affected tendon (Fig. 41-8). If bone is encountered, the needle is withdrawn into the subcutaneous tissue. The contents of the syringe are then gently injected. Little resistance to injection should be felt. If significant resistance is encountered, the needle is probably in the tendon and should be withdrawn until the injection can proceed with less resistance. The needle is then removed, and a sterile pressure dressing and ice pack are applied to the injection site.

Physical modalities, including local heat and gentle range-of-motion exercises, should be introduced several days after the patient undergoes injection for elbow pain. A Velcro band placed around the flexor tendons may also help relieve the symptoms. Occupational therapy for activities of daily living education may also be beneficial. Vigorous exercises should be avoided, because they will exacerbate the patient's symptoms, and return to play should not occur until the patient's symptoms are completely resolved.

COMPLICATIONS AND PITFALLS

The major complications associated with this injection technique are related to trauma to the inflamed and previously damaged tendon, which may rupture if it is injected directly. Therefore, the needle position should be confirmed to be outside the tendon before the clinician proceeds with the injection. Another complication of the injection technique is infection, although it should be exceedingly rare if strict aseptic technique is followed. Injection is safe if careful attention is paid to the clinically relevant anatomy; in particular, the ulnar nerve is susceptible to damage at the elbow. Approximately 25% of patients complain of a transient increase in pain after this injection technique, and patients should be warned of this possibility.

Clinical Pearls

A complete understanding of the biomechanics of overhead throwing is essential if the clinician is to diagnose and treat thrower's elbow successfully. The injection technique described is extremely effective in the treatment of pain secondary to thrower's elbow. Coexistent bursitis and tendinitis may contribute to elbow pain, thus necessitating additional treatment with more localized injection of local anesthetic and methylprednisolone. Simple analgesics and NSAIDs drugs can be used concurrently with this injection technique. Cervical radiculopathy may mimic thrower's elbow and must be excluded.

SUGGESTED READINGS

Cain EL Jr, Dugas JR: History and examination of the thrower's elbow, *Clin Sports Med* 23(4):553–566, 2004.

Ciccotti MC, Schwartz MA, Ciccotti MG: Diagnosis and treatment of medial epicondylitis of the elbow, *Clin Sports Med* 23(4):693–705, 2004.

Rineer CA, Ruch DS: Elbow tendinopathy and tendon ruptures: epicondylitis, biceps and triceps ruptures, *J Hand Surg* 34(3):566–576, 2009.

Wilk KE, Reinold MM, Andrews JR: Rehabilitation of the thrower's elbow, *Clin Sports Med* 23(4):765–801, 2004.

Chapter 42

ANCONEUS SYNDROME

ICD-9 CODE   **729.1**

ICD-10 CODE   **M79.7**

THE CLINICAL SYNDROME

The anconeus muscle is susceptible to the development of myofascial pain syndrome. Such pain is most often the result of repetitive microtrauma to the muscle caused by such activities as prolonged ironing, handshaking, or digging (Fig. 42-1). Tennis injuries caused by an improper one-handed backhand technique have also been implicated as an inciting factor in myofascial pain syndrome, as has blunt trauma to the muscle.

Myofascial pain syndrome is a chronic pain syndrome that affects a focal or regional portion of the body. The sine qua non of myofascial pain syndrome is the finding of myofascial trigger points on physical examination. Although these trigger points are generally localized to the part of the body affected, the pain is often referred to other areas. This referred pain may be misdiagnosed or attributed to other organ systems, thus leading to extensive evaluation and ineffective treatment. Patients with myofascial pain syndrome involving the anconeus often have referred pain in the ipsilateral forearm.

The trigger point is pathognomonic of myofascial pain syndrome and is characterized by a local point of exquisite tenderness in the affected muscle. Mechanical stimulation of the trigger point by palpation or stretching produces not only intense local pain but also referred pain. In addition, involuntary withdrawal of the stimulated muscle, called a jump sign, is often seen and is characteristic of myofascial pain syndrome. Patients with anconeus syndrome have a trigger point over the superior insertion of the muscle (Fig. 42-2).

Taut bands of muscle fibers are often identified when myofascial trigger points are palpated. In spite of this consistent physical finding, the pathophysiology of the myofascial trigger point remains elusive, although trigger points are believed to result from

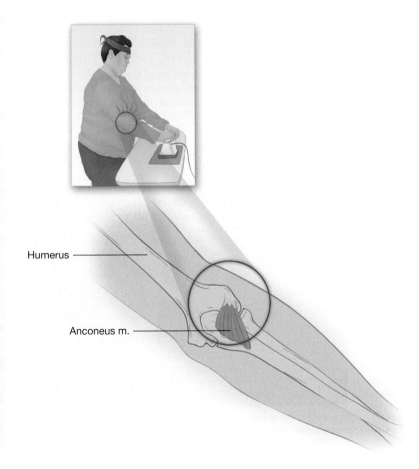

Humerus

Anconeus m.

Figure 42-1 Myofascial pain syndrome affecting the anconeus muscle usually results from repetitive microtrauma from activities such as prolonged ironing.

microtrauma to the affected muscle. This trauma may result from a single injury, repetitive microtrauma, or chronic deconditioning of the agonist and antagonist muscle unit.

In addition to muscle trauma, various other factors seem to predispose patients to develop myofascial pain syndrome. For instance, a weekend athlete who subjects his or her body to unaccustomed physical activity may develop myofascial pain syndrome. Poor posture while sitting at a computer or while watching television has also been implicated as a predisposing factor. Previous injuries may result in abnormal muscle function and lead to the development of myofascial pain syndrome. All these predisposing factors may be intensified if the patient also suffers from poor nutritional status or coexisting psychological or behavioral abnormalities, including chronic stress and depression. The anconeus muscle seems to be particularly susceptible to stress-induced myofascial pain syndrome.

Stiffness and fatigue often coexist with pain, and they increase the functional disability associated with this disease and complicate its treatment. Myofascial pain syndrome may occur as a primary disease state or in conjunction with other painful conditions, including radiculopathy and chronic regional pain syndromes. Psychological or behavioral abnormalities, including depression, frequently coexist with the muscle abnormalities, and management of these psychological disorders is an integral part of any successful treatment plan.

SIGNS AND SYMPTOMS

The trigger point is the pathologic lesion of anconeus syndrome, and it is characterized by a local point of exquisite tenderness over the superior insertion of the muscle (see Fig. 42-2). Mechanical

stimulation of the trigger point by palpation or stretching produces both intense local pain and referred pain. The jump sign is also characteristic of anconeus syndrome, as is pain over the anconeus muscle that is referred to the ipsilateral forearm.

TESTING

Biopsies of clinically identified trigger points have not revealed consistently abnormal histologic features. The muscle hosting the trigger points has been described either as "moth-eaten" or as containing "waxy degeneration." Increased plasma myoglobin has been reported in some patients with anconeus syndrome, but this finding has not been corroborated by other investigators. Electrodiagnostic testing of patients suffering from anconeus syndrome has revealed an increase in muscle tension in some patients, but again, this finding has not been reproducible. Because of the lack of objective diagnostic testing, the clinician must rule out other coexisting disease processes that may mimic anconeus syndrome (see "Differential Diagnosis").

DIFFERENTIAL DIAGNOSIS

The diagnosis of anconeus syndrome is made on the basis of clinical findings rather than specific laboratory, electrodiagnostic, or radiographic testing. For this reason, a targeted history and physical examination, with a systematic search for trigger points and identification of a positive jump sign, must be carried out in every patient suspected of suffering from anconeus syndrome. The anconeus muscle is susceptible to the development of a compartment syndrome, and this possibility should be considered in the differential diagnosis (Fig. 42-3). The clinician must rule out other coexisting disease processes that may mimic anconeus syndrome, including primary inflammatory muscle disease, multiple sclerosis, and collagen vascular disease. Electrodiagnostic and radiographic testing can help identify coexisting disorders such as bursitis, tendinitis, and epicondylitis (Fig. 42-4). The clinician must also identify coexisting psychological and behavioral abnormalities that may mask or exacerbate the symptoms associated with anconeus syndrome.

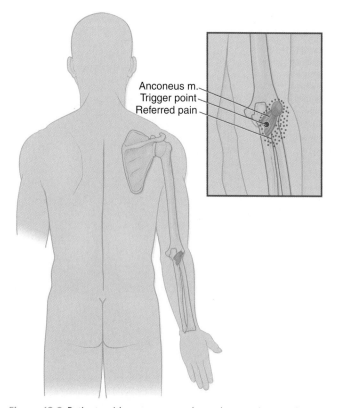

Figure 42-2 Patients with anconeus syndrome have a trigger point over the superior insertion of the muscle. *(From Waldman SD: Atlas of pain management injection techniques, ed 2, Philadelphia, 2007, Saunders, p 134.)*

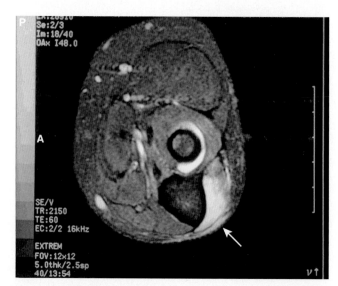

Figure 42-3 Magnetic resonance imaging indicates a signal change at the anconeus muscle consistent with edema *(arrow)*. *(From Steinmann SP, Bishop AT: Chronic anconeus compartment syndrome: a case report, J Hand Surg 25[5]:959–961, 2000.)*

TREATMENT

Treatment is focused on blocking the myofascial trigger and achieving prolonged relaxation of the affected muscle. Because the mechanism of action is poorly understood, an element of trial and error is often required when developing a treatment plan. Conservative therapy consisting of trigger point injections with local anesthetic or saline solution is the starting point. Because underlying depression and anxiety are present in many patients suffering from fibromyalgia, the administration of antidepressants is an integral part of most treatment plans. Pregabalin and gabapentin have also been shown to provide some palliation of the symptoms associated with fibromyalgia.

In addition, several adjuvant methods are available for the treatment of fibromyalgia of the cervical spine. The therapeutic use of heat and cold is often combined with trigger point injections and antidepressants to achieve pain relief. Some patients experience decreased pain with the application of transcutaneous nerve stimulation or electrical stimulation to fatigue the affected muscles. Exercise may also provide some palliation of symptoms and improve the fatigue associated with this disease. Although not currently approved by the Food and Drug Administration for this indication, the injection of minute quantities of botulinum toxin type A directly into trigger points has been used with success in patients who have not responded to traditional treatment modalities.

COMPLICATIONS AND PITFALLS

Trigger point injections are extremely safe if careful attention is paid to the clinically relevant anatomy. Sterile technique must be used to avoid infection, along with universal precautions to minimize any risk to the operator. Most complications of trigger point injection are related to needle-induced trauma at the injection site and in underlying tissues. The incidence of ecchymosis and hematoma formation can be decreased if pressure is applied to the injection site immediately after injection. The avoidance of overly long needles can decrease the incidence of trauma to underlying structures.

Clinical Pearls

Although anconeus syndrome is a common disorder, it is often misdiagnosed. Therefore, in patients suspected of suffering from anconeus syndrome, a careful evaluation to identify underlying disease processes is mandatory. Anconeus syndrome commonly coexists with various somatic and psychological disorders.

SUGGESTED READINGS

Bradley LA: Pathophysiology of fibromyalgia, *Am J Med* 122(12 Suppl 1):S22–S30, 2009.

Ge H-Y, Nie H, Madeleine P, et al: Contribution of the local and referred pain from active myofascial trigger points in fibromyalgia syndrome, *Pain* 147(1–3):233–240, 2009.

Hayter CL, Giuffre BM: Overuse and traumatic injuries of the elbow, *Magn Reson Imaging Clin N Am* 17(4):617–638, 2009.

Putnam MD, Cohen M: Painful conditions around the elbow, *Orthop Clin North Am* 30(1):109–118, 1999.

Steinmann SP, Bishop AT: Chronic anconeus compartment syndrome: a case report, *J Hand Surg* 25(5):959–961, 2000.

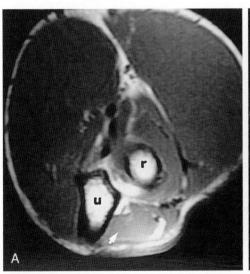 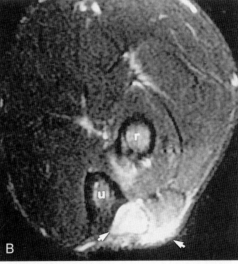

Figure 42-4 Anconeus muscle tear with edema in a 30-year-old male bodybuilder who experienced acute pain during weightlifting. Transaxial T1-weighted **(A)** and T2-weighted **(B)** spin-echo magnetic resonance images, the latter obtained with fat suppression, show altered morphology. In **B**, increased signal intensity is evident in the anconeus muscle and surrounding tissues *(arrows)*. Inflammatory changes about the biceps tendon are also seen. The radius (r) and ulna (u) are indicated. *(From Resnick D: Diagnosis of bone and joint disorders, ed 4, Philadelphia, 2002, Saunders, p 3065.)*

Chapter 43

SUPINATOR SYNDROME

ICD-9 CODE 729.1

ICD-10 CODE M79.7

THE CLINICAL SYNDROME

As its name implies, the supinator muscle supinates the forearm. Curving around the upper third of the radius, the supinator muscle is composed of a superficial and a deep layer. The superficial layer originates in a tendinous insertion from the lateral epicondyle of the humerus, the radial collateral ligament of the elbow, and the annular ligament of the supinator crest of the ulna.

The supinator muscle is susceptible to the development of myofascial pain syndrome. This pain is most often the result of repetitive microtrauma to the muscle caused by such activities as turning a screwdriver, prolonged ironing, handshaking, or digging with a trowel (Fig. 43-1). Tennis injuries caused by an improper one-handed backhand technique have also been implicated as an inciting factor in myofascial pain syndrome, as has blunt trauma to the muscle.

Myofascial pain syndrome is a chronic pain syndrome that affects a focal or regional portion of the body. The sine qua non of myofascial pain syndrome is the finding of myofascial trigger points on physical examination. Although these trigger points are generally localized to the part of the body affected, the pain is often referred to other areas. This referred pain may be misdiagnosed or attributed to other organ systems, thus leading to extensive evaluation and ineffective treatment. Patients with myofascial pain syndrome involving the supinator muscle often have referred pain in the ipsilateral forearm.

The trigger point is pathognomonic of myofascial pain syndrome and is characterized by a local point of exquisite tenderness in the affected muscle. Mechanical stimulation of the trigger point by palpation or stretching produces not only intense local pain but also referred pain. In addition, an involuntary withdrawal of the stimulated muscle, called a jump sign, is often seen and is characteristic of myofascial pain syndrome. Patients with supinator syndrome have a trigger point over the superior portion of the muscle (Fig. 43-2).

Taut bands of muscle fibers are often identified when myofascial trigger points are palpated. In spite of this consistent physical finding, the pathophysiology of the myofascial trigger point remains elusive, although trigger points are believed to result from microtrauma to the affected muscle. This trauma may result from a single injury, repetitive microtrauma, or chronic deconditioning of the agonist and antagonist muscle unit.

In addition to muscle trauma, various other factors seem to predispose patients to develop myofascial pain syndrome. For

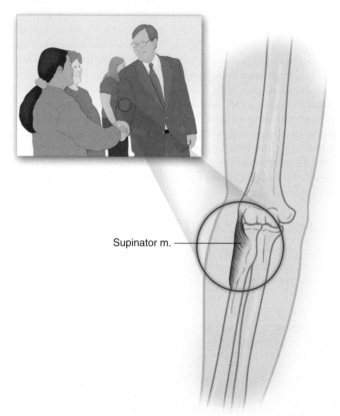

Figure 43-1 Myofascial pain syndrome affecting the supinator muscle is usually the result of repetitive microtrauma caused by activities such as turning a screwdriver, prolonged ironing, handshaking, or digging.

instance, a weekend athlete who subjects his or her body to unaccustomed physical activity may develop myofascial pain syndrome. Poor posture while sitting at a computer or while watching television has also been implicated as a predisposing factor. Previous injuries may result in abnormal muscle function and lead to the development of myofascial pain syndrome. All these predisposing factors may be intensified if the patient also suffers from poor nutritional status or coexisting psychological or behavioral abnormalities, including chronic stress and depression. The supinator muscle seems to be particularly susceptible to stress-induced myofascial pain syndrome.

Stiffness and fatigue often coexist with pain, and they increase the functional disability associated with this disease and complicate its treatment. Myofascial pain syndrome may occur as a primary disease state or in conjunction with other painful conditions, including radiculopathy and chronic regional pain syndromes. Psychological or behavioral abnormalities, including depression, frequently coexist with the muscle abnormalities, and

Supinator m.

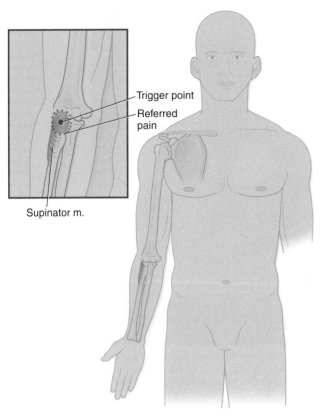

Figure 43-2 Patients with supinator syndrome have a trigger point over the superior portion of the muscle. *(From Waldman SD: Atlas of pain management injection techniques, ed 2, Philadelphia, 2007, Saunders, p 155.)*

management of these psychological disorders is an integral part of any successful treatment plan.

SIGNS AND SYMPTOMS

The trigger point is the pathologic lesion of supinator syndrome, and it is characterized by a local point of exquisite tenderness in the supinator muscle. This trigger point can best be demonstrated by having the patient supinate the forearm against active resistance. Point tenderness over the lateral epicondyle may also be present and may be amenable to injection therapy.

Mechanical stimulation of the trigger point by palpation or stretching produces both intense local pain and referred pain. The jump sign is also characteristic of supinator syndrome, as is pain over the supinator muscle that radiates from the lateral epicondyle and superior portion of the muscle into the forearm.

TESTING

Biopsies of clinically identified trigger points have not revealed consistently abnormal histologic features. The muscle hosting the trigger points has been described either as "moth-eaten" or as containing "waxy degeneration." Increased plasma myoglobin has been reported in some patients with supinator syndrome, but this finding has not been corroborated by other investigators. Electrodiagnostic testing of patients suffering from supinator syndrome has revealed an increase in muscle tension in some patients, but again, this finding has not been reproducible. Because of the lack of objective diagnostic testing, the clinician must rule out other

coexisting disease processes that may mimic supinator syndrome (see "Differential Diagnosis").

DIFFERENTIAL DIAGNOSIS

The diagnosis of supinator syndrome is made on the basis of clinical findings rather than specific laboratory, electrodiagnostic, or radiographic testing. For this reason, a targeted history and physical examination, with a systematic search for trigger points and identification of a positive jump sign, must be carried out in every patient suspected of suffering from supinator syndrome. The clinician must rule out other coexisting disease processes that may mimic supinator syndrome, including primary inflammatory muscle disease, collagen vascular disease, inflammatory arthritis, tennis elbow, radial tunnel syndrome, tumor, bursitis, tendinitis, and crystal deposition diseases (Fig. 43-3). Radiographic testing, including magnetic resonance imaging of the elbow, can help identify coexisting pathologic processes such as internal derangement of the elbow, tendinitis, and bursitis. Electromyography can rule out cubital and radial tunnel syndromes. The clinician must also identify coexisting psychological and behavioral abnormalities that may mask or exacerbate the symptoms associated with supinator syndrome.

TREATMENT

Treatment is focused on blocking the myofascial trigger and achieving prolonged relaxation of the affected muscle. Because the mechanism of action is poorly understood, an element of trial and error is often required when developing a treatment plan. Conservative therapy consisting of trigger point injections with local anesthetic or saline solution is the starting point. Because underlying depression and anxiety are present in many patients suffering from fibromyalgia, the administration of antidepressants is an integral part of most treatment plans. Pregabalin and gabapentin have also been shown to provide some palliation of the symptoms associated with fibromyalgia.

In addition, several adjuvant methods are available for the treatment of fibromyalgia of the cervical spine. The therapeutic use of heat and cold is often combined with trigger point injections and antidepressants to achieve pain relief. Some patients experience decreased pain with the application of transcutaneous nerve stimulation or electrical stimulation to fatigue the affected muscles. Exercise may also provide some palliation of symptoms and improve the fatigue associated with this disease. Although not currently approved by the Food and Drug Administration for this indication, the injection of minute quantities of botulinum toxin type A directly into trigger points has been used with success in patients who have not responded to traditional treatment modalities.

COMPLICATIONS AND PITFALLS

Trigger point injections are extremely safe if careful attention is paid to the clinically relevant anatomy. Sterile technique must be used to avoid infection, along with universal precautions to minimize any risk to the operator. Most complications of trigger point injection are related to needle-induced trauma at the injection site and in underlying tissues. The incidence of ecchymosis and hematoma formation can be decreased if pressure is applied to the injection site immediately after injection. The avoidance of overly long needles can decrease the incidence of trauma to underlying

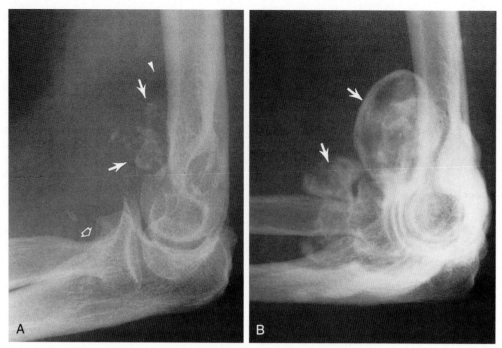

Figure 43-3 Idiopathic synovial osteochondromatosis. This 67-year-old woman reported progressive pain and swelling in her elbow over a 6-month period. **A,** The radiograph outlines irregular ossification in the joint *(solid arrows)*, with displacement of the anterior fat pad *(arrowhead)*, minor osseous erosion *(open arrow)*, and osteophytes. **B,** An arthrogram identifies multiple radiolucent filling defects *(arrows)*. The diagnosis was confirmed histologically. *(From Resnick D: Diagnosis of bone and joint disorders, ed 4, Philadelphia, 2002, Saunders, p 3067.)*

structures. Special care must be taken to avoid damage to the underlying neural structures when injecting trigger points in proximity to the elbow and forearm.

Clinical Pearls

> Although supinator syndrome is a common disorder, it is often misdiagnosed. Therefore, in patients suspected of suffering from supinator syndrome, a careful evaluation to identify underlying disease processes is mandatory. Supinator syndrome commonly coexists with various somatic and psychological disorders.

SUGGESTED READINGS

Bradley LA: Pathophysiology of fibromyalgia, *Am J Med* 122(12 Suppl 1): S22–S30, 2009.

Erak S, Day R, Wang A: The role of supinator in the pathogenesis of chronic lateral elbow pain: a biomechanical study, *J Hand Surg* 29(5):461–464, 2004.

Ge H-Y, Nie H, Madeleine P, et al: Contribution of the local and referred pain from active myofascial trigger points in fibromyalgia syndrome, *Pain* 147(1–3):233–240, 2009.

Hayter CL, Giuffre BM: Overuse and traumatic injuries of the elbow, *Magn Reson Imaging Clin N Am* 17(4):617–638, 2009.

Markiewitz AD, Merryman J: Radial nerve compression in the upper extremity, *J Am Soc Surg Hand* 5(2):87–99, 2005.

Chapter **44**

BRACHIORADIALIS SYNDROME

ICD-9 CODE **729.1**

ICD-10 CODE **M79.7**

THE CLINICAL SYNDROME

The brachioradialis muscle flexes the forearm at the elbow, pronates the forearm when supinated, and supinates the forearm when pronated. It originates at the upper lateral supracondylar ridge of the humerus and the lateral intermuscular septum of the humerus. The muscle inserts on the superior aspect of the styloid process of the radius, the lateral side of the distal radius, and the antebrachial fascia. The muscle is innervated by the radial nerve.

The brachioradialis muscle is susceptible to the development of myofascial pain syndrome. This pain is most often the result of repetitive microtrauma to the muscle from such activities as turning a screwdriver, prolonged ironing, repeated flexing of the forearm at the elbow (e.g., when using exercise equipment), handshaking, or digging with a trowel. Tennis injuries caused by an improper one-handed backhand technique have also been implicated as an inciting factor in myofascial pain syndrome, as has blunt trauma to the muscle (Fig. 44-1).

Myofascial pain syndrome is a chronic pain syndrome that affects a focal or regional portion of the body. The sine qua non of myofascial pain syndrome is the finding of myofascial trigger points on physical examination. Although these trigger points are generally localized to the part of the body affected, the pain is often referred to other areas. This referred pain may be misdiagnosed or attributed to other organ systems, thus leading to extensive evaluation and ineffective treatment. Patients with myofascial pain syndrome involving the brachioradialis muscle often have referred pain in the ipsilateral forearm and, on occasion, above the elbow.

The trigger point is the pathognomonic lesion of myofascial pain syndrome and is characterized by a local point of exquisite tenderness in the affected muscle. Mechanical stimulation of the trigger point by palpation or stretching produces not only intense local pain but also referred pain. In addition, involuntary withdrawal of the stimulated muscle, called a jump sign, is often seen and is characteristic of myofascial pain syndrome. Patients with brachioradialis syndrome have a trigger point over the superior belly of the muscle (Fig. 44-2).

Taut bands of muscle fibers are often identified when myofascial trigger points are palpated. In spite of this consistent physical finding, the pathophysiology of the myofascial trigger point remains elusive, although trigger points are believed to result from microtrauma to the affected muscle. This trauma may occur from a single injury, repetitive microtrauma, or chronic deconditioning of the agonist and antagonist muscle unit.

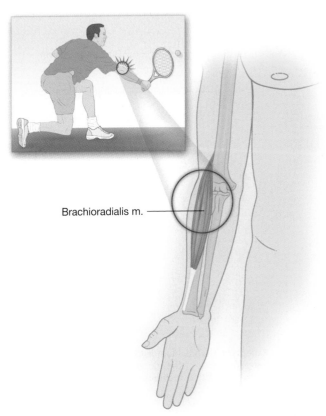

Brachioradialis m.

Figure 44-1 Tennis injuries caused by an improper one-handed backhand technique have been implicated in brachioradialis syndrome.

In addition to muscle trauma, various other factors seem to predispose patients to develop myofascial pain syndrome. For instance, a weekend athlete who subjects his or her body to unaccustomed physical activity may develop myofascial pain syndrome. Poor posture while sitting at a computer or while watching television has also been implicated as a predisposing factor. Previous injuries may result in abnormal muscle function and lead to the development of myofascial pain syndrome. All these predisposing factors may be intensified if the patient also suffers from poor nutritional status or coexisting psychological or behavioral abnormalities, including chronic stress and depression. The brachioradialis muscle seems to be particularly susceptible to stress-induced myofascial pain syndrome.

Stiffness and fatigue often coexist with pain, and they increase the functional disability associated with this disease and complicate its treatment. Myofascial pain syndrome may occur as a primary disease state or in conjunction with other painful conditions, including radiculopathy and chronic regional pain syndromes. Psychological or behavioral abnormalities, including

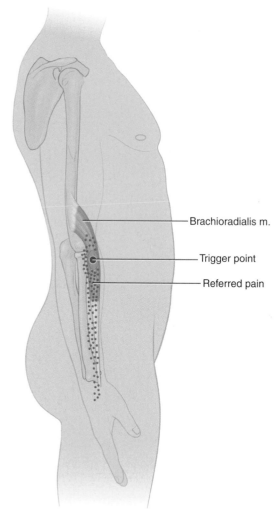

Brachioradialis m.

Trigger point

Referred pain

Figure 44-2 Patients with brachioradialis syndrome have a trigger point over the superior belly of the muscle. *(From Waldman SD: Atlas of pain management injection techniques, ed 2, Philadelphia, 2007, Saunders.)*

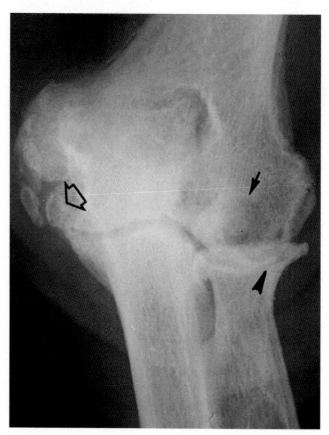

Figure 44-3 Characteristics of pyrophosphate arthropathy, including an unusual articular distribution. Changes in the elbow include joint space narrowing, subchondral cysts *(solid arrow)*, deformity of the radial head *(arrowhead)*, and fragmentation *(open arrow)*. *(From Resnick D: Diagnosis of bone and joint disorders, ed 4, Philadelphia, 2002, Saunders, p 1584.)*

depression, frequently coexist with the muscle abnormalities, and management of these psychological disorders is an integral part of any successful treatment plan.

SIGNS AND SYMPTOMS

The trigger point is the pathologic lesion of brachioradialis syndrome, and it is characterized by a local point of exquisite tenderness in the brachioradialis muscle. This trigger point can best be demonstrated by having the patient simultaneously flex and pronate the forearm against active resistance. Point tenderness over the lateral supracondylar ridge of the humerus may also be present and may be amenable to injection therapy.

Mechanical stimulation of the trigger point by palpation or stretching produces both intense local pain and referred pain. The jump sign is also characteristic of brachioradialis syndrome, as is pain over the brachioradialis muscle that radiates from the lateral epicondyle and superior portion of the muscle into the forearm.

TESTING

Biopsies of clinically identified trigger points have not revealed consistently abnormal histologic features. The muscle hosting the trigger points has been described either as "moth-eaten" or

as containing "waxy degeneration." Increased plasma myoglobin has been reported in some patients with brachioradialis syndrome, but this finding has not been corroborated by other investigators. Electrodiagnostic testing of patients suffering from brachioradialis syndrome has revealed an increase in muscle tension in some patients, but again, this finding has not been reproducible. Because of the lack of objective diagnostic testing, the clinician must rule out other coexisting disease processes that may mimic brachioradialis syndrome (see "Differential Diagnosis").

DIFFERENTIAL DIAGNOSIS

The diagnosis of brachioradialis syndrome is made on the basis of clinical findings rather than specific laboratory, electrodiagnostic, or radiographic testing. For this reason, a targeted history and physical examination, with a systematic search for trigger points and identification of a positive jump sign, must be carried out in every patient suspected of suffering from brachioradialis syndrome. The clinician must rule out other coexisting disease processes that may mimic brachioradialis syndrome, including primary inflammatory muscle disease and collagen vascular disease. Radiographic testing, including magnetic resonance imaging, can help identify coexisting pathologic processes such as internal derangement of the elbow, tumor, bursitis, tendinitis, crystal deposition diseases, and tennis elbow (Fig. 44-3). Electromyography can rule out cubital and radial tunnel syndromes. The clinician must also identify coexisting psychological and behavioral abnormalities that may mask or exacerbate the symptoms associated with brachioradialis syndrome.

TREATMENT

Treatment is focused on blocking the myofascial trigger and achieving prolonged relaxation of the affected muscle. Because the mechanism of action is poorly understood, an element of trial and error is often required when developing a treatment plan. Conservative therapy consisting of trigger point injections with local anesthetic or saline solution is the starting point. Because underlying depression and anxiety are present in many patients suffering from fibromyalgia, the administration of antidepressants is an integral part of most treatment plans. Pregabalin and gabapentin have also been shown to provide some palliation of the symptoms associated with fibromyalgia.

In addition, several adjuvant methods are available for the treatment of fibromyalgia of the cervical spine. The therapeutic use of heat and cold is often combined with trigger point injections and antidepressants to achieve pain relief. Some patients experience decreased pain with the application of transcutaneous nerve stimulation or electrical stimulation to fatigue the affected muscles. Exercise may also provide some palliation of symptoms and improve the fatigue associated with this disease. Although not currently approved by the Food and Drug Administration for this indication, the injection of minute quantities of botulinum toxin type A directly into trigger points has been used with success in patients who have not responded to traditional treatment modalities.

COMPLICATIONS AND PITFALLS

Trigger point injections are extremely safe if careful attention is paid to the clinically relevant anatomy. Sterile technique must be used to avoid infection, along with universal precautions to minimize any risk to the operator. Most complications of trigger point injection are related to needle-induced trauma at the injection site and in underlying tissues. The incidence of ecchymosis and hematoma formation can be decreased if pressure is applied to the injection site immediately after injection. The avoidance of overly long needles can decrease the incidence of trauma to underlying structures. Special care must be taken to avoid damage to the underlying neural structures when injecting trigger points in proximity to the elbow and forearm.

Clinical Pearls

Although brachioradialis syndrome is a common disorder, it is often misdiagnosed. Therefore, in patients suspected of suffering from brachioradialis syndrome, a careful evaluation to identify underlying disease processes is mandatory. Brachioradialis syndrome commonly coexists with various somatic and psychological disorders.

SUGGESTED READINGS

Bradley LA: Pathophysiology of fibromyalgia, *Am J Med* 122(12 Suppl 1): S22–S30, 2009.

Ge H-Y, Nie H, Madeleine P, et al: Contribution of the local and referred pain from active myofascial trigger points in fibromyalgia syndrome, *Pain* 147(1–3): 233–240, 2009.

Hayter CL, Giuffre BM: Overuse and traumatic injuries of the elbow, *Magn Reson Imaging Clin N Am* 17(4):617–638, 2009.

Putnam MD, Cohen M: Painful conditions around the elbow, *Orthop Clin North Am* 30(1):109–118, 1999.

Waldman SD: Brachioradialis syndrome. In Waldman SD, editor: *Atlas of pain management injection techniques*, ed 3, Philadelphia, 2009, Saunders, pp 158–161.

Chapter 45

ULNAR NERVE ENTRAPMENT AT THE ELBOW

ICD-9 CODE **354.2**

ICD-10 CODE **G65.20**

THE CLINICAL SYNDROME

Ulnar nerve entrapment at the elbow is one of the most common entrapment neuropathies encountered in clinical practice. Causes include compression of the ulnar nerve by an aponeurotic band that runs from the medial epicondyle of the humerus to the medial border of the olecranon, direct trauma to the ulnar nerve at the elbow, and repetitive elbow motion. Ulnar nerve entrapment at the elbow is also called tardy ulnar palsy, cubital tunnel syndrome, and ulnar nerve neuritis. This entrapment neuropathy manifests as pain and associated paresthesias in the lateral forearm that radiate to the wrist and to the ring and little fingers. Some patients also notice pain referred to the medial aspect of the scapula on the affected side. Untreated, ulnar nerve entrapment at the elbow can result in a progressive motor deficit and, ultimately, flexion contracture of the affected fingers. Symptoms usually begin after repetitive elbow motion or repeated pressure on the elbow, such as leaning on the elbow while lying on the floor (Fig. 45-1). Direct trauma to the ulnar nerve as it enters the cubital tunnel may result in a similar clinical presentation. Patients vulnerable to nerve syndromes, such as diabetic and alcoholic patients, are at greater risk for the development of ulnar nerve entrapment at the elbow.

SIGNS AND SYMPTOMS

Physical findings include tenderness over the ulnar nerve at the elbow. A positive Tinel sign is usually present over the ulnar nerve as it passes beneath the aponeurosis. Weakness of the intrinsic muscles of the forearm and hand that are innervated by the ulnar nerve may be identified with careful manual muscle testing; however, early in the course of cubital tunnel syndrome, the only physical finding other than tenderness over the nerve may be loss of sensation on the ulnar side of the little finger. Muscle wasting of the intrinsic muscles of the hand can best be identified by viewing the hand from above with the palm down. Patients suffering from ulnar nerve entrapment at the elbow often exhibit a positive Froment sign, which is due to weakness of the adductor pollicis brevis and flexor pollicis brevis muscles (Fig. 45-2A). Patients with significant muscle weakness secondary to ulnar nerve entrapment at the elbow also exhibit a positive Wartenberg sign, with patients often complaining that the little finger gets caught outside the pants pocket when they reach for car keys (Fig. 45-2B).

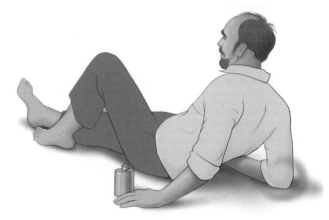

Figure 45-1 The ulnar nerve is susceptible to compression at the elbow.

TESTING

Electromyography and nerve conduction velocity studies are extremely sensitive tests, and a skilled electromyographer can diagnose ulnar nerve entrapment at the elbow with a high degree of accuracy, as well as distinguish other neuropathic causes of pain that may mimic it, including radiculopathy and plexopathy. Plain radiographs are indicated in all patients who present with ulnar nerve entrapment at the elbow to rule out occult bony disorders. If surgery is contemplated, magnetic resonance imaging (MRI) of the affected elbow may further delineate the pathologic process responsible for the nerve entrapment (e.g., bone spur, aponeurotic band thickening) (Fig. 45-3). Ultrasound imaging of the ulnar nerve may also help identify nerve disease (Fig. 45-4). If Pancoast's tumor or some other tumor of the brachial plexus is suspected, chest radiographs with apical lordotic views may be helpful. If the diagnosis is in question, screening laboratory tests consisting of a complete blood count, erythrocyte sedimentation rate, antinuclear antibody testing, and automated blood chemistry should be performed to rule out other causes of the patient's pain. The injection technique described later serves as both a diagnostic and a therapeutic maneuver.

DIFFERENTIAL DIAGNOSIS

Ulnar nerve entrapment at the elbow is often misdiagnosed as golfer's elbow, which explains why many patients with presumed golfer's elbow fail to respond to conservative measures (see Chapter 39). In patients with cubital tunnel syndrome, the maximal tenderness to palpation is over the ulnar nerve 1 inch below the medial epicondyle, whereas with golfer's elbow, the maximal tenderness to palpation is directly over the medial epicondyle. Cubital

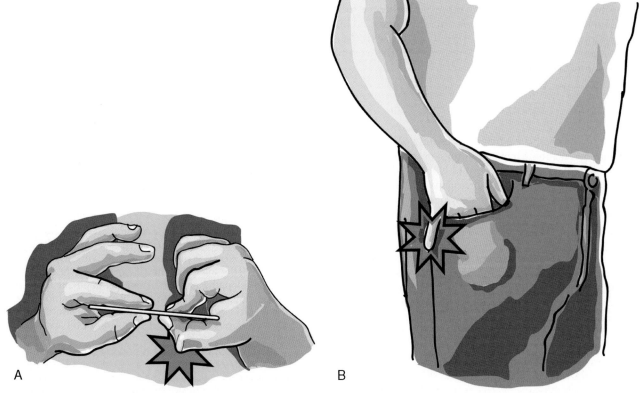

Figure 45-2 **A,** Froment's sign is elicited by asking the patient to grasp a piece of paper lightly between the thumb and index finger of each hand and monitoring flexion of the thumb interphalangeal joint on the affected side. **B,** Wartenberg's sign for ulnar nerve entrapment at the elbow. *(From Waldman SD: The little finger adduction test for ulnar nerve entrapment at the elbow. In Physical diagnosis of pain: an atlas of signs and symptoms, ed 2, Philadelphia, 2010, Saunders, pp 126, 128.)*

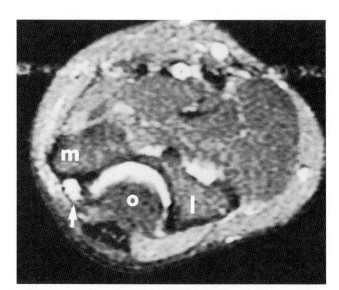

Figure 45-3 Entrapment neuropathy: cubital tunnel syndrome. A transaxial T2-weighted spin-echo magnetic resonance image, obtained with fat suppression, shows increased signal intensity in the ulnar nerve *(arrow)* within the cubital tunnel. The medial (m) and lateral (l) epicondyles of the humerus and the olecranon process (o) of the ulna are indicated. Joint effusion is present. *(From Resnick D: Diagnosis of bone and joint disorders, ed 4, Philadelphia, 2002, Saunders, p 3065.)*

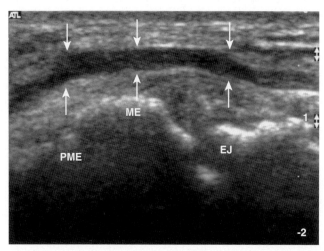

Figure 45-4 Longitudinal ultrasound image at the medial elbow demonstrating the ulnar nerve *(arrows),* which shows diffuse swelling above and below the medial epicondyle (ME). The *arrows* define the outline of the swollen nerve section. EJ, elbow joint; PME, proximal end of the medial epicondyle. *(From Park G-Y, Kim J-M, Lee S-M: The ultrasonographic and electrodiagnostic findings of ulnar neuropathy at the elbow, Arch Phys Med Rehabil 85[6]:1000–1005, 2004.)*

tunnel syndrome should also be differentiated from cervical radiculopathy involving the C7 or C8 roots. Further, cervical radiculopathy and ulnar nerve entrapment may coexist as the double-crush syndrome. The double-crush syndrome is seen most commonly with median nerve entrapment at the wrist or with carpal tunnel syndrome.

TREATMENT

A short course of conservative therapy consisting of simple analgesics, nonsteroidal antiinflammatory drugs, or cyclooxygenase-2 inhibitors, along with splinting to avoid elbow flexion, is indicated in patients who present with ulnar nerve entrapment at the elbow. If no marked improvement in symptoms occurs within 1 week, careful injection of the ulnar nerve at the elbow using the following technique is a reasonable next step.

Ulnar nerve injection at the elbow is carried out by placing the patient in the supine position with the arm fully adducted at the patient's side, the elbow slightly flexed, and the dorsum of the hand resting on a folded towel. A total of 5 to 7 mL local anesthetic is drawn up in a 12-mL sterile syringe. For the first block, 80 mg methylprednisolone is added to the local anesthetic; 40 mg depot steroid is added with subsequent blocks. The clinician identifies the olecranon process and the medial epicondyle of the humerus; the ulnar nerve sulcus is located between these two bony landmarks. After preparation of the skin with antiseptic solution, a ⅝-inch, 25-gauge needle is inserted just proximal to the sulcus and is slowly advanced with a slightly cephalad trajectory. When the needle has advanced approximately half an inch, a strong paresthesia in the distribution of the ulnar nerve will be elicited. The patient should be warned to expect this and to say "There!" as soon as the paresthesia is felt. After the paresthesia is elicited and its distribution is identified, gentle aspiration is performed to identify blood. If the aspiration test result is negative and no persistent paresthesia in the distribution of the ulnar nerve remains, 5 to 7 mL of local anesthetic solution is slowly injected while the patient is monitored closely for signs of local anesthetic toxicity. If no paresthesia can be elicited, a similar amount of solution is slowly injected in a fanlike manner just proximal to the notch, with care taken to avoid intravascular injection.

If the patient does not respond to these treatments or experiences progressive neurologic deficits, surgical decompression of the ulnar nerve is indicated. As mentioned earlier, MRI of the affected elbow can clarify the pathologic process responsible for the ulnar nerve compression.

COMPLICATIONS AND PITFALLS

Failure to identify and treat ulnar nerve entrapment at the elbow promptly can result in permanent neurologic deficit. To avoid harm to the patient, the clinician must also rule out other causes of pain and numbness that may mimic the symptoms of ulnar nerve entrapment, such as Pancoast's tumor.

Ulnar nerve block at the elbow is relatively safe. The major complications are inadvertent intravascular injection into the ulnar artery and persistent paresthesia secondary to needle-induced trauma to the nerve. Because the nerve passes through the ulnar nerve sulcus and is enclosed by a dense fibrous band, care should be taken to inject slowly, just proximal to the sulcus, to avoid additional compromise of the nerve.

Clinical Pearls

Ulnar nerve entrapment at the elbow is often misdiagnosed as golfer's elbow. It must also be differentiated from cervical radiculopathy involving the C8 spinal root; however, cervical radiculopathy and ulnar nerve entrapment may coexist in the double-crush syndrome. Pancoast's tumor invading the medial cord of the brachial plexus may also mimic ulnar nerve entrapment and must be ruled out by apical lordotic chest radiography.

If cubital tunnel syndrome is suspected, injection of the ulnar nerve at the elbow with local anesthetic and steroid provides almost instantaneous relief. This is a simple and safe technique for the evaluation and treatment of ulnar nerve entrapment. Before ulnar nerve block is performed, a careful neurologic examination should be done to identify preexisting neurologic deficits that could later be attributed to the nerve block. Persistent paresthesia tends to develop when the nerve is blocked at this level. The incidence of this complication can be decreased by blocking the nerve proximal to the ulnar nerve sulcus and injecting slowly.

SUGGESTED READINGS

Bencardino JT, Rosenberg ZS: Entrapment neuropathies of the shoulder and elbow in the athlete, *Clin Sports Med* 25(3):465–487, 2006.

Burge P: Abducted little finger in low ulnar nerve palsy, *J Hand Surg* 11(2): 234–236, 1986.

Waldman SD: Ulnar nerve entrapment at the elbow. In *Pain review*, Philadelphia, 2009, Saunders, pp 270–271.

Waldman SD: The little finger adduction test for ulnar nerve entrapment at the elbow. In *Physical diagnosis of pain: an atlas of signs and symptoms*, ed 2, Philadelphia, 2010, Saunders, pp 124–125.

Waldman SD: The Wartenberg test for ulnar nerve entrapment at the elbow. In *Physical diagnosis of pain: an atlas of signs and symptoms*, ed 2, Philadelphia, 2010, Saunders, pp 123–124.

Chapter 46

LATERAL ANTEBRACHIAL CUTANEOUS NERVE ENTRAPMENT AT THE ELBOW

ICD-9 CODE **354.8**

ICD-10 CODE **G56.80**

THE CLINICAL SYNDROME

The lateral antebrachial cutaneous nerve may be entrapped by the biceps tendon or the brachialis muscle (Fig. 46-1). Clinically, patients complain of pain and paresthesias radiating from the elbow to the base of the thumb. Dull aching of the radial aspect of the forearm is also common. The pain of lateral antebrachial cutaneous nerve entrapment at the elbow may develop after an acute twisting injury to the elbow or direct trauma to the soft tissues overlying the lateral antebrachial cutaneous nerve; in other cases, the onset of pain is more insidious, without an obvious inciting factor. The pain is constant and becomes worse with use of the elbow. Patients with lateral antebrachial cutaneous nerve entrapment often note an increase in pain when using a computer keyboard or playing the piano (Fig. 46-2). Sleep disturbance is common.

SIGNS AND SYMPTOMS

On physical examination, the patient notes tenderness to palpation of the lateral antebrachial cutaneous nerve at a point just lateral to the biceps tendon (Fig. 46-3). Elbow range of motion is normal. Patients with lateral antebrachial cutaneous nerve entrapment experience pain with active resisted flexion or rotation of the forearm.

TESTING

Electromyography and nerve conduction velocity studies are extremely sensitive tests, and a skilled electromyographer can diagnose lateral antebrachial cutaneous nerve entrapment with a high degree of accuracy, as well as distinguish other neuropathic causes of pain that may mimic it, including radiculopathy and plexopathy. Plain radiographs are indicated in all patients who present with lateral antebrachial cutaneous nerve entrapment to rule out occult bony disorders. If surgery is contemplated, magnetic resonance imaging (MRI) of the affected elbow may further delineate the pathologic process responsible for the nerve entrapment (e.g., bone spur, aponeurotic band thickening). If Pancoast's tumor or some other tumor of the brachial plexus is suspected, chest radiographs with apical lordotic views may be helpful. If the diagnosis is in question, screening laboratory tests consisting of a complete blood count, erythrocyte sedimentation rate, antinuclear antibody testing, and automated blood chemistry should be performed to

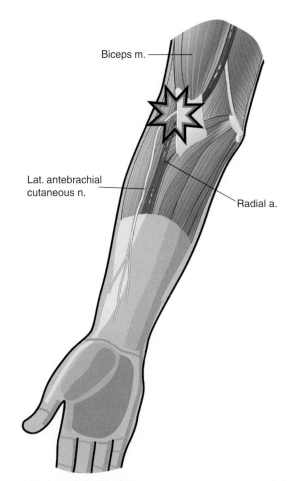

Figure 46-1 Lateral antebrachial cutaneous nerve entrapment: relevant soft tissue anatomy. *(From Waldman SD: Physical diagnosis of pain: an atlas of signs and symptoms, Philadelphia, 2006, Saunders, p 130.)*

rule out other causes of the patient's pain. Injection of the nerve serves as both a diagnostic and a therapeutic maneuver.

DIFFERENTIAL DIAGNOSIS

Cervical radiculopathy and tennis elbow can mimic nerve entrapment. In patients with lateral antebrachial cutaneous nerve entrapment, the maximal tenderness to palpation is at the level of the biceps tendon, whereas with tennis elbow, the maximal tenderness to palpation is over the lateral epicondyle (see Chapter 38). Electromyography can distinguish cervical radiculopathy and lateral antebrachial cutaneous nerve entrapment from tennis elbow. Further, cervical radiculopathy and lateral antebrachial cutaneous nerve entrapment may coexist as the double-crush

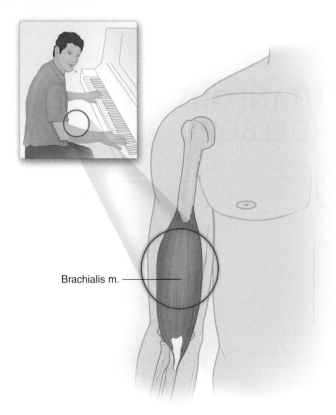

Figure 46-2 Patients with lateral antebrachial cutaneous nerve entrapment at the elbow often note increased pain when using a computer keyboard or playing the piano.

Brachialis m.

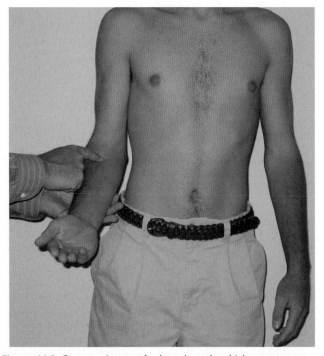

Figure 46-3 Compression test for lateral antebrachial cutaneous nerve entrapment. *(From Waldman SD: Physical diagnosis of pain: an atlas of signs and symptoms, Philadelphia, 2006, Saunders, p 131.)*

syndrome. The double-crush syndrome is seen most commonly with median nerve entrapment at the wrist or with carpal tunnel syndrome.

TREATMENT

A short course of conservative therapy consisting of simple analgesics, nonsteroidal antiinflammatory drugs, or cyclooxygenase-2 inhibitors, along with splinting to avoid elbow flexion, is indicated in patients who present with lateral antebrachial cutaneous nerve entrapment at the elbow. If no marked improvement in symptoms occurs within 1 week, careful injection of the lateral antebrachial cutaneous nerve at the elbow is a reasonable next step.

If the patient does not respond to these treatments or experiences progressive neurologic deficits, surgical decompression of the lateral antebrachial cutaneous nerve is indicated. As mentioned, MRI of the affected elbow can clarify the pathologic process responsible for nerve compression.

COMPLICATIONS AND PITFALLS

Failure to identify and treat lateral antebrachial cutaneous nerve entrapment at the elbow promptly can result in permanent neurologic deficit. To avoid harm to the patient, the clinician must rule out other causes of pain and numbness that may mimic the symptoms of lateral antebrachial cutaneous nerve entrapment, such as Pancoast's tumor.

Lateral antebrachial cutaneous nerve block at the elbow is relatively safe. The major complications are inadvertent intravascular injection into the lateral antebrachial cutaneous artery and persistent paresthesia secondary to needle-induced trauma to the nerve. Because the nerve passes through the lateral antebrachial cutaneous nerve sulcus and is enclosed by a dense fibrous band, care should be taken to inject slowly, just proximal to the sulcus, to avoid additional compromise of the nerve.

Clinical Pearls

> Lateral antebrachial cutaneous nerve entrapment at the elbow is often misdiagnosed as tennis elbow, which explains why many patients with presumed tennis elbow fail to respond to conservative measures. Lateral antebrachial cutaneous nerve block at the elbow is a simple and safe technique for the evaluation and treatment of this condition. Before the nerve block is performed, a careful neurologic examination should be done to identify preexisting neurologic deficits that could later be attributed to the nerve block. The incidence of persistent paresthesia can be decreased by blocking the nerve proximal to the lateral antebrachial cutaneous nerve sulcus and injecting slowly.

SUGGESTED READINGS

Allen DM, Nunley JA: Lateral antebrachial cutaneous neuropathy, *Oper Tech Sports Med* 9(4):222–224, 2001.

Belzile E, Cloutier D: Entrapment of the lateral antebrachial cutaneous nerve exiting through the forearm fascia, *J Hand Surg* 26(1):64–67, 2001.

Gillingham BL, Mack GR: Compression of the lateral antebrachial cutaneous nerve by the biceps tendon, *J Shoulder Elbow Surg* 5(4):330–332, 1996.

Waldman SD: The lateral antebrachial cutaneous nerve. In *Pain review*, Philadelphia, 2009, Saunders, p 99.

Chapter 47

OSTEOCHONDRITIS DISSECANS OF THE ELBOW

ICD-9 CODE 732.7

ICD-10 CODE M93.20

THE CLINICAL SYNDROME

Although osteochondritis dissecans was first described in the late 1800s, its exact etiology remains unknown. Current thinking is that osteochondritis dissecans is the result of continual microtrauma to the articular cartilage of the elbow. Studies suggested that this repetitive microtrauma causes an ischemic insult to the cartilage and supporting structures that results in the characteristic localized separation of the articular cartilage and subchondral bone. Osteochondritis dissecans most often affects the elbow of the dominant upper extremity in young male athletes. Sports most often associated with the development of osteochondritis dissecans include racquetball, baseball, weight lifting, and competitive gymnastics (Fig. 47-1). Pain on use of the affected elbow is universally present in patients suffering with osteochondritis dissecans and improves at rest. The pain is often deep, dull, and poorly defined. Loose bodies of the joint are common. Bilateral disease has been reported.

SIGNS AND SYMPTOMS

The pain of osteochondritis dissecans is generally the patient's first indication of an elbow problem. The pain is poorly localized, and the patient often rubs his or her elbow when trying to describe it. If joint mice are present, the patient may complain of grating or popping sensations with flexion and extension of the affected elbow. Sleep disturbance is common. Patients suffering from osteochondritis dissecans may exhibit a decreased ability to extend the affected elbow fully. Active compression across the radiocapitellar joint from muscular forces may reproduce the patient's pain, as will an active radiocapitellar compression test, which is performed by having the patient pronate and supinate the forearm while flexing and extending the elbow (Fig. 47-2A and B). Physical examination may also reveal tenderness to palpation of the elbow. If the patient

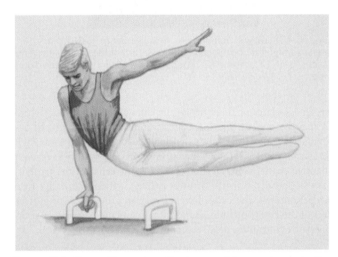

Figure 47-1 Competitive gymnastics is one of the sports most often associated with the development of osteochondritis dissecans. *(From Dorling Kindersley/Getty images, New York, 2010.)*

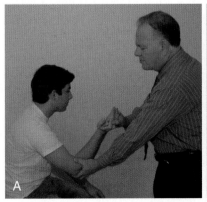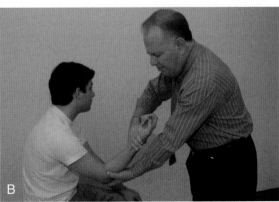

Figure 47-2 The active radiocapitellar compression test is performed by having the patient pronate and supinate the forearm while flexing and extending the elbow.

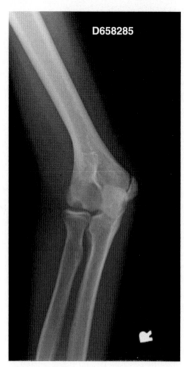

Figure 47-3 Lateral radiograph demonstrating radiolucency and rarefaction typical of osteochondritis dissecans of the capitellum. *(From Savoie FH III: Osteochondritis dissecans of the elbow,* Oper Tech Sports Med *16[4]:187–193, 2008.)*

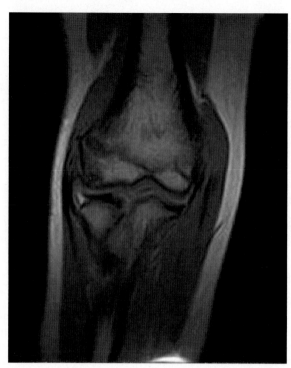

Figure 47-4 Coronal magnetic resonance image of osteochondritis dissecans of the capitellum. Increased signal intensity of the T2-weighted image indicates a detachment of the primary fragment. *(From Savoie FH III: Osteochondritis dissecans of the elbow,* Oper Tech Sports Med *16[4]:187–193, 2008.)*

has an associated acute injury to the elbow, swelling and ecchymosis may be present. Flexion contracture may also be present and results in a loss of full elbow extension (see Fig. 41-3). In some high-performing athletes, these range-of-motion abnormalities represent adaptive changes and are not often the sole cause of the patient's pain symptoms. As with thrower's elbow, patients suffering from osteochondritis dissecans often suffer from other coexisting disorders of the elbow including tendinitis, ligamentous injury, myofascial pain syndromes, nerve entrapments, and bursitis.

TESTING

Plain radiographs should be obtained in all patients who present with elbow pain, to rule out joint mice and other occult bony disorders such as avulsion fractures of the olecranon (Fig. 47-3) Based on the patient's clinical presentation, additional testing may be warranted, including a complete blood count, uric acid level, erythrocyte sedimentation rate, and antinuclear antibody testing. Magnetic resonance imaging of the elbow is indicated if joint instability is suspected or if the symptoms of osteochondritis dissecans persist (Fig. 47-4). Electromyography (EMG) is indicated to diagnose entrapment neuropathy at the elbow and to exclude cervical radiculopathy. The injection technique described later serves as both a diagnostic and a therapeutic maneuver.

DIFFERENTIAL DIAGNOSIS

Occasionally, cervical radiculopathy mimics osteochondritis dissecans; however, patients suffering from cervical radiculopathy usually have neck pain and proximal upper extremity pain in addition to symptoms below the elbow. As noted earlier, EMG can distinguish radiculopathy from osteochondritis

dissecans. Bursitis, arthritis, tendinitis, and gout may also mimic osteochondritis dissecans and confuse the diagnosis. The olecranon bursa lies in the posterior aspect of the elbow joint and may become inflamed as a result of direct trauma to the joint or its overuse. Other bursae susceptible to the development of bursitis are located between the insertion of the biceps and the head of the radius, as well as in the antecubital and cubital areas.

TREATMENT

Initial treatment of the pain and functional disability associated with osteochondritis dissecans includes a combination of nonsteroidal antiinflammatory drugs (NSAIDs) or cyclooxygenase-2 inhibitors and physical therapy. Local application of heat and cold may also be beneficial. Any repetitive activity that may exacerbate the patient's symptoms should be avoided. For patients who do not respond to these treatment modalities, injection with local anesthetic and steroid is a reasonable next step.

Injection for osteochondritis dissecans is carried out by placing the patient in the supine position with the arm fully adducted at the patient's side, the elbow fully extended, and the dorsum of the hand resting on a folded towel to relax the affected tendons. A total of 1 mL local anesthetic and 40 mg methylprednisolone is drawn up in a 5-mL sterile syringe. After sterile preparation of the skin overlying the medial aspect of the joint, the medial epicondyle is identified. Using strict aseptic technique, a 1-inch, 25-gauge needle is inserted perpendicular to the medial epicondyle through the skin and into the subcutaneous tissue overlying the affected tendon. If bone is encountered, the needle is withdrawn into the subcutaneous tissue. The contents of the syringe are then gently injected. Little resistance to injection should be felt. If significant resistance is encountered, the needle is probably in the tendon and should be withdrawn until the injection can proceed with less resistance. The needle is then removed, and a sterile pressure dressing and ice pack are applied to the injection site.

Physical modalities, including local heat and gentle range-of-motion exercises, should be introduced several days after the patient undergoes injection for elbow pain. A Velcro band placed around the flexor tendons may also help relieve the symptoms. Occupational therapy for activities of daily living education may also be beneficial. Vigorous exercises should be avoided, because they will exacerbate the patient's symptoms, and return to play should not occur until the patient's symptoms are completely resolved.

COMPLICATIONS AND PITFALLS

The major complications associated with this injection technique are related to trauma to the inflamed and previously damaged tendon, which may rupture if it is injected directly. Therefore, the needle position should be confirmed to be outside the tendon before the clinician proceeds with the injection. Another complication of the injection technique is infection, although it should be exceedingly rare if strict aseptic technique is followed. Injection is safe if careful attention is paid to the clinically relevant anatomy; in particular, the ulnar nerve is susceptible to damage at the elbow. Approximately 25%

of patients complain of a transient increase in pain after this injection technique, and patients should be warned of this possibility.

Clinical Pearls

A complete understanding of the biomechanics of overhead throwing is essential if the clinician is to diagnose and treat osteochondritis dissecans successfully. The injection technique described is extremely effective in the treatment of pain secondary to osteochondritis dissecans. Coexistent bursitis and tendinitis may contribute to elbow pain, thus necessitating additional treatment with more localized injection of local anesthetic and methylprednisolone. Simple analgesics and NSAIDs can be used concurrently with this injection technique. Cervical radiculopathy may mimic osteochondritis dissecans and must be excluded.

SUGGESTED READINGS

Birk GT, DeLee JC: Osteochondral injuries: clinical findings, *Clin Sports Med* 20(2):279–286, 2001.

Ciccotti MC, Schwartz MA, Ciccotti MG: Diagnosis and treatment of medial epicondylitis of the elbow, *Clin Sports Med* 23(4):693–705, 2004.

Jones RB, Miller RH III: Bony overuse injuries about the elbow, *Oper Tech Orthop* 11(1):55–62, 2001.

Rineer CA, Ruch DS: Elbow tendinopathy and tendon ruptures: epicondylitis, biceps and triceps ruptures, *J Hand Surg* 34(3):566–576, 2009.

Stubbs MJ, Field LD, Savoie FH III: Osteochondritis dissecans of the elbow, *Clin Sports Med* 29(1):1–9, 2001.

Chapter 48

OLECRANON BURSITIS

ICD-9 CODE `726.33`

ICD-10 CODE `M70.20`

THE CLINICAL SYNDROME

Olecranon bursitis may develop gradually as a result of repetitive irritation of the olecranon bursa or acutely as a result of trauma or infection. The olecranon bursa lies in the posterior aspect of the elbow between the olecranon process of the ulna and the overlying skin. It may exist as a single bursal sac or, in some patients, as a multisegmented series of loculated sacs. With overuse or misuse, these bursae may become inflamed, enlarged, and, on rare occasions, infected. The swelling associated with olecranon bursitis may be quite impressive, and the patient may complain about being unable to wear a long-sleeved shirt.

The olecranon bursa is vulnerable to injury from both acute trauma and repeated microtrauma. Acute injuries are often caused by direct trauma to the elbow in patients who play sports such as hockey or who fall directly onto the olecranon process. Repeated pressure from leaning on the elbow, such as when working long hours at a drafting table, may result in inflammation and swelling of the olecranon bursa (Fig. 48-1). Rarely, gout or bacterial infection precipitates acute olecranon bursitis. If inflammation of the olecranon bursa becomes chronic, calcification of the bursa may occur, resulting in residual nodules called gravel.

SIGNS AND SYMPTOMS

Patients suffering from olecranon bursitis frequently complain of swelling and pain with any movement of the elbow, but especially with extension. The pain is localized to the olecranon area, with referred pain often noted above the elbow joint. Frequently, the patient is more concerned about the swelling than about the pain. Physical examination reveals point tenderness over the olecranon and swelling of the bursa that may be extensive (Fig. 48-2). Passive extension and resisted flexion reproduce the pain, as does any pressure over the bursa. Fever and chills usually accompany infection of the bursa.

TESTING

The diagnosis of olecranon bursitis is usually made on clinical grounds alone. Plain radiographs of the posterior elbow are indicated if the patient has a history of elbow trauma or if arthritis of the elbow is suspected. Plain radiographs may also reveal calcification of the bursa and associated structures, consistent with chronic inflammation. Magnetic resonance imaging is indicated if joint instability is suspected or if the diagnosis of olecranon bursitis is in question. A complete blood count, automated chemistry profile including uric acid level, erythrocyte sedimentation rate, and antinuclear antibody testing should be performed if collagen vascular disease is suspected. If infection is suspected, aspiration, Gram stain, and culture of the bursal fluid, followed by treatment with appropriate antibiotics, are required on an emergency basis (Fig. 48-3).

DIFFERENTIAL DIAGNOSIS

Olecranon bursitis is usually a straightforward clinical diagnosis. Occasionally, rheumatoid nodules or gouty arthritis of the elbow may confuse the clinical picture. Synovial cysts of the elbow may also mimic olecranon bursitis. Coexistent tendinitis (e.g., tennis elbow, golfer's elbow) may require additional treatment.

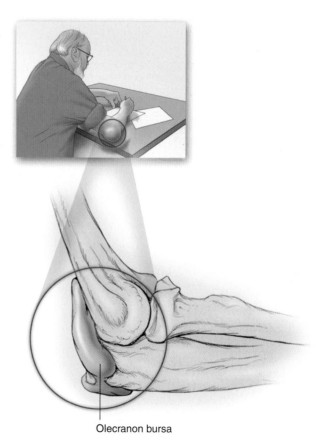

Olecranon bursa

Figure 48-1 Olecranon bursitis is often caused by repeated pressure on the elbow.

TREATMENT

A short course of conservative therapy consisting of simple analgesics, nonsteroidal antiinflammatory drugs (NSAIDs), or cyclooxygenase-2 inhibitors, along with an elbow protector to prevent further trauma, is the initial treatment for patients suffering from olecranon bursitis. If rapid improvement fails to occur, the following injection technique is a reasonable next step.

The patient is placed in the supine position with the arm fully adducted at the patient's side, the elbow flexed, and the palm of

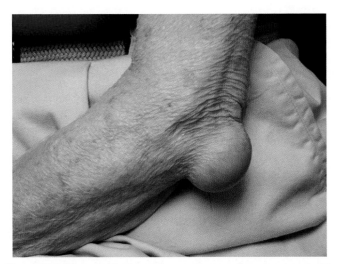

Figure 48-2 Photograph of an enlarged olecranon bursa consistent with nonseptic olecranon bursitis. *(From DeLee JC, Drez DD, Miller M, editors: Orthopaedic sports medicine: principles and practice, ed 3, Philadelphia, 2010, Saunders, p 1247.)*

the hand resting on the patient's abdomen. A total of 2 mL local anesthetic and 40 mg methylprednisolone is drawn up in a 5-mL sterile syringe. After sterile preparation of the skin overlying the posterior aspect of the joint, the olecranon process and overlying bursa are identified. Using strict aseptic technique, the clinician inserts a 1-inch, 25-gauge needle through the skin and subcutaneous tissues directly into the bursa in the midline. If bone is encountered, the needle is withdrawn into the bursa. The contents of the syringe are gently injected; little resistance to injection should be felt. The needle is removed, and a sterile pressure dressing and ice pack are applied to the injection site.

Physical modalities, including local heat and gentle range-of-motion exercises, should be introduced several days after injection for elbow pain. Vigorous exercises should be avoided, because they will exacerbate the patient's symptoms.

COMPLICATIONS AND PITFALLS

Failure to treat olecranon bursitis adequately may result in chronic pain and loss of elbow range of motion. The injection technique is safe if careful attention is paid to the clinically relevant anatomy. In particular, the ulnar nerve is susceptible to damage at the elbow; such damage can be avoided by keeping the needle trajectory in the midline. Sterile technique must be used to avoid infection, along with universal precautions to minimize any risk to the operator. The major complication of bursal injection is infection, although it should be exceedingly rare if strict aseptic technique is followed. The incidence of ecchymosis and hematoma formation can be decreased if pressure is applied to the injection site immediately after injection. Approximately 25% of patients complain of a transient increase in pain after injection of the olecranon bursa, and patients should be warned of this possibility.

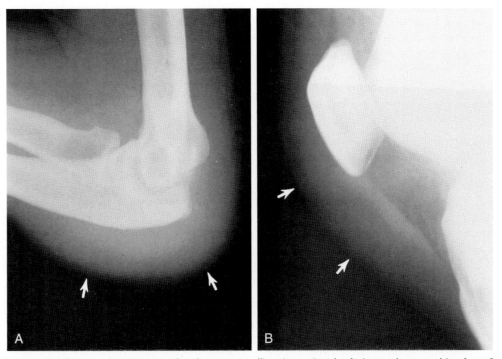

Figure 48-3 Septic bursitis. **A,** Olecranon bursitis. Note the olecranon swelling *(arrows)* and soft tissue edema resulting from *Staphylococcus aureus* infection. Previous surgery and trauma caused the adjacent bony abnormalities. **B,** Prepatellar bursitis. This 28-year-old carpenter who worked on his knees for prolonged periods developed tender swelling in front of the knee *(arrows)*. Inflammatory fluid that was culture positive for *S. aureus* was recovered from the bursa. *(From Resnick D: Diagnosis of bone and joint disorders, ed 4, Philadelphia, 2002, Saunders, p 2447.)*

Clinical Pearls

The injection technique described is extremely effective in the treatment of pain and swelling secondary to olecranon bursitis. Coexistent tendinitis and epicondylitis may contribute to elbow pain, thus necessitating additional treatment with more localized injection of local anesthetic and methylprednisolone. Simple analgesics and NSAIDs can be used concurrently with the injection technique.

SUGGESTED READINGS

Chartash EK, Good PK, Gould ES, et al: Septic subdeltoid bursitis, *Semin Arthritis Rheum* 22(1):25–29, 1992.

Matsumoto T, Fujita K, Fujioka H, et al: Massive nonspecific olecranon bursitis with multiple rice bodies, *J Shoulder Elbow Surg* 13(6):680–683, 2004.

Waldman SD: Injection technique for olecranon bursitis pain. In *Pain review,* Philadelphia, 2009, Saunders, pp 461–462.

Waldman SD: Olecranon bursitis. In *Pain review,* Philadelphia, 2009, Saunders, pp 272–273.

Chapter **49**

ARTHRITIS PAIN OF THE WRIST

ICD-9 CODE 715.93

ICD-10 CODE M19.90

THE CLINICAL SYNDROME

Arthritis of the wrist is a common complaint that can cause significant pain and suffering. The wrist joint is susceptible to the development of arthritis from various conditions that have in common the ability to damage joint cartilage. Patients with arthritis of the wrist present with pain, swelling, and decreasing function of the wrist. Decreased grip strength is also a common finding. Osteoarthritis is the most common form of arthritis that results in wrist joint pain. However, rheumatoid arthritis, posttraumatic arthritis, and psoriatic arthritis are also common causes of arthritic wrist pain. These types of arthritis can result in significant alteration in the biomechanics of the wrist because they affect not only the joint but also the tendons and other connective tissues that make up the functional unit.

SIGNS AND SYMPTOMS

Most patients presenting with wrist pain secondary to osteoarthritis or posttraumatic arthritis complain of pain that is localized around the wrist and hand. Activity makes the pain worse, whereas rest and heat provide some relief. The pain is constant and is characterized as aching; it may interfere with sleep. Some patients complain of a grating or popping sensation with use of the joint, and crepitus may be present on physical examination. If the pain and dysfunction are secondary to rheumatoid arthritis, the metacarpophalangeal joints are often involved, with characteristic deformity.

In addition to pain, patients suffering from arthritis of the wrist joint often experience a gradual reduction in functional ability because of decreasing wrist range of motion that makes simple everyday tasks such as using a computer keyboard, holding a coffee cup, turning a doorknob, or unscrewing a bottle cap quite difficult (Fig. 49-1). With continued disuse, muscle wasting may occur, and adhesive capsulitis with subsequent ankylosis may develop.

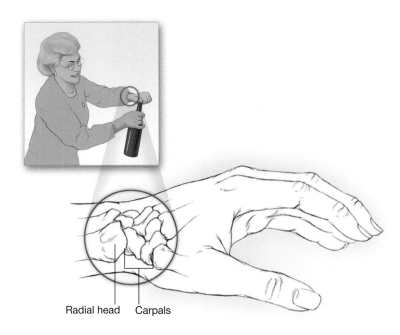

Radial head   Carpals

Figure 49-1 Arthritis of the wrist often makes simple everyday tasks such as opening a bottle painful.

TESTING

Plain radiographs are indicated in all patients who present with wrist pain (Fig. 49-2). Based on the patient's clinical presentation, additional testing may be warranted, including a complete blood count, erythrocyte sedimentation rate, and antinuclear antibody testing. Magnetic resonance imaging of the wrist is indicated if joint instability is thought to be present (Fig. 49-3). If infection is suspected, Gram stain and culture of the synovial fluid should be performed on an emergency basis, and treatment with appropriate antibiotics should be started.

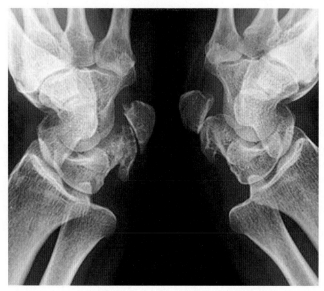

Figure 49-2 Pisotriquetral joint osteoarthritis. Comparative ulnar side radiograph shows bilateral pisotriquetral joint osteoarthritis. *(From Feydy A, Pluot E, Guerini H, Drapé J-L: Role of imaging in spine, hand, and wrist osteoarthritis,* Rheum Dis Clin North Am *35[3]:605–649, 2009.)*

DIFFERENTIAL DIAGNOSIS

Osteoarthritis is the most common form of arthritis that results in wrist joint pain. However, rheumatoid arthritis and post-traumatic arthritis are also common causes of wrist pain. Less common causes of arthritis-induced wrist pain include collagen vascular diseases, infection, villonodular synovitis, and Lyme disease. Acute infectious arthritis is usually accompanied by significant systemic symptoms, including fever and malaise, and should be easily recognized and treated with antibiotics. Collagen vascular diseases generally manifest as polyarthropathy rather than as monarthropathy limited to the wrist joint; however, wrist pain secondary to collagen vascular disease responds exceedingly well to the intraarticular injection technique described here.

TREATMENT

Initial treatment of the pain and functional disability associated with osteoarthritis of the wrist includes a combination of non-steroidal antiinflammatory drugs (NSAIDs) or cyclooxygenase-2 inhibitors and physical therapy. Local application of heat and cold may also be beneficial. Splinting the wrist in the neutral position may provide symptomatic relief and protect the joint from additional trauma. For patients who do not respond to these treatment modalities, intraarticular injection of local anesthetic and steroid is a reasonable next step.

Intraarticular injection of the wrist is performed by placing the patient in the supine position with the arm fully adducted at the patient's side, the elbow slightly flexed, and the palm of the hand resting on a folded towel. A total of 1.5 mL local anesthetic and 40 mg methylprednisolone is drawn up in a 5-mL sterile syringe. After sterile preparation of the skin overlying the dorsal joint, the midcarpus proximal to the indentation of the capitate bone is identified. Just proximal to the capitate bone is an indentation that allows easy access to the wrist joint. Using strict aseptic technique, the clinician inserts a 1-inch, 25-gauge needle in the center of the midcarpal indentation through the skin,

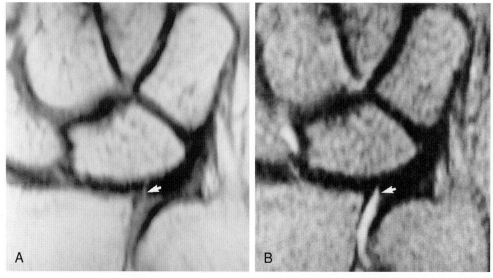

Figure 49-3 Triangular fibrocartilage complex with a communicating defect. **A,** Coronal intermediate-weighted spin-echo magnetic resonance imaging (MRI). Note the linear region of increased signal intensity *(arrow)* in the triangular fibrocartilage. **B,** T2-weighted spin-echo MRI. Fluid of high signal intensity is present in the defect *(arrow)* in the triangular fibrocartilage and in the distal radioulnar joint. Fluid is also present in the midcarpal joint. *(From Resnick D:* Diagnosis of bone and joint disorders, *ed 4, Philadelphia, 2002, Saunders, p 3033.)*

subcutaneous tissues, and joint capsule and into the joint. If bone is encountered, the needle is withdrawn into the subcutaneous tissues and is redirected superiorly. After the joint space is entered, the contents of the syringe are gently injected. Little resistance to injection should be felt. If resistance is encountered, the needle is probably in a ligament or tendon and should be advanced slightly into the joint space until the injection can proceed without significant resistance. The needle is then removed, and a sterile pressure dressing and ice pack are applied to the injection site.

Physical modalities, including local heat and gentle range-of-motion exercises, should be introduced several days after the patient begins treatment for arthritis of wrist. Vigorous exercises should be avoided, because they will exacerbate the patient's symptoms.

COMPLICATIONS AND PITFALLS

Joint protection is especially important in patients suffering from inflammatory arthritis of the wrist, because repetitive trauma can result in further damage to the joint, tendons, and connective tissues. The major complication of intraarticular injection of the wrist is infection, although it should be exceedingly rare if strict aseptic technique is followed. The injection technique is safe if careful attention is paid to the clinically relevant anatomy; the ulnar nerve is especially susceptible to damage at the wrist.

Approximately 25% of patients complain of a transient increase in pain after intraarticular injection of the wrist joint, and patients should be warned of this possibility.

Clinical Pearls

The injection technique described is extremely effective in the treatment of pain secondary to arthritis of the wrist joint. Simple analgesics and NSAIDs can be used concurrently with the injection technique. Coexistent bursitis and tendinitis may contribute to wrist pain and necessitate additional treatment with more localized injection of local anesthetic and methylprednisolone.

SUGGESTED READINGS

Feydy A, Pluot E, Guerini H, et al: Osteoarthritis of the wrist and hand, and spine, *Radiol Clin North Am* 47(4):723–759, 2009.

Feydy A, Pluot E, Guerini H, et al: Role of imaging in spine, hand, and wrist osteoarthritis, *Rheum Dis Clin North Am* 35(3):605–649, 2009.

Waldman SD: Functional anatomy of the wrist. In *Pain review*, Philadelphia, 2009, Saunders, pp 100–102.

Waldman SD: Painful conditions of the wrist and hand. In *Physical diagnosis of pain: an atlas of signs and symptoms,* ed 2, Philadelphia, 2010, Saunders, pp 153–154.

Weiss KE, Rodner CM: Osteoarthritis of the wrist, *J Hand Surg* 32(5):725–746, 2007.

Chapter 50

CARPAL TUNNEL SYNDROME

ICD-9 CODE `354.0`

ICD-10 CODE `G56.00`

THE CLINICAL SYNDROME

Carpal tunnel syndrome is the most common entrapment neuropathy encountered in clinical practice. It is caused by compression of the median nerve as it passes through the carpal canal at the wrist. The most common causes of compression of the median nerve at this location include flexor tenosynovitis, rheumatoid arthritis, pregnancy, amyloidosis, and other space-occupying lesions that compromise the median nerve as it passes through this closed space. This entrapment neuropathy presents as pain, numbness, paresthesias, and associated weakness in the hand and wrist that radiate to the thumb, index finger, middle finger, and radial half of the ring finger. These symptoms may also radiate proximal to the entrapment into the forearm. Untreated, progressive motor deficit and, ultimately, flexion contracture of the affected fingers can result. Symptoms usually begin after repetitive wrist motions or repeated pressure on the wrist, such as resting the wrists on the edge of a computer keyboard (Fig. 50-1). Direct trauma to the median nerve as it enters the carpal tunnel may result in a similar clinical presentation.

SIGNS AND SYMPTOMS

Physical findings include tenderness over the median nerve at the wrist. A positive Tinel sign is usually present over the median nerve as it passes beneath the flexor retinaculum (Fig. 50-2). A positive Phalen maneuver is highly suggestive of carpal tunnel syndrome. Phalen's maneuver is performed by having the patient place the wrists in complete unforced flexion for at least 30 seconds (Fig. 50-3). If the median nerve is entrapped at the wrist, this

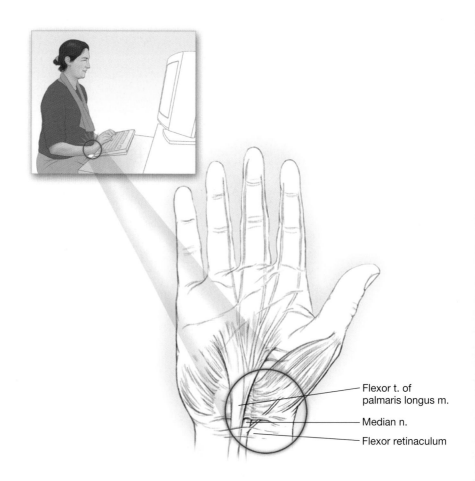

Flexor t. of palmaris longus m.

Median n.

Flexor retinaculum

Figure 50-1 Poor positioning of the hand and wrist during keyboarding can result in carpal tunnel syndrome.

maneuver reproduces the symptoms of carpal tunnel syndrome. Weakness of thumb opposition and wasting of the thenar eminence are often seen in advanced cases of carpal tunnel syndrome; however, because of the complex motion of the thumb, subtle motor deficits can easily be missed (Fig. 50-4). Early in the course of carpal tunnel syndrome, the only physical finding other than tenderness over the median nerve may be the loss of sensation in the foregoing fingers.

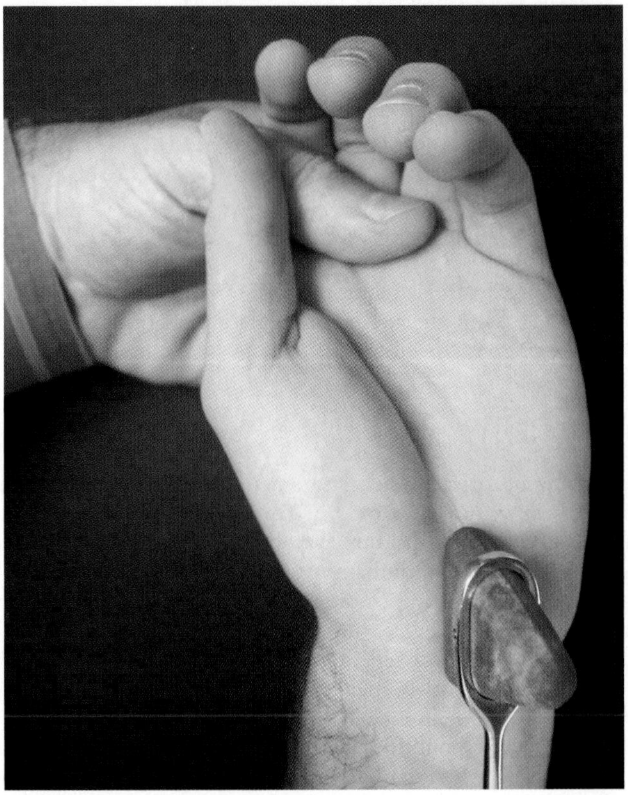

TESTING

Electromyography can distinguish cervical radiculopathy and diabetic polyneuropathy from carpal tunnel syndrome. Plain radiographs are indicated in all patients who present with carpal tunnel syndrome, to rule out occult bony disorders. Based on the patient's clinical presentation, additional testing may be warranted, including a complete blood count, uric acid level,

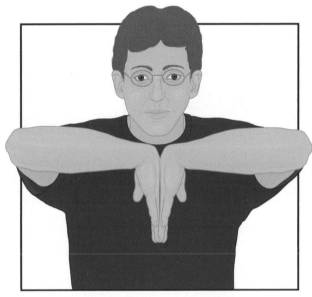

Figure 50-2 Tinel's sign for carpal tunnel syndrome. *(From Waldman SD: Physical diagnosis of pain: an atlas of signs and symptoms, Philadelphia, 2006, Saunders, p 178.)*

Figure 50-3 A positive Phalen maneuver is highly indicative of carpal tunnel syndrome. *(From Waldman SD: Atlas of pain management injection techniques, Philadelphia, 2000, Saunders.)*

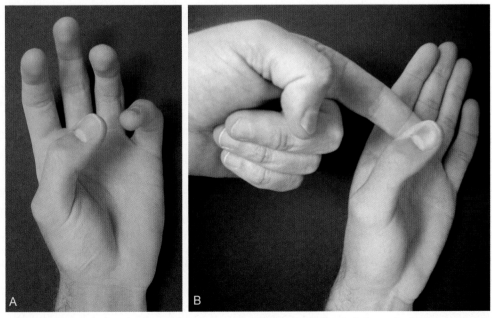

Figure 50-4 The opponens weakness test for carpal tunnel syndrome. *(From Waldman SD: Physical diagnosis of pain: an atlas of signs and symptoms, Philadelphia, 2006, Saunders, p 180.)*

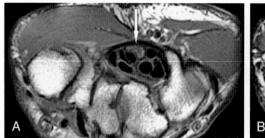
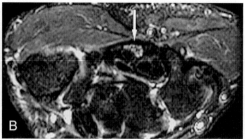

Figure 50-5 Axial T1-weighted **(A)** and short tau inversion recovery **(B)** magnetic resonance images of a patient with carpal tunnel syndrome without marked nerve enlargement. *(From Edelman RR, Hesselink JR, Zlatkin MB, Crues JV, editors:* Clinical magnetic resonance imaging, *ed 3, Philadelphia, 2006, Saunders, p 2381.)*

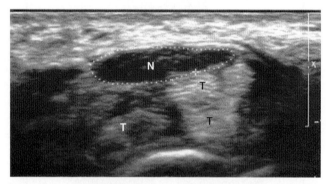

Figure 50-6 In this ultrasound image from a patient with carpal tunnel syndrome, the measurement of the cross-sectional area of the median nerve is shown by the *dots* encircling the nerve. A cross-sectional area of 32 mm² was recorded. N, median nerve; TT, flexor digitorum tendons. *(From Wiesler ER, Chloros GD, Cartwright MS, et al: The use of diagnostic ultrasound in carpal tunnel syndrome,* J Hand Surg 31[5]:726–732, 2006.)

erythrocyte sedimentation rate, and antinuclear antibody testing. Magnetic resonance imaging of the wrist is indicated if joint instability or a space-occupying lesion is suspected or to confirm the actual cause of median nerve compression (Fig. 50-5). Ultrasound imaging may also be useful in the evaluation of the median nerve as it passes through the carpal tunnel. Studies have suggested a strong correlation between the cross-sectional area of the nerve and clinical carpal tunnel syndrome (Fig. 50-6). The injection technique described later serves as both a diagnostic and a therapeutic maneuver.

DIFFERENTIAL DIAGNOSIS

Carpal tunnel syndrome is often misdiagnosed as arthritis of the carpometacarpal joint of the thumb, cervical radiculopathy, or diabetic polyneuropathy. Patients with arthritis of the carpometacarpal joint of the thumb have a positive Watson test and radiographic evidence of arthritis. Most patients suffering from cervical radiculopathy have reflex, motor, and sensory changes associated with neck pain; in contrast, patients with carpal tunnel syndrome have no reflex changes, and motor and sensory changes are limited to the distal median nerve. Diabetic polyneuropathy generally manifests as a symmetrical sensory deficit involving the entire hand, rather than being limited to the distribution of the median nerve. Cervical radiculopathy and median nerve entrapment may coexist as the double-crush syndrome.

Further, carpal tunnel syndrome is commonly seen in patients with diabetes, and it is not uncommon for diabetic polyneuropathy to be present as well.

TREATMENT

Mild cases of carpal tunnel syndrome usually respond to conservative therapy; surgery should be reserved for more severe cases. Initial treatment of carpal tunnel syndrome consists of simple analgesics, nonsteroidal antiinflammatory drugs, or cyclooxygenase-2 inhibitors and splinting of the wrist. At a minimum, the splint should be worn at night, but wearing it for 24 hours a day is ideal. Avoidance of the repetitive activities that are thought to be responsible for carpal tunnel syndrome (e.g., keyboarding, hammering) can also help ameliorate the patient's symptoms. If the patient fails to respond to these conservative measures, a next reasonable step is injection of the carpal tunnel with local anesthetic and steroid.

Carpal tunnel injection is performed by placing the patient in the supine position with the arm fully abducted at the patient's side, the elbow slightly flexed, and the dorsum of the hand resting on a folded towel. A total of 3 mL local anesthetic and 49 mg methylprednisolone is drawn up in a 5-mL sterile syringe. The patient is then told to make a fist and at the same time flex his or her wrist to aid in identifying the palmaris longus tendon. After preparation of the skin with antiseptic solution, a ⅝-inch, 25-gauge needle is inserted just medial to the tendon and just proximal to the crease of the wrist at a 30-degree angle (Fig. 50-7). The needle is slowly advanced until the tip is just beyond the tendon. Paresthesia in the distribution of the median nerve is often elicited, and the patient should be warned to expect this and to say "There!" as soon as the paresthesia is felt. If a paresthesia is elicited, the needle is withdrawn slightly away from the median nerve. Gentle aspiration is then carried out to identify blood. If the aspiration test result is negative and no persistent paresthesia is noted in the distribution of the median nerve, 3 mL of solution is slowly injected while the patient is monitored closely for signs of local anesthetic toxicity. If no paresthesia is elicited and the needle tip hits bone, the needle is withdrawn out of the periosteum, and, after careful aspiration, 3 mL of solution is slowly injected.

When these treatment modalities fail, surgical release of the median nerve at the carpal tunnel is indicated. Endoscopic techniques are showing promise and appear to result in less postoperative pain and dysfunction.

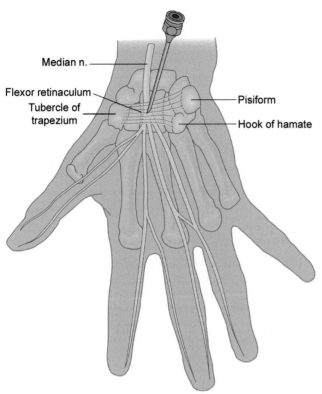

Median n.

Flexor retinaculum

Tubercle of trapezium

Pisiform

Hook of hamate

Figure 50-7 Proper needle placement for injection of the carpal tunnel. *(From Waldman SD:* Atlas of pain management injection techniques, *Philadelphia, 2000, Saunders.)*

COMPLICATIONS AND PITFALLS

Failure to treat carpal tunnel syndrome adequately can result in permanent pain, numbness, and functional disability. The problem can be exacerbated if coexistent reflex sympathetic dystrophy is not aggressively treated with sympathetic neural blockade. Injection of the carpal tunnel is a relatively safe technique. The major complications are inadvertent intravascular injection and persistent paresthesia secondary to needle-induced trauma to the nerve. This technique can be safely performed in the presence of anticoagulation by using a 25- or 27-gauge needle, albeit with an increased risk of hematoma formation. The incidence of this complication can be decreased if manual pressure is applied to the area immediately after injection. The application of cold packs for 20 minutes after injection can also decrease the amount of postprocedure pain and bleeding.

Clinical Pearls

Carpal tunnel syndrome should always be differentiated from cervical radiculopathy involving the cervical nerve roots, which may mimic median nerve compression. Further, cervical radiculopathy and median nerve entrapment may coexist in the double-crush syndrome.

Carpal tunnel injection is a simple and safe technique. Before median nerve block at the wrist is initiated, a careful neurologic examination should be performed to identify preexisting neurologic deficits that may later be attributed to the nerve block, especially in patients with clinical symptoms of diabetes or clinically significant carpal tunnel syndrome.

Care should be taken to place the needle just beyond the flexor retinaculum and to inject slowly, to allow the solution to flow easily into the carpal tunnel without further compromising the median nerve.

SUGGESTED READINGS

Martins RS, Siqueira MG, Simplício H, et al: Magnetic resonance imaging of idiopathic carpal tunnel syndrome: correlation with clinical findings and electrophysiological investigation, *Clin Neurol Neurosurg* 110(1):38–45, 2008.

Seror P: Sonography and electrodiagnosis in carpal tunnel syndrome diagnosis: an analysis of the literature, *Eur J Radiol* 67(1):146–152, 2008.

Waldman SD: Carpal tunnel syndrome. In *Pain review*, Philadelphia, 2009, Saunders, pp 273–275.

Waldman SD: Functional anatomy of the wrist. In *Pain review*, Philadelphia, 2009, Saunders, pp 100–102.

Watts AC, McEachan J: Carpal tunnel syndrome in men, *Curr Orthop* 20(4): 294–298, 2006.

Chapter 51

DE QUERVAIN'S TENOSYNOVITIS

ICD-9 CODE 727.04

ICD-10 CODE M65.4

THE CLINICAL SYNDROME

de Quervain's tenosynovitis is caused by inflammation and swelling of the tendons of the abductor pollicis longus and extensor pollicis brevis at the level of the radial styloid process. It is usually the result of trauma to the tendon from repetitive twisting motions. If the inflammation and swelling become chronic, the tendon sheath thickens, resulting in its constriction. A triggering phenomenon may occur, with the tendon catching within the sheath and causing the thumb to lock, or "trigger." Arthritis and gout of the first metacarpal joint may coexist with de Quervain's tenosynovitis and exacerbate the associated pain and disability.

de Quervain's tenosynovitis occurs in patients engaged in repetitive activities such as handshaking or high-torque wrist turning (e.g., when scooping ice cream). De Quervain's tenosynovitis may also develop without obvious antecedent trauma.

The pain of de Quervain's tenosynovitis is localized to the region of the radial styloid. It is constant and is made worse with active pinching activities of the thumb or ulnar deviation of the wrist (Fig. 51-1). Patients note an inability to hold a coffee cup or turn a screwdriver. Sleep disturbance is common.

SIGNS AND SYMPTOMS

On physical examination, the patient has tenderness and swelling over the tendons and tendon sheaths along the distal radius, with point tenderness over the radial styloid. Many patients with de Quervain's tenosynovitis note a creaking sensation with flexion and extension of the thumb. Range of motion of the thumb may be decreased by the pain, and a trigger thumb phenomenon may be noted. Patients with de Quervain's tenosynovitis demonstrate a positive Finkelstein test result (Fig. 51-2). The Finkelstein test is performed by stabilizing the patient's forearm, having the patient fully flex his or her thumb into the palm, and then actively forcing the wrist toward the ulna. Sudden severe pain is highly suggestive of de Quervain's tenosynovitis.

TESTING

The diagnosis is generally made on clinical grounds, but magnetic resonance imaging (MRI) can confirm the presence of tenosynovitis (Fig. 51-3). Electromyography can distinguish de Quervain's tenosynovitis from neuropathic processes such as cervical radiculopathy

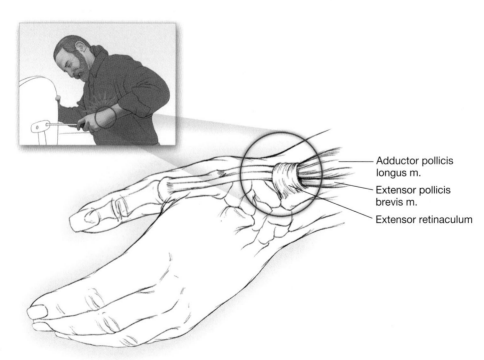

Adductor pollicis longus m.

Extensor pollicis brevis m.

Extensor retinaculum

Figure 51-1 Repetitive microtrauma to the wrist can result in de Quervain's tenosynovitis.

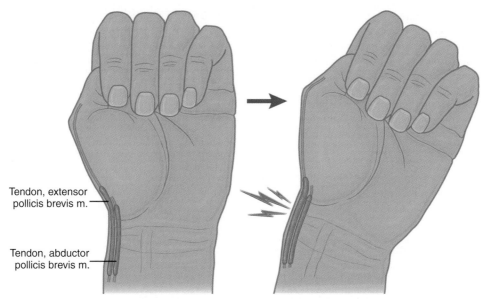

Tendon, extensor
pollicis brevis m.

Tendon, abductor
pollicis brevis m.

Figure 51-2 A positive Finkelstein test is indicative of de Quervain's tenosynovitis. *(From Waldman SD:* Atlas of pain management injection techniques, *Philadelphia, 2000, Saunders.)*

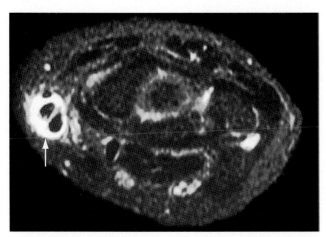

Figure 51-3 Axial short tau inversion recovery magnetic resonance image demonstrating de Quervain's tenosynovitis. Note the thickened first extensor compartment tendons, with prominent tendon sheath fluid *(arrow). (From Edelman RR, Hesselink JR, Zlatkin MB, Crues JV, editors:* Clinical magnetic resonance imaging, *ed 3, Philadelphia, 2006, Saunders, p 3357.)*

and cheiralgia paresthetica. Plain radiographs are indicated in all patients who present with de Quervain's tenosynovitis, to rule out occult bony disease. Based on the patient's clinical presentation, additional testing may be warranted, including a complete blood count, uric acid level, erythrocyte sedimentation rate, and antinuclear antibody testing. MRI of the wrist is also indicated if joint instability is suspected. The injection technique described later serves as both a diagnostic and a therapeutic maneuver.

DIFFERENTIAL DIAGNOSIS

Entrapment of the lateral antebrachial cutaneous nerve, arthritis of the first metacarpal joint, gout, cheiralgia paresthetica (caused by entrapment of the superficial branch of the radial nerve at the wrist), and occasionally C6-7 radiculopathy can mimic de Quervain's tenosynovitis. All these painful conditions can also coexist with de Quervain's tenosynovitis.

TREATMENT

Initial treatment of the pain and functional disability associated with de Quervain's tenosynovitis includes a combination of nonsteroidal antiinflammatory drugs (NSAIDs) or cyclooxygenase-2 inhibitors and physical therapy. Local application of heat and cold may also be beneficial. Any repetitive activity that may exacerbate the patient's symptoms should be avoided. Nighttime splinting of the affected thumb may help avoid the trigger phenomenon that can occur on awakening in many patients suffering from this condition. For patients who do not respond to these treatment modalities, the following injection technique is a reasonable next step.

Injection for de Quervain's tenosynovitis is carried out by placing the patient in the supine position with the arm fully adducted at the patient's side and the ulnar surface of the wrist and hand resting on a folded towel to relax the affected tendons. A total of 2 mL local anesthetic and 40 mg methylprednisolone is drawn up in a 5-mL sterile syringe. After sterile preparation of the skin overlying the affected tendons, the radial styloid is identified. Using strict aseptic technique, the clinician inserts a 1-inch, 25-gauge needle at a 45-degree angle toward the radial styloid through the skin and into the subcutaneous tissue overlying the affected tendon. If bone is encountered, the needle is withdrawn into the subcutaneous tissue. The contents of the syringe are then gently injected. Little resistance to injection should be felt. If resistance is encountered, the needle is probably in the tendon and should be withdrawn until the injection can proceed without significant resistance. The needle is then removed, and a sterile pressure dressing and ice pack are applied to the injection site.

Physical modalities, including local heat and gentle range-of-motion exercises, should be introduced several days after the patient undergoes injection. Vigorous exercises should be avoided, because they will exacerbate the patient's symptoms.

COMPLICATIONS AND PITFALLS

The injection technique is safe if careful attention is paid to the clinically relevant anatomy. The radial artery and superficial branch of the radial nerve are susceptible to damage if the needle is placed too medially, so care must be taken to avoid these structures. The major complications associated with injection are related to trauma to the inflamed and previously damaged tendons. These tendons may rupture if they are injected directly, so the needle position should be confirmed to be outside the tendon before injection. Another complication of injection is infection, although it should be exceedingly rare if strict aseptic technique is followed, as well as universal precautions to minimize any risk to the operator. The incidence of ecchymosis and hematoma formation can be decreased if pressure is applied to the injection site immediately after injection. Approximately 25% of patients complain of a transient increase in pain after injection, and patients should be warned of this possibility.

Clinical Pearls

> The injection technique described is extremely effective in the treatment of pain secondary to de Quervain's tenosynovitis. A hand splint to immobilize the thumb may also help relieve the symptoms. Simple analgesics and NSAIDs can be used concurrently with the injection technique. Coexistent arthritis and gout may contribute to the pain, thus necessitating additional treatment with more localized injection of local anesthetic and methylprednisolone. Arthritis of the first metacarpal joint, gout, cheiralgia paresthetica, and cervical radiculopathy may mimic de Quervain's tenosynovitis and must be excluded.

SUGGESTED READINGS

Cannon DE, Dillingham TR, Miao H, et al: Musculoskeletal disorders in referrals for suspected cervical radiculopathy, *Arch Phys Med Rehabil* 88(10):1256–1259, 2007.

Ilyas AM: Nonsurgical treatment for de Quervain's tenosynovitis, *J Hand Surg* 34(5):928–929, 2009.

Waldman SD: de Quervain's tenosynovitis. In *Pain review,* Philadelphia, 2009, Saunders, pp 276–277.

Waldman SD: Functional anatomy of the wrist. In *Pain review,* Philadelphia, 2009, Saunders, pp 100–102.

Waldman SD: Painful conditions of the wrist and hand. In *Physical diagnosis of pain: an atlas of signs and symptoms,* ed 2, Philadelphia, 2010, Saunders, pp 153–154.

Wolf JM, Sturdivant RX, Owens BD: Incidence of de Quervain's tenosynovitis in a young, active population, *J Hand Surg* 34(1):112–115, 2009.

Chapter 52

ARTHRITIS PAIN AT THE CARPOMETACARPAL JOINTS

ICD-9 CODE `715.94`

ICD-10 CODE `M18.9`

The Clinical Syndrome

The carpometacarpal joints of the fingers are synovial plane joints that serve as the articulation between the carpals and the metacarpals and allow the bases of the metacarpal bones to articulate with one another. Movement of the joints is limited to a slight gliding motion, with the carpometacarpal joint of the little finger possessing the greatest range of motion. The primary function of these joints is to optimize the grip function of the hand. Most patients have a common joint space.

Pain and dysfunction from arthritis of the carpometacarpal joints are common complaints. These joints are susceptible to the development of arthritis from various conditions that share the ability to damage joint cartilage. Osteoarthritis is the most common form of arthritis that results in carpometacarpal joint pain. It occurs more often in female patients, and although the thumb is most frequently affected, arthritis may develop in the other carpometacarpal joints as well, especially after trauma. Rheumatoid arthritis, posttraumatic arthritis, and psoriatic arthritis are also common causes of carpometacarpal pain. Less frequent causes of arthritis-induced carpometacarpal pain include collagen vascular diseases, infection, and Lyme disease. Acute infectious arthritis is usually accompanied by significant systemic symptoms, including fever and malaise, and should be easily recognized; it is treated with culture and antibiotics rather than injection therapy. Collagen vascular diseases generally manifest as polyarthropathy rather than as monarthropathy limited to the carpometacarpal joint; however, carpometacarpal pain secondary to collagen vascular disease responds exceedingly well to the intraarticular injection technique described here.

Signs and Symptoms

Most patients presenting with carpometacarpal pain secondary to osteoarthritis or posttraumatic arthritis complain of pain that is localized to the dorsum of the wrist. Activity associated with flexion, extension, and ulnar deviation of the carpometacarpal joints exacerbates the pain, whereas rest and heat provide some relief. The pain is constant and is characterized as aching; it may interfere with sleep. Some patients complain of a grating or popping sensation with use of the joint, and crepitus may be present on physical examination.

In addition to pain, patients suffering from arthritis of the carpometacarpal joint often experience a gradual reduction in functional ability because of decreasing pinch and grip strength that makes everyday tasks such as using a pencil or opening a jar quite difficult (Fig. 52-1). With continued disuse, muscle wasting may occur, and adhesive capsulitis with subsequent ankylosis may develop.

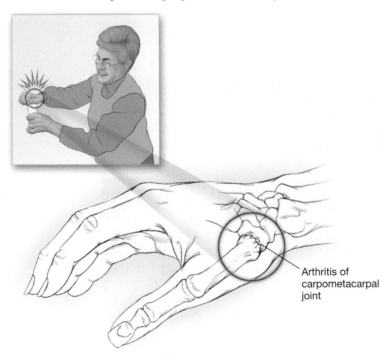

Arthritis of carpometacarpal joint

Figure 52-1 Arthritis of the carpometacarpal joints may cause pain and decreased grip strength.

TESTING

Plain radiographs are indicated in all patients who present with carpometacarpal pain. Based on the patient's clinical presentation, additional testing may be warranted, including a complete blood count, erythrocyte sedimentation rate, and antinuclear antibody testing. Magnetic resonance imaging (MRI) of the carpometacarpal joint is indicated if joint instability is thought to be present. If infection is suspected, Gram stain and culture of the synovial fluid should be performed on an emergency basis, and treatment with appropriate antibiotics should be started. If the patient has a history of trauma, MRI or radionuclide bone scanning may be useful (Fig. 52-2), because fractures of the navicular bone are often missed on plain radiographs of the wrist.

DIFFERENTIAL DIAGNOSIS

Arthritis pain of the carpometacarpal joints is usually diagnosed on clinical grounds, and plain radiographs confirm the clinical findings (Fig. 52-3). Occasionally, arthritis pain of the carpometacarpal

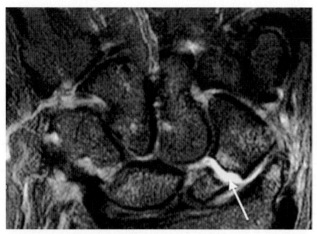

Figure 52-2 Coronal long TR/TE (repetition time/echo time) fast spin-echo magnetic resonance image with fat saturation shows nonunion of a proximal pole scaphoid fracture *(arrow)*, outlined by fluid signal in the fracture. *(From Edelman RR, Hesselink JR, Zlatkin MB, Crues JV, editors:* Clinical magnetic resonance imaging, *ed 3, Philadelphia, 2006, Saunders, p 3344.)*

joints may be confused with de Quervain's tenosynovitis or other forms of tendinitis involving the wrist and fingers. These painful conditions, as well as gout, may coexist and make the diagnosis more difficult. If the patient has a history of trauma, occult fractures of the metacarpals should always be considered.

TREATMENT

Initial treatment of the pain and functional disability associated with osteoarthritis of the carpometacarpal joints includes a combination of nonsteroidal antiinflammatory drugs (NSAIDs) or cyclooxygenase-2 inhibitors and physical therapy. Local application of heat and cold may also be beneficial. Splinting the wrist in the neutral position may provide symptomatic relief and protect the joint from additional trauma. For patients who do not respond to these treatment modalities, intraarticular injection of local anesthetic and steroid is a reasonable next step.

Intraarticular injection of the carpometacarpal joint is performed by placing the patient in the supine position with the arm fully adducted at the patient's side and the hand in a neutral position, with the palmar aspect resting on a folded towel. A total of 1.5 mL local anesthetic and 40 mg methylprednisolone is drawn up in a 5-mL sterile syringe. After sterile preparation of the skin overlying the affected carpometacarpal joint, the space between the carpal and metacarpal joints is identified. The joint can be more easily identified by gliding it back and forth. Using strict aseptic technique, the clinician inserts a 1-inch, 25-gauge needle through the skin, subcutaneous tissues, and joint capsule and into the center of the joint (Fig. 52-4). If bone is encountered, the needle is withdrawn into the subcutaneous tissues and is redirected medially. After entering the joint space, the contents of the syringe are gently injected. Little resistance to injection should be felt. If resistance is encountered, the needle is probably in a tendon and should be advanced slightly into the joint space until the injection can proceed without significant resistance. The needle is then removed, and a sterile pressure dressing and ice pack are applied to the injection site.

Physical modalities, including local heat and gentle range-of-motion exercises, should be introduced several days after the patient begins treatment for arthritis of the carpometacarpal joints. Vigorous exercises should be avoided, because they will exacerbate the patient's symptoms.

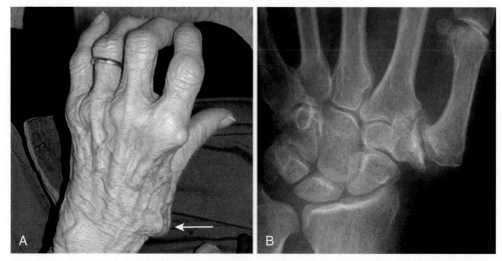

Figure 52-3 First carpometacarpal arthritis. **A,** Radial subluxation of the base of the first metacarpal giving the "shoulder sign" *(arrow)*. **B,** Anteroposterior radiograph of the same hand. *(From Young D, Papp S, Giachino A: Physical examination of the wrist,* Orthop Clin North Am *38[2]:149–165, 2007.)*

COMPLICATIONS AND PITFALLS

Joint protection is especially important in patients suffering from inflammatory arthritis of the carpometacarpal joints, because repetitive trauma can result in further damage to the joints, tendons, and connective tissues. The major complication associated with the intraarticular injection technique is infection, although it should be exceedingly rare if strict aseptic technique is followed. Approximately 25% of patients complain of a transient increase in pain after intraarticular injection of the carpometacarpal joints, and patients should be warned of this possibility.

Clinical Pearls

The injection technique described is extremely effective in the treatment of arthritis pain of the carpometacarpal joints, and it is safe as long as careful attention is paid to the clinically relevant anatomy. Simple analgesics and NSAIDs can be used concurrently with the injection technique. Coexistent bursitis and tendinitis may contribute to the patient's pain, thus necessitating additional treatment with more localized injection of local anesthetic and methylprednisolone.

SUGGESTED READINGS

Feydy A, Pluot E, Guerini H, et al: Osteoarthritis of the wrist and hand, and spine, *Radiol Clin North Am* 47(4):723–759, 2009.

Feydy A, Pluot E, Guerini H, et al: Role of imaging in spine, hand, and wrist osteoarthritis, *Rheum Dis Clin North Am* 35(3):605–649, 2009.

Fumagalli M, Sarzi-Puttini P, Atzeni F: Hand osteoarthritis, *Semin Arthritis Rheum* 34(6 Suppl 2):47–52, 2004.

Mahendira D, Towheed TE: Systematic review of non-surgical therapies for osteoarthritis of the hand: an update, *Osteoarthritis Cartilage* 17(10):1263–1268, 2009.

Waldman SD: Painful conditions of the wrist and hand. In *Physical diagnosis of pain: an atlas of signs and symptoms*, ed 2, Philadelphia, 2010, Saunders, pp 153–154.

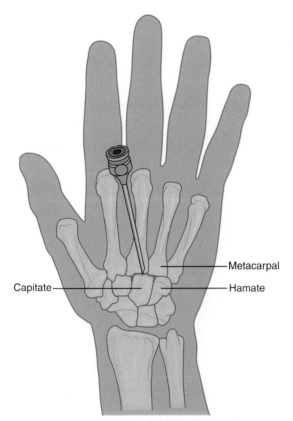

Capitate — Metacarpal — Hamate

Figure 52-4 Proper needle placement for injection of the carpometacarpal joints. *(From Waldman SD: Atlas of pain management injection techniques, Philadelphia, 2000, Saunders.)*

Chapter 53

GANGLION CYSTS OF THE WRIST

ICD-9 CODE **727.43**

ICD-10 CODE **M67.40**

THE CLINICAL SYNDROME

The dorsum of the wrist is especially susceptible to the development of ganglion cysts in the area overlying the extensor tendons or the joint space, with a predilection for the joint space of the lunate or from the tendon sheath of the extensor carpi radialis (Fig. 53-1). These cysts are thought to form as the result of herniation of synovial-containing tissues from joint capsules or tendon sheaths. This tissue may then become irritated and begin producing increased amounts of synovial fluid, which can pool in cystlike cavities overlying the tendons and joint space. A one-way valve phenomenon may cause these cystlike cavities to expand, because the fluid cannot flow freely back into the synovial cavity. Ganglion cysts may also occur on the volar aspect of the wrist. Occurring three times more commonly in women than in men, ganglion cysts of the wrist represent 65% to 70% of all soft tissue tumors of the hand and wrist. Ganglion cysts occur in all age groups, with a peak incidence in fourth to sixth decades.

SIGNS AND SYMPTOMS

Activity, especially extreme flexion and extension, makes the pain worse; rest and heat provide some relief (Fig. 53-2). The pain is constant and is characterized as aching. Often, the unsightly nature of the ganglion cyst, rather than the pain, causes the patient to seek medical attention. The ganglion is smooth to palpation and transilluminates with a penlight, in contradistinction to solid tumors, which do not transilluminate. Palpation of the ganglion may increase the pain.

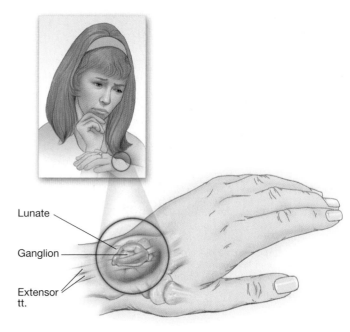

Figure 53-2 Ganglion cysts usually appear on the dorsum of the wrist, overlying the extensor tendon or joint space. Patients often seek medical attention out of a fear of cancer.

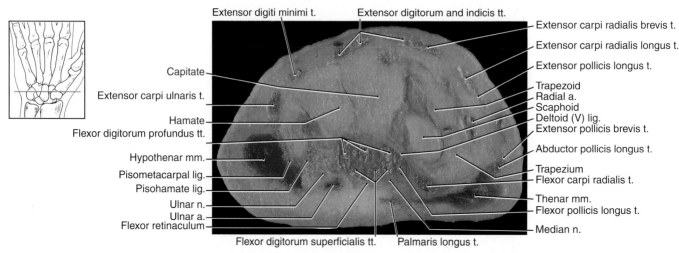

Figure 53-1 Ganglion cysts of the wrists are thought to form as the result of herniation of synovial-containing tissues from joint capsules or tendon sheaths. (From Kang HS, Ahn JM, Resnick D: MRI of the extremities: an anatomic atlas, ed 2, Philadelphia, 2002, Saunders, p 178.)

TESTING

Plain radiographs of the wrist are indicated in all patients who present with ganglion cysts, to rule out bony abnormalities, including tumors. Ultrasound imaging will help determine whether a soft tissue mass of the wrist is cystic or solid (Fig. 53-3). Based on the patient's clinical presentation, additional testing may be indicated, including complete blood count, sedimentation rate, and antinuclear antibody testing. Magnetic resonance imaging (MRI) scan of the wrist is indicated if the cause of the wrist mass is suspect (Figs. 53-4 and 53-5).

DIFFERENTIAL DIAGNOSIS

Although ganglion cysts are the most common soft tissue tumor of the wrist, many other pathologic processes can mimic this disorder (Table 53-1). Infection, tenosynovitis, lipomas, and carpal bosses are among the more common diseases that may mimic ganglion cysts of the wrist. Less commonly, malignant tumors including sarcomas and metastatic disease may confuse the diagnosis (Fig. 53-6).

TREATMENT

Initial treatment of the pain and functional disability associated with osteoarthritis of the wrist includes a combination of nonsteroidal antiinflammatory drugs (NSAIDs) or cyclooxy-genase-2 inhibitors and physical therapy. Local application of heat and cold may also be beneficial. Splinting the wrist in the neutral position may provide symptomatic relief and protect the joint from additional trauma. For patients who do not respond to these treatment modalities, injection of the ganglion cyst with local anesthetic and steroid is a reasonable next step. If symptoms persist, surgical excision of the ganglion is recommended.

To inject a ganglion cyst of the wrist, the patient is placed in a supine position with the arm fully adducted at the patient's side and the elbow slightly flexed with the palm of the hand resting on a folded towel. A total of 1.5 mL of local anesthetic and 40 mg of methylprednisolone is drawn up in a 5-mL sterile syringe.

After sterile preparation of skin overlying the ganglion, a 1-inch, 22-gauge needle is inserted in the center of the ganglion, and the contents of the cyst are aspirated (Fig. 53-7). If bone is encountered, the needle is withdrawn back into the ganglion cyst and aspiration is performed. After the ganglion cyst is aspirated, the contents of the syringe are gently injected. Little resistance to injection should be felt. The needle is then removed, and a sterile pressure dressing and ice pack are placed at the injection site. If the ganglion reappears, surgical treatment ultimately may be required.

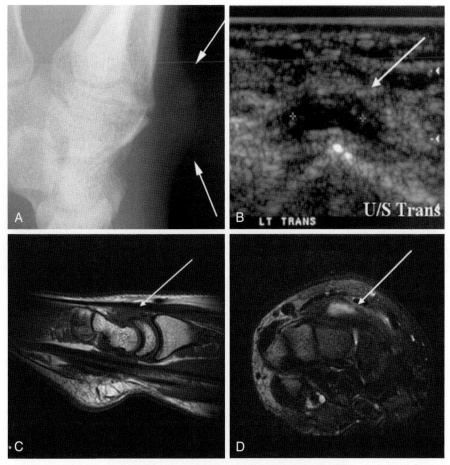

Figure 53-3 Dorsal wrist ganglion *(arrows)*. Lateral radiograph **(A)** demonstrates a soft-tissue mass on the dorsum of the wrist. Ultrasound **(B)** in a second patient shows the typical anechoic cystic appearance of a ganglion. Sagittal T1-weighted **(C)** and axial T2-weighted fat-saturation **(D)** magnetic resonance images through the distal carpal row in a third patient show a circumscribed cystic mass. *(From Nguyen V, Choi J, Davis KW: Imaging of wrist masses, Curr Probl Diagn Radiol 33[4]:147–160, 2004.)*

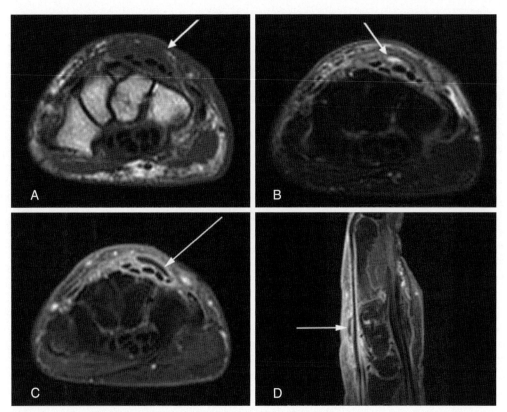

Figure 53-4 Abscess. Axial T1-weighted **(A)** and axial T2-weighted fat-saturation **(B)** magnetic resonance imaging (MRI) scans demonstrate a small focus of fluid *(arrows)* dorsal to the extensor tendons. Postgadolinium axial **(C)** and sagittal T1-weighted **(D)** fat-saturation MRI scans show rim enhancement. *(From Nguyen V, Choi J, Davis KW: Imaging of wrist masses,* Curr Probl Diagn Radiol *33[4]:147–160, 2004.)*

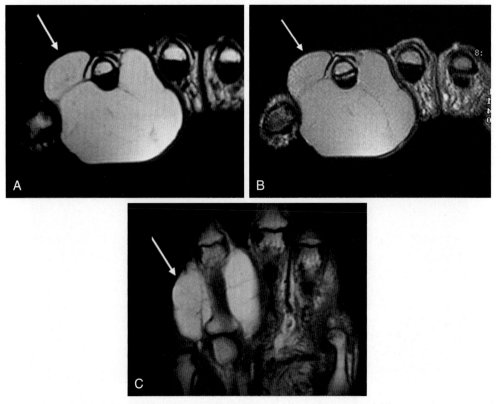

Figure 53-5 Lipoma *(arrows)*. Axial T1-weighted **(A)**, axial T2-weighted **(B)**, and coronal T1-weighted **(C)** magnetic resonance images demonstrate a large mass surrounding the index finger. The lesion has identical signal to fat on all sequences. *(From Nguyen V, Choi J, Davis KW: Imaging of wrist masses,* Curr Probl Diagn Radiol *33[4]:147–160, 2004.)*

TABLE 53-1

Diseases That May Mimic Ganglion Cyst of the Wrist

- Infection
- Lipoma
- Tenosynovitis
- Carpal boss
- Neuroma
- Hypertrophied extensor digitorum brevis manus muscle belly
- Instability of the scaphoid
- Instability of the lunate
- Scaphotrapezial arthritis
- Vascular aneurysm
- Sarcoma

COMPLICATIONS AND PITFALLS

The injection technique described here is safe if careful attention is paid to the clinically relevant anatomy; the ulnar nerve is especially susceptible to damage at the wrist. Care must be taken to avoid injecting directly into tendons that may already be inflamed from irritation caused by rubbing of the ganglion against the tendon. Approximately 25% of patients complain of a transient increase in pain after this injection technique, and patients should be warned of this possibility.

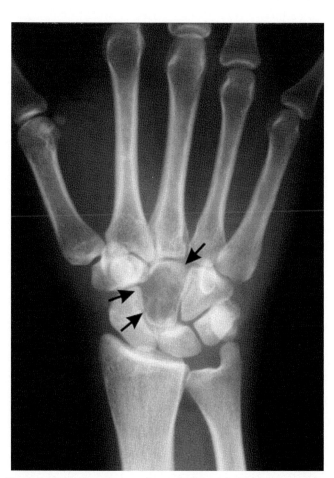

Figure 53-6 Posteroanterior radiograph of the right hand demonstrating a lytic lesion of the capitate *(arrows)* with cortical destruction secondary to metastatic malignant melanoma. *(From Tomas X, Conill C, Combalia A, et al: Malignant melanoma with metastasis into the capitate,* Eur J Radiol *56[3]:362–364, 2005.)*

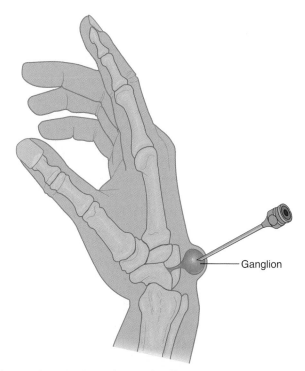

Figure 53-7 Injection technique for the treatment of ganglion cysts of the wrist. *(From Waldman SD:* Atlas of pain management injection techniques, *ed 2, Philadelphia, 2007, Saunders, p 273.)*

Clinical Pearls

The injection technique described is extremely effective in the treatment of pain secondary to arthritis of the wrist joint. Simple analgesics and NSAIDs can be used concurrently with the injection technique. Coexistent bursitis and tendinitis may contribute to wrist pain and necessitate additional treatment with more localized injection of local anesthetic and methylprednisolone.

SUGGESTED READING

Young D, Papp S, Giachino A: Physical examination of the wrist, *Hand Clin* 26(1):21–36, 2007.

Chapter **54**

TRIGGER THUMB

ICD-9 CODE **727.03**

ICD-10 CODE **M65.30**

THE CLINICAL SYNDROME

Trigger thumb is caused by inflammation and swelling of the tendon of the flexor pollicis longus as a result of compression by the head of the first metacarpal bone. Sesamoid bones in this region may also compress and cause trauma to the tendon. Trauma is usually caused by repetitive motion or pressure on the tendon as it passes over these bony prominences. If the inflammation and swelling become chronic, the tendon sheath may thicken, resulting in constriction (Fig. 54-1). Frequently, nodules develop on the tendon, and they can often be palpated when the patient flexes and extends the thumb. Such nodules may catch in the tendon sheath and produce a triggering phenomenon that causes the thumb to catch or lock. Pathologic changes of the pulley mechanism also contribute to the triggering phenomenon (Fig. 54-2). Trigger thumb occurs in patients engaged in repetitive activities, such as handshaking by politicians, or activities that require repetitive pinching movements of the thumb, such as playing video games or frequent card playing (Fig. 54-3).

SIGNS AND SYMPTOMS

The pain of trigger thumb is localized to the palmar aspect of the base of the thumb (unlike the pain of de Quervain's tenosynovitis, which is most pronounced more proximally, over the radial styloid). The pain of trigger thumb is constant and is made worse with active pinching of the thumb. Patients note the inability to hold a coffee cup or a pen. Sleep disturbance is common, and patients often awaken to find that the thumb has become locked in a flexed position.

On physical examination, tenderness and swelling are noted over the tendon, with maximal point tenderness over the base of the thumb. Many patients with trigger thumb experience a creaking sensation with flexion and extension of the thumb. Range of motion of the thumb may be decreased because of pain, and a triggering phenomenon may be present. As mentioned earlier,

patients with trigger thumb often have nodules on the flexor pollicis longus tendon.

TESTING

Plain radiographs are indicated in all patients who present with trigger thumb, to rule out occult bony disease (Fig. 54-4). Based on the patient's clinical presentation, additional testing may be warranted, including a complete blood count, uric acid level, erythrocyte sedimentation rate, and antinuclear antibody testing. Magnetic resonance imaging of the hand is indicated if first metacarpal joint instability is suspected or if the diagnosis of trigger finger is in question. The injection technique described later serves as both a diagnostic and a therapeutic maneuver.

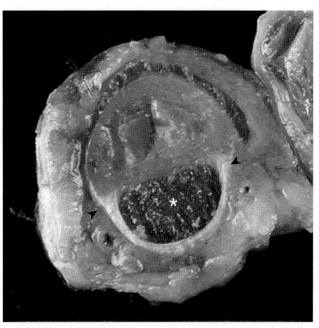

Figure 54-1 Axial specimen photograph demonstrated the flexor tendon *(asterisk)* as it resides in a fibro-osseous canal, anchored to the bones of the fingers by thickened fibrous sheaths called the annular pulleys *(arrowheads)*. *(From Ragheb D, Stanley A, Gentili A, et al: MR imaging of the finger tendons: normal anatomy and commonly encountered pathology, Eur J Radiol 56[3]:296–306, 2005.)*

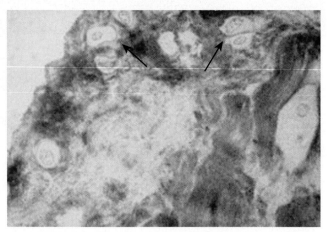

Figure 54-2 Specimen from a pathologic pulley showing chondroid metaplasia *(arrows)* with cells that look like cartilaginous cells organized in nests. (Semithin section, toluidine blue stain; original magnification ×250.) *(From Sbernardori MC, Bandiera P: Histopathology of the A1 pulley in adult trigger fingers,* J Hand Surg Eur Vol 32[5]:556–559, 2007.)

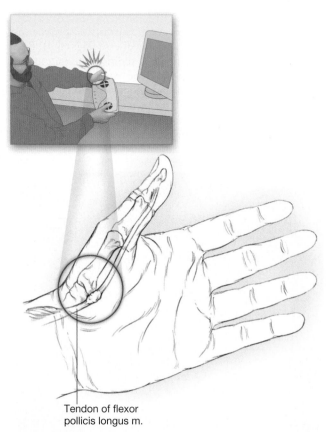

Tendon of flexor
pollicis longus m.

Figure 54-3 Trigger thumb is caused by microtrauma from repetitive pinching movements of the thumb.

DIFFERENTIAL DIAGNOSIS

The diagnosis of trigger thumb is usually made on clinical grounds. Arthritis or gout of the first metacarpal joint may accompany trigger thumb and exacerbate the patient's pain. The nidus of pain from trigger thumb is the flexor pollicis longus tendon at the level of the base of the first metacarpal; occasionally, this may be confused with de Quervain's tenosynovitis.

TREATMENT

Initial treatment of the pain and functional disability associated with trigger thumb includes a combination of nonsteroidal anti-inflammatory drugs or cyclooxygenase-2 inhibitors and physical therapy. A quilter's glove to protect the thumb may also help relieve the patient's symptoms. If these treatments fail, the following injection technique is a reasonable next step.

Injection of trigger thumb is carried out by placing the patient in the supine position with the arm fully adducted at the patient's side and the dorsal surface of the hand resting on a folded towel. A total of 2 mL local anesthetic and 40 mg methylprednisolone is drawn up in a 5-mL sterile syringe. After sterile preparation of the skin overlying the affected tendon, the metacarpophalangeal joint of the thumb is identified. Using strict aseptic technique, at a point just proximal to the joint, the clinician inserts a 1-inch, 25-gauge needle at a 45-degree angle parallel to the affected tendon through the skin and into the subcutaneous tissue overlying the tendon. If bone is encountered, the needle is withdrawn into the subcutaneous tissue. The contents of the syringe are then gently injected. The tendon sheath should distend as the injection proceeds. Little resistance to injection should be felt; if resistance is encountered, the needle is probably in the tendon and should be withdrawn until the injection can be accomplished without significant resistance. The needle is then removed, and a sterile pressure dressing and ice pack are applied to the injection site.

Physical modalities, including local heat and gentle range-of-motion exercises, should be introduced several days after the patient undergoes injection. Vigorous exercises should be avoided, because they will exacerbate the patient's symptoms.

COMPLICATIONS AND PITFALLS

Failure to treat trigger thumb early adequately in its course can result in permanent pain and functional disability caused by continued trauma to the tendon and tendon sheath. The major complications associated with injection are related to trauma to the inflamed and previously damaged tendon. The tendon may rupture if it is injected directly, so a needle position outside the tendon should be confirmed before proceeding with the injection. Further, the radial artery and superficial branch of the radial nerve are susceptible to damage if the needle is placed too far medially. Another complication of injection is infection, although it should be exceedingly rare if strict aseptic technique is followed. Approximately 25% of patients complain of a transient increase in pain after injection, and patients should be warned of this possibility.

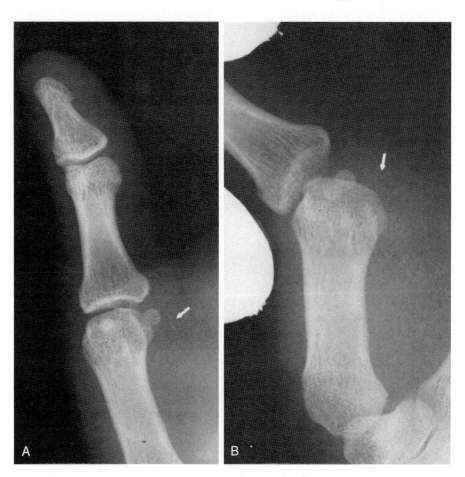

Figure 54-4 Gamekeeper's thumb. **A,** The initial radiograph outlines small osseous fragments adjacent to the first metacarpophalangeal joint *(arrow).* **B,** A radiograph obtained during radial stress reveals subluxation of the phalanx on the metacarpal bone. The fracture fragments are shown *(arrow). (From Resnick D: Diagnosis of bone and joint disorders, ed 4, Philadelphia, 2002, Saunders, p 2583.)*

Clinical Pearls

The injection technique described is extremely effective in the treatment of pain secondary to trigger thumb. Coexistent arthritis and gout may contribute to the patient's pain, thus necessitating additional treatment with more localized injection of local anesthetic and methylprednisolone. The injection technique is safe if careful attention is paid to the clinically relevant anatomy, including the radial artery and the superficial branch of the radial nerve. De Quervain's tenosynovitis may be confused with trigger thumb, but it can be distinguished by the location of the pain and the motions that cause the triggering phenomenon.

SUGGESTED READINGS

Ragheb D, Stanley A, Gentili A, et al: MR imaging of the finger tendons: normal anatomy and commonly encountered pathology, *Eur J Radiol* 56(3):296–306, 2005.

Waldman SD: Trigger finger. In *Atlas of pain management injection techniques,* ed 2, Philadelphia, 2007, Saunders, pp 244–247.

Waldman SD: Painful conditions of the wrist and hand. In *Physical diagnosis of pain: an atlas of signs and symptoms,* ed 2, Philadelphia, 2010, Saunders, pp 153–154.

Wang AA, Hutchinson DT: The effect of corticosteroid injection for trigger finger on blood glucose level in diabetic patients, *J Hand Surg* 31(6):979–981, 2006.

Chapter 55

TRIGGER FINGER

ICD-9 CODE **727.03**

ICD-10 CODE **M65.30**

THE CLINICAL SYNDROME

Trigger finger is caused by inflammation and swelling of the tendon of the flexor digitorum superficialis resulting from compression by the head of the metacarpal bone. Sesamoid bones in this region may also compress and cause trauma to the tendon. Trauma is usually the result of repetitive motion or pressure on the tendon as it passes over these bony prominences. If the inflammation and swelling become chronic, the tendon sheath may thicken, resulting in constriction. Frequently, nodules develop on the tendon, and they can often be palpated when the patient flexes and extends the fingers. Such nodules may catch in the tendon sheath as they pass under a restraining tendon pulley, thus producing a triggering phenomenon that causes the finger to catch or lock. Trigger finger occurs in patients engaged in repetitive activities such as hammering, gripping a steering wheel, or holding a horse's reins too tightly (Fig. 55-1).

SIGNS AND SYMPTOMS

The pain of trigger finger is localized to the distal palm, and tender nodules can often be palpated. The pain is constant and is made worse with active gripping motions of the hand. Patients note significant stiffness when flexing the fingers. Sleep disturbance is common, and patients often awaken to find that the finger has become locked in a flexed position.

On physical examination, tenderness and swelling are noted over the tendon, with maximal point tenderness over the head of the metacarpal. Many patients with trigger finger experience a creaking sensation with flexion and extension of the fingers. Range of motion of the fingers may be decreased because of pain, and a triggering phenomenon may be noted. A catching tendon sign may also be elicited by having the patient clench the affected hand for 30 seconds and then relax but not open the hand. The examiner then passively extends the affected finger, and if he or she appreciates a locking, popping, or catching of the tendon as the finger is straightened, the sign is positive (Fig. 55-2).

TESTING

Plain radiographs are indicated in all patients who present with trigger finger, to rule out occult bony disease (Fig. 55-3). Based on the patient's clinical presentation, additional testing may be warranted, including a complete blood count, uric acid level, erythrocyte sedimentation rate, and antinuclear antibody testing.

Magnetic resonance imaging of the hand is indicated if joint instability or some other abnormality is suspected. The injection technique described later serves as both a diagnostic and a therapeutic maneuver.

DIFFERENTIAL DIAGNOSIS

The diagnosis of trigger finger is usually made on clinical grounds. Arthritis or gout of the metacarpal or interphalangeal joints may accompany trigger finger and exacerbate the patient's pain. Occult fractures occasionally confuse the clinical presentation.

TREATMENT

Initial treatment of the pain and functional disability associated with trigger finger includes a combination of nonsteroidal anti-inflammatory drugs (NSAIDs) or cyclooxygenase-2 inhibitors

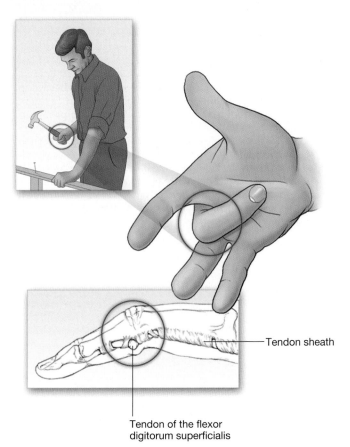

Tendon sheath

Tendon of the flexor
digitorum superficialis

Figure 55-1 Trigger finger is caused by repetitive microtrauma from repeated clenching of the hand.

and physical therapy. A nighttime splint to protect the fingers may also help relieve the symptoms. If these treatments fail, the following injection technique is a reasonable next step.

Injection of trigger finger is carried out by placing the patient in the supine position with the arm fully adducted at the patient's side and the dorsal surface of the hand resting on a folded towel. A total of 2 mL local anesthetic and 40 mg methylprednisolone is drawn up in a 5-mL sterile syringe. After sterile preparation of the skin overlying the affected tendon, the head of the metacarpal beneath the tendon is identified. Using strict aseptic technique, at a point just proximal to the joint,

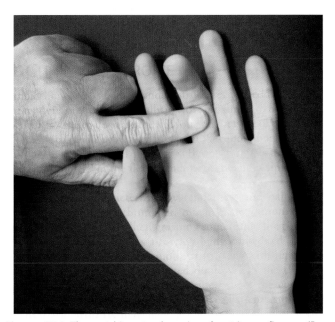

Figure 55-2 The catching tendon sign for trigger finger. *(From Waldman SD:* Physical diagnosis of pain: an atlas of signs and symptoms, *Philadelphia, 2006, Saunders, p 195.)*

a 1-inch, 25-gauge needle at a 45-degree angle parallel to the affected tendon through the skin and into the subcutaneous tissue overlying the tendon. If bone is encountered, the needle is withdrawn into the subcutaneous tissue. The contents of the syringe are then gently injected. The tendon sheath should distend as the injection proceeds. Little resistance to injection should be felt; if resistance is encountered, the needle is probably in the tendon and should be withdrawn until the injection can be accomplished without significant resistance. The needle is then removed, and a sterile pressure dressing and ice pack are applied to the injection site.

Physical modalities, including local heat and gentle range-of-motion exercises, should be introduced several days after the patient undergoes injection. Vigorous exercises should be avoided, because they will exacerbate the patient's symptoms.

Surgical treatment should be considered for patients who fail to respond to the aforementioned treatment modalities.

COMPLICATIONS AND PITFALLS

Failure to treat trigger finger early adequately in its course can result in permanent pain and functional disability because of continued trauma to the tendon and tendon sheath. The major complications associated with injection are related to trauma to the inflamed and previously damaged tendon. The tendon may rupture if it is injected directly, so a needle position outside the tendon should be confirmed before proceeding with the injection. Further, the radial artery and superficial branch of the radial nerve are susceptible to damage if the needle is placed too far medially. Another complication of injection is infection, although it should be exceedingly rare if strict aseptic technique is used, along with universal precautions to minimize any risk to the operator. The incidence of ecchymosis and hematoma formation can be decreased if pressure is applied to the injection site immediately after injection. Approximately 25% of patients complain of a transient increase in pain after injection, and patients should be warned of this possibility.

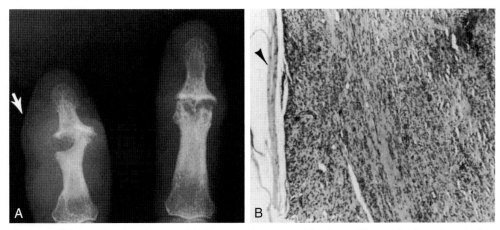

Figure 55-3 Giant cell tumor of the tendon sheath. **A,** In this 55-year-old woman with a 2-year history of pain and gradual swelling of the fingers, a soft tissue mass *(arrow)* can be identified at one distal interphalangeal joint. Underlying inflammatory osteoarthritis of the articulations is evident, and this combination of findings would suggest that the mass is a mucous cyst. However, biopsy of the affected joint demonstrated a giant cell tumor of the tendon sheath. **B,** Photomicrograph (×86) in a different patient reveals a tendon capsule tumor *(arrowhead)* associated with moderately vascularized stroma, plump spindle-shaped or ovoid cells, and multinucleated giant cells. *(From Resnick D:* Diagnosis of bone and joint disorders, *ed 4, Philadelphia, 2002, Saunders, p 4248.)*

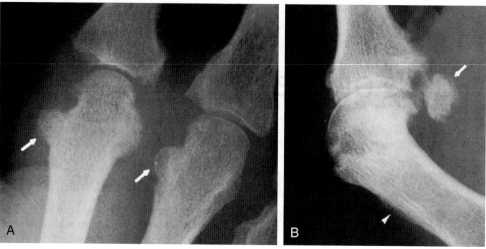

Figure 56-2 Radiographic abnormalities of the metacarpophalangeal joints. **A,** Startling osseous excrescences *(arrows)* around the metacarpal heads are associated with soft tissue swelling, joint space narrowing, and bony erosion and proliferation in the phalanges. **B,** At the first metacarpophalangeal joint, irregular bone formation in the metacarpal head, proximal phalanx, and adjacent sesamoid *(arrow)* can be seen. Periostitis of the metacarpal diaphysis is also evident *(arrowhead)*. *(From Resnick D:* Diagnosis of bone and joint disorders, *ed 4, Philadelphia, 2002, Saunders, p 1087.)*

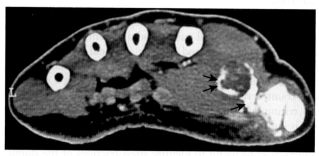

Figure 56-3 Computed tomography image of a chondroma *(double arrows)* and the ulnar sesamoid bone *(single arrow)*. *(From Louaste J, Amhajji L, Eddine EC, Rachid K: Chondroma in a sesamoid bone of the thumb: case report,* J Hand Surg *33[8]:1378–1379, 2008.)*

affected digit until the needle tip rests against the sesamoid bone (see Fig. 56-1). The needle is then withdrawn slightly out of the periosteum and substance of the tendon. Once the needle is in the correct position next to the affected sesamoid bone and aspiration for blood is negative, the contents of the syringe are gently injected. Slight resistance to injection may be felt, given the closed nature of the space. If significant resistance is encountered, the needle is probably in a ligament or tendon and should be advanced or withdrawn slightly until the injection can proceed without significant resistance. The needle is then removed, and a sterile pressure dressing and ice pack are applied to the injection site. The ice should not be left on for longer than 10 minutes to avoid freezing injuries.

Physical modalities, including local heat and gentle range-of-motion exercises, should be introduced several days after the patient undergoes injection. Vigorous exercises should be avoided, because they will exacerbate the patient's symptoms.

COMPLICATIONS AND PITFALLS

The injection technique is safe if careful attention is paid to the clinically relevant anatomy. The major complication of injection is infection, which should be exceedingly rare if strict aseptic technique is followed; in addition, universal precautions should be used to minimize any risk to the operator. The incidence of ecchymosis and hematoma formation can be decreased if pressure is applied to the injection site immediately after injection. Approximately 25% of patients complain of a transient increase in pain after injection of sesamoid bones, and patients should be warned of this possibility.

Clinical Pearls

Pain emanating from the hand is a common problem. Sesamoiditis must be distinguished from stress fractures and other occult disease of the phalanges, as well as fractures of the sesamoid bones. Although the injection technique described provides pain relief, patients often require resting hand splints to aid in rehabilitation of the affected finger. Padded gloves may be useful to take pressure off the affected sesamoid bone and overlying soft tissue. Coexisting bursitis and tendinitis may contribute to the patient's pain, thus necessitating additional treatment with more localized injection of local anesthetic and steroid. Simple analgesics and NSAIDs can be used concurrently with the injection technique.

SUGGESTED READINGS

Lang CJ, Lourie GM: Sesamoiditis of the index finger presenting as acute suppurative flexor tenosynovitis, *J Hand Surg* 24(6):1327–1330, 1999.

Louaste J, Amhajji L, Eddine EC, et al: Chondroma in a sesamoid bone of the thumb: case report, *J Hand Surg* 33(8):1378–1379, 2008.

Patel MR, Pearlman HS, Bassini L, et al: Fractures of the sesamoid bones of the thumb, *J Hand Surg* 15(5):776–781, 1990.

Waldman SD: Sesamoiditis pain syndrome of the hand. In *Atlas of pain management injection techniques,* ed 2, Philadelphia, 2007, Saunders, pp 236–239.

Waldman SD: Painful conditions of the wrist and hand. In *Physical diagnosis of pain: an atlas of signs and symptoms,* ed 2, Philadelphia, 2010, Saunders, pp 153–154.

and physical therapy. A nighttime splint to protect the fingers may also help relieve the symptoms. If these treatments fail, the following injection technique is a reasonable next step.

Injection of trigger finger is carried out by placing the patient in the supine position with the arm fully adducted at the patient's side and the dorsal surface of the hand resting on a folded towel. A total of 2 mL local anesthetic and 40 mg methylprednisolone is drawn up in a 5-mL sterile syringe. After sterile preparation of the skin overlying the affected tendon, the head of the metacarpal beneath the tendon is identified. Using strict aseptic technique, at a point just proximal to the joint,

a 1-inch, 25-gauge needle at a 45-degree angle parallel to the affected tendon through the skin and into the subcutaneous tissue overlying the tendon. If bone is encountered, the needle is withdrawn into the subcutaneous tissue. The contents of the syringe are then gently injected. The tendon sheath should distend as the injection proceeds. Little resistance to injection should be felt; if resistance is encountered, the needle is probably in the tendon and should be withdrawn until the injection can be accomplished without significant resistance. The needle is then removed, and a sterile pressure dressing and ice pack are applied to the injection site.

Physical modalities, including local heat and gentle range-of-motion exercises, should be introduced several days after the patient undergoes injection. Vigorous exercises should be avoided, because they will exacerbate the patient's symptoms.

Surgical treatment should be considered for patients who fail to respond to the aforementioned treatment modalities.

COMPLICATIONS AND PITFALLS

Failure to treat trigger finger early adequately in its course can result in permanent pain and functional disability because of continued trauma to the tendon and tendon sheath. The major complications associated with injection are related to trauma to the inflamed and previously damaged tendon. The tendon may rupture if it is injected directly, so a needle position outside the tendon should be confirmed before proceeding with the injection. Further, the radial artery and superficial branch of the radial nerve are susceptible to damage if the needle is placed too far medially. Another complication of injection is infection, although it should be exceedingly rare if strict aseptic technique is used, along with universal precautions to minimize any risk to the operator. The incidence of ecchymosis and hematoma formation can be decreased if pressure is applied to the injection site immediately after injection. Approximately 25% of patients complain of a transient increase in pain after injection, and patients should be warned of this possibility.

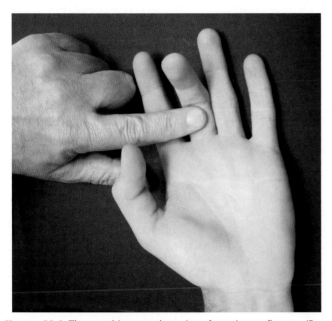

Figure 55-2 The catching tendon sign for trigger finger. *(From Waldman SD: Physical diagnosis of pain: an atlas of signs and symptoms, Philadelphia, 2006, Saunders, p 195.)*

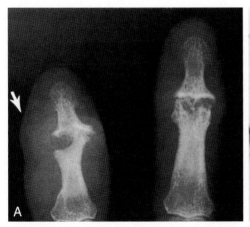
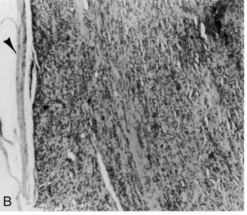

Figure 55-3 Giant cell tumor of the tendon sheath. **A,** In this 55-year-old woman with a 2-year history of pain and gradual swelling of the fingers, a soft tissue mass *(arrow)* can be identified at one distal interphalangeal joint. Underlying inflammatory osteoarthritis of the articulations is evident, and this combination of findings would suggest that the mass is a mucous cyst. However, biopsy of the affected joint demonstrated a giant cell tumor of the tendon sheath. **B,** Photomicrograph (×86) in a different patient reveals a tendon capsule tumor *(arrowhead)* associated with moderately vascularized stroma, plump spindle-shaped or ovoid cells, and multinucleated giant cells. *(From Resnick D: Diagnosis of bone and joint disorders, ed 4, Philadelphia, 2002, Saunders, p 4248.)*

Clinical Pearls

The injection technique described is extremely effective in the treatment of pain secondary to trigger finger. Coexistent arthritis or gout may contribute to the patient's pain, thus necessitating additional treatment with more localized injection of local anesthetic and methylprednisolone. A hand splint to protect the fingers may also help relieve the symptoms of trigger finger. Simple analgesics and NSAIDs can be used concurrently with the injection technique.

SUGGESTED READINGS

Ragheb D, Stanley A, Gentili A, et al: MR imaging of the finger tendons: normal anatomy and commonly encountered pathology, *Eur J Radiol* 56(3):296–306, 2005.

Waldman SD: Trigger finger. In *Atlas of pain management injection techniques,* ed 2, Philadelphia, 2007, Saunders, pp 244–247.

Waldman SD: Painful conditions of the wrist and hand. In *Physical diagnosis of pain: an atlas of signs and symptoms,* ed 2, Philadelphia, 2010, Saunders, pp 153–154.

Wang AA, Hutchinson DT: The effect of corticosteroid injection for trigger finger on blood glucose level in diabetic patients, *J Hand Surg* 31(6):979–981, 2006.

Chapter 56

SESAMOIDITIS OF THE HAND

ICD-9 CODE `733.99`

ICD-10 CODES `M89.8x9`

THE CLINICAL SYNDROME

Sesamoid bones are small, rounded structures embedded in the flexor tendons of the hand, usually in close proximity to the joints. These bones serve to decrease the friction and pressure of the flexor tendon as it passes in proximity to a joint. Sesamoid bones of the thumb occur in almost all patients suffering from sesamoiditis, and they are present in the flexor tendons of the index finger in a few patients.

Sesamoiditis is characterized by tenderness and pain over the flexor aspect of the thumb or, much less commonly, the index finger (Fig. 56-1). When grasping something, the patient often feels that he or she has a foreign body embedded in the affected digit. The pain of sesamoiditis worsens with repeated flexion and extension of the affected digit. When the thumb is affected, it is usually on the radial side, where the condyle of the adjacent metacarpal is less obtrusive. Patients suffering from psoriatic arthritis may have a higher incidence of sesamoiditis of the hand.

SIGNS AND SYMPTOMS

On physical examination, pain can be reproduced by pressure on the sesamoid bone. In patients with sesamoiditis, the tender area moves with the flexor tendon when the patient actively flexes the thumb or finger, whereas with occult bony disease of the phalanges, the tender area remains over the pathologic area. With acute trauma to the sesamoid, ecchymosis over the flexor surface of the affected digit may be present.

TESTING

Plain radiographs (Fig. 56-2) and magnetic resonance imaging (MRI) are indicated in all patients who present with sesamoiditis, to rule out fractures and identify sesamoid bones that may have become inflamed. Based on the patient's clinical presentation, additional testing may be warranted, including a complete blood count, erythrocyte sedimentation rate, and antinuclear antibody testing. MRI or computed tomography of the fingers and wrist is indicated if joint instability, occult mass, occult fracture, infection, or tumor is suspected (Fig. 56-3). Radionuclide bone scanning may be useful to identify stress fractures of the thumb and fingers or sesamoid bones that may be missed on plain radiographs of the hand.

DIFFERENTIAL DIAGNOSIS

The tentative diagnosis of sesamoiditis is made on clinical grounds and is confirmed by radiographic testing. Arthritis, tenosynovitis, or gout of the affected digit may accompany sesamoiditis and exacerbate the patient's pain. Occult fractures occasionally confuse the clinical presentation. Occasionally, osseous neoplasm can occur within a sesamoid bone and can further confuse the diagnosis.

TREATMENT

Initial treatment of the pain and functional disability associated with sesamoiditis of the hand includes a combination of nonsteroidal antiinflammatory drugs (NSAIDs) or cyclooxygenase-2 inhibitors and physical therapy. A nighttime splint to protect the fingers may also help relieve the symptoms. If the patient does not respond to these conservative measures, a trial of injection therapy with local anesthetic and steroid is a reasonable next step.

To perform injection of the sesamoid bone, the patient is placed in the supine position with the palmar surface of the hand exposed. The skin overlying the tender sesamoid bone is prepared with antiseptic solution. A sterile syringe containing 2 mL of 0.25% preservative-free bupivacaine and 40 mg methylprednisolone is attached to a ⅝-inch, 25-gauge needle using strict aseptic technique. The needle is carefully advanced through the palmar surface of the

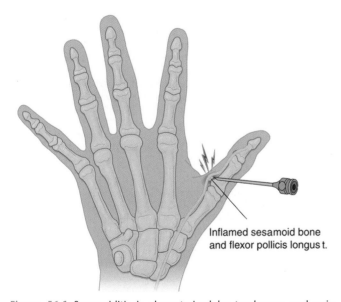

Inflamed sesamoid bone and flexor pollicis longus t.

Figure 56-1 Sesamoiditis is characterized by tenderness and pain over the flexor aspect of the thumb. *(From Waldman SD: Atlas of pain management injection techniques, ed 2, Philadelphia, 2007, Saunders, p 238.)*

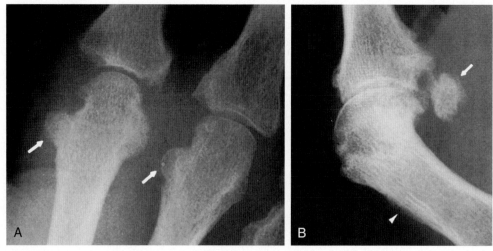

Figure 56-2 Radiographic abnormalities of the metacarpophalangeal joints. **A,** Startling osseous excrescences *(arrows)* around the metacarpal heads are associated with soft tissue swelling, joint space narrowing, and bony erosion and proliferation in the phalanges. **B,** At the first metacarpophalangeal joint, irregular bone formation in the metacarpal head, proximal phalanx, and adjacent sesamoid *(arrow)* can be seen. Periostitis of the metacarpal diaphysis is also evident *(arrowhead). (From Louaste J:* Diagnosis of bone and joint disorders, *ed 4, Philadelphia, 2002, Saunders, p 1087.)*

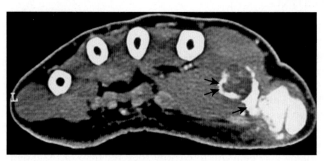

Figure 56-3 Computed tomography image of a chondroma *(double arrows)* and the ulnar sesamoid bone *(single arrow). (From Louaste J, Amhajji L, Eddine EC, Rachid K: Chondroma in a sesamoid bone of the thumb: case report,* J Hand Surg *33[8]:1378–1379, 2008.)*

affected digit until the needle tip rests against the sesamoid bone (see Fig. 56-1). The needle is then withdrawn slightly out of the periosteum and substance of the tendon. Once the needle is in the correct position next to the affected sesamoid bone and aspiration for blood is negative, the contents of the syringe are gently injected. Slight resistance to injection may be felt, given the closed nature of the space. If significant resistance is encountered, the needle is probably in a ligament or tendon and should be advanced or withdrawn slightly until the injection can proceed without significant resistance. The needle is then removed, and a sterile pressure dressing and ice pack are applied to the injection site. The ice should not be left on for longer than 10 minutes to avoid freezing injuries.

Physical modalities, including local heat and gentle range-of-motion exercises, should be introduced several days after the patient undergoes injection. Vigorous exercises should be avoided, because they will exacerbate the patient's symptoms.

COMPLICATIONS AND PITFALLS

The injection technique is safe if careful attention is paid to the clinically relevant anatomy. The major complication of injection is infection, which should be exceedingly rare if strict aseptic

technique is followed; in addition, universal precautions should be used to minimize any risk to the operator. The incidence of ecchymosis and hematoma formation can be decreased if pressure is applied to the injection site immediately after injection. Approximately 25% of patients complain of a transient increase in pain after injection of sesamoid bones, and patients should be warned of this possibility.

Clinical Pearls

Pain emanating from the hand is a common problem. Sesamoiditis must be distinguished from stress fractures and other occult disease of the phalanges, as well as fractures of the sesamoid bones. Although the injection technique described provides pain relief, patients often require resting hand splints to aid in rehabilitation of the affected finger. Padded gloves may be useful to take pressure off the affected sesamoid bone and overlying soft tissue. Coexisting bursitis and tendinitis may contribute to the patient's pain, thus necessitating additional treatment with more localized injection of local anesthetic and steroid. Simple analgesics and NSAIDs can be used concurrently with the injection technique.

SUGGESTED READINGS

Lang CJ, Lourie GM: Sesamoiditis of the index finger presenting as acute suppurative flexor tenosynovitis, *J Hand Surg* 24(6):1327–1330, 1999.
Louaste J, Amhajji L, Eddine EC, et al: Chondroma in a sesamoid bone of the thumb: case report, *J Hand Surg* 33(8):1378–1379, 2008.
Patel MR, Pearlman HS, Bassini L, et al: Fractures of the sesamoid bones of the thumb, *J Hand Surg* 15(5):776–781, 1990.
Waldman SD: Sesamoiditis pain syndrome of the hand. In *Atlas of pain management injection techniques,* ed 2, Philadelphia, 2007, Saunders, pp 236–239.
Waldman SD: Painful conditions of the wrist and hand. In *Physical diagnosis of pain: an atlas of signs and symptoms,* ed 2, Philadelphia, 2010, Saunders, pp 153–154.

Chapter 57

PLASTIC BAG PALSY

ICD-9 CODE `354.9`

ICD-10 CODE `G56.90`

THE CLINICAL SYNDROME

Plastic bag palsy is an entrapment neuropathy of the digital nerves caused by compression of the nerves against the bony phalanges by the handles of a plastic bag. The common digital nerves arise from fibers of the median and ulnar nerves. The thumb also has contributions from superficial branches of the radial nerve. The common digital nerves pass along the metacarpal bones and divide as they reach the distal palm. The volar digital nerves supply the majority of sensory innervation to the fingers and run along the ventrolateral aspect of the finger beside the digital vein and artery. The smaller dorsal digital nerves contain fibers from the ulnar and radial nerves and supply the dorsum of the fingers as far as the proximal joints.

Plastic bag palsy has increased in frequency as stores have switched from paper to plastic bags. Compression by the handles of a heavy plastic bag is the inciting cause, and the most common clinical feature is the presence of painful digital nerves at the point of compression (Fig. 57-1). Plastic bag palsy may present in either an acute or a chronic form. Pain may develop from an acute injury to the nerves after carrying a heavy bag on too few fingers, or it may occur from direct trauma to the soft tissues overlying the digital nerves if the fingers become caught in a bag handle twisted around them. Plastic bag palsy is occasionally seen in homeless people who carry their possessions around in bags and who use the same hand day after day. The affected nerves may be thickened, and inflammation of the nerve and overlying soft tissues may be seen. In addition to pain, patients may complain of paresthesias and numbness just below the point of nerve compromise.

SIGNS AND SYMPTOMS

The pain of plastic bag palsy is constant and is made worse with compression of the affected digital nerves. Patients often note the inability to hold objects with the affected fingers. Sleep disturbance is common.

On physical examination, the patient has tenderness to palpation of the affected digital nerves. Palpation can also cause paresthesias, and continued pressure on the nerves may induce numbness distal to the point of compression. Range of motion of the thumb is normal. With acute trauma to the sesamoid, ecchymosis of the skin overlying the affected digital nerves may be present.

TESTING

Plain radiographs are indicated in all patients who present with plastic bag palsy, to rule out occult bony disorders such as bone spurs or cysts that may be compressing the digital nerves. Electromyography can distinguish other causes of hand numbness. Based on the patient's clinical presentation, additional testing may be indicated, including a complete blood count, uric acid level, erythrocyte sedimentation rate, and antinuclear antibody testing. Magnetic resonance imaging of the hand can rule out soft tissue abnormalities including tumors that may be compressing the digital nerves (Fig. 57-2). Injection of the nerve serves as both a diagnostic and a therapeutic maneuver.

DIFFERENTIAL DIAGNOSIS

The tentative diagnosis of plastic bag palsy is made on clinical grounds and is confirmed by electromyography. Arthritis, tenosynovitis, or gout of the affected digits may accompany plastic bag

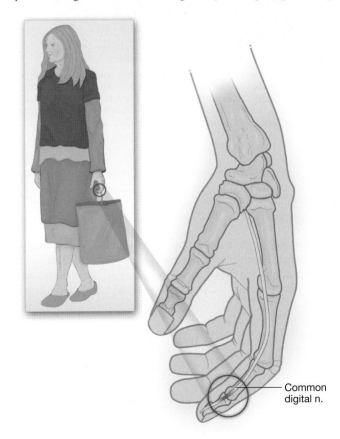

Common digital n.

Figure 57-1 Compression by the handles of a heavy plastic bag can cause plastic bag palsy.

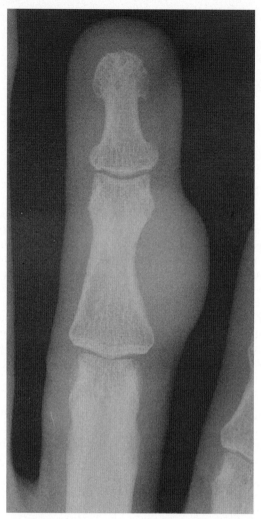

Figure 57-2 Fibrous xanthoma. A soft tissue mass adjacent to the middle phalanx has produced erosion of the adjacent bone. This pattern of bony resorption is indicative of pressure atrophy and is not a sign of malignancy. *(From Resnick D: Diagnosis of bone and joint disorders, ed 4, Philadelphia, 2002, Saunders, p 4190.)*

palsy and exacerbate the patient's pain. Occult fractures occasionally confuse the clinical presentation.

TREATMENT

The first step in the treatment of the pain and functional disability associated with plastic bag palsy is to remove the offending compression of the digital nerves. Nonsteroidal antiinflammatory drugs, simple analgesics, or cyclooxygenase-2 inhibitors may be prescribed as well. If the patient complains of significant dysesthesias or paresthesias, the addition of gabapentin should be considered. Gabapentin is started at a bedtime dose of 300 mg; it is then titrated upward to 3600 mg in divided doses, as side effects allow. Physical modalities, including local heat and gentle range-of-motion exercises, should be introduced to avoid loss of function. Vigorous exercises should be avoided, because they will exacerbate the patient's symptoms. A nighttime splint to protect the fingers may be helpful, and wearing padded gloves can take pressure off the affected digital nerves and overlying soft tissue. If sleep disturbance is present, low-dose tricyclic antidepressants are indicated. If the patient does not respond to these conservative modalities, a trial of injection therapy with local anesthetic and steroid is a reasonable next step. Rarely, surgical exploration and neuroplasty of the affected nerves are required for symptomatic relief.

COMPLICATIONS AND PITFALLS

Injection of the affected digital nerves is safe if careful attention is paid to the clinically relevant anatomy. Sterile technique must be used to avoid infection, as well as universal precautions to minimize any risk to the operator. The incidence of ecchymosis and hematoma formation can be decreased if pressure is applied to the injection site immediately after injection. The major complication of injection is infection, which should be exceedingly rare if strict aseptic technique is followed. Approximately 25% of patients complain of a transient increase in pain after injection of the affected digital nerves, and patients should be warned of this possibility.

Clinical Pearls

Pain emanating from the hand is a common problem. Plastic bag palsy must be distinguished from stress fractures and other occult disorders of the phalanges, as well as sesamoiditis and occult fractures of the sesamoid bones. Coexistent bursitis and tendinitis may contribute to the patient's pain, thus necessitating additional treatment with more localized injection of local anesthetic and steroid.

SUGGESTED READINGS

De Smet L: Compression of the common digital nerve in the palm of the hand: a case report, *J Hand Surg* 22(6):1047–1048, 1997.

Hug U, Burg D, Baldi SV, et al: Compression neuropathy of the radial palmar thumb nerve, *Chir Main* 23(1):49–51, 2004.

Izzi J, Dennison D, Noerdlinger M, et al: Nerve injuries of the elbow, wrist, and hand in athletes, *Clin Sports Med* 20(1):203–217, 2001.

Waldman SD: Painful conditions of the wrist and hand. In *Physical diagnosis of pain: an atlas of signs and symptoms,* ed 2, Philadelphia, 2010, Saunders, pp 153–154.

Chapter 58

CARPAL BOSS SYNDROME

ICD-9 CODE **726.91**

ICD-10 CODE **M25.70**

THE CLINICAL SYNDROME

Carpal boss syndrome, or os styloideum, is characterized by localized tenderness and sharp pain over the junction of the second and third carpometacarpal joints. The pain of carpal boss results from exostosis of the second and third carpometacarpal joints or, more uncommonly, a loose body involving the intraarticular space (Fig. 58-1). Patients often report that the pain is worse *after* rigorous physical activity involving the hand rather than during the activity itself. The pain of carpal boss may also radiate locally, thus confusing the clinical presentation. Carpal boss syndrome has a slight male predominance and a peak incidence in the middle of the third decade of life. Trauma is often the common denominator in the development of carpal boss.

SIGNS AND SYMPTOMS

On physical examination, the carpal boss appears as a bony protuberance that can be seen more easily by having the patient flex his or her wrist (Fig. 58-2). The pain associated with can be reproduced by applying pressure to the soft tissue overlying the carpal boss. Patients with carpal boss demonstrate a positive hunchback sign; that is, the examiner can appreciate a bony prominence when he or she palpates the carpal boss (Fig. 58-3). With acute trauma to the dorsum of the hand, ecchymosis over the carpal boss of the affected joint or joints may be present.

TESTING

Plain radiographs are indicated in all patients who present with carpal boss, to rule out fractures and to identify exostoses responsible for the symptoms (see Fig. 58-1). Based on the patient's clinical presentation, additional testing may be warranted to exclude inflammatory arthritis, including a complete blood count,

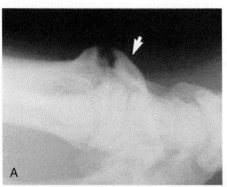

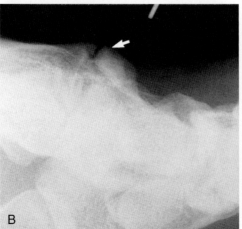

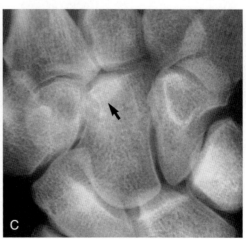

Figure 58-1 Radiographic manifestations of os styloideum. A lateral radiograph of the hand **(A)** demonstrates the osteophytic appearance of the extra ossification center *(arrow)*. Clinically, a painless soft tissue lump is often evident. In another patient, a similar outgrowth *(arrows)* is evident on lateral **(B)** and frontal **(C)** radiographs. *(From Resnick D:* Diagnosis of bone and joint disorders, *ed 4, Philadelphia, 2002, Saunders, p 1312.)*

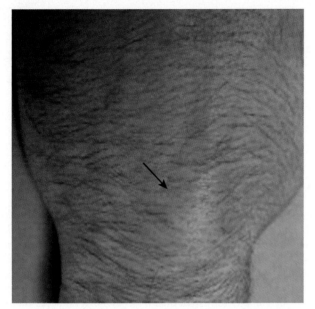

Figure 58-2 The carpal boss is frequently confused initially with a dorsal ganglion on viewing the dorsal wrist. It generally feels harder with palpation, is positioned more distally than wrist ganglion, and overlies the index and middle finger carpometacarpal joints *(arrow)*. *(From Park MJ, Namdari S, Weiss A-P: The carpal boss: review of diagnosis and treatment,* J Hand Surg *33[3]:446–449, 2008.)*

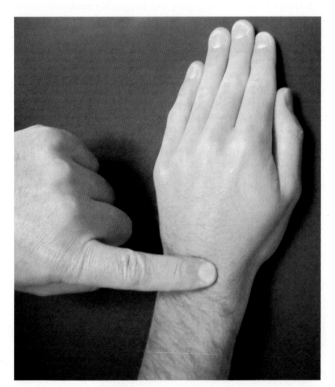

Figure 58-3 The hunchback sign for carpal boss. *(From Waldman SD: Painful conditions of the wrist and hand. In* Physical diagnosis of pain: an atlas of signs and symptoms, *ed 2, Philadelphia 2010, Saunders, p 189.)*

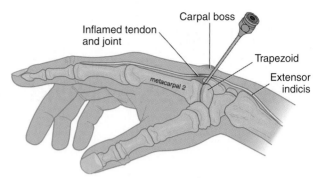

Figure 58-4 Injection technique for carpal boss, or os styloideum. *(From Waldman SD: Carpal boss. In* Atlas of pain management injection techniques, *ed 2, Philadelphia, 2007, Saunders, p 268.)*

erythrocyte sedimentation rate, uric acid level, and antinuclear antibody testing. Magnetic resonance imaging of the fingers and wrist is indicated if joint instability, occult mass, occult fracture, infection, or tumor is suspected. Radionuclide bone scanning may be useful to identify stress fractures.

DIFFERENTIAL DIAGNOSIS

The tentative diagnosis of carpal boss is made on clinical grounds and is confirmed by radiographic testing. Arthritis, tenosynovitis, or gout of the affected digits may accompany carpal boss and exacerbate the patient's pain. Occult fractures occasionally confuse the clinical presentation.

TREATMENT

Initial treatment of the pain and functional disability associated with carpal boss consists of nonsteroidal antiinflammatory drugs, simple analgesics, or cyclooxygenase-2 inhibitors. Physical modalities, including local heat and gentle range-of-motion exercises, should be introduced to avoid loss of function. Vigorous exercises should be avoided, because they will exacerbate the patient's symptoms. A nighttime splint to protect the fingers may be helpful. If sleep disturbance is present, low-dose tricyclic antidepressants are indicated. If the patient does not respond to these conservative modalities, a trial of injection therapy with local anesthetic and steroid is a reasonable next step (Fig. 58-4). Rarely, surgical exploration and removal of the carpal boss are required for symptomatic relief.

COMPLICATIONS AND PITFALLS

The major complication of injection with local anesthetic and steroid is infection, which should be exceedingly rare if strict aseptic technique is followed. Approximately 25% of patients complain of a transient increase in pain after injection, and patients should be warned of this possibility. The clinician should always keep in mind that occult fracture or tumor may mimic the clinical symptoms of carpal boss.

Clinical Pearls

Pain emanating from the hand is a common problem. Carpal boss must be distinguished from stress fracture, arthritis, and other occult disorders of the wrist and hand. Although injection with local anesthetic and steroid palliates the pain of carpal boss, patients may ultimately require surgical removal of the exostosis to obtain long-lasting relief. Coexistent bursitis and tendinitis may contribute to the patient's pain, thus necessitating additional treatment with more localized injection of local anesthetic and steroid.

SUGGESTED READINGS

Alemohammad AM, Nakamura K, El-Sheneway M, et al: Incidence of carpal boss and osseous coalition: an anatomic study, *J Hand Surg* 34(1):1–6, 2009.

Fusi S, Watson HK, Cuono CB: The carpal boss: a 20-year review of operative management, *J Hand Surg* 20(3):405–408, 1995.

Melone CP Jr, Polatsch DB, Beldner S: Disabling hand injuries in boxing: boxer's knuckle and traumatic carpal boss, *Clin Sports Med* 28(4):609–621, 2009.

Park MJ, Namdari S, Weiss A-P: The carpal boss: review of diagnosis and treatment, *J Hand Surg* 33(3):446–449, 2008.

Waldman SD: Carpal boss. In *Atlas of pain management injection techniques*, ed 2, Philadelphia, 2007, Saunders, pp 267–279.

Waldman SD: Painful conditions of the wrist and hand. In *Physical diagnosis of pain: an atlas of signs and symptoms*, ed 2, Philadelphia, 2010, Saunders, pp 153–154.

Chapter 59

DUPUYTREN'S CONTRACTURE

ICD-9 CODE 728.6

ICD-10 CODE M72.0

THE CLINICAL SYNDROME

Dupuytren's contracture is a common complaint. Although it is initially painful, the pain seems to decrease as the condition progresses. As a result, patients suffering from Dupuytren's contracture generally seek medical attention for functional disability rather than for pain.

Dupuytren's contracture is caused by progressive fibrosis of the palmar fascia. Initially, the patient may notice fibrotic nodules along the course of the flexor tendons of the hand that are tender to palpation. As the disease advances, these nodules coalesce and form fibrous bands that gradually thicken and contract around the flexor tendons; this has the effect of drawing the affected fingers into flexion. Although any finger can develop Dupuytren's contracture, the ring and little fingers are most commonly affected (Fig. 59-1). If untreated, the fingers can develop permanent flexion contractures. The plantar fascia may be affected concurrently.

Dupuytren's contracture is thought to have a genetic basis and occurs most frequently in male patients of northern Scandinavian descent. The disease may also be associated with trauma to the palm, diabetes, alcoholism, and long-term barbiturate use. The disease rarely occurs before the fourth decade.

SIGNS AND SYMPTOMS

In the early stages of the disease, hard fibrotic nodules along the path of the flexor tendons can be palpated. These nodules are often misdiagnosed as calluses or warts. At this early stage, pain is invariably present. As the disease progresses, taut fibrous

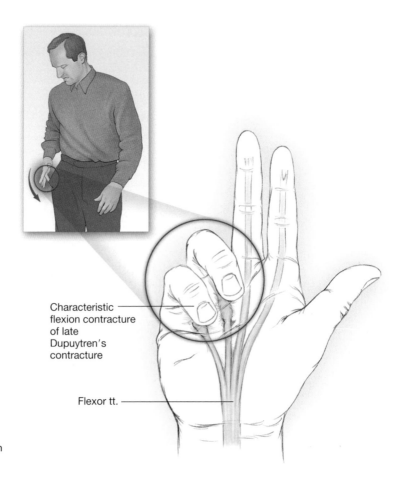

Characteristic flexion contracture of late Dupuytren's contracture

Flexor tt.

Figure 59-1 Dupuytren's contracture usually affects the fourth and fifth digits in men older than 40 years.

bands form; they may cross the metacarpophalangeal joint and ultimately the proximal interphalangeal joint (Fig. 59-2). These bands are not painful to palpation, and although they limit finger extension, finger flexion remains relatively normal. At this point, patients often seek medical advice because of difficulty putting on gloves and reaching into their pockets. In the final stages of the disease, flexion contracture develops, with its negative impact on function. Arthritis, gout of the metacarpal and interphalangeal joints, and trigger finger may coexist with Dupuytren's contracture and may exacerbate the patient's pain and disability.

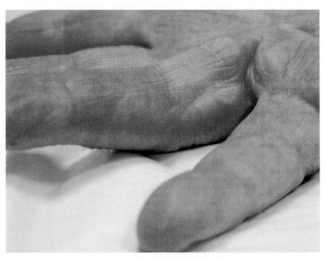

Figure 59-2 Dupuytren's contracture of the ring finger. Pitting of the skin and a longitudinal cord can be seen causing metacarpophalangeal joint flexion. *(From Hochberg MC, Silman AJ, Smolen JS, et al, editors: Rheumatology, ed 5, Philadelphia, 2011, Mosby, p 717.)*

TESTING

Plain radiographs are indicated for all patients who present with Dupuytren's contracture, to rule out occult bony disease (Fig. 59-3). Based on the patient's clinical presentation, additional testing may be warranted, including a complete blood count, uric acid level, erythrocyte sedimentation rate, and antinuclear antibody testing. Magnetic resonance imaging of the hand is indicated if joint instability or tumor is suspected. Electromyography is indicated if coexistent ulnar or carpal tunnel syndrome is a possibility.

DIFFERENTIAL DIAGNOSIS

Dupuytren's contracture is a clinically distinct entity that is rarely misdiagnosed once the syndrome is well established. Coexisting flexor tendinitis or trigger finger may be confused with Dupuytren's contracture early in the course of the disease.

TREATMENT

Initial treatment of the pain and functional disability associated with Dupuytren's contracture includes a combination of nonsteroidal antiinflammatory drugs (NSAIDs) or cyclooxygenase-2 inhibitors and physical therapy. A nighttime splint to protect the fingers may be helpful. If greater symptomatic relief is required, the following injection technique is a reasonable next step.

Injection of Dupuytren's contracture is carried out by placing the patient in the supine position with the arm fully adducted at the patient's side and the dorsal surface of the hand resting on a folded towel. A total of 2 mL local anesthetic and 40 mg methylprednisolone is drawn up in a 5-mL sterile syringe. The skin overlying the fibrous band or nodule is prepared with antiseptic solution. At a point just lateral to the fibrosis, a 1-inch, 25-gauge needle is inserted at a 45-degree angle parallel to the fibrosis,

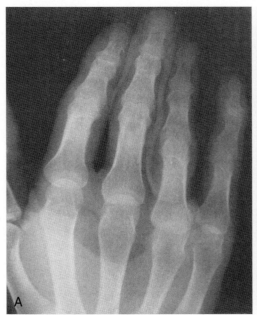
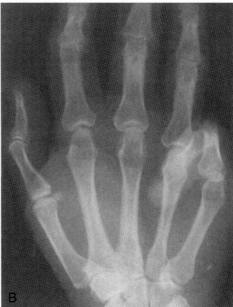

Figure 59-3 Radiographic manifestations of Dupuytren's contracture. **A,** Flexion deformities of the metacarpophalangeal joints of the four ulnar digits are demonstrated. **B,** Severe flexion contracture is evident in the fifth finger, with minor changes in the other digits. *(From Resnick D: Diagnosis of bone and joint disorders, ed 4, Philadelphia, 2002, Saunders, p 4667.)*

through the skin, and into the subcutaneous tissue overlying the fibrotic area. If bone is encountered, the needle is withdrawn into the subcutaneous tissue and is advanced again in proximity to the fibrosis. The contents of the syringe are then gently injected. The clinician may feel some resistance to injection because of fibrosis of the surrounding tissue. If significant resistance is encountered, the needle is probably in the tendon or nodule and should be withdrawn until the injection can proceed without significant resistance. The needle is then removed, and a sterile pressure dressing and ice pack are applied to the injection site.

Physical modalities, including local heat and gentle range-of-motion exercises, should be introduced several days after the patient undergoes injection. Vigorous exercises should be avoided, because they will exacerbate the patient's symptoms.

Although the foregoing treatment modalities provide symptomatic relief, Dupuytren's contracture usually requires surgical treatment.

COMPLICATIONS AND PITFALLS

The injection technique is safe if careful attention is paid to the clinically relevant anatomy. Sterile technique must be used to avoid infection, as well as universal precautions to minimize any risk to the operator. The incidence of ecchymosis and hematoma formation can be decreased if pressure is applied to the injection site immediately after injection. The major complications associated with injection are related to trauma to an inflamed or previously damaged tendon. Such tendons may rupture if they are injected

directly, so a needle position outside the tendon should be confirmed before the clinician proceeds with the injection. Another complication of injection is infection, although it should be exceedingly rare if strict aseptic technique is followed. Approximately 25% of patients complain of a transient increase in pain after injection, and patients should be warned of this possibility.

Clinical Pearls

The aforementioned treatment modalities are useful in providing symptomatic relief of the pain and disability of Dupuytren's contracture. However, most patients ultimately require surgical treatment. Coexistent arthritis or gout may contribute to the patient's pain, thus necessitating additional treatment with more localized injection of local anesthetic and methylprednisolone. Simple analgesics and NSAIDs can be used concurrently with this injection technique.

SUGGESTED READINGS

Geoghegan JM, Forbes J, Clark DI, et al: Dupuytren's disease risk factors, *J Hand Surg* 29(5):423–426, 2004.

Hughes TB Jr, Mechrefe A, Littler JW, et al: Dupuytren's disease, *J Am Soc Surg Hand* 3(1):27–40, 2003.

Reilly RM, Stern PJ, Goldfarb CA: A retrospective review of the management of Dupuytren's nodules, *J Hand Surg* 30(5):1014–1018, 2005.

Waldman SD: Dupuytren's contracture. In *Atlas of pain management injection techniques,* ed 2, Philadelphia, 2007, Saunders, pp 275–277.

Waldman SD: Dupuytren's contracture. In *Pain review,* Philadelphia, 2009, Saunders, pp 277–278.

Chapter 60

COSTOSTERNAL SYNDROME

ICD-9 CODE   786.50

ICD-10 CODE   R07.9

THE CLINICAL SYNDROME

Many patients with noncardiogenic chest pain are suffering from costosternal joint pain. Most commonly, the costosternal joints become painful in response to inflammation as a result of overuse or misuse or in response to trauma secondary to acceleration-deceleration injuries or blunt trauma to the chest wall (Fig. 60-1). With severe trauma, the joints may subluxate or dislocate. The costosternal joints are susceptible to the development of osteoarthritis, rheumatoid arthritis, ankylosing spondylitis, Reiter's syndrome, and psoriatic arthritis. The joints are also subject to invasion by tumor from primary malignant tumors, including thymoma, or from metastatic disease.

SIGNS AND SYMPTOMS

Physical examination reveals that the patient vigorously attempts to splint the joints by keeping the shoulders stiffly in a neutral position. Pain is reproduced with active protraction or retraction of the shoulder, deep inspiration, and full elevation of the arm. Shrugging of the shoulder may also reproduce the pain. Coughing may be difficult, leading to inadequate pulmonary toilet in patients who have sustained trauma to the anterior chest wall. The costosternal joints and adjacent intercostal muscles may be tender to palpation. The patient may also complain of a clicking sensation with movement of the joint.

TESTING

Plain radiographs are indicated for all patients who present with pain that is thought to be emanating from the costosternal joints, to rule out occult bony disorders, including tumor (Fig. 60-2). If trauma is present, radionuclide bone scanning may be useful to exclude occult fractures of the ribs or sternum. Based on the patient's

clinical presentation, additional testing may be indicated, including a complete blood count, prostate-specific antigen level, erythrocyte sedimentation rate, and antinuclear antibody testing. Laboratory evaluation for collagen vascular disease is indicated in patients suffering from costosternal joint pain if other joints are involved. Magnetic resonance imaging of the joints is indicated if joint instability or occult mass is suspected or to elucidate the cause of the pain further. The injection technique described later serves as both a diagnostic and a therapeutic maneuver.

DIFFERENTIAL DIAGNOSIS

As mentioned, the pain of costosternal syndrome is often mistaken for pain of cardiac origin, and it leads to visits to the emergency department and unnecessary cardiac workups. If trauma has occurred, costosternal syndrome may coexist with fractured ribs or fractures of the sternum itself, which can be missed on plain radiographs and may require radionuclide bone scanning for proper identification. Tietze's syndrome, which is painful enlargement of the upper costochondral cartilage associated with viral infection, may be confused with costosternal syndrome.

Neuropathic pain involving the chest wall may also be confused or coexist with costosternal syndrome. Examples of such neuropathic pain syndromes include diabetic polyneuropathies and acute herpes zoster involving the thoracic nerves. Diseases of the structures of the mediastinum are possible and may be difficult to diagnose. Pathologic processes that inflame the pleura, such as pulmonary embolus, infection, and Bornholm disease, may also confuse the diagnosis and complicate treatment.

TREATMENT

Initial treatment of the pain and functional disability associated with costosternal syndrome includes a combination of nonsteroidal antiinflammatory drugs (NSAIDs) or cyclooxygenase-2 inhibitors. The local application of heat and cold may also be beneficial. Use of an elastic rib belt may provide symptomatic relief and protect the costosternal joints from additional trauma. For patients who do not respond to these treatment modalities, injection with local anesthetic and steroid is a reasonable next step.

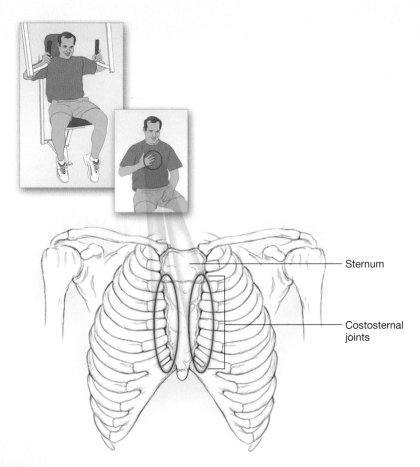

Figure 60-1 Irritation of the costosternal joints from overuse of exercise equipment can cause costosternal syndrome.

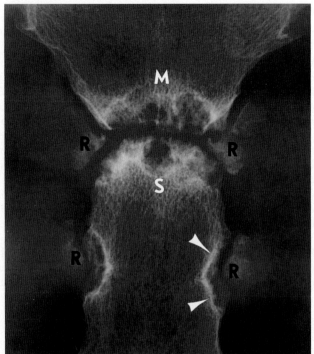

Figure 60-2 Abnormalities of manubriosternal and sternocostal joints in rheumatoid arthritis. Radiograph of a sternum from a cadaver with rheumatoid arthritis shows large erosions of the articular surface of both the manubrium (M) and the body of the sternum (S). Subtle irregularities of the second and third sternocostal joints are evident, most prominently in the sternal facet of the left third sternocostal joint (*arrowheads*). R, ossified costal cartilage. (*From Resnick D:* Diagnosis of bone and joint disorders, *ed 4, Philadelphia, 2002, Saunders, p 854.*)

Intraarticular injection of the costosternal joint is performed by placing the patient in the supine position. The skin overlying the affected costosternal joints is prepared with antiseptic solution. A sterile syringe containing 1 mL of 0.25% preservative-free bupivacaine for each joint to be injected and 40 mg methylprednisolone is attached to a 1½-inch, 25-gauge needle using strict aseptic technique. The costosternal joints are identified; they should be easily palpable as a slight bulging at the point where the rib attaches to the sternum. The needle is then carefully advanced through the skin and subcutaneous tissues medially, with a slight cephalad trajectory, into proximity with the joint (Fig. 60-3). If bone is encountered, the needle is withdrawn from the periosteum. After the needle is in proximity to the joint, 1 mL of solution is gently injected. The clinician should feel limited resistance to injection. If significant resistance is encountered, the needle should be withdrawn slightly until the injection can proceed with only limited resistance. This procedure is repeated for each affected joint. The needle is then removed, and a sterile pressure dressing and ice pack are applied to the injection site.

Physical modalities, including local heat and gentle range-of-motion exercises, should be introduced several days after the patient undergoes injection for costosternal joint pain. Vigorous exercises should be avoided, because they will exacerbate the patient's symptoms. Simple analgesics and NSAIDs may be used concurrently with this injection technique.

COMPLICATIONS AND PITFALLS

Because many pathologic processes can mimic the pain of costosternal syndrome, the clinician must carefully rule out underlying cardiac disease and diseases of the lung and structures of the

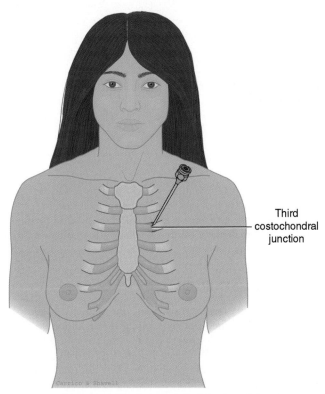

Third costochondral junction

Figure 60-3 Correct needle placement for injection of the costosternal joints. *(From Waldman SD: Atlas of pain management injection techniques, Philadelphia, 2000, Saunders.)*

mediastinum. Failure to do so could lead to disastrous results. The major complication of the injection technique is pneumothorax if the needle is placed too laterally or deeply and invades the pleural space. Infection, although rare, can occur if strict aseptic technique is not followed. Trauma to the contents of the mediastinum is also a possibility. The risk of this complication can be greatly decreased with strict attention to accurate needle placement.

Clinical Pearls

Patients suffering from pain emanating from the costosternal joints often believe that they are having a heart attack. Reassurance is required, but the clinician should remember that musculoskeletal pain syndromes and coronary artery disease can coexist. Tietze's syndrome may be confused with costosternal syndrome, although both respond to the aforementioned injection technique.

SUGGESTED READINGS

Baldry PE: The chest wall. In Baldry PE, Baldry P, Muhammad B, editors: *Myofascial pain and fibromyalgia syndromes,* New York, 2001, Churchill Livingstone, pp 303–327.

Hillen TJ, Wessell DE: Multidetector CT scan in the evaluation of chest pain of nontraumatic musculoskeletal origin, *Thorac Surg Clin* 20(1):167–173, 2010.

Stochkendahl MJ, Christensen HW: Chest pain in focal musculoskeletal disorders, *Med Clin North Am* 94(2):259–273, 2010.

Waldman SD: Costosternal joint injection. In *Pain review,* Philadelphia, 2009, Saunders, pp 495–496.

Waldman SD: Costosternal syndrome. In *Pain review,* Philadelphia, 2009, Saunders, pp 246–247.

Chapter 61

MANUBRIOSTERNAL SYNDROME

ICD-9 CODE 786.52

ICD-10 CODE R07.2

The Clinical Syndrome

The manubrium articulates with the body of the sternum by way of the manubriosternal joint at the angle of Louis. The manubriosternal joint is a fibrocartilaginous joint or synchondrosis, which lacks a true joint cavity. The joint allows protraction and retraction of the thorax.

Pain originating from the manubriosternal joint can mimic pain of cardiac origin. The manubriosternal joint is susceptible to the development of osteoarthritis, rheumatoid arthritis, ankylosing spondylitis, Reiter's syndrome, and psoriatic arthritis. The joint can also be traumatized during acceleration-deceleration injuries and blunt trauma to the chest (Fig. 61-1). With severe trauma, the joint may subluxate or dislocate. Overuse or misuse can result in acute inflammation of the manubriosternal joint, which can be quite debilitating. The joint is also subject to invasion by tumor from primary malignant tumors, including thymoma, or from metastatic disease.

Signs and Symptoms

Physical examination reveals that the patient vigorously attempts to splint the joint by keeping the shoulders stiffly in a neutral position. Pain is reproduced with active protraction or retraction of the shoulder, deep inspiration, and full elevation of the arm. Shrugging of the shoulder may also reproduce the pain. Coughing may be difficult, leading to inadequate pulmonary toilet in patients who have sustained trauma to the anterior chest wall. The manubriosternal joint may be tender to palpation. The patient may also complain of a clicking sensation with movement of the joint.

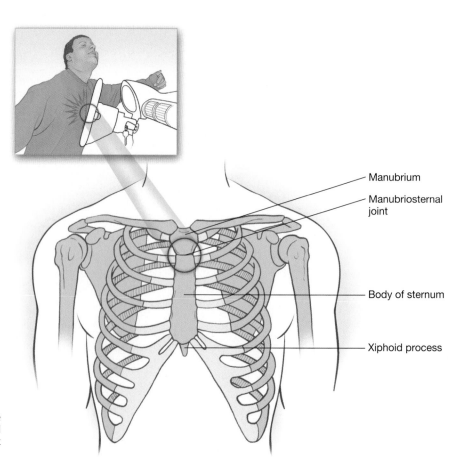

- Manubrium
- Manubriosternal joint
- Body of sternum
- Xiphoid process

Figure 61-1 The manubriosternal joint is susceptible to the development of arthritis. It is often traumatized during acceleration-deceleration injuries and blunt trauma to the chest.

TESTING

Plain radiographs are indicated for all patients who present with pain thought to be emanating from the manubriosternal joint, to rule out occult bony disorders, including tumor. If trauma is present, radionuclide bone scanning may be useful to exclude occult fractures of the ribs or sternum. Based on the patient's clinical presentation, additional testing may be indicated, including a complete blood count, prostate-specific antigen level, erythrocyte sedimentation rate, and antinuclear antibody testing. Laboratory evaluation for collagen vascular disease is indicated in patients suffering from manubriosternal joint pain if other joints are involved. Magnetic resonance imaging or computed tomography (CT) of the joint is indicated if joint instability, infection, or occult mass is suspected or to further elucidate the cause of the pain further (Figs. 61-2 and 61-3). The use of multidetector CT for patients presenting to the emergency room with acute chest pain has led to more rapid and accurate diagnosis of chest wall pain syndromes. The injection technique described later serves as both a diagnostic and a therapeutic maneuver.

DIFFERENTIAL DIAGNOSIS

As mentioned, the pain of manubriosternal syndrome is often mistaken for pain of cardiac origin, and it leads to visits to the emergency department and unnecessary cardiac workups. If trauma has occurred, manubriosternal syndrome may coexist with fractured ribs or fractures of the sternum itself, which can be missed on plain radiographs and may require radionuclide bone scanning for proper identification. Tietze's syndrome, which is painful enlargement of the upper costochondral cartilage associated with viral infection, may be confused with manubriosternal syndrome.

Neuropathic pain involving the chest wall may also be confused or coexist with manubriosternal syndrome. Examples of such neuropathic pain syndromes include diabetic polyneuropathies and acute herpes zoster involving the thoracic nerves. Diseases of the structures of the mediastinum are possible and can be difficult to diagnose. Pathologic processes that inflame the pleura, such as pulmonary embolus, infection, and Bornholm disease, may also confuse the diagnosis and complicate treatment.

TREATMENT

Initial treatment of the pain and functional disability associated with manubriosternal syndrome includes a combination of nonsteroidal antiinflammatory drugs (NSAIDs) or cyclooxygenase-2 inhibitors. The local application of heat and cold may also be beneficial. Use of an elastic rib belt may also provide symptomatic relief and protect the manubriosternal joint from additional trauma. For patients who do not respond to these treatment modalities, injection with local anesthetic and steroid is a reasonable next step.

The patient is placed in the supine position, and the skin overlying the angle of the sternum is prepared with antiseptic solution. A sterile syringe containing 1 mL of 0.25% preservative-free bupivacaine and 40 mg methylprednisolone is attached to a 1½-inch, 25-gauge needle using strict aseptic technique. The angle of the sternum is identified; the manubriosternal joint should be easily palpable as a slight indentation at this point. The needle is then carefully advanced through the skin and subcutaneous tissues medially, with a slight cephalad trajectory, into the joint (Fig. 61-4). If bone is encountered, the needle is withdrawn into the subcutaneous tissues and is redirected slightly more cephalad. After the needle enters the joint, the contents of the syringe are gently injected. The clinician should feel some resistance to injection because of the fibrocartilaginous nature of the joint. If significant resistance is encountered, the needle should be advanced or withdrawn slightly into the joint until the injection can proceed with only limited resistance. The needle is then removed, and a sterile pressure dressing and ice pack are applied to the injection site.

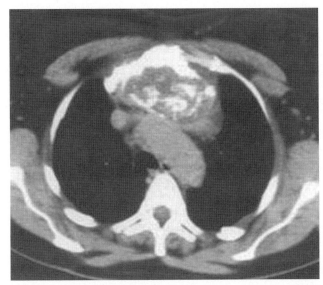

Figure 61-2 Chondrosarcoma of the sternum. Computed tomography clearly demonstrates manubrial irregularity and a preaortic soft tissue mass with chondral calcification. Nearly all sternal tumors are malignant. *(From Grainger RG, Allison DJ, Adam A, Dixon AK: Grainger & Allison's diagnostic radiology: a textbook of medical imaging, ed 4, Philadelphia, 2002, Churchill Livingstone, p 253.)*

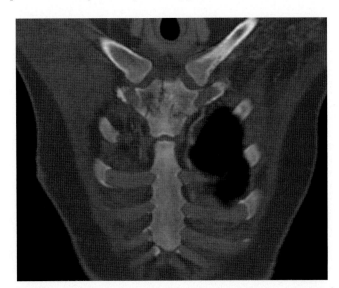

Figure 61-3 Pulmonary embolus (PE) protocol multidetector computed tomography (MDCT) examination for acute chest pain in a patient with lung cancer metastatic to the manubrium with a pathologic fracture. The patient had a known history of lung cancer, and the MDCT examination was obtained to evaluate for suspected PE. Although the presence of the lesion was evident on the straight transverse (axial) images, the extent of the lesion and the associated pathologic fracture are better elucidated on the coronal reformats. *(From Hillen TJ, Wessell DE: Multidetector CT scan in the evaluation of chest pain of nontraumatic musculoskeletal origin,* Thorac Surg Clin *20[1]:167–173, 2010.)*

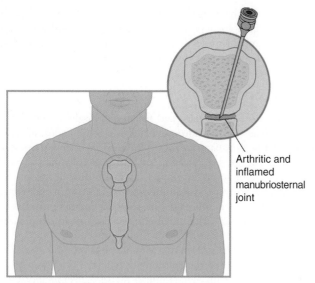

Arthritic and
inflamed
manubriosternal
joint

Figure 61-4 Correct needle placement for injection of the manubriosternal joint. *(From Waldman SD: Atlas of pain management injection techniques, ed 2, Philadelphia, 2000, Saunders.)*

Physical modalities, including local heat and gentle range-of-motion exercises, should be introduced several days after the patient undergoes injection for manubriosternal joint pain. Vigorous exercises should be avoided, because they will exacerbate the patient's symptoms. Simple analgesics and NSAIDs may be used concurrently with this injection technique.

COMPLICATIONS AND PITFALLS

Because many pathologic processes can mimic the pain of manubriosternal syndrome, the clinician must carefully rule out underlying cardiac disease and diseases of the lung and structures of the mediastinum. Failure to do so could lead to disastrous results. The major complication of the injection technique is pneumothorax if the needle is placed too laterally or deeply and invades the pleural space. Infection, although rare, can occur if strict aseptic technique is not followed. Trauma to the contents of the mediastinum is also a possibility. The incidence of complication can be greatly decreased with strict attention to accurate needle placement.

Clinical Pearls

Patients suffering from pain emanating from the manubriosternal joint often believe that they are having a heart attack. Reassurance is required, but the clinician should remember that musculoskeletal pain syndromes and coronary artery disease can coexist. Tietze's syndrome may be confused with manubriosternal syndrome, although both respond to the aforementioned injection technique.

SUGGESTED READINGS

Baldry PE: The chest wall. In Baldry PE, Baldry P, Muhammad B, editors: *Myofascial pain and fibromyalgia syndromes,* New York, 2001, Churchill Livingstone, pp 303–327.
Shukla PC: Primary sternal osteomyelitis, *J Emerg Med* 12(3):293–297, 1994.
Stochkendahl MJ, Christensen HW: Chest pain in focal musculoskeletal disorders, *Med Clin North Am* 94(2):259–273, 2010.
Waldman SD: Manubriosternal joint syndrome. In *Pain review,* Philadelphia, 2009, Saunders, pp 247–248.

Chapter **62**

INTERCOSTAL NEURALGIA

ICD-9 CODE `353.8`

ICD-10 CODE `G54.8`

THE CLINICAL SYNDROME

Whereas most other causes of chest wall pain are musculoskeletal, the pain of intercostal neuralgia is neuropathic. As with costosternal joint pain, Tietze's syndrome, and rib fractures, many patients who suffer from intercostal neuralgia seek medical attention because they believe they are having a heart attack. If the subcostal nerve is involved, gallbladder disease may be suspected. The pain of intercostal neuralgia is the result of damage to or inflammation of the intercostal nerves. The pain is constant and burning, and it may involve any of the intercostal nerves, as well as the subcostal nerve of the twelfth rib. The pain usually begins at the posterior axillary line and radiates anteriorly into the distribution of the affected intercostal or subcostal nerves, or both (Fig. 62-1). Deep inspiration or movement of the chest wall may slightly increase the pain of intercostal neuralgia, but to a much lesser extent than with musculoskeletal causes of chest wall pain.

SIGNS AND SYMPTOMS

Physical examination generally reveals minimal findings unless the patient has a history of previous thoracic or subcostal surgery or cutaneous evidence of herpes zoster involving the thoracic dermatomes. Unlike patients with musculoskeletal causes of chest wall and subcostal pain, those with intercostal neuralgia do not attempt to splint or protect the affected area. Careful sensory examination of the affected dermatomes may reveal decreased sensation or allodynia. When motor involvement of the subcostal nerve is significant, the patient may complain that his or her abdomen bulges outward.

TESTING

Plain radiographs are indicated for all patients who present with pain thought to be emanating from the intercostal nerve, to rule out occult bony disorders, including tumor (Fig. 62-2). If trauma is present, radionuclide bone scanning may be useful to exclude occult fractures of the ribs or sternum. Based on the patient's clinical presentation, additional testing may be indicated, including a complete blood count, prostate-specific antigen level, erythrocyte sedimentation rate, and antinuclear antibody testing. Computed tomography of the thoracic contents is indicated if an occult mass is suspected. The injection technique described later serves as both a diagnostic and a therapeutic maneuver.

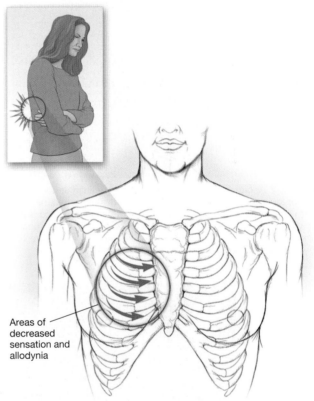

Areas of decreased sensation and allodynia

Figure 62-1 The pain of intercostal neuralgia is neuropathic rather than musculoskeletal in origin.

DIFFERENTIAL DIAGNOSIS

As mentioned, the pain of intercostal neuralgia is often mistaken for pain of cardiac or gallbladder origin, and it leads to visits to the emergency department and unnecessary cardiac and gastrointestinal workups. If trauma has occurred, intercostal neuralgia may coexist with fractured ribs or fractures of the sternum itself, which can be missed on plain radiographs and may require radionuclide bone scanning for proper identification. Tietze's syndrome, which is painful enlargement of the upper costochondral cartilage associated with viral infection, may be confused with intercostal neuralgia.

Other types of neuropathic pain involving the chest wall may be confused or coexist with intercostal neuralgia. Examples of such neuropathic pain syndromes include diabetic polyneuropathies and acute herpes zoster involving the thoracic nerves. Diseases of the structures of the mediastinum and thoracic aorta are possible and can be difficult to diagnose (Fig. 62-3). Pathologic processes that inflame the pleura, such as pulmonary embolus, infection, and Bornholm disease, may also confuse the diagnosis and complicate treatment.

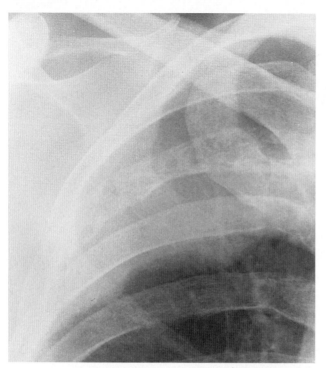

Figure 62-2 Angiosarcoma of the ribs. An ill-defined lesion of the posterior aspect of the fourth rib is associated with a coarsened trabecular pattern and a large soft tissue mass. The osseous changes are consistent with a vascular lesion. The extent of the soft tissue involvement suggests an aggressive process. *(From Resnick D:* Diagnosis of bone and joint disorders, *ed 4, Philadelphia, 2002, Saunders, p 4006.)*

TREATMENT

Initial treatment of intercostal neuralgia includes a combination of simple analgesics and nonsteroidal antiinflammatory drugs or cyclooxygenase-2 inhibitors. If these medications do not adequately control the patient's symptoms, a tricyclic antidepressant or gabapentin should be added.

Traditionally, tricyclic antidepressants have been a mainstay in the palliation of pain caused by intercostal neuralgia. Controlled studies have demonstrated the efficacy of amitriptyline, and nortriptyline and desipramine have also proved to be clinically useful. Unfortunately, this class of drugs is associated with significant anticholinergic side effects, including dry mouth, constipation, sedation, and urinary retention. These drugs should be used with caution in patients suffering from glaucoma, cardiac arrhythmia, and prostatism. To minimize side effects and encourage compliance, the physician should start amitriptyline or nortriptyline at a 10-mg dose at bedtime; the dose can then be titrated upward to 25 mg at bedtime, as side effects allow. Subsequently, upward titration in 25-mg increments can be carried out each week, as side effects allow. Even at lower doses, patients generally report a rapid improvement in sleep disturbance and begin to experience some pain relief in 10 to 14 days. If the patient does not show any improvement in pain as the dose is being titrated upward, the addition of gabapentin alone or in combination with nerve blocks is recommended (see later). The selective serotonin reuptake inhibitors such as fluoxetine have also been used to treat the pain of intercostal neuralgia, and although these drugs are better tolerated than are the tricyclic antidepressants, they appear to be less efficacious.

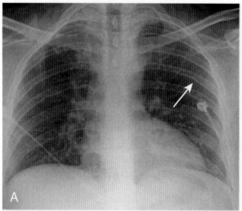

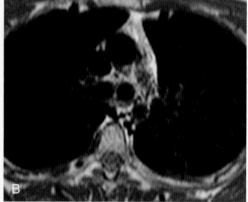

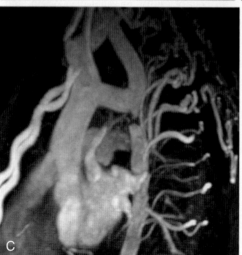

Figure 62-3 Coarctation of the thoracic aorta with intercostal collateral vessels in a 27-year-old man evaluated for a ruptured aneurysm. **A,** Frontal chest radiograph shows rib notching *(arrow)* and abnormal contour of the thoracic aorta. **B,** Axial T1-weighted magnetic resonance imaging (MRI) shows large paraspinous and intercostal collateral vessels with associated flow-related signal voids. **C,** Oblique sagittal maximum-intensity projected MRI shows severe coarctation of the thoracic aorta with large intercostal and internal thoracic collateral vessels. *(From Lee TJ, Collins J: MR imaging evaluation of disorders of the chest wall,* Magn Reson Imaging Clin N Am *16[2]:355–379, 2008.)*

If the antidepressant compounds are ineffective or contraindicated, gabapentin is a reasonable alternative. Gabapentin is started at a 300-mg dose at bedtime for 2 nights. The patient should be cautioned about potential side effects, including dizziness, sedation, confusion, and rash. The drug is then increased in 300-mg increments given in equally divided doses over 2 days, as side effects allow, until pain relief is obtained or a total dose of 2400 mg/day is reached. At this point, if the patient has experienced partial pain relief, blood values are measured, and the drug is carefully titrated upward using 100-mg tablets. Rarely is a dose greater than 3600 mg/day required.

The local application of heat and cold or the use of an elastic rib belt may also provide symptomatic relief. For patients who do not respond to these treatment modalities, injection using local anesthetic and steroid is a reasonable next step.

The patient is placed in the prone position with the arms hanging loosely off the sides of the table. Alternatively, this block can be done with the patient in the sitting or lateral position. The rib to be blocked is identified by palpating its path at the posterior axillary line. The operator's index and middle fingers are then placed on the rib, thus bracketing the site of needle insertion, and the skin is prepared with antiseptic solution. A 1½-inch, 22-gauge needle is attached to a 12-mL syringe and is advanced perpendicular to the skin while aiming for the middle of the rib between the operator's index and middle fingers. The needle should impinge on bone after being advanced approximately ¾ inch. Once bony contact is made, the needle is withdrawn into the subcutaneous tissues, and the skin and subcutaneous tissues are retracted with the operator's palpating fingers inferiorly. This technique allows the needle to be walked off the inferior margin of the rib. As soon as bony contact is lost, the needle is slowly advanced approximately 2 mm deeper. This maneuver places the needle in proximity to the costal groove, which contains the intercostal nerve as well as the intercostal artery and vein. After careful aspiration reveals no blood or air, the operator injects 3 to 5 mL of 1% preservative-free lidocaine. If the pain has an inflammatory component, the local anesthetic is combined with 80 mg methylprednisolone and injected in incremental doses. Subsequent daily nerve blocks are carried out in a similar manner, substituting 40 mg methylprednisolone for the initial 80-mg dose. Because of the overlapping innervation of the chest and upper abdominal wall, the intercostal nerves above and below the nerve suspected of causing the pain must also be blocked.

COMPLICATIONS AND PITFALLS

The major problem in the treatment of patients thought to be suffering from intercostal neuralgia is failure to identify potentially serious disease of the thorax or upper abdomen. Given the proximity of the pleural space, pneumothorax after intercostal nerve block is a distinct possibility. The incidence of this complication is less than 1%, but it occurs with greater frequency in patients with chronic obstructive pulmonary disease. Owing to the proximity to the intercostal nerve and artery, the clinician must carefully calculate the total dosage of local anesthetic administered, because vascular uptake through these vessels is high. Although uncommon, infection is always a possibility, especially in immunocompromised patients with cancer. Early detection of infection is crucial to avoid potentially life-threatening sequelae.

Clinical Pearls

Intercostal neuralgia is a commonly encountered cause of chest wall and thoracic pain. Correct diagnosis is necessary to treat this painful condition properly and to avoid overlooking serious intrathoracic or intraabdominal disease. Pharmacologic agents generally provide adequate pain control. If necessary, intercostal nerve block is a simple technique that can produce dramatic pain relief, but the proximity of the intercostal nerve to the pleural space makes careful attention to technique mandatory.

SUGGESTED READINGS

Hardy PA: Post-thoracotomy intercostal neuralgia, *Lancet* 327(8481):626–627, 1986.

Waldman SD: Intercostal nerve block. In *Atlas of interventional pain management*, ed 3, Philadelphia, 2009, Saunders, pp 295–297.

Waldman SD: Intercostal neuralgia. In *Pain review*, Philadelphia, 2009, Saunders, pp 244–245.

Waldman SD: Post-thoracotomy pain syndrome. In *Pain review*, Philadelphia, 2009, Saunders, pp 283–284.

Chapter **63**

DIABETIC TRUNCAL NEUROPATHY

ICD-9 CODE `354.5`

ICD-10 CODE `G58.7`

THE CLINICAL SYNDROME

Diabetic neuropathy is a term used by clinicians to describe a heterogeneous group of diseases that affect the autonomic and peripheral nervous systems of patients suffering from diabetes mellitus. Diabetic neuropathy is now thought to be the most common form of peripheral neuropathy that afflicts humankind, with an estimated 220 million people worldwide suffering from this malady.

One of the most commonly encountered forms of diabetic neuropathy is diabetic truncal neuropathy. In this condition, pain and motor dysfunction are often incorrectly attributed to intrathoracic or intraabdominal disorders and lead to extensive workups for appendicitis, cholecystitis, renal calculi, and so on. The onset of symptoms frequently coincides with periods of extreme hypoglycemia or hyperglycemia or with weight loss or gain. Patients who present with diabetic truncal neuropathy complain of severe dysesthetic pain with patchy sensory deficits in the distribution of the lower thoracic or upper thoracic dermatomes. The pain is often worse at night and causes significant sleep disturbance. The symptoms of diabetic truncal neuropathy often resolve spontaneously over 6 to 12 months. However, because of the severity of symptoms, aggressive treatment with pharmacotherapy and neural blockade is indicated.

SIGNS AND SYMPTOMS

Physical examination generally reveals minimal findings unless the patient has a history of previous thoracic or subcostal surgery or cutaneous evidence of herpes zoster involving the thoracic dermatomes. Unlike patients with musculoskeletal causes of chest wall and subcostal pain, patients with diabetic truncal neuropathy do not attempt to splint or protect the affected area. Careful sensory examination of the affected dermatomes may reveal decreased sensation or allodynia. With significant motor involvement of the subcostal nerve, the patient may complain that his or her abdomen bulges outward (Fig. 63-1).

TESTING

The presence of diabetes should lead to a high index of suspicion for diabetic truncal neuropathy. If the diagnosis of diabetic truncal neuropathy is suspected based on the targeted history and physical examination, screening laboratory tests, including a complete blood count, chemistry profile, erythrocyte sedimentation rate, thyroid function studies, antinuclear antibody testing, and urinalysis, should rule out most other peripheral neuropathies

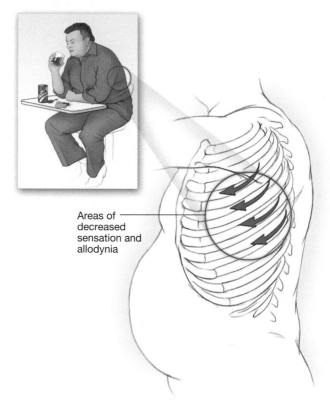

Areas of decreased sensation and allodynia

Figure 63-1 The pain of diabetic truncal neuropathy is neuropathic and is often made worse by poorly controlled blood glucose levels.

that are easily treatable. Electromyography and nerve conduction velocity testing are indicated in all patients suffering from peripheral neuropathy, to identify treatable entrapment neuropathies and further delineate the type of peripheral neuropathy present; these tests may also be able to quantify the severity of peripheral or entrapment neuropathy. Additional laboratory testing is indicated as the clinical situation dictates (e.g., Lyme disease titers, heavy metal screens). Magnetic resonance imaging of the spinal canal and cord should be performed if myelopathy is suspected. Nerve or skin biopsy is occasionally indicated if no cause of the peripheral neuropathy can be ascertained. Lack of response to the therapies discussed later should lead to a reconsideration of the diagnosis and the repetition of testing, as clinically indicated.

DIFFERENTIAL DIAGNOSIS

Diseases other than diabetic neuropathy may cause peripheral neuropathies in diabetic patients. These diseases may exist alone or may coexist with diabetic truncal neuropathy, thus making identification and treatment difficult.

Although uncommon in the United States, Hansen's disease is a common cause of peripheral neuropathy worldwide that may mimic or coexist with diabetic truncal neuropathy. Other infectious causes of peripheral neuropathies include Lyme disease and human immunodeficiency virus infection. Substances that are toxic to nerves, including alcohol, heavy metals, chemotherapeutic agents, and hydrocarbons, may also cause peripheral neuropathies that are indistinguishable from diabetic neuropathy on clinical grounds. Heritable disorders such as Charcot-Marie-Tooth disease and other familial diseases of the peripheral nervous system must also be considered, although treatment options are somewhat limited. Metabolic and endocrine causes of peripheral neuropathy that must be ruled out include vitamin deficiencies, pernicious anemia, hypothyroidism, uremia, and acute intermittent porphyria. Other causes of peripheral neuropathy that may confuse the clinical picture include Guillain-Barré syndrome, amyloidosis, entrapment neuropathies, carcinoid syndrome, paraneoplastic syndromes, and sarcoidosis. Because many of these diseases are treatable, it is imperative that the clinician exclude them before attributing a patient's symptoms solely to diabetes.

Intercostal neuralgia and musculoskeletal causes of chest wall and subcostal pain may also be confused with diabetic truncal neuropathy. In all these conditions, the patient's pain may be erroneously attributed to cardiac or upper abdominal disease, thus leading to unnecessary testing and treatment.

TREATMENT

Control of Blood Glucose Levels

Current thinking is that the better the patient's glycemic control is, the less severe the symptoms of diabetic truncal neuropathy will be. Significant swings in blood glucose levels seem to predispose diabetic patients to the development of clinically significant diabetic truncal neuropathy. Some investigators believe that although oral hypoglycemic agents control blood glucose levels, they do not protect patients from diabetic truncal neuropathy as well as does insulin. In fact, some patients taking hypoglycemic agents experience an improvement in the symptoms of diabetic truncal neuropathy when they are switched to insulin.

Pharmacologic Treatment

Antidepressants

Traditionally, tricyclic antidepressants have been a mainstay in the palliation of pain caused by diabetic truncal neuropathy. Controlled studies have demonstrated the efficacy of amitriptyline, and nortriptyline and desipramine have also proved to be clinically useful. Unfortunately, this class of drugs is associated with significant anticholinergic side effects, including dry mouth, constipation, sedation, and urinary retention. These drugs should be used with caution in patients suffering from glaucoma, cardiac arrhythmia, and prostatism. To minimize side effects and encourage compliance, the physician should start amitriptyline or nortriptyline at a 10-mg dose at bedtime; the dose can then be titrated upward to 25 mg at bedtime, as side effects allow. Subsequently, upward titration in 25-mg increments can be carried out each week, as side effects allow. Even at lower doses, patients generally report a rapid improvement in sleep disturbance and begin to experience some pain relief in 10 to 14 days. If the patient does not show any improvement in pain as the dose is being titrated upward, the addition of gabapentin alone or in combination with nerve blocks is recommended (see later). The selective serotonin reuptake inhibitors such as fluoxetine have also been used to treat the pain of diabetic truncal neuropathy, and although these drugs are better tolerated than are the tricyclic antidepressants, they appear to be less efficacious.

Anticonvulsants

Anticonvulsants have long been used to treat neuropathic pain, including that of diabetic truncal neuropathy. Both phenytoin and carbamazepine have been used with varying degrees of success, either alone or in combination with antidepressants. Unfortunately, the side effects of these drugs have limited their clinical usefulness.

The anticonvulsant gabapentin is highly efficacious in the treatment of various painful neuropathic conditions, including postherpetic neuralgia and diabetic truncal neuropathy. Used properly, gabapentin is extremely well tolerated, and in most pain centers, it has become the adjuvant analgesic of choice in the treatment of diabetic truncal neuropathy. Gabapentin has a large therapeutic window, but the physician is cautioned to start at the low end of the dosage spectrum and titrate upward slowly to avoid central nervous system side effects, including sedation and fatigue. The following recommended dosage schedule can minimize side effects and encourage compliance: A single bedtime dose of 300 mg for 2 nights is followed by 300 mg twice a day for an additional 2 days. If the patient is tolerating this twice-daily dosing, the dosage may be increased to 300 mg three times a day. Most patients begin to experience pain relief at this dosage. Additional titration upward can be carried out in 300-mg increments, as side effects allow. A total greater than 3600 mg/day in divided doses is not currently recommended. The use of 600- or 800-mg tablets can simplify maintenance dosing after titration has been completed.

Pregabalin represents a reasonable alternative to gabapentin and is better tolerated in some patients. Pregabalin is started at 50 mg three times a day and may be titrated upward to 100 mg three times a day as side effects allow. Because pregabalin is excreted primarily by the kidneys, the dosage should be decreased in patients with compromised renal function.

Antiarrhythmics

Mexiletine is an antiarrhythmic drug that may be effective in the management of diabetic truncal neuropathy. Some pain specialists believe that mexiletine is especially useful in patients with primarily sharp, lancinating pain or burning pain. Unfortunately, this drug is poorly tolerated by most patients and should be reserved for those who do not respond to first-line pharmacologic treatments such as gabapentin or nortriptyline alone or in combination with neural blockade.

Topical Agents

Some clinicians have reported the successful treatment of diabetic truncal neuropathy with topical application of capsaicin. An extract of chili peppers, capsaicin is thought to relieve neuropathic pain by depleting substance P. The side effects of capsaicin include significant burning and erythema, however, and thus limit its use.

Topical lidocaine administered by transdermal patch or in a gel can also provide short-term relief of the pain of diabetic truncal neuropathy. This drug should be used with caution in patients taking mexiletine, because of the potential for cumulative local anesthetic toxicity. Whether topical lidocaine has a role in the long-term treatment of diabetic truncal neuropathy remains to be seen.

Analgesics

In general, neuropathic pain responds poorly to analgesic compounds. The simple analgesics, including acetaminophen and aspirin, can be used in combination with antidepressants and anticonvulsants, but care must be taken not to exceed the recommended daily dose, because renal or hepatic side effects may occur. The nonsteroidal antiinflammatory drugs may also provide a modicum of pain relief when they are used with antidepressants and anticonvulsants. Because of the nephrotoxicity of this class of drugs, however, they should be used with extreme caution in diabetic patients, given the high incidence of diabetic nephropathy even early in the course of the disease. The role of cyclooxygenase-2 inhibitors in the palliation of the pain of diabetic truncal neuropathy has not been adequately studied.

The pain of diabetic truncal neuropathy responds poorly to treatment with opioid analgesics. Given the significant central nervous system and gastrointestinal side effects, coupled with the problems of tolerance, dependence, and addiction, opioid analgesics should rarely, if ever, be used as a primary treatment for the pain of diabetic truncal neuropathy. If an opioid analgesic is being considered, however, tramadol may be a reasonable choice; it binds weakly to the opioid receptors and may provide some symptomatic relief. Tramadol should be used with care in combination with antidepressants to avoid the increased risk of seizures.

Neural Blockade

Neural blockade with local anesthetic alone or in combination with steroid can be useful in the management of both acute and chronic pain associated with diabetic truncal neuropathy. Thoracic epidural or intercostal nerve block with local anesthetic, steroid, or both may be beneficial. Occasionally, neuroaugmentation by spinal cord stimulation may provide significant pain relief in patients who have not been helped by more conservative measures. Neurodestructive procedures are rarely, if ever, indicated to treat the pain of diabetic truncal neuropathy; they often worsen the patient's pain and cause functional disability.

COMPLICATIONS AND PITFALLS

The major problem in the care of patients thought to be suffering from diabetic truncal neuropathy is failure to identify potentially serious disorders of the thorax or upper abdomen. Given the proximity of the pleural space, pneumothorax after intercostal nerve block is a distinct possibility. The incidence of the complication is less than 1%, but it occurs with greater frequency in patients with chronic obstructive pulmonary disease. Owing to the proximity to the intercostal nerve and artery, the clinician must carefully calculate the total dosage of local anesthetic administered, because vascular uptake by these vessels is high. Although uncommon, infection is always a possibility, especially in immunocompromised patients with cancer. Early detection of infection is crucial to avoid potentially life-threatening sequelae.

Clinical Pearls

Diabetic truncal neuropathy is a commonly encountered cause of thoracic and subcostal pain. Correct diagnosis is necessary to treat this painful condition properly and to avoid overlooking serious intrathoracic or intraabdominal disease. Pharmacologic agents generally provide adequate pain control. If necessary, intercostal or epidural nerve block is a simple technique that can produce dramatic pain relief, but the proximity of the intercostal nerve to the pleural space makes careful attention to technique mandatory.

SUGGESTED READINGS

Brewer R: Diabetic thoracic radiculopathy: an unusual cause of post-thoracotomy pain, *Pain* 103(1–2):221–223, 2003.
Longstreth GF: Diabetic thoracic polyradiculopathy, *Best Pract Res Clin Gastroenterol* 19(2):275–281, 2005.
Pascuzzi RM: Peripheral neuropathy, *Med Clin North Am* 93(2):317–342, 2009.
Waldman SD: Diabetic truncal neuropathy. In *Pain review*, Philadelphia, 2009, Saunders, pp 279–281.

Chapter 64

TIETZE'S SYNDROME

ICD-9 CODE 733.6

ICD-10 CODE M94.0

THE CLINICAL SYNDROME

Tietze's syndrome is a frequent cause of chest wall pain. Distinct from the more common costosternal syndrome, Tietze's syndrome was first described in 1921 and is characterized by acute, painful swelling of the costal cartilage. In fact, painful swelling of the second and third costochondral joints is the sine qua non of Tietze's syndrome (Fig. 64-1); such swelling is absent in costosternal syndrome. Also distinguishing the two syndromes is the age of onset: whereas costosternal syndrome usually occurs no earlier than the fourth decade of life, Tietze's syndrome is a disease of the second and third decades. The onset is acute and is often associated with a concurrent viral infection of the respiratory tract.

Investigators have postulated that microtrauma to the costosternal joints from serve coughing or heavy labor may be the cause of Tietze's syndrome.

SIGNS AND SYMPTOMS

Physical examination reveals that patients suffering from Tietze's syndrome vigorously attempt to splint the joints by keeping the shoulders stiffly in a neutral position. Pain is reproduced with active protraction or retraction of the shoulder, deep inspiration, and full elevation of the arm. Shrugging of the shoulder may also reproduce the pain. Coughing may be difficult, leading to inadequate pulmonary toilet in some patients. The costosternal joints, especially the second and third, are swollen and exquisitely tender to palpation. This swollen costochondral joint sign is pathognomonic for Tietze's syndrome (Fig. 64-2). The adjacent intercostal muscles may also be tender to palpation. The patient may complain of a clicking sensation with movement of the joint.

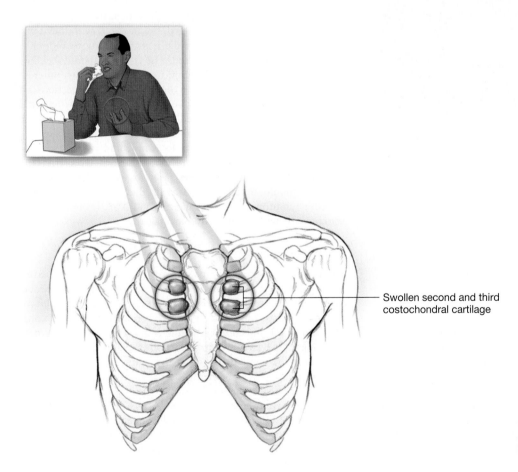

Swollen second and third costochondral cartilage

Figure 64-1 Swelling of the second and third costochondral joints is pathognomonic of Tietze's syndrome.

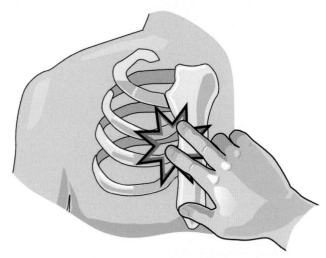

Figure 64-2 Inspection of the costosternal joint for swelling indicative of Tietze's syndrome. *(From Waldman SD: Physical diagnosis of pain: an atlas of signs and symptoms, Philadelphia, 2006, Saunders, p 209.)*

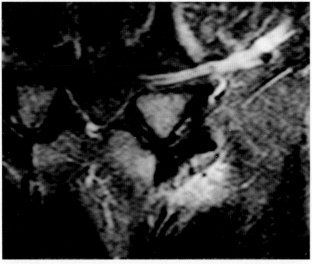

Figure 64-3 Tietze's syndrome. Coronal, short tau inversion recovery, magnetic resonance image of the thorax shows high signal intensity below the sternoclavicular joint at the costosternal junction in a 45-year-old man with pain and tenderness in this region. *(From Resnick D: Diagnosis of bone and joint disorders, ed 4, Philadelphia, 2002, Saunders, p 2605.)*

TESTING

Plain radiographs are indicated for all patients who present with pain thought to be emanating from the costosternal joints, to rule out occult bony disorders, including tumor. If trauma is present, radionuclide bone scanning should be considered to exclude occult fractures of the ribs or sternum. Based on the patient's clinical presentation, additional testing may be indicated, including a complete blood count, prostate-specific antigen level, erythrocyte sedimentation rate, and antinuclear antibody testing. Laboratory evaluation for collagen vascular disease is indicated in patients suffering from costosternal joint pain if other joints are involved. Magnetic resonance imaging of the joints is indicated if joint instability or occult mass is suspected or to confirm the diagnosis (Fig. 64-3). The injection technique described later serves as both a diagnostic and a therapeutic maneuver.

DIFFERENTIAL DIAGNOSIS

Many other painful conditions that affect the costosternal joints are much more common than Tietze's syndrome. For instance, the costosternal joints are susceptible to osteoarthritis, rheumatoid arthritis, ankylosing spondylitis, Reiter's syndrome, and psoriatic arthritis. The joints are often traumatized during acceleration-deceleration injuries and blunt trauma to the chest; with severe trauma, the joints may subluxate or dislocate. Overuse or misuse can result in acute inflammation of the costosternal joint, which can be quite debilitating. The joints are also subject to invasion by tumor from primary malignant tumors, including thymoma, or from metastatic disease.

TREATMENT

Initial treatment of the pain and functional disability associated with Tietze's syndrome includes nonsteroidal antiinflammatory drugs (NSAIDs) or cyclooxygenase-2 inhibitors. The local application of heat and cold may also be beneficial. Use of an elastic rib belt may provide symptomatic relief and protect the costosternal joints from additional trauma. For patients who do not respond to these treatment modalities, injection using local anesthetic and steroid is a reasonable next step.

Injection for Tietze's syndrome is performed by placing the patient in the supine position. The skin overlying the affected costosternal joints is prepared with antiseptic solution. A sterile syringe containing 1 mL of 0.25% preservative-free bupivacaine for each joint to be injected and 40 mg methylprednisolone is attached to a 1½-inch, 25-gauge needle using strict aseptic technique. The costosternal joints are identified; they should be easily palpable as a slight bulging at the point where the rib attaches to the sternum. The needle is carefully advanced through the skin and subcutaneous tissues medially, with a slight cephalad trajectory, in proximity to the joint. If bone is encountered, the needle is withdrawn out of the periosteum. After the needle is in proximity to the joint, 1 mL of solution is gently injected. The clinician should feel limited resistance to injection. If significant resistance is encountered, the needle should be withdrawn slightly until the injection can proceed with only limited resistance. This procedure is repeated for each affected joint. The needle is then removed, and a sterile pressure dressing and ice pack are applied to the injection site.

Physical modalities, including local heat and gentle range-of-motion exercises, should be introduced several days after the patient undergoes injection for Tietze's syndrome. Vigorous exercises should be avoided, because they will exacerbate the patient's symptoms. Simple analgesics and NSAIDs may be used concurrently with this injection technique.

COMPLICATIONS AND PITFALLS

Because many pathologic processes can mimic the pain of Tietze's syndrome, the clinician must carefully rule out underlying cardiac disease and diseases of the lung and structures of the mediastinum. Failure to do so could lead to disastrous results. The major complication of the injection technique is pneumothorax if the needle is placed too laterally or deeply and invades the pleural space. Trauma to the contents of the mediastinum is also a possibility. This complication can be greatly decreased with strict attention to accurate needle placement. Infection, although rare, can occur if strict aseptic technique is not followed, and universal precautions should be used to minimize risk to the operator. The incidence of ecchymosis and hematoma formation can be decreased if pressure is applied to the injection site immediately after injection.

Clinical Pearls

Patients suffering from pain emanating from the costosternal joint often believe that they are having a heart attack. Reassurance is required, but clinicians should remember that musculoskeletal pain syndromes and coronary artery disease can coexist. Tietze's syndrome may be confused with the more common costosternal syndrome, although both respond to the aforementioned injection technique.

SUGGESTED READINGS

Achem SR: Noncardiac chest pain: treatment approaches, *Gastroenterol Clin North Am* 37(4):859–878, 2008.

De Filippo M, Albini A, Castaldi V, et al: MRI findings of Tietze's syndrome mimicking mediastinal malignancy on MDCT, *Eur J Radiol Extra* 65(1):33–35, 2008.

Stochkendahl MJ, Christensen HW: Chest pain in focal musculoskeletal disorders, *Med Clin North Am* 94(2):259–273, 2010.

Waldman SD: Tietze's syndrome. In *Pain review,* Philadelphia, 2009, Saunders, p 282.

Chapter 65

PRECORDIAL CATCH SYNDROME

ICD-9 CODE **786.51**

ICD-10 CODE **R07.2**

THE CLINICAL SYNDROME

Precordial catch syndrome, also known as Texidor's twinge, is a common cause of chest wall pain. Occurring most frequently in adolescents and young adults, precordial catch syndrome is the cause of anxiety among patients and clinicians alike, given the intensity of the pain and its frequent attribution to the heart. Precordial catch syndrome almost always occurs at rest, often while the patient is sitting in a slumped position on an old couch (Fig. 65-1).

Distinct from other causes of chest wall pain, precordial catch syndrome is characterized by sharp, stabbing, needle-like pain that is well localized in the precordial region. Symptoms begin without warning, only adding to the patient's anxiety, and they go away as suddenly as they came. The pain lasts from 30 seconds to 3 minutes, and it is often made worse by deep inspiration. Patients suffering from precordial catch syndrome usually outgrow the syndrome by the third decade of life.

SIGNS AND SYMPTOMS

No physical findings (e.g., flushing, pallor, diaphoresis) are associated with the onset of pain, although some patients suffering from precordial catch syndrome may demonstrate tenderness to palpation in the anterior intercostal muscles overlying the painful area. Because the pain is made worse with deep inspiration, the patient may become lightheaded from prolonged shallow breathing.

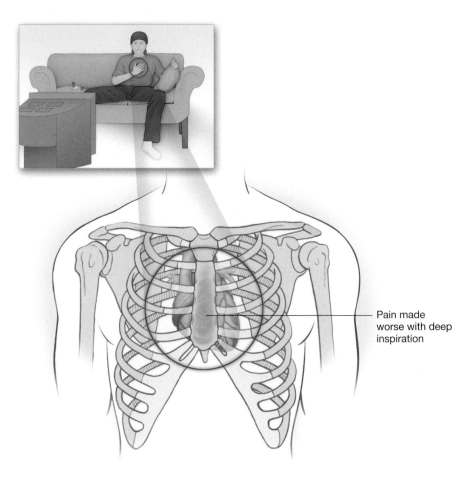

Pain made worse with deep inspiration

Figure 65-1 Precordial catch syndrome can be caused by prolonged sitting in a slumped position.

TESTING

Plain radiographs are indicated for all patients who present with pain thought to be emanating from the chest wall, to rule out occult bony disorders, including tumor. If trauma is present, radionuclide bone scanning should be considered to exclude occult fractures of the ribs or sternum. Given the location of the pain, an electrocardiogram and an echocardiogram are indicated, but in patients with precordial catch syndrome, the results are expected to be normal. Based on the patient's clinical presentation, additional testing may be indicated, including a complete blood count, prostate-specific antigen level, erythrocyte sedimentation rate, and antinuclear antibody testing. Magnetic resonance imaging of the joints is indicated if joint instability or an occult mass is suspected or to confirm the diagnosis.

DIFFERENTIAL DIAGNOSIS

Many other painful conditions that affect the chest wall occur with much greater frequency than does precordial catch syndrome. The costosternal joints are susceptible to osteoarthritis, rheumatoid arthritis, ankylosing spondylitis, Reiter's syndrome, and psoriatic arthritis. The joints are often traumatized during acceleration-deceleration injuries and blunt trauma to the chest; with severe trauma, the joints may subluxate or dislocate. Overuse or misuse can result in acute inflammation of the costosternal joint, which can be quite debilitating. The joints are also subject to invasion by tumor from primary malignant tumors, including thymoma, or from metastatic disease. Sharp pleuritic chest pain may be associated with devil's grip, pleurisy, pneumonia, or pulmonary embolus. Occult cardiac disease can also mimic the pain of precordial catch syndrome (Fig. 65-2).

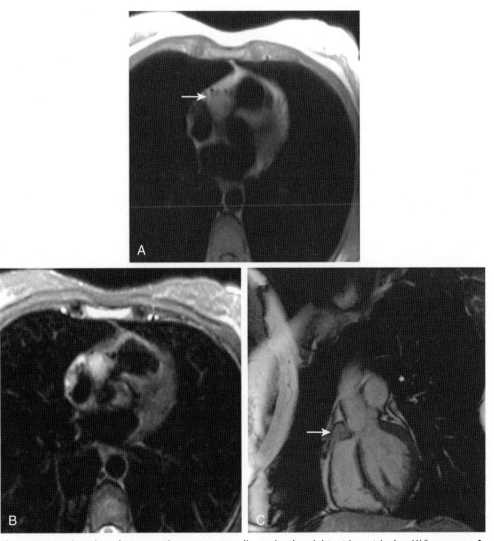

Figure 65-2 Magnetic resonance imaging demonstrating a paraganglioma in the right atrioventricular (AV) groove. **A,** Axial T1-weighted image demonstrates an isointense mass (*arrow*) in the right AV groove, immediately subjacent to the right coronary artery. Many of the imaging features of paragangliomas are a result of their high vascularity. **B,** This vascularity gives them a characteristic lightbulb bright appearance on T2-weighted images. **C,** Coronal steady-state free precession image shows a hyperintense mass in the right AV groove (*arrow*), again a result of hypervascularity.

Continued

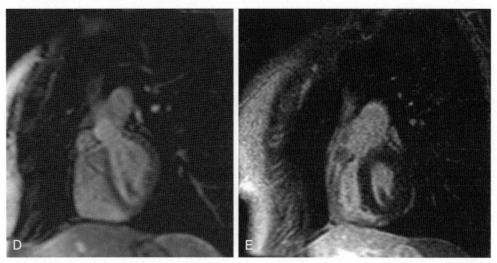

Figure 65-2—cont'd **D,** Paragangliomas appear as hypervascular structures on first-pass perfusion imaging. **E,** Delayed enhancement (DE) inversion recovery image demonstrates mild contrast retention but no real DE. *(From Syed IS, Feng D, Harris SR, et al: MR imaging of cardiac masses,* Magn Reson Imaging Clin N Am *16[2]:137–164, 2008.)*

TREATMENT

Treatment of precordial catch syndrome consists of a combination of reassurance and instructing the patient to take a deep breath as soon as the pain begins, even though this produces a sharp, stabbing pain. Improving one's posture and changing position frequently while resting or watching television should also help decrease the frequency of attacks. Pharmacologic treatment is not indicated, given the rapid onset and offset of the pain.

COMPLICATIONS AND PITFALLS

Because many pathologic processes may mimic the pain of precordial catch syndrome, the clinician must carefully rule out underlying cardiac disease and diseases of the lung and structures of the mediastinum. Failure to do so could lead to disastrous results. The greatest risk in patients suffering from precordial catch syndrome is related to unnecessary testing (e.g., cardiac catheterization) to rule out cardiac disease.

Clinical Pearls

Patients suffering from precordial catch syndrome often believe that they are having a heart attack. Reassurance is required, although the clinician should remember that musculoskeletal pain syndromes and coronary artery disease can coexist.

SUGGESTED READINGS

Baldry PE, Baldry P, Yunus M, (eds): The chest wall. In *Myofascial pain and fibromyalgia syndromes,* New York, 2001, Churchill Livingstone, pp 303–327.

Hillen TJ, Wessell DE: Multidetector CT scan in the evaluation of chest pain of nontraumatic musculoskeletal origin, *Thorac Surg Clin* 20(1):167–173, 2010.

Sampson JL, Cheitlin MD: Pathophysiology and differential diagnosis of cardiac pain, *Prog Cardiovasc Dis* 13(6):507–531, 1971.

Sigman GS: Chest pain. In Kliegman RM, Greenbaum L, Lye P, editors: *Practical strategies in pediatric diagnosis and therapy,* ed 2, Philadelphia, 2004, Saunders, pp 148–162.

Stochkendahl MJ, Christensen HW: Chest pain in focal musculoskeletal disorders, *Med Clin North Am* 94(2):259–273, 2010.

Chapter 66

FRACTURED RIBS

ICD-9 CODE **807.01**

ICD-10 CODE **S22.39xA**

THE CLINICAL SYNDROME

Fractured ribs are among the most common causes of chest wall pain, and they are usually associated with trauma to the chest wall (Fig. 66-1). In osteoporotic patients or in patients with primary tumors or metastatic disease involving the ribs, fractures may occur with coughing (tussive fractures) or spontaneously.

The pain and functional disability associated with fractured ribs are largely determined by the severity of the injury (e.g., number of ribs involved), the nature of the injury (e.g., partial or complete fracture, free-floating fragments), and the amount of damage to surrounding structures, including the intercostal nerves and pleura. The pain associated with fractured ribs ranges from a dull, deep ache with partial osteoporotic fractures to severe, sharp, stabbing pain that may lead to inadequate pulmonary toilet.

SIGNS AND SYMPTOMS

Rib fractures are aggravated by deep inspiration, coughing, and any movement of the chest wall. Palpation of the affected ribs may elicit pain and reflex spasm of the musculature of the chest wall. Ecchymosis overlying the fractures may be present. The clinician should be aware of the possibility of pneumothorax or hemopneumothorax. Damage to the intercostal nerves may produce severe pain and result in reflex splinting of the chest wall that further compromises the patient's pulmonary status. Failure to treat this pain and splinting aggressively may result in a negative cycle of hypoventilation, atelectasis, and, ultimately, pneumonia.

TESTING

Plain radiographs or computed tomography (CT) scans of the ribs and chest are indicated for all patients who present with pain from fractured ribs, to rule out occult fractures and other bony disorders, including tumor, as well as pneumothorax and hemopneumothorax (Fig. 66-2). If trauma is present, radionuclide bone scanning may be useful to exclude occult fractures of the ribs or sternum. If no trauma is present, bone density testing to rule out osteoporosis is appropriate, as are serum protein electrophoresis and testing for hyperparathyroidism. Based on the patient's clinical presentation,

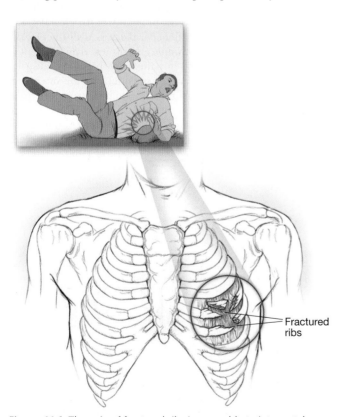

Figure 66-1 The pain of fractured ribs is amenable to intercostal nerve block with local anesthetic and steroid.

Fractured ribs

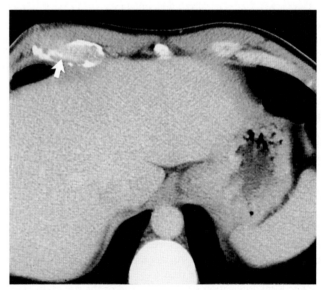

Figure 66-2 Nonunion of rib fracture. Contrast-enhanced axial computed tomography scan shows expansile right rib lesion with questionable chondroid matrix *(arrow)*. (From Haaga JR, Lanzieri CF, Gilkeson RC, editors: CT and MR imaging of the whole body, ed 4, Philadelphia, 2003, Mosby, p 1009.)

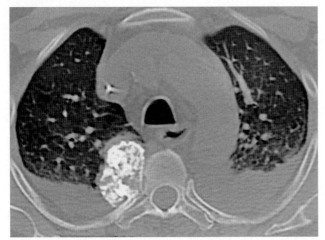

Figure 66-3 Noncontrast computed tomography scan reveals a heterogeneous, lobulated, calcified mass with a cartilaginous cap arising from the right third rib, a finding consistent with osteochondroma. *(From Haaga JR, Lanzieri CF, Gilkeson RC, editors: CT and MR imaging of the whole body, ed 4, Philadelphia, 2003, Mosby, p 1008.)*

additional testing may be warranted, including a complete blood count, prostate-specific antigen level, erythrocyte sedimentation rate, and antinuclear antibody testing. CT scanning of the thoracic contents is indicated if an occult mass or significant trauma to the thoracic contents is suspected (Fig. 66-3). Electrocardiography, to exclude cardiac contusion, is recommended for all patients with traumatic sternal fractures or significant anterior chest wall trauma. The injection technique described later should be used early to avoid pulmonary complications.

DIFFERENTIAL DIAGNOSIS

In the setting of trauma, the diagnosis of fractured ribs is usually straightforward. In the setting of spontaneous rib fracture secondary to osteoporosis or metastatic disease, the diagnosis may be less clear-cut. In this case, the pain of occult rib fracture is often mistaken for pain of cardiac or gallbladder origin, and it leads to visits to the emergency department and unnecessary cardiac and gastrointestinal workups. Tietze's syndrome, which is painful enlargement of the upper costochondral cartilage associated with viral infection, may be confused with fractured ribs, especially if the patient has been coughing.

TREATMENT

Initial treatment of rib fracture pain includes a combination of simple analgesics and nonsteroidal antiinflammatory drugs or cyclooxygenase-2 inhibitors. If these medications do not adequately control the patient's symptoms, short-acting opioid analgesics such as hydrocodone are a reasonable next step. Because opioid analgesics have the potential to suppress the cough reflex and respiration, the patient must be closely monitored and instructed in adequate pulmonary toilet techniques. Transdermal lidocaine patches may also be used in conjunction with pharmacologic management of rib fracture pain.

The local application of heat and cold or the use of an elastic rib belt may also provide symptomatic relief. For patients who do not respond to these treatment modalities, injection using local anesthetic and steroid should be implemented to avoid pulmonary complications.

The patient is placed in the prone position with the arms hanging loosely off the sides of the table. Alternatively, this injection technique can be performed with the patient in the sitting or lateral position. The rib to be blocked is identified by palpating its path at the posterior axillary line. The operator's index and middle fingers are placed on the rib, thus bracketing the site of needle insertion. The skin is prepared with antiseptic solution. A 1½-inch, 22-gauge needle is attached to a 12-mL syringe and is advanced perpendicular to the skin while aiming for the middle of the rib, between the operator's index and middle fingers. The needle should impinge on bone after being advanced approximately ¾ inch. Once bony contact is made, the needle is withdrawn into the subcutaneous tissues, and the skin and subcutaneous tissues are retracted with the palpating fingers inferiorly. This maneuver allows the needle to be walked off the inferior margin of the rib. As soon as bony contact is lost, the needle is slowly advanced approximately 2 mm deeper. This places the needle in proximity to the costal groove, which contains the intercostal nerve as well as the intercostal artery and vein. After careful aspiration reveals no blood or air, 3 to 5 mL of 1% preservative-free lidocaine is injected. If the pain has an inflammatory component, the local anesthetic is combined with 80 mg methylprednisolone and is injected in incremental doses. Subsequent daily nerve blocks are carried out in a similar manner, substituting 40 mg methylprednisolone for the initial 80-mg dose. Because of the overlapping innervation of the chest and upper abdominal wall, the intercostal nerves above and below the nerve suspected of causing the pain must also be blocked.

COMPLICATIONS AND PITFALLS

The major problem in the care of patients thought to be suffering from rib fracture is failure to identify potentially serious disorders of the thorax or upper abdomen, such as tumor, pneumothorax, or hemopneumothorax. Given the proximity of the pleural space, pneumothorax after intercostal nerve block is a distinct possibility. The incidence of this complication is less than 1%, but it occurs with greater frequency in patients with chronic obstructive pulmonary disease. Given the proximity to the intercostal nerve and artery, the clinician must carefully calculate the total dosage of local anesthetic administered, because vascular uptake by these vessels is high. Although uncommon, infection is always a possibility, especially in immunocompromised patients with cancer. Early detection of infection is crucial to avoid potentially life-threatening sequelae.

Clinical Pearls

Rib fracture is a common cause of chest wall and thoracic pain. Correct diagnosis is necessary to treat this painful condition properly and to avoid overlooking serious intrathoracic or intraabdominal disorders. Pharmacologic agents, including opioid analgesics, are usually adequate to control the pain of rib fracture. If necessary, intercostal nerve block is a simple technique that can produce dramatic pain relief. However, because of the proximity of the intercostal nerve to the pleural space, strict attention to technique is mandatory. The clinician should be aware of the direct correlation between the number of fractured ribs identified following trauma and mortality and morbidity (Fig. 66-4).

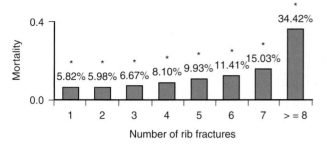

MORTALITY BY NUMBER OF FRACTURED RIBS

Figure 66-4 Mortality rate for patients with a specific number of fractured ribs. The increase in mortality was statistically (*P* < .02) greater with each successive rib fracture. The mortality rate for patients with more than six rib fractures dramatically increased in comparison with the patients sustaining fractures of six or fewer ribs. *(From Flagel BT, Luchette FA, Reed RL, et al: Half-a-dozen ribs: the breakpoint for mortality, Surgery 138[4]:717–725, 2005.)*

SUGGESTED READINGS

Boyle RK: Cough stress rib fractures in two obstetric patients: case report and pathophysiology, *Int J Obstet Anesth* 7(1):54–58, 1998.

Flagel BT, Luchette FA, Reed RL, et al: Half-a-dozen ribs: the breakpoint for mortality, *Surgery* 138(4):717–725, 2005.

Ingalls NK, Horton ZA, Bettendorf M, et al: Randomized, double-blind, placebo-controlled trial using lidocaine patch 5% in traumatic rib fractures, *J Am Coll Surg* 210(2):205–209, 2010.

Waldman SD: Intercostal nerve block. In *Pain review*, Philadelphia, 2009, Saunders, pp 487–488.

Waldman SD: The intercostal nerves. In *Pain review*, Philadelphia, 2009, Saunders, pp 109–110.

Chapter 67

POSTTHORACOTOMY PAIN SYNDROME

ICD-9 CODE 786.52

ICD-10 CODE R07.1

THE CLINICAL SYNDROME

Essentially all patients who undergo thoracotomy suffer from acute postoperative pain. This acute pain syndrome invariably responds to the rational use of systemic and spinal opioids, as well as intercostal nerve block. Unfortunately, in a few patients who undergo thoracotomy, the pain persists beyond the postoperative period and can be difficult to treat. The causes of postthoracotomy pain syndrome are listed in Table 67-1 and include direct surgical trauma, fractured ribs, compressive neuropathy, neuroma, and stretch injuries. When the syndrome is caused by fractured ribs, it produces local pain that is worse with deep inspiration, coughing, or movement of the affected ribs. The other causes of the syndrome result in moderate to severe pain that is constant and follows the distribution of the affected intercostal nerves. The pain may be characterized as neuritic and may occasionally have a dysesthetic quality.

SIGNS AND SYMPTOMS

Physical examination generally reveals tenderness along the healed thoracotomy incision (Fig. 67-1). Occasionally, palpation of the scar elicits paresthesias, a finding suggestive of neuroma

TABLE 67-1

Causes of Postthoracotomy Pain Syndrome

Direct surgical trauma to the intercostal nerves
Fractured ribs resulting from use of the rib spreader
Compressive neuropathy of the intercostal nerves resulting from direct compression by retractors
Cutaneous neuroma formation
Stretch injuries to the intercostal nerves at the costovertebral junction

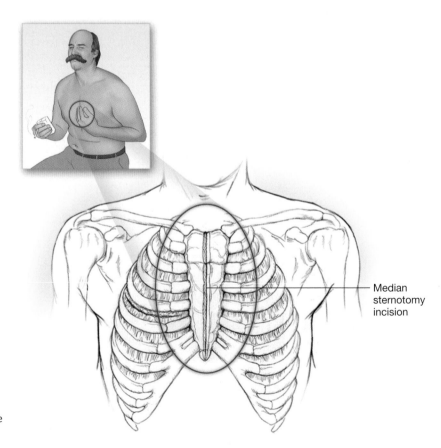

Median sternotomy incision

Figure 67-1 Patients with postthoracotomy syndrome exhibit tenderness to palpation of the scar.

formation. Patients suffering from postthoracotomy syndrome may attempt to splint or protect the affected area. Careful sensory examination of the affected dermatomes may reveal decreased sensation or allodynia. With significant motor involvement of the subcostal nerve, patients may complain that the abdomen bulges outward. Occasionally, patients suffering from postthoracotomy syndrome develop reflex sympathetic dystrophy of the ipsilateral upper extremity that, if left untreated, may result in a frozen shoulder.

TESTING

For all patients who present with pain that is thought to be emanating from the intercostal nerve, plain radiographs are indicated to rule out occult bony disorders, including unsuspected fracture or tumor. Radionuclide bone scanning may be useful to exclude occult fractures of the ribs or sternum. Based on the patient's clinical presentation, additional testing may be warranted, including a complete blood count, prostate-specific antigen level, erythrocyte sedimentation rate, and antinuclear antibody testing. Computed tomography scanning of the thoracic contents is indicated if an occult mass or pleural disease is suspected (Fig. 67-2). The injection technique described later serves as both a diagnostic and a therapeutic maneuver. Electromyography is useful in distinguishing injury of the distal intercostal nerve from stretch injuries of the intercostal nerve at the costovertebral junction.

DIFFERENTIAL DIAGNOSIS

The pain of postthoracotomy syndrome may be mistaken for pain of cardiac or gallbladder origin, thus leading to visits to the emergency department and unnecessary cardiac and gastrointestinal workups. In the presence of trauma, postthoracotomy syndrome may coexist with fractured ribs or fractures of the sternum itself, which can be missed on plain radiographs and may require radionuclide bone scanning for proper identification. Tietze's syndrome,

which is painful enlargement of the upper costochondral cartilage associated with viral infection, may be confused with postthoracotomy syndrome.

Neuropathic pain involving the chest wall may also be confused or coexist with postthoracotomy syndrome. Examples of such neuropathic pain syndromes include diabetic polyneuropathies and acute herpes zoster involving the thoracic nerves. Diseases of the structures of the mediastinum are possible and may be difficult to diagnose. Pathologic processes that inflame the pleura, such as pulmonary embolus, infection, and Bornholm disease, may also confuse the diagnosis and complicate treatment (Fig. 67-3).

TREATMENT

Initial treatment of postthoracotomy syndrome includes a combination of simple analgesics and nonsteroidal antiinflammatory drugs or cyclooxygenase-2 inhibitors. If these medications do not adequately control the patient's symptoms, a tricyclic antidepressant or gabapentin should be added.

Traditionally, tricyclic antidepressants have been a mainstay in the palliation of pain caused by postthoracotomy syndrome. Controlled studies have demonstrated the efficacy of amitriptyline, and nortriptyline and desipramine have also proved to be clinically useful. Unfortunately, this class of drugs is associated with significant anticholinergic side effects, including dry mouth, constipation, sedation, and urinary retention. These drugs should be used with caution in patients suffering from glaucoma, cardiac arrhythmia, and prostatism. To minimize side effects and encourage compliance, the physician should start amitriptyline or nortriptyline at a 10-mg dose at bedtime; the dose can then be titrated upward to 25 mg at bedtime, as side effects allow. Subsequently, upward titration in 25-mg increments can be carried out each week, as side effects allow. Even at lower doses, patients generally report a rapid improvement in sleep disturbance and begin to experience some pain relief in 10 to 14 days. If the patient does

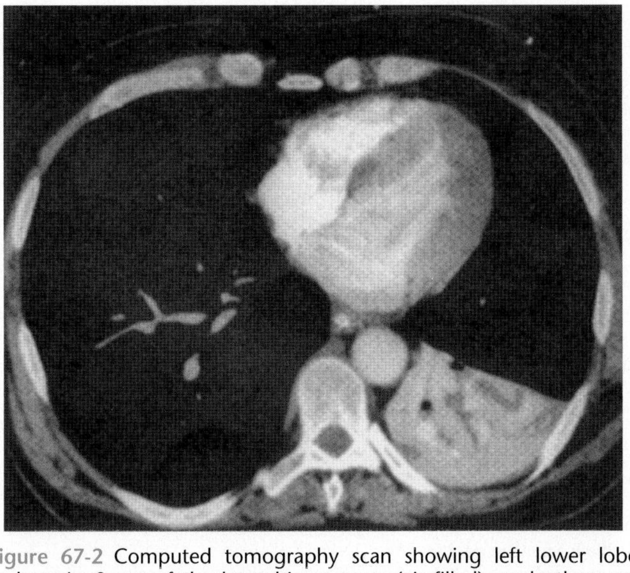

Figure 67-2 Computed tomography scan showing left lower lobe atelectasis. Some of the bronchi are open (air filled), and others are plugged (mucus filled). (*From Grainger RG, Allison DJ, Adam A, Dixon AK: Grainger & Allison's diagnostic radiology: a textbook of medical imaging, ed 4, Philadelphia, 2002, Churchill Livingstone.*)

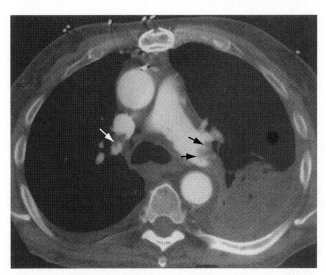

Figure 67-3 Computed tomography demonstrates bilateral pulmonary emboli in the presence of left lower lobe consolidation and bilateral pleural effusions. A large embolus is visible in the left main pulmonary artery (*black arrows*), and a small embolus is evident in the proximal right upper lobe pulmonary artery (*white arrow*). (*From Grainger RG, Allison DJ, Adam A, Dixon AK: Grainger & Allison's diagnostic radiology: a textbook of medical imaging, ed 4, Philadelphia, 2002, Churchill Livingstone.*)

not show any improvement in pain as the dose is being titrated upward, the addition of gabapentin alone or in combination with nerve blocks is recommended (see later). The selective serotonin reuptake inhibitors such as fluoxetine have also been used to treat the pain of postthoracotomy syndrome, and although these drugs are better tolerated than are the tricyclic antidepressants, they appear to be less efficacious.

If the antidepressant compounds are ineffective or contraindicated, gabapentin is a reasonable alternative. Gabapentin is started at a 300-mg dose at bedtime for 2 nights. The patient should be cautioned about potential side effects, including dizziness, sedation, confusion, and rash. The drug is then increased in 300-mg increments given in equally divided doses over 2 days, as side effects allow, until pain relief is obtained or a total dosage of 2400 mg/day is reached. At this point, if the patient has experienced partial pain relief, blood values are measured, and the drug is carefully titrated upward using 100-mg tablets. Rarely is a dose greater than 3600 mg/day required. Pregabalin represents a reasonable alternative to gabapentin and is better tolerated in some patients. Pregabalin is started at 50 mg three times a day and may be titrated upward to 100 mg three times a day as side effects allow. Because pregabalin is excreted primarily by the kidneys, the dosage should be decreased in patients with compromised renal function.

The local application of heat and cold or the use of an elastic rib belt may also provide symptomatic relief. Concurrent use of a transdermal lidocaine patch may also offer additional pain relief in patients suffering from postthoracotomy pain. For patients who do not respond to these treatment modalities, injection using local anesthetic and steroid is a reasonable next step.

The patient is placed in the prone position with the arms hanging loosely off the sides of the table. Alternatively, this block can be done with the patient in the sitting or lateral position. The rib to be blocked is identified by palpating its path at the posterior axillary line. The operator's index and middle fingers are placed on the rib, thus bracketing the site of needle insertion. The skin is prepared with antiseptic solution. A 1½-inch, 22-gauge needle is attached to a 12-mL syringe and is advanced perpendicular to the skin while aiming for the middle of the rib between the operator's index and middle fingers. The needle should impinge on bone after being advanced approximately ¾ inch. Once bony contact is made, the needle is withdrawn into the subcutaneous tissues, and the skin and subcutaneous tissues are retracted with the palpating fingers inferiorly. This maneuver allows the needle to be walked off the inferior margin of the rib. As soon as bony contact is lost, the needle is slowly advanced approximately 2 mm deeper. This places the needle in proximity to the costal groove, which contains the intercostal nerve as well as the intercostal artery and vein. After careful aspiration reveals no blood or air, 3 to 5 mL of 1% preservative-free lidocaine is injected. If the pain has an inflammatory component, the local anesthetic is combined with 80 mg methylprednisolone and is injected in incremental doses. Subsequent daily nerve blocks are carried out in a similar manner, substituting 40 mg methylprednisolone for the initial 80-mg dose. Because of the overlapping innervation of the chest and upper abdominal wall, the intercostal nerves above and below the nerve suspected of causing the pain must also be blocked. For persistent pain, cryoneurolysis of the intercostal nerves can be considered (Fig. 67-4).

If postthoracotomy pain syndrome is caused by stretch injury of the intercostal nerve (identified by electromyography), it may respond to thoracic epidural nerve block with steroid.

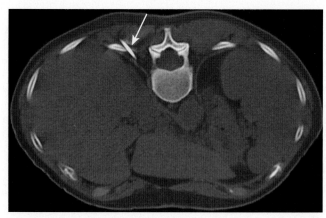

Figure 67-4 Axial computed tomographic image of a 45-year-old woman with history of postthoracotomy pain syndrome. The interprocedural computed tomographic image shows a cryoablation probe *(arrow)* placed just inferior to the twelfth right posterior rib. *(From Moore W, Kolnick D, Tan J, Yu HS: CT guided percutaneous cryoneurolysis for post-thoracotomy pain syndrome: early experience and effectiveness,* Acad Radiol *17[5]:603–606, 2010.)*

COMPLICATIONS AND PITFALLS

The major problem in the care of patients thought to be suffering from postthoracotomy syndrome is failure to identify potentially serious disorders of the thorax or upper abdomen. Given the proximity of the pleural space, pneumothorax after intercostal nerve block is a distinct possibility. The incidence of this complication is less than 1%, but it occurs with greater frequency in patients with chronic obstructive pulmonary disease. Given the proximity to the intercostal nerve and artery, the clinician must carefully calculate the total dosage of local anesthetic administered, because vascular uptake by these vessels is high. Although uncommon, infection is always a possibility, especially in immunocompromised patients with cancer. Early detection of infection is crucial to avoid potentially life-threatening sequelae.

Clinical Pearls

> Postthoracotomy syndrome is a common cause of chest wall and thoracic pain. Correct diagnosis is necessary to treat this painful condition properly and to avoid overlooking serious intrathoracic or intraabdominal disorders. Pharmacologic agents are usually adequate to control the pain of postthoracotomy syndrome. If necessary, intercostal nerve block is a simple technique that can produce dramatic pain relief. However, because of the proximity of the intercostal nerve to the pleural space, strict attention to technique is mandatory.

SUGGESTED READINGS

Moore W, Kolnick D, Tan J, et al: CT guided percutaneous cryoneurolysis for post-thoracotomy pain syndrome: early experience and effectiveness, *Acad Radiol* 17(5):603–606, 2010.

Solak O, Metin M, Esme H, et al: Effectiveness of gabapentin in the treatment of chronic post-thoracotomy pain, *Eur J Cardiothorac Surg* 32(1):9–12, 2007.

Waldman SD: Post-thoracotomy pain syndrome. In *Pain review,* Philadelphia, 2009, Saunders, pp 283–284.

Wildgaard K, Ravn J, Kehlet H: Chronic post-thoracotomy pain: a critical review of pathogenic mechanisms and strategies for prevention, *Eur J Cardiothorac Surg* 36(1):170–180, 2009.

Chapter **68**

ACUTE HERPES ZOSTER OF THE THORACIC DERMATOMES

ICD-9 CODE `053.9`

ICD-10 CODE `B02.9`

THE CLINICAL SYNDROME

Herpes zoster is an infectious disease caused by the varicella-zoster virus (VZV). Primary infection with VZV in a nonimmune host manifests clinically as the childhood disease chickenpox. Investigators have postulated that during the course of the primary infection, the virus migrates to the dorsal root of the thoracic nerves, where it remains dormant in the ganglia and produces no clinically evident disease. In some individuals, the virus reactivates and travels along the sensory pathways of the thoracic nerves, to produce the pain and skin lesions characteristic of herpes zoster, or shingles. Although the thoracic nerve roots are the most common site for the development of acute herpes zoster, the first division of the trigeminal nerve may also be affected.

Why reactivation occurs in some individuals but not in others is not fully understood. Investigators have theorized, however, that a decrease in cell-mediated immunity may play an important role in the evolution of this disease by allowing the virus to multiply in the ganglia and spread to the corresponding sensory nerves, thus producing clinical disease. Patients who are suffering from malignant (particularly lymphoma) or chronic disease and those receiving immunosuppressive therapy (chemotherapy, steroids, radiation) are generally debilitated and thus are much more likely than the healthy population to develop acute herpes zoster. These patients all have in common a decreased cell-mediated immune response, which may also explain why the incidence of shingles increases dramatically in patients older than 60 years and is relatively uncommon in those younger than 20 years.

SIGNS AND SYMPTOMS

As viral reactivation occurs, ganglionitis and peripheral neuritis cause pain that may be accompanied by flulike symptoms. The pain generally progresses from a dull, aching sensation to dysesthetic or

neuritic pain in the distribution of the thoracic nerve roots (Fig. 68-1). In most patients, the pain of acute herpes zoster precedes the eruption of rash by 3 to 7 days, and this delay often leads to an erroneous diagnosis (see "Differential Diagnosis"). However, in most patients, the clinical diagnosis of shingles is readily made when the characteristic rash appears. As in chickenpox, the rash of herpes zoster appears in crops of macular lesions, which rapidly progress to papules and then to vesicles (Fig. 68-2). Eventually, the vesicles coalesce, and crusting occurs. The affected area can

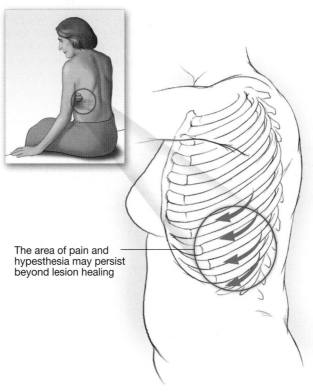

The area of pain and hypesthesia may persist beyond lesion healing

Figure 68-1 Acute herpes zoster occurs most commonly in the thoracic dermatomes.

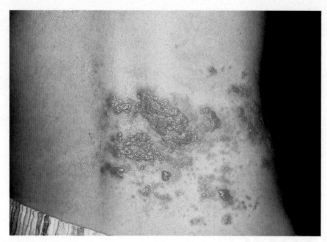

Figure 68-2 Herpes zoster involving the lumbar dermatome. *(From Mandell GL, Bennett JE, Dolin R, editors: Principles and practice of infectious diseases, ed 7, Philadelphia, 2010, Churchill Livingstone, p 1965.)*

be extremely painful, and the pain tends to be exacerbated by any movement or contact (e.g., with clothing or sheets). As the lesions heal, the crust falls away, leaving pink scars that gradually become hypopigmented and atrophic.

In most patients, the hyperesthesia and pain resolve as the skin lesions heal. In some patients, however, pain persists beyond lesion healing. This common and feared complication of acute herpes zoster is called postherpetic neuralgia, and older patients are affected at a higher rate than is the general population suffering from acute herpes zoster. The symptoms of postherpetic neuralgia can vary from a mild, self-limited condition to a debilitating, constantly burning pain that is exacerbated by light touch, movement, anxiety, or temperature change. This unremitting pain may be so severe that it completely devastates the patient's life; ultimately, it can lead to suicide. To avoid this disastrous sequela to a usually benign, self-limited disease, the clinician must use all possible therapeutic efforts in patients with acute herpes zoster of the thoracic nerve roots.

TESTING

Although in most instances the diagnosis of acute herpes zoster involving the thoracic nerve roots is easily made on clinical grounds, confirmatory testing is occasionally required. Such testing may be desirable in patients with other skin lesions that confuse the clinical picture, such as patients with human immunodeficiency virus infection who are suffering from Kaposi's sarcoma. In such patients, the diagnosis of acute herpes zoster may be confirmed by obtaining a Tzanck smear from the base of a fresh vesicle that reveals multinucleated giant cells and eosinophilic inclusions. To differentiate acute herpes zoster from localized herpes simplex infection, the clinician can obtain fluid from a fresh vesicle and submit it for immunofluorescent testing.

DIFFERENTIAL DIAGNOSIS

A careful initial evaluation, including a thorough history and physical examination, is indicated in all patients suffering from acute herpes zoster involving the thoracic nerve roots. The goal is to rule out occult malignant or systemic disease that may be responsible

for the patient's immunocompromised state. A prompt diagnosis allows early recognition of changes in clinical status that may presage the development of complications, including myelitis or dissemination of the disease. Other causes of pain in the distribution of the thoracic nerve roots include thoracic radiculopathy and peripheral neuropathy. Intrathoracic and intraabdominal disorders may also mimic the pain of acute herpes zoster involving the thoracic dermatomes.

TREATMENT

The therapeutic challenge in patients presenting with acute herpes zoster involving the thoracic nerve roots is twofold: (1) the immediate relief of acute pain and other symptoms and (2) the prevention of complications, including postherpetic neuralgia. Most pain specialists agree that the earlier treatment is initiated, the less likely postherpetic neuralgia will be to develop. Further, because older individuals are at highest risk for developing postherpetic neuralgia, early and aggressive treatment of this group of patients is mandatory.

Nerve Block

Thoracic epidural nerve block with local anesthetic and steroid is the treatment of choice to relieve the symptoms of acute herpes zoster involving the thoracic nerve roots, as well as to prevent the occurrence of postherpetic neuralgia. As vesicular crusting occurs, the steroid may also reduce neural scarring. Neural blockade is thought to achieve these goals by blocking the profound sympathetic stimulation that results from viral inflammation of the nerve and dorsal root ganglion. If untreated, this sympathetic hyperactivity can cause ischemia secondary to decreased blood flow to the intraneural capillary bed. If this ischemia is allowed to persist, endoneural edema will form. Endoneural edema increases endoneural pressure and further reduces endoneural blood flow, with resulting irreversible nerve damage.

These sympathetic blocks should be continued aggressively until the patient is pain free and should be reimplemented if the pain returns. Failure to use sympathetic neural blockade immediately and aggressively, especially in older patients, may sentence the patient to a lifetime of suffering from postherpetic neuralgia. Occasionally, some patients with acute herpes zoster of the thoracic nerve roots do not experience pain relief from thoracic epidural nerve block but may respond to blockade of the thoracic sympathetic nerves.

Opioid Analgesics

Opioid analgesics can be useful to relieve the aching pain that is common during the acute stages of herpes zoster while sympathetic nerve blocks are being implemented. Opioids are less effective in relieving neuritic pain, which is also common. Careful administration of potent, long-acting opioid analgesics (e.g., oral morphine elixir, methadone) on a time-contingent rather than an as-needed basis may be a beneficial adjunct to the pain relief provided by sympathetic neural blockade. Because many patients suffering from acute herpes zoster are older or have severe multisystem disease, close monitoring for the potential side effects of potent opioid analgesics (e.g., confusion or dizziness, which may cause a patient to fall) is warranted. Daily dietary fiber supplementation and Milk of Magnesia should be started along with opioid analgesics to prevent constipation.

Adjuvant Analgesics

The anticonvulsant gabapentin represents a first-line treatment for the neuritic pain of acute herpes zoster of the thoracic nerve roots. Studies suggest that gabapentin may also help prevent postherpetic neuralgia. Treatment with gabapentin should begin early in the course of the disease; this drug may be used concurrently with neural blockade, opioid analgesics, and other adjuvant analgesics, including antidepressants, if care is taken to avoid central nervous system side effects. Gabapentin is started at a bedtime dose of 300 mg and is titrated upward in 300-mg increments to a maximum of 3600 mg/day given in divided doses, as side effects allow.

Pregabalin represents a reasonable alternative to gabapentin and is better tolerated in some patients. Pregabalin is started at 50 mg three times a day and may be titrated upward to 100 mg three times a day as side effects allow. Because pregabalin is excreted primarily by the kidneys, the dosage should be decreased in patients with compromised renal function.

Carbamazepine should be considered in patients suffering from severe neuritic pain who fail to respond to nerve blocks and gabapentin. If this drug is used, strict monitoring of hematologic parameters is indicated, especially in patients receiving chemotherapy or radiation therapy. Phenytoin may also be beneficial to treat neuritic pain, but it should not be used in patients with lymphoma; the drug may induce a pseudolymphoma-like state that is difficult to distinguish from the actual lymphoma.

Antidepressants

Antidepressants may also be useful adjuncts in the initial treatment of patients suffering from acute herpes zoster. On a short-term basis, these drugs help alleviate the significant sleep disturbance that is commonly seen. In addition, antidepressants may be valuable in ameliorating the neuritic component of the pain, which is treated less effectively with opioid analgesics. After several weeks of treatment, antidepressants may exert a mood-elevating effect, which may be desirable in some patients. Care must be taken to observe closely for central nervous system side effects in this patient population. In addition, these drugs may cause urinary retention and constipation, which may mistakenly be attributed to herpes zoster myelitis.

Antiviral Agents

A limited number of antiviral agents, including famciclovir and acyclovir, can shorten the course of acute herpes zoster and may even help prevent its development. These drugs are probably useful in attenuating the disease in immunosuppressed patients. These antiviral agents can be used in conjunction with the aforementioned treatment modalities. Careful monitoring for side effects is mandatory.

Adjunctive Treatments

The application of ice packs to the lesions of acute herpes zoster may provide relief in some patients. Application of heat increases pain in most patients, presumably because of the increased conduction of small fibers; however, it is beneficial in an occasional patient and may be worth trying if the application of cold is ineffective. Transcutaneous electrical nerve stimulation and vibration may also be effective in a limited number of patients. The use of transdermal lidocaine may be effective, but its utility is limited on nonintact skin. The favorable risk-to-benefit ratio of these modalities makes them reasonable alternatives for patients who cannot or will not undergo sympathetic neural blockade or who cannot tolerate pharmacologic interventions.

Topical application of aluminum sulfate as a tepid soak provides excellent drying of the crusting and weeping lesions of acute herpes zoster, and most patients find these soaks soothing. Zinc oxide ointment may also be used as a protective agent, especially during the healing phase, when temperature sensitivity is a problem. Disposable diapers can be used as absorbent padding to protect healing lesions from contact with clothing and sheets.

COMPLICATIONS AND PITFALLS

In most patients, acute herpes zoster involving the thoracic nerve roots is a self-limited disease. In older and immunosuppressed patients, however, complications may occur. Cutaneous and visceral dissemination may range from a mild rash resembling chickenpox to an overwhelming, life-threatening infection in patients already suffering from severe multisystem disease. Myelitis may cause bowel, bladder, and lower extremity paresis.

Clinical Pearls

Because the pain of herpes zoster usually precedes the eruption of skin lesions by 3 to 7 days, some other painful condition (e.g., thoracic radiculopathy, cholecystitis) may erroneously be diagnosed. In this setting, an astute clinician should advise the patient to call immediately if a rash appears, because acute herpes zoster is a possibility. Some pain specialists believe that in a few immunocompetent patients, when reactivation of VZV occurs, a rapid immune response attenuates the natural course of the disease, and the characteristic rash of acute herpes zoster may not appear. In this case, pain in the distribution of the thoracic nerve roots without an associated rash is called zoster sine herpete and is, by necessity, a diagnosis of exclusion. Therefore, other causes of thoracic and subcostal pain must be ruled out before this diagnosis is invoked.

SUGGESTED READINGS

McKendrick MW, Ogan P, Care CC: A 9 year follow up of post herpetic neuralgia and predisposing factors in elderly patients following herpes zoster, *J Infect* 59(6):416–420, 2009.

Tyring SK: Management of herpes zoster and postherpetic neuralgia, *J Am Acad Dermatol* 57(6 Suppl 1):S136-S142.

Waldman SD: Acute herpes zoster of the thoracic dermatomes. In *Pain review*, Philadelphia, 2009, Saunders, pp 286–288.

Waldman SD: Postherpetic neuralgia. In *Pain review*, Philadelphia, 2009, Saunders, pp 289–290.

Wu CL, Marsh A, Dworkin RH: The role of sympathetic nerve blocks in herpes zoster and postherpetic neuralgia, *Pain* 87(2):121–129, 2000.

Chapter 69

COSTOVERTEBRAL JOINT SYNDROME

ICD-9 CODE **719.48**

ICD-10 CODE **M25.50**

THE CLINICAL SYNDROME

The costovertebral joint is a true joint and is susceptible to osteoarthritis, rheumatoid arthritis, psoriatic arthritis, Reiter's syndrome, and, in particular, ankylosing spondylitis (Figs. 69-1 and 69-2). The joint is often traumatized during acceleration-deceleration injuries and blunt trauma to the chest; with severe trauma, the joint may subluxate or dislocate. Overuse or misuse can result in acute inflammation of the costovertebral joint that can be quite debilitating. The joint is also subject to invasion by tumor from primary malignant disease, including lung cancer, or from metastatic disease. Pain emanating from the costovertebral joint can mimic pain of pulmonary or cardiac origin.

SIGNS AND SYMPTOMS

On physical examination, patients attempt to splint the affected joint or joints by avoiding flexion, extension, and lateral bending of the spine; they may also retract the scapulae in an effort to relieve the pain. The costovertebral joint may be tender to palpation and feel hot and swollen if it is acutely inflamed. Patients may also complain of a "clicking" sensation with movement of the joint. Because ankylosing spondylitis commonly affects both the costovertebral joint and the sacroiliac joint, many patients assume a stooped posture, which should alert the clinician to the possibility of this disease as the cause of costovertebral joint pain.

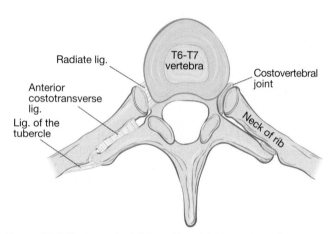

Figure 69-1 Costovertebral joint. *(From Waldman SD: Atlas of pain management injection techniques, ed 2, Philadelphia, 2007, Saunders.)*

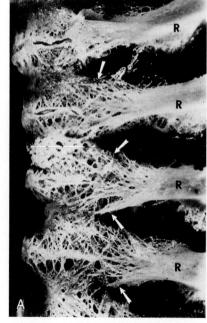

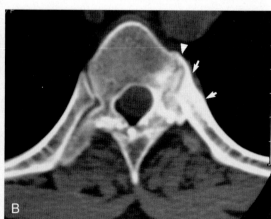

Figure 69-2 Costovertebral joint ankylosis. **A,** Photograph of the lateral aspect of the macerated thoracic spine of a spondylitic cadaver demonstrates extensive bony ankylosis *(arrows)* of the head of the ribs (R) and vertebral bodies. Disk ossification is also seen. **B,** Transaxial computed tomography scan of a thoracic vertebra in a patient with ankylosing spondylitis reveals bone erosions and partial ankylosis *(arrowhead)* of the costovertebral joints on one side. Note the involvement of the ipsilateral rib with cortical thickening *(arrows).* *(From Resnick D: Diagnosis of bone and joint disorders, ed 4, Philadelphia, 2002, Saunders, p 1045.)*

TESTING

Plain radiographs or computed tomography scans are indicated for all patients who present with pain that is thought to be emanating from the costovertebral joint, to rule out occult bony disorders, including tumor (Fig. 69-3). If trauma is present, radionuclide bone scanning may be useful to exclude occult fractures of the ribs or sternum. Laboratory evaluation for collagen vascular disease and other joint diseases, including ankylosing spondylitis, is indicated for patients with costovertebral joint pain, especially if other joints are involved. Because of the high incidence of costovertebral joint abnormalities in patients with ankylosing spondylitis, human leukocyte antigen (HLA)-B27 testing should also be considered. Based on the patient's clinical presentation, additional testing may be warranted, including a complete blood count, prostate-specific antigen level, erythrocyte sedimentation rate, and antinuclear antibody testing. Magnetic resonance imaging of the joints is indicated if joint instability or occult mass is suspected or to elucidate the cause of the pain further.

DIFFERENTIAL DIAGNOSIS

As mentioned earlier, the pain of costovertebral joint syndrome is often mistaken for pain of pulmonary or cardiac origin, and it leads to visits to the emergency department and unnecessary pulmonary or cardiac workups. If trauma has occurred, costovertebral joint syndrome may coexist with fractured ribs or fractures of the spine or sternum itself, injuries that can be missed on plain radiographs and may require radionuclide bone scanning for proper identification.

Neuropathic pain involving the chest wall may also be confused or coexist with costovertebral joint syndrome. Examples of such neuropathic pain include diabetic polyneuropathies and acute herpes zoster involving the thoracic nerves. Diseases of the structures of the mediastinum are possible and can be difficult to diagnose. Pathologic processes that inflame the pleura, such as pulmonary embolus, infection, and Bornholm disease, may also confuse the diagnosis and complicate treatment.

TREATMENT

Initial treatment of the pain and functional disability associated with costovertebral joint syndrome is with nonsteroidal anti-inflammatory drugs (NSAIDs) or cyclooxygenase-2 inhibitors. The local application of heat and cold may also be beneficial. Use of an elastic rib belt may provide symptomatic relief and protect the costovertebral joints from additional trauma. For patients who do not respond to these treatment modalities, injection of the costovertebral joint with local anesthetic and steroid is a reasonable next step (Fig. 69-4). Physical modalities, including local heat and

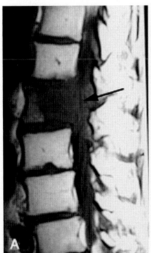
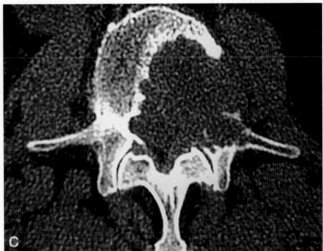
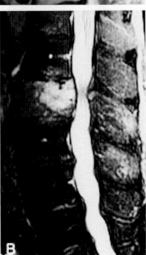

Figure 69-3 Metastatic renal carcinoma. Sagittal T1-weighted **(A)** and short tau inversion recovery **(B)** magnetic resonance images show an expansile, destructive mass replacing a lumbar vertebra, with remodeling of the posterior margin and an epidural component *(arrow)*. Axial computed tomography scan **(C)** shows the lesion involving the pedicle and transverse process, with a significant intraspinal component. *(From Edelman RR, Hesselink JR, Zlatkin MB, Crues JV, editors:* Clinical magnetic resonance imaging, *ed 3, Philadelphia, 2006, Saunders, p 2324.)*

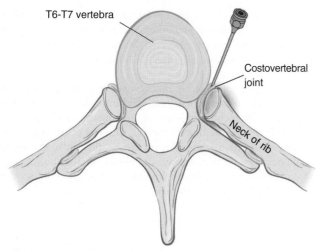

T6-T7 vertebra

Costovertebral joint

Neck of rib

Figure 69-4 Needle placement for costovertebral joint injection. *(From Waldman SD: Atlas of pain management injection techniques, ed 2, Philadelphia, 2007, Saunders.)*

gentle range-of-motion exercises, should be introduced several days after injection for costovertebral joint pain. Vigorous exercises should be avoided, because they will exacerbate the patient's symptoms. Simple analgesics and NSAIDs can be used concurrently with the injection technique.

COMPLICATIONS AND PITFALLS

Because many pathologic processes can mimic the pain of costovertebral joint syndrome, the clinician must carefully rule out underlying diseases of the lung, heart, and structures of the spine and mediastinum. Failure to do so could lead to disastrous results.

The major complication of the injection technique is pneumothorax if the needle is placed too laterally or deeply and invades the pleural space. Infection, although rare, can occur if strict aseptic technique is not followed. Trauma to the contents of the mediastinum is also a possibility. This complication can be greatly reduced with strict attention to accurate needle placement.

Clinical Pearls

Patients with pain emanating from the costovertebral joint may believe that they are suffering from pneumonia or having a heart attack. Reassurance is required.

SUGGESTED READINGS

Arslan G, Cevikol C, Karaali K, et al: Single rib sclerosis as a sequel of compression fracture of adjacent vertebra and costovertebral joint ankylosis, *Eur J Radiol Extra* 51(1):43–46, 2004.

Duprey S, Subit D, Guillemot H, et al: Biomechanical properties of the costovertebral joint, *Med Eng Phys* 32(2):222–227, 2010.

Erwin WM, Jackson PC, Homonko DA: Innervation of the human costovertebral joint: implications for clinical back pain syndromes, *J Manipulative Physiol Ther* 23(6):395–403, 2000.

Illiasch H, Likar R, Stanton-Hicks M: CT use in pain management, *Tech Reg Anesth Pain Manag* 11(2):103–112, 2007.

Waldman SD: Costovertebral joint pain. In *Atlas of pain management injection techniques,* ed 2, Philadelphia, 2007, Saunders, pp 304–308.

Chapter 70

POSTHERPETIC NEURALGIA

ICD-9 CODE 053.13

ICD-10 CODE B02.23

THE CLINICAL SYNDROME

Postherpetic neuralgic is one of the most difficult pain syndromes to treat. It affects 10% of patients with acute herpes zoster. Although the reason that this painful condition occurs in some patients but not in others is unknown, postherpetic neuralgia is more common in older individuals and appears to occur more frequently after acute herpes zoster involving the trigeminal nerve, as opposed to the thoracic dermatomes. Conditions that cause vulnerable nerve syndrome, such as diabetes, may also predispose patients to develop postherpetic neuralgia. Pain specialists agree that aggressive treatment of acute herpes zoster can help prevent postherpetic neuralgia.

SIGNS AND SYMPTOMS

As the lesions of acute herpes zoster heal, the crust falls away, leaving pink scars that gradually become hypopigmented and atrophic. The affected cutaneous areas are often allodynic, although hypesthesia and, rarely, anesthesia may occur. In most patients, the sensory abnormalities and pain resolve as the skin lesions heal. In some patients, however, pain persists beyond lesion healing.

The pain of postherpetic neuralgia is characterized as a constant dysesthetic pain that may be exacerbated by movement or stimulation of the affected cutaneous regions (Fig. 70-1). Sharp, shooting neuritic pain may be superimposed on the constant dysesthetic pain. Some patients suffering from postherpetic neuralgia also note a burning component, reminiscent of reflex sympathetic dystrophy.

TESTING

In most cases, the diagnosis of postherpetic neuralgia is made on clinical grounds. Testing is generally used to evaluate other treatable coexisting conditions, such as vertebral compression fractures, or to identify any underlying disease responsible for the patient's immunocompromised state. Such testing includes basic laboratory screening, rectal examination, mammography, and testing for collagen vascular diseases and human immunodeficiency virus infection. Skin biopsy may confirm the presence of previous infection with herpes zoster if the history is in question.

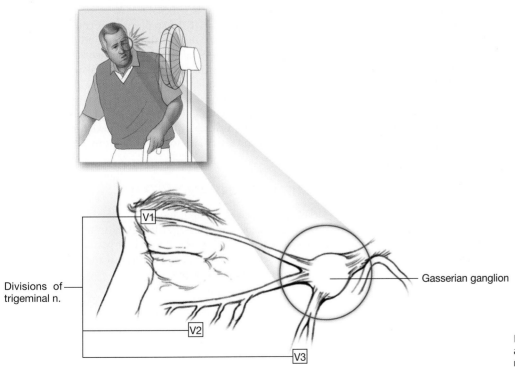

Divisions of trigeminal n.

V1

V2

V3

Gasserian ganglion

Figure 70-1 Allodynia and dysesthesia are characteristic of postherpetic neuralgia.

DIFFERENTIAL DIAGNOSIS

A careful initial evaluation, including a thorough history and physical examination, is indicated for all patients suffering from postherpetic neuralgia, to rule out an occult malignant or systemic disease that may be responsible for the patient's immunocompromised state. This evaluation also allows early recognition of changes in clinical status that may presage the development of complications, including myelitis or dissemination of the disease. Other causes of pain in the distribution of the thoracic nerve roots include thoracic radiculopathy and peripheral neuropathy. Intrathoracic and intraabdominal disorders may also mimic the pain of acute herpes zoster involving the thoracic dermatomes. For pain in the distribution of the first division of the trigeminal nerve, the clinician must exclude diseases of the eye, ear, nose, and throat, as well as intracranial disorders.

TREATMENT

Ideally, rapid and aggressive treatment of acute herpes zoster is instituted in every patient, because most pain specialists believe that the earlier treatment is initiated, the less likely postherpetic neuralgia will be to develop. This approach is especially important in older individuals, who are at greatest risk for postherpetic neuralgia. If, despite everyone's best efforts, postherpetic neuralgia occurs, the following treatment regimens are appropriate.

Analgesics

The anticonvulsant gabapentin is first-line treatment for the pain of postherpetic neuralgia. Treatment with gabapentin should begin early in the course of the disease, and this drug may be used concurrently with neural blockade, opioid analgesics, and other analgesics, including antidepressants, if care is taken to avoid central nervous system side effects. Gabapentin is started at a dose of 300 mg at bedtime and is titrated upward in 300-mg increments to a maximum of 3600 mg/day in divided doses, as side effects allow.

Pregabalin represents a reasonable alternative to gabapentin and is better tolerated in some patients. Pregabalin is started at 50 mg three times a day and may be titrated upward to 100 mg three times a day as side effects allow. Because pregabalin is excreted primarily by the kidneys, the dosage should be decreased in patients with compromised renal function.

Carbamazepine should be considered in patients suffering from severe neuritic pain in whom nerve blocks and gabapentin fail to provide relief. If this drug is used, rigid monitoring of hematologic parameters is indicated, especially in patients receiving chemotherapy or radiation therapy. Phenytoin may also be beneficial to treat neuritic pain, but it should not be used in patients with lymphoma; the drug may induce a pseudolymphoma-like state that is difficult to distinguish from actual lymphoma.

Antidepressants

Antidepressants may be useful adjuncts in the initial treatment of postherpetic neuralgia. On a short-term basis, these drugs help alleviate the significant sleep disturbance that is common in this setting. In addition, antidepressants may be valuable in ameliorating the neuritic component of the pain, which is treated less effectively with opioid analgesics. After several weeks of treatment, antidepressants may exert a mood-elevating effect that is desirable in some patients. Care must be taken to observe closely for central nervous system side effects in this patient population. These drugs may cause urinary retention and constipation that may mistakenly be attributed to herpes zoster myelitis.

Nerve Block

Neural blockade with local anesthetic and steroid through either epidural nerve block or blockade of the sympathetic nerves subserving the painful area is a reasonable next step if the aforementioned pharmacologic modalities fail to control the pain of postherpetic neuralgia. Although the exact mechanism of pain relief is unknown, it may be related to modulation of pain transmission at the spinal cord level. In general, neurodestructive procedures have a very low success rate and should be used only after all other treatments have failed, if at all.

Opioid Analgesics

Opioid analgesics have a limited role in the management of postherpetic neuralgia and may do more harm than good. Careful administration of potent, long-acting opioid analgesics (e.g., oral morphine elixir, methadone) on a time-contingent rather than an as-needed basis may be a beneficial adjunct to the pain relief provided by sympathetic neural blockade. Because many patients suffering from postherpetic neuralgia are older or have severe multisystem disease, close monitoring for the potential side effects of opioid analgesics (e.g., confusion or dizziness, which may cause a patient to fall) is warranted. Daily dietary fiber supplementation and Milk of Magnesia should be started along with opioid analgesics to prevent constipation.

Adjunctive Treatments

The application of ice packs to the affected area may provide relief in some patients. The application of heat increases pain in most patients, presumably because of increased conduction of small fibers; however, it is beneficial in an occasional patient and may be worth trying if the application of cold is ineffective. Transcutaneous electrical nerve stimulation and vibration may also be effective in a limited number of patients. The favorable risk-to-benefit ratio of all these modalities makes them reasonable alternatives for patients who cannot or will not undergo sympathetic neural blockade or who cannot tolerate pharmacologic interventions. The topical application of capsaicin may be beneficial in some patients suffering from postherpetic neuralgia; however, this substance tends to burn when applied, thus limiting its usefulness.

COMPLICATIONS AND PITFALLS

Although no specific complications are associated with postherpetic neuralgia itself, the consequences of the unremitting pain can be devastating. Failure to treat the pain of postherpetic neuralgia and the associated symptoms of sleep disturbance and depression aggressively can result in suicide.

Clinical Pearls

> Because the pain of postherpetic neuralgia is so severe, the clinician must make every effort to avoid its occurrence by rapidly and aggressively treating acute herpes zoster. If postherpetic neuralgia develops, the aggressive treatment outlined here, with special attention to the insidious onset of severe depression, should be undertaken. If serious depression occurs, hospitalization with suicide precautions is mandatory.

SUGGESTED READINGS

Delaney A, Colvin LA, Fallon MT, et al: Postherpetic neuralgia: from preclinical models to the clinic, *Neurotherapeutics* 6(4):630–637, 2009.

Schmader KE, Dworkin RH: Natural history and treatment of herpes zoster, *J Pain* 9(1 Suppl 1):3–9, 2008.

Stacey BR, Barrett JA, Whalen E, et al: Pregabalin for postherpetic neuralgia: placebo-controlled trial of fixed and flexible dosing regimens on allodynia and time to onset of pain relief, *J Pain* 9(11):1006–1017, 2008.

Waldman SD: Postherpetic neuralgia. In *Pain review,* Philadelphia, 2009, Saunders, pp 289–290.

Chapter 71

THORACIC VERTEBRAL COMPRESSION FRACTURE

ICD-9 CODES	805.2	Traumatic
	733.13	Pathologic

ICD-10 CODES	S22.009A	Traumatic
	M84.48xA	Pathologic

THE CLINICAL SYNDROME

Thoracic vertebral compression fracture is one of the most common causes of dorsal spine pain. Vertebral compression fractures are most often the result of osteoporosis (Fig. 71-1), but they may also occur with trauma to the dorsal spine caused by acceleration-deceleration injuries. In osteoporotic patients or in those with primary tumors or metastatic disease involving the

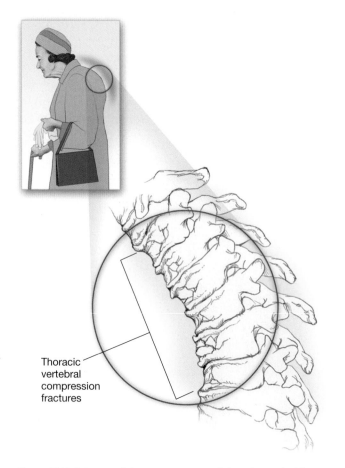

Thoracic vertebral compression fractures

Figure 71-1 Osteoporosis is a common cause of thoracic vertebral fractures.

224

thoracic vertebrae, fracture may occur with coughing (tussive fractures) or spontaneously.

The pain and functional disability associated with fractured vertebrae are determined largely by the severity of the injury (e.g., number of vertebrae involved) and the nature of the injury (e.g., whether the fracture causes impingement on the spinal nerves or spinal cord). The pain associated with thoracic vertebral compression fracture may range from a dull, deep ache (with minimal compression of the vertebrae and no nerve impingement) to severe, sharp, stabbing pain that limits the patient's ability to ambulate and cough.

SIGNS AND SYMPTOMS

Compression fractures of the thoracic vertebrae are aggravated by deep inspiration, coughing, and any movement of the dorsal spine. Palpation of the affected vertebra may elicit pain and reflex spasm of the paraspinous musculature of the dorsal spine. If trauma has occurred, hematoma and ecchymosis may be present overlying the fracture site, and the clinician should be aware of the possibility of damage to the bony thorax and the intraabdominal and intrathoracic contents. Damage to the spinal nerves may produce abdominal ileus and severe pain, resulting in splinting of the paraspinous muscles and further compromise to the patient's pulmonary status and ability to ambulate. Failure to treat this pain and splinting aggressively may result in a negative cycle of hypoventilation, atelectasis, and, ultimately, pneumonia.

TESTING

Plain radiographs of the vertebrae are indicated to rule out other occult fractures and other bony disorders, including tumor. Magnetic resonance imaging may help characterize the nature of the fracture and distinguish benign from malignant causes of pain (Fig. 71-2). If trauma is present, radionuclide bone scanning may be useful to exclude occult fractures of the vertebrae or sternum. If no trauma is present, bone density testing to evaluate for osteoporosis is appropriate, as are serum protein electrophoresis and testing for hyperparathyroidism. Based on the patient's clinical presentation, additional testing may be warranted, including a complete blood count, prostate-specific antigen level, erythrocyte sedimentation rate, and antinuclear antibody testing. Computed tomography of the thoracic contents is indicated if an occult mass or significant trauma is suspected. Electrocardiography to rule out cardiac contusion is indicated in all patients with traumatic sternal fractures or significant anterior dorsal spine trauma. The injection technique described later should be used early to avoid pulmonary complications.

DIFFERENTIAL DIAGNOSIS

In the setting of trauma, the diagnosis of thoracic vertebral compression fracture is usually straightforward. In the setting of spontaneous vertebral fracture secondary to osteoporosis or metastatic disease, the diagnosis may be less clear-cut. In this case, the pain of occult vertebral compression fracture is often mistaken for pain of cardiac or gallbladder origin, and it leads to visits to the emergency department and unnecessary cardiac and gastrointestinal workups. Acute sprain of the thoracic paraspinous muscles may be confused with thoracic vertebral compression fracture, especially if the patient has been coughing. Because the pain of acute herpes zoster may precede the rash by 3 to 7 days, it may erroneously be attributed to vertebral compression fracture.

TREATMENT

The initial treatment of pain secondary to compression fracture of the thoracic spine includes a combination of simple analgesics and nonsteroidal antiinflammatory drugs or cyclooxygenase-2 inhibitors. If these medications do not adequately control the patient's symptoms, a short-acting opioid analgesic such as hydrocodone is a reasonable next step. Because the opioid analgesics have the potential to suppress the cough reflex and respiration, the patient must be closely monitored and instructed in adequate pulmonary toilet techniques.

The local application of heat and cold or the use of an orthotic device (e.g., the Cash brace) may provide symptomatic relief. For patients who do not respond to these treatment modalities, thoracic epidural block with local anesthetic and steroid is a reasonable next step. Kyphoplasty with cement fixation of the fracture is also a good option if pain and decreased mobility become a problem (Figs. 71-3 and 71-4).

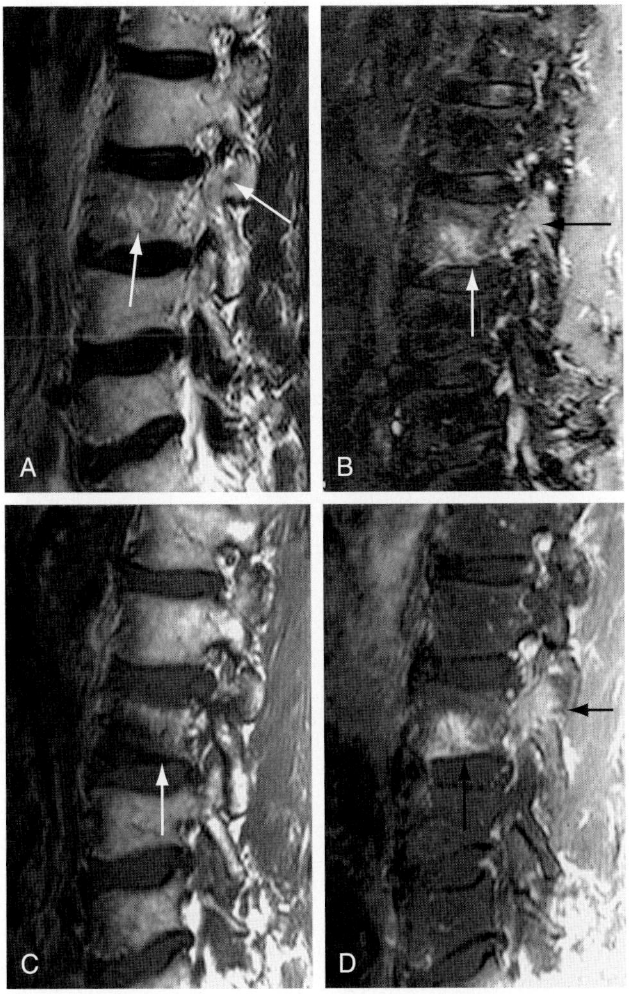

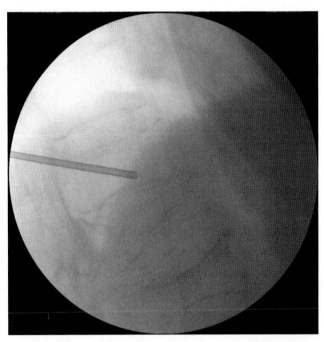

Figure 71-3 Trocar in the proper position to inject polymethyl methacrylate. Note the relative degree of demineralization of the vertebral body.

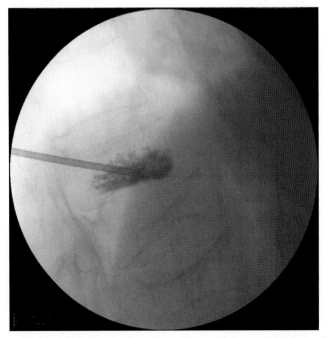

Figure 71-4 Fluoroscopy image showing satisfactory injection of polymethyl methacrylate into the vertebral body. Note the relative degree of demineralization of the vertebral body.

Figure 71-2 Metastasis. **A,** Parasagittal fast spin-echo T2-weighted magnetic resonance imaging (MRI) shows an ill-defined, heterogeneous signal abnormality involving the L3 vertebral body and the pedicle *(arrows)*. **B,** The lesion is more conspicuous on sagittal short tau inversion recovery MRI *(arrows)*. **C,** The lesion *(arrow)* is predominantly hypointense on sagittal T1-weighted MRI. **D,** The lesion *(arrows)* enhances on postgadolinium T1-weighted MRI with fat saturation. *(From Edelman RR, Hesselink JR, Zlatkin MB, Crues JV, editors: Clinical magnetic resonance imaging, ed 3, Philadelphia, 2006, Saunders, p 2315.)*

COMPLICATIONS AND PITFALLS

The major problem in the care of patients thought to be suffering from compression fractures of the thoracic vertebrae is failure to identify compression of the spinal cord or to recognize that the fracture is caused by metastatic disease. In patients with thoracic vertebral compression fractures resulting from osteoporosis, rapid pain control and early ambulation are mandatory to avoid complications such as pneumonia and thrombophlebitis.

Clinical Pearls

Compression fractures of the thoracic vertebrae are a common cause of dorsal spine pain. Correct diagnosis is necessary to treat this painful condition properly and to avoid overlooking serious intrathoracic or upper intraabdominal disorders. Pharmacologic agents usually provide adequate pain control. If necessary, thoracic epidural block is a simple technique that can produce dramatic pain relief.

SUGGESTED READINGS

Habib M, Serhan H, Marchek C, et al: Cement leakage and filling pattern study of low viscous vertebroplastic versus high viscous confidence cement, *SAS J* 4(1):26–33, 2010.

Majumdar SR, Villa-Roel C, Lyons KJ, et al: Prevalence and predictors of vertebral fracture in patients with chronic obstructive pulmonary disease, *Respir Med* 104(2):260–266, 2010.

Ortiz O, Mathis JM: Vertebral body reconstruction: techniques and tools, *Neuroimaging Clin North Am* 20(2):145–158, 2010.

Waldman SD: Percutaneous kyphoplasty. In *Atlas of interventional pain management,* ed 3, Philadelphia, 2009, Saunders, pp 654–658.

Waldman SD: Percutaneous vertebroplasty. In *Atlas of interventional pain management,* ed 3, Philadelphia, 2009, Saunders, pp 650–653.

Waldman SD: Vertebral compression fracture. In *Pain review,* Philadelphia, 2009, Saunders, pp 249–250.

Chapter 72

ACUTE PANCREATITIS

ICD-9 CODE **577.0**

ICD-10 CODE **R85.9**

THE CLINICAL SYNDROME

Acute pancreatitis is one of the most common causes of abdominal pain, with an incidence of approximately 0.5% among the general population. The mortality rate is 1% to 1.5%. In the United States, acute pancreatitis is most commonly caused by excessive alcohol consumption (Fig. 72-1); gallstones are the most frequent cause in most European countries. Acute pancreatitis has many other causes, however, including viral infection, tumor, and medications Table 72-1.

Abdominal pain is a common feature of acute pancreatitis. It may range from mild to severe and is characterized by steady, boring epigastric pain that radiates to the flanks and chest. The pain is worse in the supine position, and patients with acute pancreatitis often prefer to sit with the dorsal spine flexed and the knees

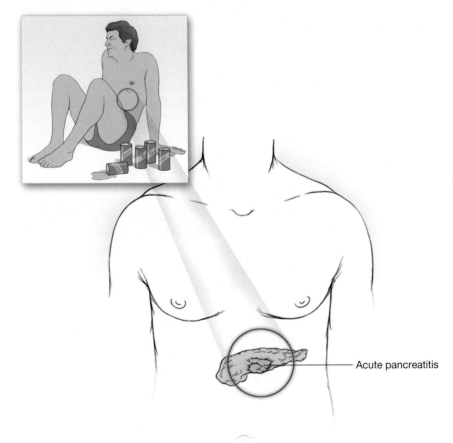

Acute pancreatitis

Figure 72-1 Excessive consumption of alcohol is one of the causes of acute pancreatitis.

227

TABLE 72-1

Common Causes of Acute Pancreatitis

Alcohol
Gallstones
Viral infections
Medications
Metabolic causes
Connective tissue diseases
Tumor obstructing the ampulla of Vater
Hereditary causes

drawn up to the abdomen. Nausea, vomiting, and anorexia are other common features.

SIGNS AND SYMPTOMS

Patients with acute pancreatitis appear ill and anxious. Tachycardia and hypotension resulting from hypovolemia are common, as is low-grade fever. Saponification of subcutaneous fat is seen in approximately 15% of patients suffering from acute pancreatitis; a similar percentage of patients experiences pulmonary complications, including pleural effusion and pleuritic pain that may compromise respiration. Diffuse abdominal tenderness with peritoneal signs is invariably present. A pancreatic mass or pseudocyst secondary to pancreatic edema may be palpable. If hemorrhage occurs, periumbilical ecchymosis (Cullen's sign) and flank ecchymosis (Turner's sign) may be present. Both these findings suggest severe necrotizing pancreatitis and indicate a poor prognosis. If the patient has hypocalcemia, Chvostek's or Trousseau's sign may be present.

TESTING

Elevation of serum amylase levels is the sine qua non of acute pancreatitis. Levels tend to peak at 48 to 72 hours and then begin to drift toward normal. Serum lipase remains elevated and may correlate better with actual disease severity. Because serum amylase levels may be elevated in other diseases, such as parotitis, amylase isozymes may be necessary to confirm a pancreatic basis for this finding. Plain radiographs of the chest are indicated for all patients who present with acute pancreatitis, to identify pulmonary complications, including pleural effusion. Given the extrapancreatic manifestations (e.g., acute renal or hepatic failure), serial complete blood counts, serum calcium and glucose levels, liver function tests, and electrolytes are indicated in all patients with acute pancreatitis. Computed tomography (CT) or magnetic resonance imaging of the abdomen can identify pancreatic pseudocyst and edema and may help the clinician gauge the severity and progress of the disease (Figs. 72-2 and 72-3). Gallbladder evaluation with radionuclides is indicated if gallstones may be the cause of acute pancreatitis. Arterial blood gas analysis can identify respiratory failure and metabolic acidosis.

DIFFERENTIAL DIAGNOSIS

The differential diagnosis includes perforated peptic ulcer, acute cholecystitis, bowel obstruction, renal calculi, myocardial infarction, mesenteric infarction, diabetic ketoacidosis, and pneumonia. Rarely, the collagen vascular diseases, including systemic lupus erythematosus and polyarteritis nodosa, may mimic pancreatitis. Because the pain of acute herpes zoster may precede the rash by 3 to 5 days, it may erroneously be attributed to acute pancreatitis.

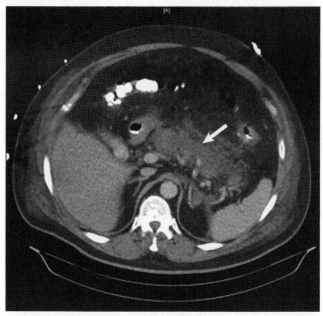

Figure 72-2 Contrast-enhanced computed tomography scan on hospital day 1 that demonstrates interstitial pancreatitis *(arrow). (From Wu BU, Conwell DL: Acute pancreatitis. Part I. Approach to early management,* Clin Gastroenterol Hepatol *8[5]:410–416, 2010.)*

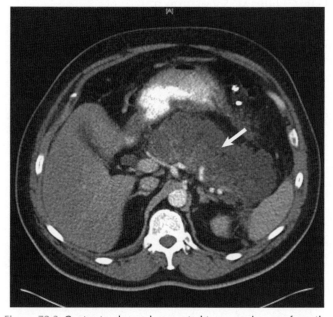

Figure 72-3 Contrast-enhanced computed tomography scan from the same patient as in Figure 72-2 on hospital day 5. The scan demonstrates extensive pancreatic necrosis *(arrow). (From Wu BU, Conwell DL: Acute pancreatitis. Part I. Approach to early management,* Clin Gastroenterol Hepatol *8[5]:410–416, 2010.)*

TREATMENT

Most cases of acute pancreatitis are self-limited and resolve within 5 to 7 days. Initial treatment is aimed primarily at allowing the pancreas to rest, which is accomplished by giving the patient nothing by mouth to decrease serum gastrin secretion and, if ileus is present, by instituting nasogastric suction. Short-acting opioid analgesics such as hydrocodone are a reasonable next step if conservative measures do not control the patient's pain. If ileus is provide adequate pain control and allow the patient to avoid the respiratory depression associated with systemic opioid analgesics.

Hypovolemia following celiac plexus block should be treated aggressively with crystalloid and colloid infusions. For prolonged cases of acute pancreatitis, parenteral nutrition is indicated to avoid malnutrition. Surgical drainage and removal of necrotic tissue may be required if severe necrotizing pancreatitis fails to respond to these treatment modalities.

COMPLICATIONS AND PITFALLS

The major pitfall is failure to recognize the severity of the patient's condition and to identify and aggressively treat the extrapancreatic manifestations of acute pancreatitis. Hypovolemia, hypocalcemia, and renal and respiratory failure occur with sufficient frequency that the clinician must actively seek these potentially fatal complications and treat them aggressively.

Clinical Pearls

> Acute pancreatitis is a common cause of abdominal pain. Correct diagnosis is necessary to treat this painful condition properly and to avoid overlooking serious extrapancreatic complications associated with this disease. Opioid analgesics generally provide adequate pain control. If necessary, celiac plexus block and thoracic epidural block are straightforward techniques that can produce dramatic pain relief.

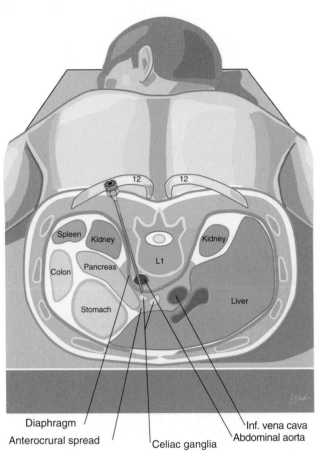

Figure 72-4 Celiac plexus block using the single-needle transaortic approach. *(From Waldman SD: Atlas of interventional pain management, ed 2, Philadelphia, 2004, Saunders, p 286.)*

present, a parenteral opioid such as meperidine is a good alternative. Because the opioid analgesics have the potential to suppress the cough reflex and respiration, the patient must be closely monitored and instructed in pulmonary toilet techniques. If symptoms persist, CT-guided celiac plexus block with local anesthetic and steroid is indicated and may decrease the mortality and morbidity associated with the disease (Fig. 72-4). Alternatively, continuous thoracic epidural block with local anesthetic, opioid, or both may

SUGGESTED READINGS

Abela JE, Carter CR: Acute pancreatitis: a review, *Surgery (Oxford)* 28(5): 205–211, 2010.

Waldman SD: Celiac plexus block. In *Pain review,* Philadelphia, 2009, Saunders, pp 502–509.

Waldman SD: Celiac plexus block: single needle transaortic approach. In *Atlas of interventional pain management,* ed 3, Philadelphia, 2009, Saunders, pp 338–342.

Waldman SD: The celiac plexus. In *Pain review,* Philadelphia, 2009, Saunders, pp 113–114.

Waldman SD: The splanchnic nerves. In *Pain review,* Philadelphia, 2009, Saunders, pp 112–113.

Wu BU, Conwell DL: Acute pancreatitis. Part I. Approach to early management, *Clin Gastroenterol Hepatol* 8(5):410–416, 2010.

Wu BU, Conwell DL: Acute pancreatitis. Part II. Approach to follow-up, *Clin Gastroenterol Hepatol* 8(5):417–422, 2010.

Chapter 73

CHRONIC PANCREATITIS

ICD-9 CODE **577.1**

ICD-10 CODE **K86.1**

THE CLINICAL SYNDROME

Chronic pancreatitis may manifest as recurrent episodes of acute inflammation of the pancreas superimposed on chronic pancreatic dysfunction, or it may be a more constant problem. As the exocrine function of the pancreas deteriorates, malabsorption with steatorrhea and azotorrhea develops. In the United States, chronic pancreatitis is most commonly caused by alcohol consumption, followed by cystic fibrosis and malignant pancreatic tumors. Hereditary causes such as alpha₁-antitrypsin deficiency are also common. In developing countries, the most common cause of chronic pancreatitis is severe protein-calorie malnutrition. Chronic pancreatitis can also result from acute pancreatitis.

Abdominal pain is a common feature of chronic pancreatitis, and it mimics the pain of acute pancreatitis; it ranges from mild to severe and is characterized by steady, boring epigastric pain that radiates to the flanks and chest. The pain is worse after the consumption of alcohol and fatty meals. Nausea, vomiting, and anorexia are also common features. With chronic pancreatitis, the clinical symptoms are often subject to periods of exacerbation and remission.

SIGNS AND SYMPTOMS

Patients with chronic pancreatitis present similarly to those with acute pancreatitis but may appear more chronically ill than acutely ill (Fig. 73-1). Tachycardia and hypotension resulting from hypovolemia are much less common in chronic pancreatitis and are ominous prognostic indicators, or they may suggest the presence of another pathologic process, such as perforated peptic ulcer. Diffuse abdominal tenderness with peritoneal signs may be noted if the patient has acute inflammation. A pancreatic mass or pseudocyst secondary to pancreatic edema may be palpable.

TESTING

Although serum amylase levels are always elevated in acute pancreatitis, they may be only mildly elevated or even within normal limits in chronic pancreatitis. Serum lipase levels are also attenuated in chronic, compared with acute, pancreatitis, although lipase may remain elevated longer than amylase in this setting and be more indicative of actual disease severity. Because serum amylase may be elevated in other diseases, such as parotitis, amylase isozymes may be necessary to confirm a pancreatic basis for this finding.

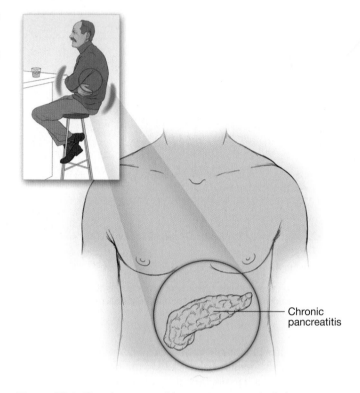

Figure 73-1 Chronic pancreatitis may present similarly to acute pancreatitis, but it can be more challenging to treat.

Plain radiographs of the chest are indicated in all patients with chronic pancreatitis to identify pulmonary complications, including pleural effusion. Given its extrapancreatic manifestations (e.g., acute renal or hepatic failure), serial complete blood counts, serum calcium and glucose levels, liver function tests, and electrolytes are indicated in all patients with chronic pancreatitis. Computed tomography (CT) of the abdomen can identify pancreatic pseudocyst or pancreatic tumor that may have been overlooked, and it may help the clinician gauge the severity and progress of the disease (Figs. 73-2 and 73-3). Gallbladder evaluation with radionuclides is indicated if gallstones are a possible cause of chronic pancreatitis. Arterial blood gas analysis can identify respiratory failure and metabolic acidosis.

DIFFERENTIAL DIAGNOSIS

The differential diagnosis includes perforated peptic ulcer, acute cholecystitis, bowel obstruction, renal calculi, myocardial infarction, mesenteric infarction, diabetic ketoacidosis, and pneumonia. Rarely, the collagen vascular diseases, including systemic lupus

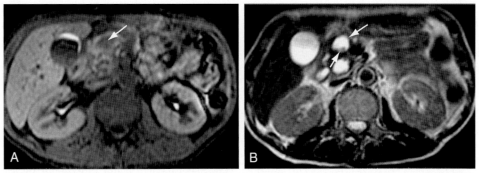

Figure 73-2 Chronic pancreatic pseudocyst. **A,** Axial T1-weighted postgadolinium magnetic resonance imaging (MRI) shows a low-signal collection anterior to the pancreas *(arrow)*. **B,** Axial T2-weighted MRI shows a high-signal collection *(long arrow)*. In a patient with a prior history of pancreatitis, this finding is consistent with a pseudocyst. Debris is noted within the pseudocyst *(short arrow)*. *(From Edelman RR, Hesselink JR, Zlatkin MB, Crues JV, editors: Clinical magnetic resonance imaging, ed 3, Philadelphia, 2006, Saunders, p 2666.)*

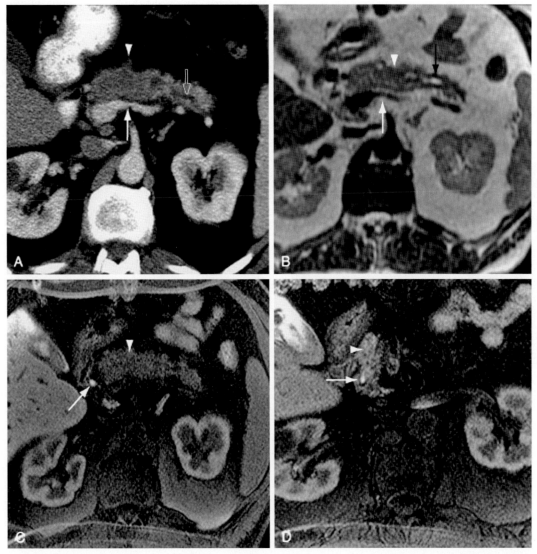

Figure 73-3 Pancreatic cancer. **A,** Axial contrast-enhanced computed tomography scan shows a large pancreatic body mass *(arrowhead)* with distal ductal dilation *(open arrow)*. The splenic vein *(arrow)* is not involved. **B,** Axial T1-weighted magnetic resonance imaging (MRI) shows similar findings: pancreatic body mass *(arrowhead)*, distal ductal dilation *(black arrow)*, and a clear fat plane from the splenic vein *(white arrow)*. **C** and **D,** Postmanganese T1-weighted fat-saturated MRI. The pancreatic mass does not enhance *(arrowhead)*. The common bile duct is enhanced and is seen as a high-signal structure *(arrow)*. *(From Edelman RR, Hesselink JR, Zlatkin MB, Crues JV, editors: Clinical magnetic resonance imaging, ed 3, Philadelphia, 2006, Saunders, p 2672.)*

erythematosus and polyarteritis nodosa, may mimic chronic pancreatitis. Because the pain of acute herpes zoster may precede the rash by 3 to 7 days, it may erroneously be attributed to chronic pancreatitis in patients who have had previous bouts of the disease. In addition, the clinician should always consider the possibility of malignant pancreatic disease.

TREATMENT

The initial management of chronic pancreatitis focuses on alleviating pain and treating malabsorption. As with acute pancreatitis, the pancreas is allowed to rest by giving the patient nothing by mouth to decrease serum gastrin secretion and, if ileus is present, instituting nasogastric suction. Short-acting opioid analgesics such as hydrocodone are a reasonable next step if conservative measures do not control the patient's pain. If ileus is present, a parenteral opioid such as meperidine is a good alternative. Because the opioid analgesics have the potential to suppress the cough reflex and respiration, the patient must be closely monitored and instructed in pulmonary toilet techniques. The use of opioid analgesics must be monitored carefully, because the potential for misuse and dependence is high.

If symptoms persist, CT-guided celiac plexus block with local anesthetic and steroid is indicated and may decrease the mortality and morbidity associated with this disease (Fig. 73-4). If the relief from this technique is short-lived, neurolytic CT-guided celiac plexus block with alcohol or phenol is a reasonable next step. Alternatively, continuous thoracic epidural block with local

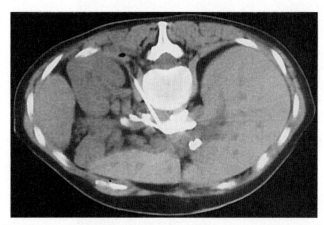

Figure 73-4 Computed tomography–guided celiac plexus block. *(From Waldman SD:* Atlas of interventional pain management, *ed 2, Philadelphia, 2004, Saunders, p 288.)*

anesthetic, opioid, or both may provide adequate pain control and allow the patient to avoid the respiratory depression associated with systemic opioid analgesics.

Hypovolemia should be treated aggressively with crystalloid and colloid infusions. For prolonged cases of chronic pancreatitis, parenteral nutrition is indicated to avoid malnutrition. Surgical drainage and removal of necrotic tissue may be required if severe necrotizing pancreatitis fails to respond to these treatment modalities.

COMPLICATIONS AND PITFALLS

The major pitfall is failure to recognize the severity of the patient's condition and to identify and aggressively treat the extrapancreatic manifestations of chronic pancreatitis. Hypovolemia, hypocalcemia, and renal and respiratory failure occur with sufficient frequency that the clinician must actively seek these potentially fatal complications and treat them aggressively. If opioids are used, the clinician must constantly watch for overuse and dependence, especially if the underlying cause of the chronic pancreatitis is alcohol abuse.

Clinical Pearls

Chronic pancreatitis is a common cause of abdominal pain. Correct diagnosis is necessary to treat this painful condition properly and to avoid overlooking serious extrapancreatic complications. The judicious use of opioid analgesics is usually adequate to control the pain of acute exacerbations. If necessary, celiac plexus block and thoracic epidural block are straightforward techniques that can produce dramatic pain relief.

SUGGESTED READINGS

Fernandez HJ, Barkin JS: Chronic pancreatitis. In McNally PR, editor: *GI/liver secrets plus,* ed 4 Philadelphia, 2010, Saunders, pp 274–281.

French JJ, Charnley RM: Chronic pancreatitis, *Surgery (Oxford)* 28(5):212–217, 2010.

Waldman SD: Celiac plexus block. In *Pain review,* Philadelphia, 2009, Saunders, pp 502–509.

Waldman SD: Celiac plexus block: single needle transaortic approach. In *Atlas of interventional pain management,* ed 3, Philadelphia, 2009, Saunders, pp 338–342.

Waldman SD: Chronic pancreatitis. In *Pain review,* Philadelphia, 2009, Saunders, pp 297–298.

Waldman SD: The celiac plexus. In *Pain review,* Philadelphia, 2009, Saunders, pp 113–114.

Waldman SD: The splanchnic nerves. In *Pain review,* Philadelphia, 2009, Saunders, pp 112–113.

Chapter 74

ILIOINGUINAL NEURALGIA

ICD-9 CODE **355.8**

ICD-10 CODE **G57.90**

THE CLINICAL SYNDROME

Ilioinguinal neuralgia is one of the most common causes of lower abdominal and pelvic pain encountered in clinical practice. Ilioinguinal neuralgia is caused by compression of the ilioinguinal nerve, and the most common causes of compression are traumatic injury to the nerve, including direct blunt trauma and damage during inguinal herniorrhaphy and pelvic surgery. Rarely, ilioinguinal neuralgia occurs spontaneously.

The ilioinguinal nerve is a branch of the L1 nerve root, with a contribution from T12 in some patients. The nerve follows a curvilinear course that takes it from its origin at the L1 (or occasionally T12) somatic nerves to inside the concavity of the ileum. The ilioinguinal nerve continues anteriorly to perforate the transverse abdominal muscle at the level of the anterior superior iliac spine. The nerve may interconnect with the iliohypogastric nerve as it continues to pass along its course medially and inferiorly, where it accompanies the spermatic cord through the inguinal ring and into the inguinal canal. The distribution of the sensory innervation of the ilioinguinal nerves varies from patient to patient, and overlap with the iliohypogastric nerve may be considerable. In general, the ilioinguinal nerve provides sensory innervation to the skin of the upper inner thigh and the root of the penis and upper scrotum in men or the mons pubis and lateral labia in women.

SIGNS AND SYMPTOMS

Ilioinguinal neuralgia manifests as paresthesias, burning pain, and occasionally numbness over the lower abdomen that radiates into the scrotum or labia and occasionally into the upper inner thigh; pain does not radiate below the knee. The pain of ilioinguinal neuralgia is made worse by extension of the lumbar spine, which puts traction on the nerve; thus, patients often assume a bent-forward, novice skier's position (Fig. 74-1). If the condition remains untreated, progressive motor deficit, consisting of bulging of the anterior abdominal wall muscles, may occur. This bulging may be confused with inguinal hernia.

Physical findings include sensory deficit in the inner thigh, scrotum, or labia in the distribution of the ilioinguinal nerve. Weakness of the anterior abdominal wall musculature may be present. Tinel's sign may be elicited by tapping over the ilioinguinal nerve at the point where it pierces the transverse abdominal muscle.

TESTING

Electromyography (EMG) can distinguish ilioinguinal nerve entrapment from lumbar plexopathy, lumbar radiculopathy, and diabetic polyneuropathy. Plain radiographs of the hip and pelvis are indicated in all patients who present with ilioinguinal neuralgia, to rule out occult bony disease. Based on the patient's clinical presentation, additional testing may be warranted, including a complete blood count, uric acid level, erythrocyte sedimentation rate, and antinuclear antibody testing. Magnetic resonance imaging (MRI) of the lumbar plexus is indicated if tumor or hematoma is suspected. The injection technique described later serves as both a diagnostic and a therapeutic maneuver.

DIFFERENTIAL DIAGNOSIS

Lesions of the lumbar plexus caused by trauma, hematoma, tumor, diabetic neuropathy, or inflammation can mimic the pain, numbness, and weakness of ilioinguinal neuralgia and must be excluded. Further, significant variability exists in the anatomy of

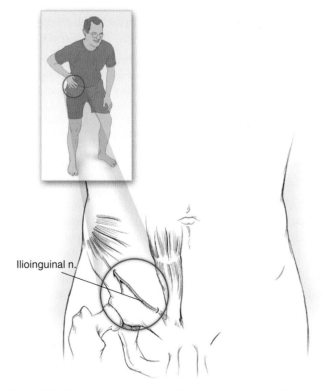

Ilioinguinal n.

Figure 74-1 Patients suffering from ilioinguinal neuralgia often bend forward in the novice skier's position to relieve the pain.

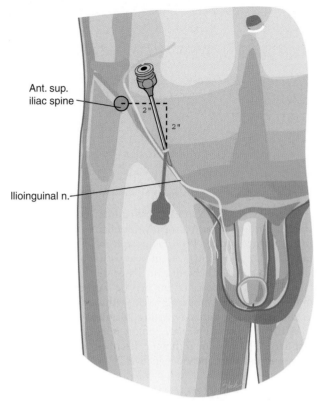

Figure 74-2 Correct needle placement for ilioinguinal nerve block. *(From Waldman SD:* Atlas of interventional pain management, *Philadelphia, 1998, Saunders.)*

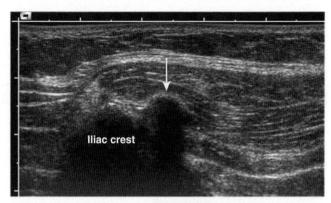

Figure 74-3 Ultrasound image demonstrating an ice ball *(arrow)* formed during cryoanalgesia of the ilioinguinal nerve. The ultrasound waves cannot cross the ice. Therefore, the ice ball produces a white (hyperechoic) surface reflex and a shadow behind it. *(From Curatolo M, Eichenberger U: Ultrasound-guided blocks for the treatment of chronic pain,* Tech Reg Anesth Pain Manag *11[2]:95–102, 2007.)*

the ilioinguinal nerve and can result in significant variation in the clinical presentation.

TREATMENT

Initial treatment of ilioinguinal neuralgia consists of simple analgesics, nonsteroidal antiinflammatory drugs, or cyclooxygenase-2 inhibitors. Avoidance of repetitive activities thought to exacerbate the pain (e.g., squatting or sitting for prolonged periods) may also ameliorate the patient's symptoms. Pharmacologic treatment is usually disappointing, however, in which case ilioinguinal nerve block with local anesthetic and steroid is required.

Ilioinguinal nerve block is performed with the patient in the supine position; a pillow can be placed under the patient's knees if lying with the legs extended increases the pain because of traction on the nerve. The anterior superior iliac spine is identified by palpation, and a point 2 inches medial and 2 inches inferior to it is identified and prepared with antiseptic solution. A 1½-inch, 25-gauge needle is advanced at an oblique angle toward the pubic symphysis (Fig. 74-2). A total of 5 to 7 mL of 1% preservative-free lidocaine in solution with 40 mg methylprednisolone is injected in a fanlike manner as the needle pierces the fascia of the external oblique muscle. Care must be taken not to insert the needle too deeply, which risks entering the peritoneal cavity and perforating the abdominal viscera. Because of the overlapping innervation of the ilioinguinal and iliohypogastric nerves, it is usually not necessary to block branches of each nerve. After injection of the solution, pressure is applied to the injection site to decrease the incidence of ecchymosis and hematoma formation, which can be quite dramatic, especially in anticoagulated patients. If anatomic landmarks are unclear, the use of fluoroscopic or ultrasound guidance should be considered (Fig. 74-3).

For patients who do not rapidly respond to ilioinguinal nerve block, consideration should be given to epidural steroid injection of the T12-L1 segments.

COMPLICATIONS AND PITFALLS

Because of the anatomy of the ilioinguinal nerve, damage to or entrapment of the nerve anywhere along its course can produce a similar clinical syndrome. Therefore, a careful search for pathologic processes at the T12-L1 spinal segments and along the path of the nerve in the pelvis is mandatory in all patients who present with ilioinguinal neuralgia without a history of inguinal surgery or trauma to the region.

The major complications of ilioinguinal nerve block are ecchymosis and hematoma formation. If the needle is too deep and enters the peritoneal cavity, perforation of the colon may result in the formation of an intraabdominal abscess and fistula. Early detection of infection is crucial to avoid potentially life-threatening sequelae.

Clinical Pearls

Ilioinguinal neuralgia is a common cause of lower abdominal and pelvic pain, and ilioinguinal nerve block is a simple technique that can produce dramatic pain relief. If a patient presents with pain suggestive of ilioinguinal neuralgia and does not respond to ilioinguinal nerve block, a lesion more proximal in the lumbar plexus or an L1 radiculopathy should be considered. Such patients often respond to epidural steroid blocks. EMG and MRI of the lumbar plexus are indicated in this patient population to rule out other causes of ilioinguinal pain, including malignant disease invading the lumbar plexus or epidural or vertebral metastatic disease at T12-L1.

SUGGESTED READINGS

Bellingham GA, Peng PWH: Ultrasound-guided interventional procedures for chronic pelvic pain, *Tech Reg Anesth Pain Manag* 13(3):171–178, 2009.

Curatolo M, Eichenberger U: Ultrasound-guided blocks for the treatment of chronic pain, *Tech Reg Anesth Pain Manag* 11(2):95–102, 2007.

Waldman SD: Ilioinguinal nerve block. In *Atlas of interventional pain management*, ed 3, Philadelphia, 2009, Saunders, pp 359–361.

Waldman SD: Ilioinguinal neuralgia. In *Pain review*, Philadelphia, 2009, Saunders, pp 298–299.

Waldman SD: The ilioinguinal nerve. In *Pain review*, Philadelphia, 2009, Saunders, p 124.

Chapter **75**

GENITOFEMORAL NEURALGIA

ICD-9 CODE **355.8**

ICD-10 CODE **G57.90**

THE CLINICAL SYNDROME

Genitofemoral neuralgia is one of the most common causes of lower abdominal and pelvic pain encountered in clinical practice. It may be caused by compression of or damage to the genitofemoral nerve anywhere along its path. The most common causes of genitofemoral neuralgia involve traumatic injury to the nerve, including direct blunt trauma and damage during inguinal herniorrhaphy and pelvic surgery. Rarely, genitofemoral neuralgia occurs spontaneously.

The genitofemoral nerve arises from fibers of the L1 and L2 nerve roots and passes through the substance of the psoas muscle, where it divides into a genital and a femoral branch. The femoral branch passes beneath the inguinal ligament, along with the femoral artery, and provides sensory innervation to a small area of skin on the inner thigh. The genital branch passes through the inguinal canal to provide innervation to the round ligament of the uterus and labia majora in women. In men, the genital branch passes with the spermatic cord to innervate the cremasteric muscles and provide sensory innervation to the bottom of the scrotum.

SIGNS AND SYMPTOMS

Genitofemoral neuralgia manifests as paresthesias, burning pain, and occasionally numbness over the lower abdomen that radiates to the inner thigh in both men and women and into the labia majora in women and the bottom of the scrotum and cremasteric muscles in men (Fig. 75-1); the pain does not radiate below the knee. The pain of genitofemoral neuralgia is made worse by extension of the lumbar spine, which puts traction on the nerve. Therefore, patients with genitofemoral neuralgia often assume a bent-forward, novice skier's position (see Fig. 75-1).

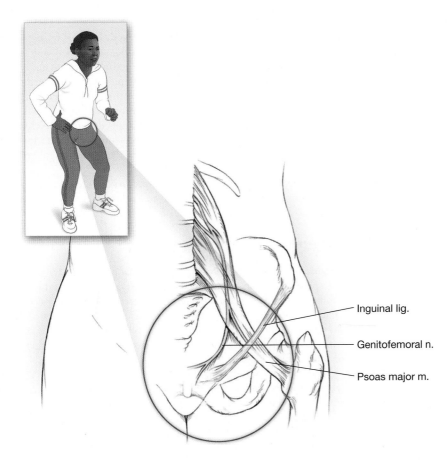

Inguinal lig.

Genitofemoral n.

Psoas major m.

Figure 75-1 The pain of genitofemoral neuralgia radiates into the inner thigh of men and women and into the labia majora in women and the inferior scrotum in men.

Physical findings include sensory deficit in the inner thigh, base of the scrotum, or labia majora in the distribution of the genitofemoral nerve. Weakness of the anterior abdominal wall musculature may be present. Tinel's sign may be elicited by tapping over the genitofemoral nerve at the point where it passes beneath the inguinal ligament.

TESTING

Electromyography (EMG) can distinguish genitofemoral nerve entrapment from lumbar plexopathy, lumbar radiculopathy, and diabetic polyneuropathy. Plain radiographs of the hip and pelvis are indicated in all patients who present with genitofemoral neuralgia, to rule out occult bony disease. Based on the patient's clinical presentation, additional testing may be warranted, including a complete blood count, uric acid level, erythrocyte sedimentation rate, and antinuclear antibody testing. Magnetic resonance imaging (MRI) of the lumbar plexus is indicated if tumor or hematoma is suspected. The injection technique described later serves as both a diagnostic and a therapeutic maneuver.

DIFFERENTIAL DIAGNOSIS

Lesions of the lumbar plexus caused by trauma, hematoma, tumor, diabetic neuropathy, or inflammation can mimic the pain, numbness, and weakness of genitofemoral neuralgia and must be excluded. Further, significant variability exists in the anatomy of the genitofemoral nerve and can result in significant variation in the clinical presentation.

TREATMENT

Initial treatment of genitofemoral neuralgia consists of simple analgesics, nonsteroidal antiinflammatory drugs, or cyclooxygenase-2 inhibitors. Avoidance of repetitive activities thought to exacerbate the pain (e.g., squatting or sitting for prolonged periods) may also ameliorate the patient's symptoms. Pharmacologic treatment is usually disappointing, however, in which case genitofemoral nerve block with local anesthetic and steroid is required.

Genitofemoral nerve block is performed with the patient in the supine position; a pillow can be placed under the patient's knees if lying with the legs extended increases the pain because of traction on the nerve. The genital branch of the genitofemoral nerve is blocked as follows: The pubic tubercle is identified by palpation, and a point just lateral to it is identified and prepared with antiseptic solution. A 1½-inch, 25-gauge needle is advanced at an oblique angle toward the pubic symphysis (Fig. 75-2). A total of 3 to 5 mL of 1% preservative-free lidocaine in solution with 80 mg methylprednisolone is injected in a fanlike manner as the needle pierces the inguinal ligament. Care must be taken not to insert the needle deeply enough to enter the peritoneal cavity and perforate the abdominal viscera.

The femoral branch of the genitofemoral nerve is blocked by identifying the middle third of the inguinal ligament. After preparation of the skin with antiseptic solution, 3 to 5 mL of 1% lidocaine is infiltrated subcutaneously just below the ligament (see Fig. 75-2). Care must be taken not to enter the femoral artery or vein or to block the femoral nerve inadvertently. The needle must be kept in a subcutaneous position to avoid entering the peritoneal cavity and perforating the abdominal viscera. If the patient has an inflammatory component to the pain, the local anesthetic is

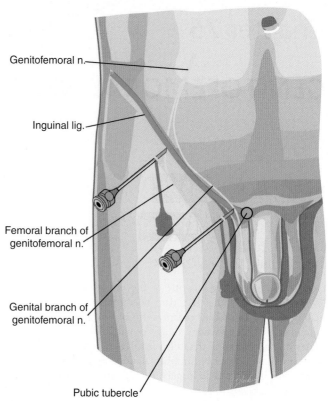

Figure 75-2 Correct needle placement for genitofemoral nerve block. *(From Waldman SD: Atlas of interventional pain management, Philadelphia, 1998, Saunders, p 374.)*

combined with 80 mg methylprednisolone and injected in incremental doses. Subsequent daily nerve blocks are carried out in a similar manner, by substituting 40 mg methylprednisolone for the initial 80-mg dose. Because of overlapping innervation of the ilioinguinal and iliohypogastric nerves, it is usually not necessary to block branches of each nerve during genitofemoral nerve block. After injection of the solution, pressure is applied to the injection site to decrease the incidence of ecchymosis and hematoma formation, which can be quite dramatic, especially in anticoagulated patients.

For patients who do not rapidly respond to genitofemoral nerve block, consideration should be given to epidural steroid injection of the L1-2 segments.

COMPLICATIONS AND PITFALLS

Because of the anatomy of the genitofemoral nerve, damage to or entrapment of the nerve anywhere along its course can produce a similar clinical syndrome. Therefore, a careful search for pathologic processes at the L1-2 spinal segments and along the path of the nerve in the pelvis is mandatory in all patients who present with genitofemoral neuralgia without a history of inguinal surgery or trauma to the region.

The major complications of genitofemoral nerve block are ecchymosis and hematoma formation. If the needle is too deep and enters the peritoneal cavity, perforation of the colon may result in the formation of an intraabdominal abscess and fistula. Early detection of infection is crucial to avoid potentially life-threatening sequelae.

Clinical Pearls

Genitofemoral neuralgia is a common cause of lower abdominal and pelvic pain, and genitofemoral nerve block is a simple technique that can produce dramatic pain relief. If a patient presents with pain suggestive of genitofemoral neuralgia and does not respond to genitofemoral nerve block, lesions more proximal in the lumbar plexus or an L1 radiculopathy should be considered. Such patients often respond to epidural steroid blocks. EMG and MRI of the lumbar plexus are indicated in this patient population to rule out other causes of genitofemoral pain, including malignant disease invading the lumbar plexus or epidural or vertebral metastatic disease at T12-L1.

SUGGESTED READINGS

Bellingham GA, Peng PWH: Ultrasound-guided interventional procedures for chronic pelvic pain, *Tech Reg Anesth Pain Manag* 13(3):171–178, 2009.

Curatolo M, Eichenberger U: Ultrasound-guided blocks for the treatment of chronic pain, *Tech Reg Anesth Pain Manag* 11(2):95–102, 2007.

Waldman SD: Genitofemoral nerve block. In *Atlas of interventional pain management,* ed 3, Philadelphia, 2009, Saunders, pp 366–370.

Waldman SD: Genitofemoral neuralgia. In *Pain review,* Philadelphia, 2009, Saunders, pp 299–300.

Waldman SD: The genitofemoral nerve. In *Pain review,* Philadelphia, 2009, Saunders, p 127.

Chapter **76**

LUMBAR RADICULOPATHY

ICD-9 CODE **724.4**

ICD-10 CODE **M54.16**

THE CLINICAL SYNDROME

Lumbar radiculopathy is a constellation of symptoms including neurogenic back and lower extremity pain emanating from the lumbar nerve roots. In addition to pain, patients may experience numbness, weakness, and loss of reflexes. The causes of lumbar radiculopathy include herniated disk, foraminal stenosis, tumor, osteophyte formation, and, rarely, infection. Many patients and their physicians refer to lumbar radiculopathy as *sciatica*.

SIGNS AND SYMPTOMS

Patients suffering from lumbar radiculopathy complain of pain, numbness, tingling, and paresthesias in the distribution of the affected nerve root or roots (Table 76-1). Patients may also note weakness and lack of coordination in the affected extremity. Muscle spasms and back pain, as well as pain referred into the buttocks, are common. Decreased sensation, weakness, and reflex changes are demonstrated on physical examination. Patients with lumbar radiculopathy commonly experience a reflex shifting of the trunk to one side, called *list* (Fig. 76-1). Lasègue's straight leg raising sign is almost always positive in patients with lumbar radiculopathy (Fig. 76-2). Occasionally, patients suffering from lumbar radiculopathy experience compression of the lumbar spinal nerve roots and cauda equina that results in lumbar myelopathy or cauda equina syndrome; if so, they experience varying degrees of lower extremity weakness and bowel and bladder symptoms. This condition represents a neurosurgical emergency and should be treated as such.

TESTING

Magnetic resonance imaging (MRI) provides the best information about the lumbar spine and its contents and should be performed in all patients suspected of suffering from lumbar radiculopathy (Fig. 76-3). MRI is highly accurate and can identify abnormalities that may put the patient at risk for the development of lumbar myelopathy. In patients who cannot undergo MRI (e.g., those with pacemakers), computed tomography (CT) or myelography is a reasonable alternative. Diskography may also help clarify the diagnosis in difficult cases (Fig. 76-4). Radionuclide bone scanning and plain radiography are indicated if fracture or a bony abnormality, such as metastatic disease, is being considered.

Although MRI, CT, and myelography can supply useful neuroanatomic information, electromyography (EMG) and nerve conduction velocity testing provide neurophysiologic information about the actual status of each individual nerve root and the lumbar plexus. EMG can also distinguish plexopathy from radiculopathy and can identify a coexistent entrapment neuropathy, such as tarsal tunnel syndrome, which may confuse the diagnosis.

If the diagnosis of lumbar radiculopathy is in question, laboratory testing consisting of a complete blood count, erythrocyte sedimentation rate, antinuclear antibody testing, human leukocyte

TABLE 76-1				
Clinical Features of Lumbar Radiculopathy				
Lumbar Root	**Pain**	**Sensory Changes**	**Weakness**	**Reflex Changes**
L4	Back, shin, thigh, and leg	Shin numbness	Ankle dorsiflexors	Knee jerk
L5	Back, posterior thigh, and leg	Numbness of top of foot and first web space	Extensor hallucis longus	None
S1	Back, posterior calf, and leg	Numbness of lateral foot	Gastrocnemius and soleus	Ankle jerk

antigen (HLA)-B27 antigen screening, and automated blood chemistry should be performed to rule out other causes of the patient's pain.

DIFFERENTIAL DIAGNOSIS

Lumbar radiculopathy is a clinical diagnosis supported by a combination of clinical history, physical examination, radiography, and MRI. Pain syndromes that may mimic lumbar radiculopathy include low back strain, lumbar bursitis, lumbar fibromyositis, inflammatory arthritis, and disorders of the lumbar spinal cord, roots, plexus, and nerves.

TREATMENT

Lumbar radiculopathy is best treated with a multimodality approach. Physical therapy, including heat modalities and deep sedative massage, combined with nonsteroidal antiinflammatory drugs and

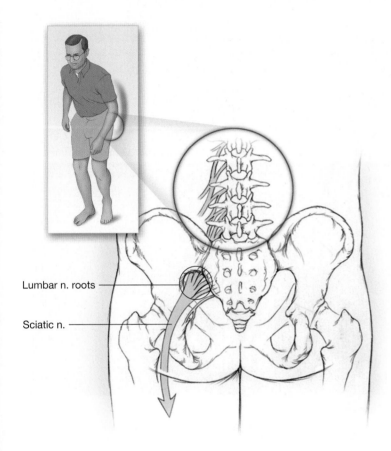

Lumbar n. roots

Sciatic n.

Figure 76-1 Patients suffering from lumbar radiculopathy often assume an unnatural posture in an attempt to take pressure off the affected nerve root and relieve pain.

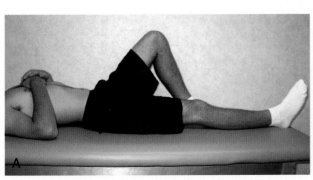
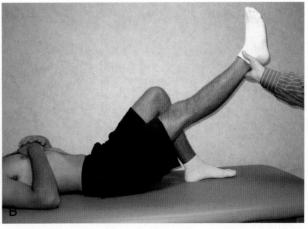

Figure 76-2 Lasègue's straight leg raising test. **A,** With the patient in the supine position, the unaffected leg is flexed 45 degrees at the knee, and the affected leg is placed flat against the table. **B,** With the ankle of the affected leg placed at 90 degrees of flexion, the affected leg is slowly raised toward the ceiling while the knee is kept fully extended. *(From Waldman SD: Physical diagnosis of pain: an atlas of signs and symptoms, Philadelphia, 2006, Saunders, pp 243–244)*

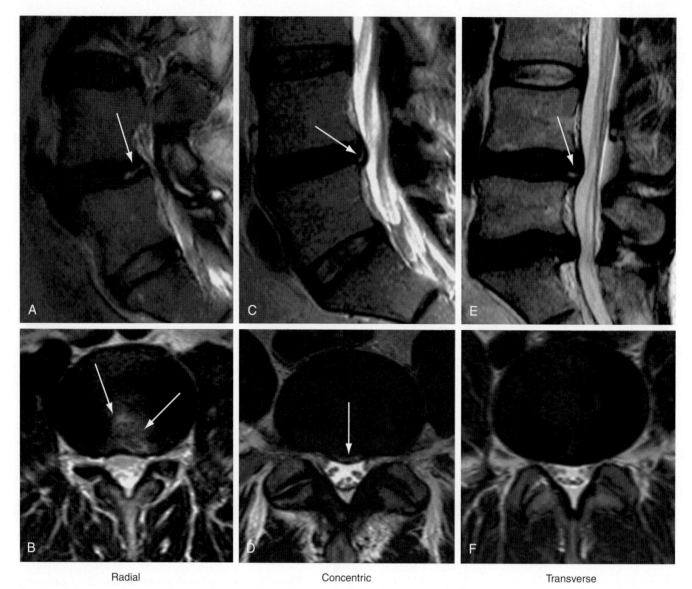

Radial   Concentric   Transverse

Figure 76-3 Magnetic resonance appearance of annular tears on sagittal **(A, C, E)** and axial **(B, D, F)** T2-weighted scans. **A** and **B,** Radial tear *(arrows).* **C** and **D,** Concentric tear *(arrows).* **E** and **F,** Transverse tear, visible only on the sagittal image *(arrow). (From Edelman RR, Hesselink JR, Zlatkin MB, Crues JV, editors:* Clinical magnetic resonance imaging, *ed 3, Philadelphia, 2006, Saunders, p 2203.)*

skeletal muscle relaxants is a good starting point. If necessary, caudal or lumbar epidural nerve blocks can be added; nerve blocks with local anesthetic and steroid are extremely effective in the treatment of lumbar radiculopathy. Underlying sleep disturbance and depression are best treated with a tricyclic antidepressant such as nortriptyline, which can be started at a single bedtime dose of 25 mg.

COMPLICATIONS AND PITFALLS

Failure to diagnosis lumbar radiculopathy accurately may put the patient at risk for the development of lumbar myelopathy, which, if untreated, may progress to paraparesis or paraplegia.

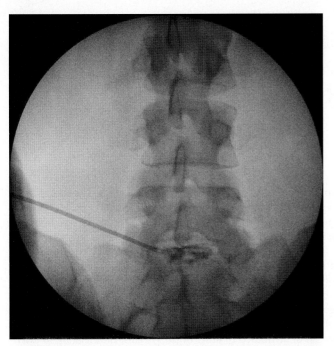

Figure 76-4 Diskography may help identify if a specific disk is responsible for the patient's pain and is useful in the diagnosis of lumbar radiculopathy.

Clinical Pearls

Tarsal tunnel syndrome must be differentiated from lumbar radiculopathy involving the lumbar nerve roots, which may also mimic tibial nerve compression. Further, lumbar radiculopathy and tibial nerve entrapment may coexist in the double-crush syndrome.

SUGGESTED READINGS

Datta S, Benyamin RM, Manchikanti L: Evidence-based practice of lumbar epidural injections, *Tech Reg Anesth Pain Manag* 13(4):281–287, 2009.

Saboeiro GR: Lumbar discography, *Radiol Clin North Am* 47(3):421–433, 2009.

Waldman SD: Caudal epidural block: prone. In *Atlas of interventional pain management,* ed 3, Philadelphia, 2009, Saunders, pp 441–448.

Waldman SD: Lumbar epidural nerve block: prone. In *Atlas of interventional pain management,* ed 3, Philadelphia, 2009, Saunders, pp 400–406.

Waldman SD: Lumbar radiculopathy. In *Pain review,* Philadelphia, 2009, Saunders, pp 250–251.

Chapter 77

LATISSIMUS DORSI SYNDROME

ICD-9 CODE **729.1**

ICD-10 CODE **M79.7**

THE CLINICAL SYNDROME

The latissimus dorsi muscle is a broad, sheetlike muscle whose primary function is to extend, adduct, and medially rotate the arm; its secondary function is to aid in deep inspiration and expiration. The latissimus dorsi muscle originates on the spine of T7; the spinous processes and supraspinous ligaments of all lower thoracic, lumbar, and sacral vertebrae; the lumbar fascia; the posterior third iliac crest; the last four ribs; and the inferior angle of the scapula. The muscle inserts on the bicipital groove of the humerus and is innervated by the thoracodorsal nerve.

The latissimus dorsi muscle is susceptible to myofascial pain syndrome, which most often results from repetitive microtrauma to the muscle during such activities as vigorous use of exercise equipment or tasks that require reaching in a forward and upward motion (Fig. 77-1). Blunt trauma to the muscle may also incite latissimus dorsi myofascial pain syndrome.

Myofascial pain syndrome is a chronic pain syndrome that affects a focal or regional portion of the body. The sine qua non of myofascial pain syndrome is the finding of myofascial trigger points on physical examination. Although these trigger points are generally localized to the part of the body affected, the pain is often referred to other areas. This referred pain may be misdiagnosed or attributed to other organ systems, thus leading to extensive evaluation and ineffective treatment.

The trigger point is pathognomonic of myofascial pain syndrome and is characterized by a local point of exquisite tenderness in the affected muscle. Mechanical stimulation of the trigger point by palpation or stretching produces not only intense local pain but also referred pain. In addition, involuntary withdrawal of the stimulated muscle, called a jump sign, often occurs and is also characteristic of myofascial pain syndrome.

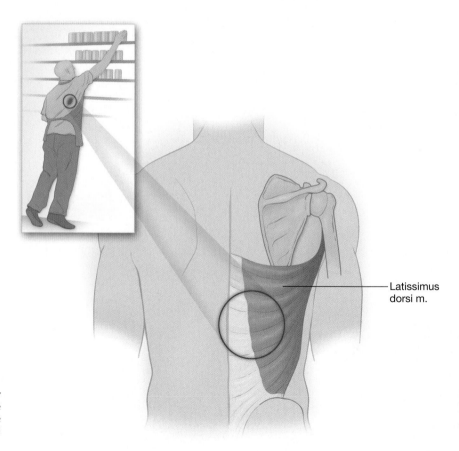

Latissimus dorsi m.

Figure 77-1 Latissimus dorsi syndrome is usually caused by repetitive microtrauma to the muscle during such activities as vigorous use of exercise equipment or tasks that require reaching forward and upward.

Taut bands of muscle fibers are often identified when myofascial trigger points are palpated. In spite of this consistent physical finding, the pathophysiology of the myofascial trigger point remains elusive, although trigger points are believed to be the result of microtrauma to the affected muscle. This trauma may result from a single injury, repetitive microtrauma, or chronic deconditioning of the agonist and antagonist muscle unit.

In addition to muscle trauma, various other factors seem to predispose patients to develop myofascial pain syndrome. For instance, a weekend athlete who subjects his or her body to unaccustomed physical activity may develop myofascial pain syndrome. Poor posture while sitting at a computer or while watching television has also been implicated as a predisposing factor. Previous injuries may result in abnormal muscle function and lead to the development of myofascial pain syndrome. All these predisposing factors may be intensified if the patient also suffers from poor nutritional status or coexisting psychological or behavioral abnormalities, including chronic stress and depression. The latissimus dorsi muscle seems to be particularly susceptible to stress-induced myofascial pain syndrome.

Stiffness and fatigue often coexist with pain, and they increase the functional disability associated with this disease and complicate its treatment. Myofascial pain syndrome may occur as a primary disease state or in conjunction with other painful conditions, including radiculopathy and chronic regional pain syndromes. Psychological or behavioral abnormalities, including depression, frequently coexist with the muscle abnormalities, and management of these psychological disorders is an integral part of any successful treatment plan.

SIGNS AND SYMPTOMS

The trigger point is the pathologic lesion of latissimus dorsi syndrome, and it is characterized by a local point of exquisite tenderness at the inferior angle of the scapula; this pain is referred to the axilla and the back of the ipsilateral upper extremity into the dorsal aspect of the ring and little fingers (Fig. 77-2). Mechanical stimulation of the trigger point by palpation or stretching produces both intense local pain and referred pain. In addition, the jump sign is often present.

TESTING

Biopsies of clinically identified trigger points have not revealed consistently abnormal histologic features. The muscle hosting the trigger points has been described either as "moth-eaten" or as containing "waxy degeneration." Increased plasma myoglobin has been reported in some patients with latissimus dorsi syndrome, but this finding has not been corroborated by other investigators. Electrodiagnostic testing has revealed an increase in muscle tension in some patients, but again, this finding has not been reproducible. Because of the lack of objective diagnostic testing, the clinician must rule out other coexisting disease processes that may mimic latissimus dorsi syndrome (see "Differential Diagnosis").

DIFFERENTIAL DIAGNOSIS

The diagnosis of latissimus dorsi syndrome is based on clinical findings rather than specific laboratory, electrodiagnostic, or radiographic testing. For this reason, a targeted history and physical examination, with a systematic search for trigger points and

identification of a positive jump sign, must be carried out in every patient suspected of suffering from latissimus dorsi syndrome. The clinician must rule out other coexisting disease processes that may mimic latissimus dorsi syndrome, including primary inflammatory muscle disease, multiple sclerosis, and collagen vascular disease. The use of electrodiagnostic and radiographic testing can identify coexisting pathologic processes such as subscapular bursitis, cervical radiculopathy, herniated nucleus pulposus, and rotator cuff tear. The clinician must also identify coexisting psychological and behavioral abnormalities that may mask or exacerbate the symptoms of latissimus dorsi syndrome.

TREATMENT

Treatment is focused on eliminating the myofascial trigger and achieving relaxation of the affected muscle. It is hoped that interrupting the pain cycle in this way will allow the patient to obtain prolonged pain relief. The mechanism of action of the treatment modalities used is poorly understood, so an element of trial and error is involved in developing a treatment plan.

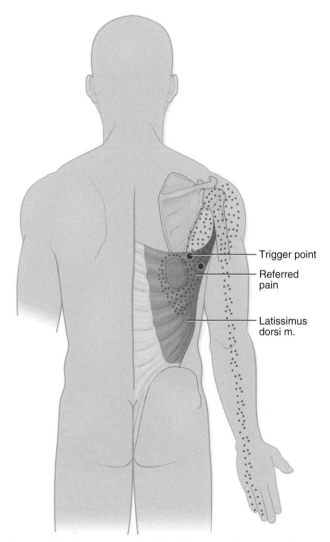

— Trigger point

— Referred pain

— Latissimus dorsi m.

Figure 77-2 The trigger point of latissimus dorsi syndrome is at the inferior angle of the scapula, with pain referred to the axilla and the back of the ipsilateral upper extremity into the dorsal aspect of the ring and little fingers. *(From Waldman SD: Atlas of pain management injection techniques, ed 2, Philadelphia, 2007, Saunders, p 299.)*

Conservative therapy consisting of trigger point injection with local anesthetic or saline solution is the initial treatment of latissimus dorsi syndrome. Because underlying depression and anxiety are present in many patients, antidepressants are an integral part of most treatment plans. Other therapies, including transcutaneous nerve stimulation and electrical stimulation, may be helpful on a case-by-case basis. For patients who do not respond to these traditional measures, consideration should be given to the use of botulinum toxin type A; although not currently approved by the Food and Drug Administration for this indication, the injection of minute quantities of botulinum toxin type A directly into trigger points has been successful in the treatment of persistent latissimus dorsi syndrome.

COMPLICATIONS AND PITFALLS

Trigger point injections are extremely safe if careful attention is paid to the clinically relevant anatomy. Sterile technique must be used to avoid infection, along with universal precautions to minimize any risk to the operator. Most complications of trigger point injection are related to needle-induced trauma at the injection site and in underlying tissues. The incidence of ecchymosis and hematoma formation can be decreased if pressure is applied to the injection site immediately after injection. The avoidance of overly long needles can decrease the incidence of trauma to underlying structures. Special care must be taken to avoid pneumothorax during injection of trigger points in proximity to the underlying pleural space.

Clinical Pearls

Although latissimus dorsi syndrome is a common disorder, it is often misdiagnosed. Therefore, in patients suspected of suffering from latissimus dorsi syndrome, a careful evaluation to identify underlying disease processes is mandatory. Latissimus dorsi syndrome often coexists with various somatic and psychological disorders.

SUGGESTED READINGS

Arnold LM: The pathophysiology, diagnosis and treatment of fibromyalgia, *Psychiatr Clin North Am* 33(2):375–408, 2010.

Bradley LA: Pathophysiology of fibromyalgia, *Am J Med* 122(12 Suppl 1): S22–S30, 2009.

Imamura M, Cassius DA, Fregni F: Fibromyalgia: from treatment to rehabilitation, *Eur J Pain Suppl* 3(2):117–122, 2009.

Chapter 78

SPINAL STENOSIS

ICD-9 CODE **724.02**

ICD-10 CODE **M48.06**

THE CLINICAL SYNDROME

Spinal stenosis is the result of congenital or acquired narrowing of the spinal canal. Clinically, spinal stenosis usually manifests in a characteristic manner as pain and weakness in the legs when walking. This neurogenic pain is called pseudoclaudication or neurogenic claudication (Fig. 78-1). These symptoms are usually accompanied by lower extremity pain emanating from the lumbar nerve roots. In addition, patients with spinal stenosis may experience numbness, weakness, and loss of reflexes. The causes of spinal stenosis include bulging or herniated disk, facet arthropathy, and thickening and buckling of the interlaminar ligaments. All these inciting factors tend to worsen with age.

SIGNS AND SYMPTOMS

Patients suffering from spinal stenosis complain of calf and leg pain and fatigue when walking, standing, or lying supine. These symptoms disappear if they flex the lumbar spine or assume the sitting position. Frequently, patients suffering from spinal stenosis exhibit a simian posture, with a forward-flexed trunk and slightly bent knees when walking, to decrease the symptoms of pseudoclaudication (Fig. 78-2). Extension of the spine may cause an increase in symptoms. Patients also complain of pain, numbness, tingling, and paresthesias in the distribution of the affected nerve root or roots. Weakness and lack of coordination in the affected extremity may be noted. Patients often have a positive stoop test for spinal stenosis (Fig. 78-3). Muscle spasms and back pain, as well as pain referred to the trapezius and interscapular region, are common. Decreased sensation, weakness, and reflex changes are demonstrated on physical examination.

Occasionally, patients suffering from spinal stenosis experience compression of the lumbar spinal nerve roots and cauda equina,

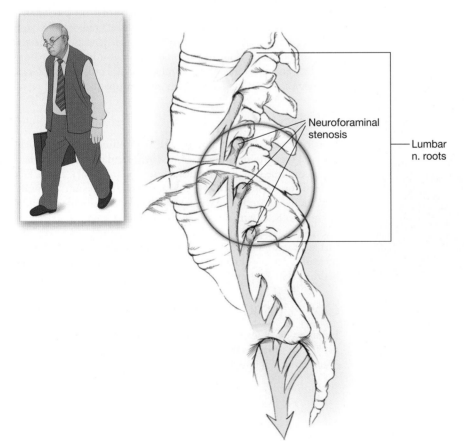

Neuroforaminal stenosis

Lumbar n. roots

Figure 78-1 Pseudoclaudication is the sine qua non of spinal stenosis.

with resulting lumbar myelopathy or cauda equina syndrome. These patients experience varying degrees of lower extremity weakness and bowel and bladder symptoms. This condition represents a neurosurgical emergency and should be treated as such, although the onset of symptoms is often insidious.

TESTING

Magnetic resonance imaging (MRI) provides the best information about the lumbar spine and its contents and should be performed in all patients suspected of having spinal stenosis. MRI is highly accurate and can identify abnormalities that may put the patient at risk for lumbar myelopathy (Fig. 78-4). In patients who cannot undergo MRI (e.g., those with pacemakers), computed tomography (CT) or myelography is a reasonable alternative. Radionuclide bone scanning and plain radiography are indicated if a coexistent fracture or bony abnormality, such as metastatic disease, is being considered.

Although MRI, CT, and myelography can supply useful neuroanatomic information, electromyography (EMG) and nerve conduction velocity testing provide neurophysiologic information about the actual status of each individual nerve root and the lumbar plexus. EMG can also distinguish plexopathy from radiculopathy and can identify a coexistent entrapment neuropathy that may confuse the diagnosis.

If the diagnosis is in question, laboratory tests consisting of a complete blood count, erythrocyte sedimentation rate, antinuclear antibody testing, human leukocyte antigen (HLA)-B27 antigen screening, and automated blood chemistry should be performed to rule out other causes of the patient's pain.

DIFFERENTIAL DIAGNOSIS

Spinal stenosis is a clinical diagnosis supported by a combination of clinical history, physical examination, radiography, and MRI. Pain syndromes that may mimic spinal stenosis include low back strain, lumbar bursitis, lumbar fibromyositis, inflammatory arthritis, and disorders of the lumbar spinal cord, roots, plexus, and nerves, including diabetic femoral neuropathy.

TREATMENT

Spinal stenosis is best treated with a multimodality approach. Physical therapy, including heat modalities and deep sedative massage, combined with nonsteroidal antiinflammatory drugs and skeletal muscle relaxants is a reasonable starting point. If necessary, caudal or lumbar epidural nerve blocks can be added. Caudal epidural blocks with local anesthetic and steroid are extremely effective in the treatment of spinal stenosis. Underlying sleep disturbance and depression are best treated with a tricyclic antidepressant such as nortriptyline, which can be started at a single bedtime dose of 25 mg.

COMPLICATIONS AND PITFALLS

Failure to diagnosis spinal stenosis accurately may put the patient at risk for the development of lumbar myelopathy or cauda equina syndrome, which, if untreated, may progress to paraparesis or paraplegia.

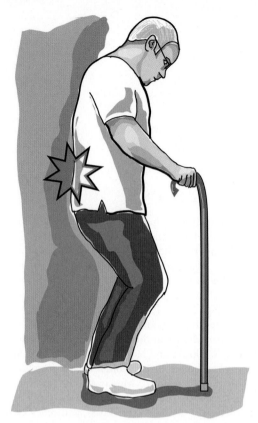

Figure 78-2 Patients suffering from spinal stenosis often assume a simian posture, with a forward-flexed trunk and slightly bent knees when walking, to decrease the symptoms of pseudoclaudication. *(From Waldman SD: Physical diagnosis of pain: an atlas of signs and symptoms, Philadelphia, 2006, Saunders, p 260.)*

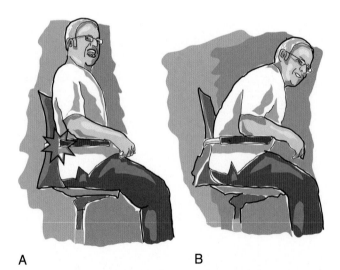

A   B

Figure 78-3 Stoop test for spinal stenosis. **A,** Extension of the lumbar spine exacerbates the pain of spinal stenosis. **B,** Flexion of the lumbar spine relieves the pain of spinal stenosis. *(From Waldman SD: Physical diagnosis of pain: an atlas of signs and symptoms, Philadelphia, 2006, Saunders, p 261.)*

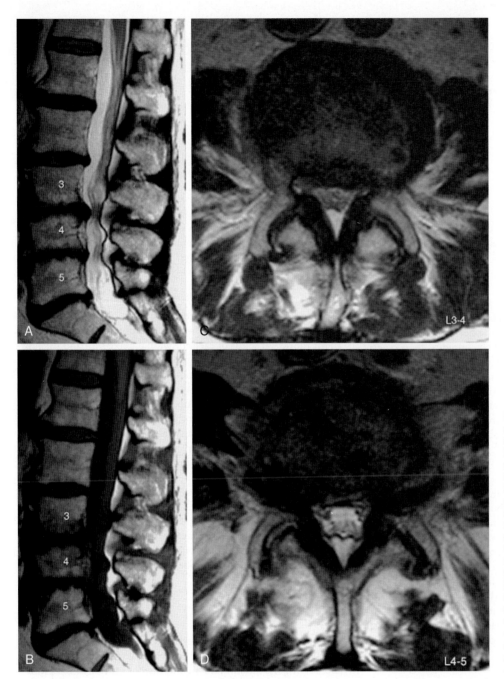

Figure 78-4 Acquired degenerative spinal stenosis. **A** and **B,** Sagittal T2- and T1-weighted magnetic resonance imaging (MRI) demonstrates severe disk degeneration at L3-4 and L4-5, with disk desiccation, disk space narrowing, irregularity of the adjacent vertebral end plates, and posterior bulging disks. The nerve roots of the cauda equina have an undulating or wavy appearance because of the marked constriction at L3-4. **C** and **D,** On axial T2-weighted MRI, the combination of posterior bulging disks, facet hypertrophy, and thickened ligamenta flava causes severe spinal canal stenosis at L3-4 and moderate stenosis at L4-5. Also note severe compromise of the lateral recesses at L3-4 bilaterally. *(From Edelman RR, Hesselink JR, Zlatkin MB, Crues JV, editors:* Clinical magnetic resonance imaging, *ed 3, Philadelphia, 2006, Saunders, p 2228.)*

Clinical Pearls

Spinal stenosis is a common cause of back and lower extremity pain, and the finding of pseudoclaudication should point the clinician toward this diagnosis. This syndrome tends to worsen with age. The onset of lumbar myelopathy or cauda equina syndrome may be insidious, so careful questioning and physical examination are required to avoid missing these complications.

SUGGESTED READINGS

Genevay S, Atlas SJ: Lumbar spinal stenosis, *Best Pract Res Clin Rheumatol* 24(2):253–265, 2010.

Waldman SD: Caudal epidural block: prone. In *Atlas of interventional pain management,* ed 3, Philadelphia, 2009, Saunders, pp 441–448.

Waldman SD: Lumbar epidural nerve block: prone. In *Atlas of interventional pain management,* ed 3, Philadelphia, 2009, Saunders, pp 400–406.

Waldman SD: Spinal stenosis. In *Pain review,* Philadelphia, 2009, Saunders, pp 202–203.

Chapter 79

ARACHNOIDITIS

ICD-9 CODE 322.9

ICD-10 CODE G03.9

The Clinical Syndrome

Arachnoiditis consists of thickening, scarring, and inflammation of the arachnoid membrane. These abnormalities may be self-limited or may lead to compression of the nerve roots and spinal cord. In addition to pain, patients with arachnoiditis may experience numbness, weakness, loss of reflexes, and bowel and bladder symptoms. The exact cause of arachnoiditis is unknown, but it may be related to herniated disk, infection, tumor, myelography, spinal surgery, or intrathecal administration of drugs. Anecdotal reports of arachnoiditis after epidural and subarachnoid administration of methylprednisolone have surfaced.

Signs and Symptoms

Patients suffering from arachnoiditis complain of pain, numbness, tingling, and paresthesias in the distribution of the affected nerve root or roots (Table 79-1). Weakness and lack of coordination in the affected extremity may be noted; muscle spasms, back pain, and pain referred to the buttocks are common. Decreased sensation, weakness, and reflex changes are demonstrated on physical examination. Occasionally, patients with arachnoiditis experience compression of the lumbar spinal cord, nerve roots, and cauda equina, with resulting lumbar myelopathy or cauda equina syndrome (Fig. 79-1). These patients experience varying degrees of lower extremity weakness and bowel and bladder symptoms.

Testing

Magnetic resonance imaging (MRI) provides the best information about the lumbar spine and its contents and should be performed in all patients suspected of suffering from arachnoiditis (Fig. 79-2). MRI is highly accurate and can identify abnormalities that may put the patient at risk for the development of lumbar myelopathy or cauda equina syndrome. In patients who cannot undergo MRI (e.g., those with pacemakers), computed tomography (CT) or myelography is a reasonable alternative (Fig. 79-3). Radionuclide bone scanning and plain radiography are indicated if a fracture or bony abnormality, such as metastatic disease, is being considered.

Although MRI, CT, and myelography can supply useful neuroanatomic information, electromyography (EMG) and nerve conduction velocity testing provide neurophysiologic information about the actual status of each individual nerve root and the lumbar plexus. EMG and somatosensory evoked potentials can also distinguish plexopathy from arachnoiditis and can identify a coexistent entrapment neuropathy that may confuse the diagnosis.

If the diagnosis is in question, laboratory tests consisting of a complete blood count, erythrocyte sedimentation rate, antinuclear antibody testing, human leukocyte antigen (HLA)-B27 screening, and automated blood chemistry should be performed to rule out other causes of the patient's pain.

Differential Diagnosis

Arachnoiditis is a clinical diagnosis supported by a combination of clinical history, physical examination, radiography, and MRI. Conditions that may mimic arachnoiditis include tumor, infection, and disorders of the lumbar spinal cord, roots, plexus, and nerves.

Treatment

Little consensus exists on the best treatment of arachnoiditis; most efforts are aimed at decompressing the nerve roots and spinal cord and treating the inflammatory component of the disease. Epidural neurolysis or the caudal administration of steroids may decompress the nerve roots if the pathologic process is localized. More generalized arachnoiditis often requires surgical decompressive laminectomy. The results of these treatment modalities are disappointing at best.

TABLE 79-1				
Clinical Features of Arachnoiditis				
Lumbar Root	**Pain**	**Sensory Changes**	**Weakness**	**Reflex Changes**
L4	Back, shin, thigh, and leg	Shin numbness	Ankle dorsiflexors	Knee jerk
L5	Back, posterior thigh, and leg	Numbness of top of foot and first web space	Extensor hallucis longus	None
S1	Back, posterior calf, and leg	Numbness of lateral foot	Gastrocnemius and soleus	Ankle jerk

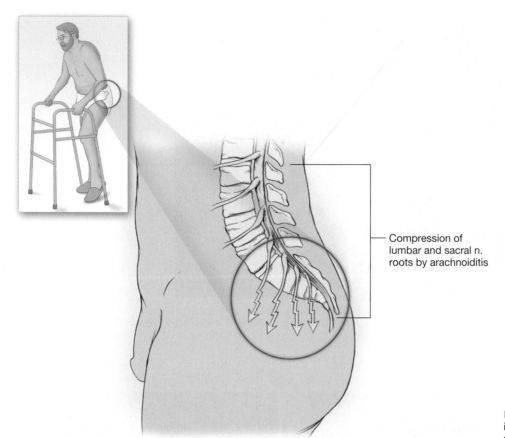

Compression of
lumbar and sacral n.
roots by arachnoiditis

Figure 79-1 Arachnoiditis may result in lumbar myelopathy or cauda equina syndrome.

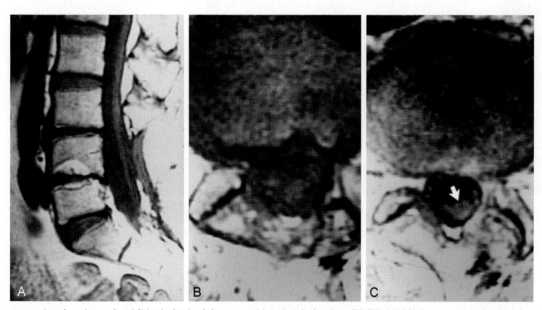

Figure 79-2 Postoperative chronic arachnoiditis. **A,** Sagittal short repetition time/echo time (TR/TE) (600/15) conventional spin-echo image magnetic resonance imaging (MRI) demonstrates degeneration of the L4-5 intervertebral disk. **B,** Axial short TR/TE (600/15) conventional spin-echo MRI at the level of L3 demonstrates spondylosis with no associated abnormality. **C,** Axial short TR/TE (600/15) conventional spin-echo MRI after gadolinium administration shows enhancement of matted nerve roots forming a thickened cord *(arrow),* indicating the presence of adhesive arachnoiditis.

Continued

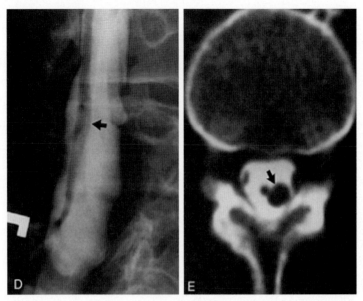

Figure 79-2—cont'd **D,** Oblique view from a water-soluble contrast myelogram shows the partially empty sac and the cordlike matting of the nerve roots *(arrow).* **E,** Axial computed tomography scan obtained through L3 shows matting of the nerve roots into a cordlike structure *(arrow). (From Edelman RR, Hesselink JR, Zlatkin MB, Crues JV, editors:* Clinical magnetic resonance imaging, *ed 3, Philadelphia, 2006, Saunders, p 2274.)*

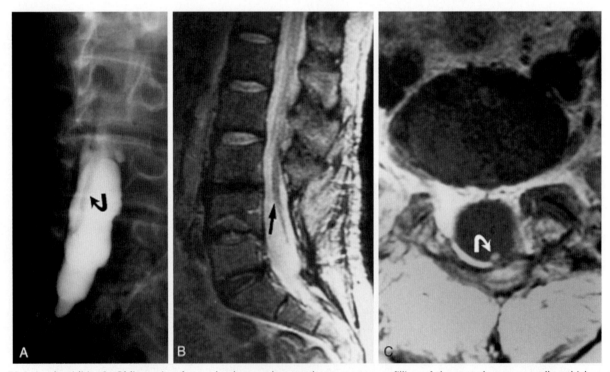

Figure 79-3 Arachnoiditis. **A,** Oblique view from a lumbar myelogram demonstrates nonfilling of the root sleeves, as well as thickened nerve roots *(arrow).* **B,** Sagittal T2-weighted magnetic resonance imaging (MRI) shows clumped, thickened nerve roots *(arrow).* **C,** Axial T1-weighted MRI after contrast administration reveals a nearly empty sac with a single thickened, slightly enhanced nerve root *(arrow)* adherent to the dorsal aspect of the dura. *(From Edelman RR, Hesselink JR, Zlatkin MB, Crues JV, editors:* Clinical magnetic resonance imaging, *ed 3, Philadelphia, 2006, Saunders, p 2186.)*

Underlying sleep disturbance and depression are treated with a tricyclic antidepressant such as nortriptyline, which can be started at a single bedtime does of 25 mg. Neuropathic pain associated with arachnoiditis may respond to gabapentin. Spinal cord stimulation may also provide symptomatic relief. Opioid analgesics should be used with caution, if at all.

COMPLICATIONS AND PITFALLS

Failure to diagnosis arachnoiditis accurately may put the patient at risk for the development of lumbar myelopathy or cauda equina syndrome, which, if untreated, may progress to paraparesis or paraplegia.

Clinical Pearls

Arachnoiditis is a potentially devastating disease that may erroneously be attributed to the clinician's efforts to diagnose and treat low back and lower extremity pain. For this reason, MRI and EMG should be obtained early in patients who have no clear cause of their symptoms.

SUGGESTED READINGS

Babar S, Saifuddin A: MRI of the post-discectomy lumbar spine, *Clin Radiol* 57(11):969–981, 2002.
Crum BA, Strommen JA: Nerve root assessment with SEP and MEP, *Handb Clin Neurophysiol* 8:455–463, 2008.
Waldman SD: Arachnoiditis. In *Pain review,* Philadelphia, 2009, Saunders, pp 303–304.

Chapter 80

DISKITIS

ICD-9 CODE **722.93**

ICD-10 CODE **M46.47**

THE CLINICAL SYNDROME

Diskitis is an often misdiagnosed cause of spine pain that, if undiagnosed, can result in paralysis or life-threatening complications. Although diskitis can occur anywhere in the spine, the lumbar spine is affected most often, followed by the cervical spine. Diskitis can occur spontaneously by hematogenous seeding, most frequently as a result of urinary tract infections that spread to the spinal epidural space through Batson's plexus. More commonly, diskitis occurs after instrumentation of the spine, including surgery, diskography, and epidural nerve blocks. Not surprisingly, the infectious agents most frequently responsible for diskitis are the same agents that cause urinary tract infections. The literature has suggested that the administration of steroids into the epidural space causes immunosuppression, with a resultant increase in the incidence of diskitis. Although this suggestion is theoretically plausible, the statistical evidence given the thousands of epidural steroid injections performed around the United States on a daily basis calls this concept into question. Diskitis has a 2:1 male predominance in adult patients. The average age of occurrence in children is approximately 7 years, and in adults it is the fifth decade of life. Untreated, the mortality associated with diskitis approaches 10%.

The patient with diskitis initially presents with ill-defined pain and spasm of the paraspinous musculature in the segment of the spine affected (e.g., cervical, thoracic, or lumbar) (Fig. 80-1). This pain becomes more intense and localized as the infection involves more of the disks and adjacent vertebral bodies and compresses neural structures. Low-grade fever and vague constitutional symptoms including malaise and anorexia progress to frank sepsis with high-grade fever, rigors, and chills. At this point, the patient begins to experience sensory and motor deficits, as well as bowel and bladder symptoms as a result of neural compromise. As the infection continues to expand into the epidural space, compromise of the vascular supply to the affected spinal cord and nerve occurs, with resultant ischemia and, if untreated, spinal cord infarction and permanent neurologic deficits.

SIGNS AND SYMPTOMS

The patient with diskitis initially presents with ill-defined pain in the general area of the infection. At this point, the patient may have mild pain on range of motion of the affected segments. The neurologic examination is within normal limits. A low-grade fever

or night sweats may be noted. Theoretically, if the patient has received steroids, these constitutional symptoms may be attenuated or their onset may be delayed. As the abscess increases in size, the patient appears acutely ill, with fever, rigors, and chills. The clinician may be able to identify neurologic findings suggestive of spinal nerve root or spinal cord compression. Subtle findings that point to the development of myelopathy (e.g., Babinski's sign, clonus, and decreased perineal sensation) may be overlooked if not carefully sought. As compression of the involved neural structures continues, the patient's neurologic status may deteriorate rapidly. If the correct diagnosis is not made, irreversible motor and sensory deficit will result.

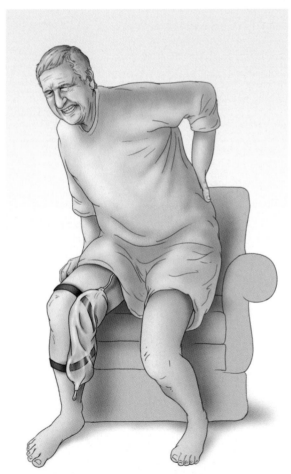

Figure 80-1 If diskitis is not promptly diagnosed, compression of the involved neural structures may continue, and the patient's neurologic status may deteriorate rapidly. If diagnosis is not made and treatment initiated, irreversible motor and sensory deficit will result.

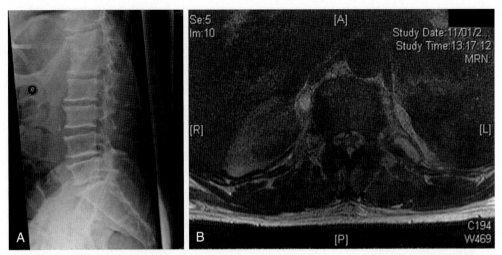

Figure 80-2 **A,** Plain film shows loss of disk space and end-plate destruction at T12-L1. This appearance is highly suggestive of infection. **B,** Axial magnetic resonance imaging at the same level indicates a paravertebral collection. *(From Cottle L, Riordan T: Infectious spondylodiscitis,* J Infect *56[6]:402–412, 2008.)*

TESTING

Plain radiographs often reveal the evidence of disk space narrowing and end-plate changes that are suggestive of diskitis; however, these changes may not be present early in the course of the disease (Fig. 80-2). Early diagnosis is best made with the use of radionucleotide scanning with gallium-67 and technetium-99m (Fig. 80-3). Both magnetic resonance imaging (MRI) and computed tomography (CT) are highly accurate in the diagnosis of diskitis and are probably more accurate than myelography in the diagnosis of intrinsic disease of the spinal cord and spinal tumor, among other disorders (Fig. 80-4). Needle or open surgical biopsy for culture should strongly be considered in all patients thought to be suffering from diskitis, but antibiotic treatment should not be delayed if these procedures are not readily available (Fig. 80-5).

All patients suspected of suffering from diskitis should undergo laboratory testing consisting of complete blood cell count, sedimentation rate, and automated blood chemistries. Blood and urine cultures should be immediately obtained in all patients thought to have diskitis, to allow immediate implementation of antibiotic therapy while the workup is in progress. Gram stains and cultures of the abscess material should also be obtained, but antibiotic treatment should not be delayed while waiting for this information. Echocardiography to rule out subacute bacterial endocarditis should also be considered, especially in intravenous drug abusers.

TREATMENT

The rapid initiation of treatment of diskitis is mandatory if the patient is to avoid the sequelae of permanent neurologic deficit or death. The treatment of diskitis is aimed at two goals: (1) treatment of the infection with antibiotics and (2) drainage of any abscess formation to relieve compression on neural structures. Because most cases of diskitis are caused by *Staphylococcus aureus,* antibiotics such as vancomycin that treat staphylococcal infection should be started immediately after blood and urine culture samples are taken. Antibiotic therapy can be tailored to the culture and sensitivity reports as they become available (Fig. 80-6). As mentioned, antibiotic therapy should not be delayed while waiting for definitive diagnosis if diskitis is being considered as part

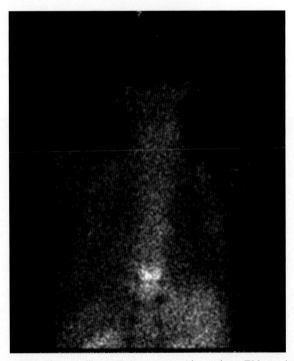

Figure 80-3 Planar gallium-67 citrate scan with uptake at T11 consistent with diskitis and osteomyelitis. *(From Stieber JR, Schweitzer ME, Errico TJ: The imaging of spinal infections,* Semin Spine Surg *19[2]:106–112, 2007.)*

of the differential diagnosis. Many atypical infectious agents (e.g., Mycobacterium tuberculosis, fungi) can cause diskitis, especially in immunocompromised patients, and such pathogens should be considered in the patient who does not respond to treatment with traditional antibiotic regimens. Bed rest and use of orthotic devices to stabilize affected spinal segments should help improve the long-term outcome of patients suffering from diskitis.

Antibiotics alone are rarely successfully in the treatment of diskitis unless the diagnosis is made very early in the course of the disease. Therefore, drainage of any epidural abscess is required to effect full recovery. Drainage is usually accomplished

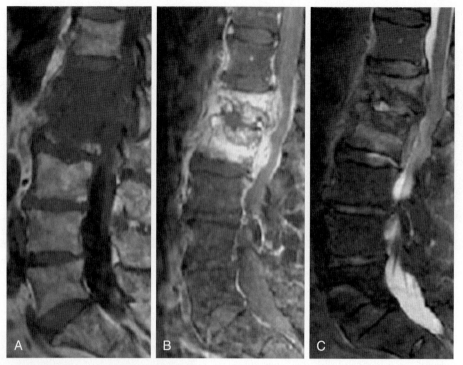

Figure 80-4 Magnetic resonance imaging scan, sagittal sections: T1-weighted sequence **(A)**, T1-weighted fat saturation sequence after gadolinium injection **(B)**, and T2-weighted fat saturation sequence **(C)**. The findings are typical of L1–L2 diskitis with epidural involvement. *(From Millot F, Bonnaire B, Clavel G, et al: Hematogenous Staphylococcus aureus discitis in adults can start outside the vertebral body,* Joint Bone Spine *77[1]:76–77, 2010.)*

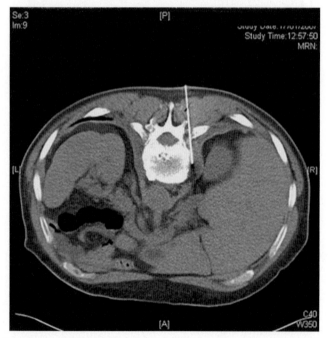

Figure 80-5 Paravertebral fluid collection being aspirated under computed tomography guidance in a patient with diskitis. *(From Cottle L, Riordan T: Infectious spondylodiscitis,* J Infect *56[6]:402–412, 2008.)*

by decompression laminectomy and evacuation of the abscess. More recently, interventional radiologists have been successful in draining epidural abscess percutaneously by using drainage catheters placed under CT or MRI guidance. Serial CT or MRI scans are useful in following the resolution of diskitis and should

be repeated immediately at the first sign of negative change in the patient's neurologic status. If compression of the spinal cord and of associated neural structures is suspected, the clinician should follow the emergency treatment algorithm set forth in Table 80-1.

DIFFERENTIAL DIAGNOSIS

The diagnosis of diskitis should be strongly considered in any patient with spine pain and fever, especially if the patient has undergone spinal instrumentation or epidural nerve blocks for either surgical anesthesia or pain control. Other pathologic processes that must be considered in the differential diagnosis include intrinsic disease of the spinal cord (e.g., demyelinating disease and syringomyelia), as well as other processes that can result in compression of the spinal cord and exiting nerve roots (e.g., metastatic tumor, Paget's disease, and neurofibromatosis). As a general rule, unless the patient has concomitant infection, none of these diseases will routinely be associated with fever, just with back pain.

COMPLICATIONS AND PITFALLS

Failure to diagnosis and treat diskitis rapidly and accurately can result only in disaster for the clinician and the patient alike. The insidious onset of neurologic deficit associated with diskitis can lull the clinician into a sense of false security. If abscesses or other causes of spinal cord compression are suspected, a heightened index of suspicion for subtle change in neurologic status must be considered.

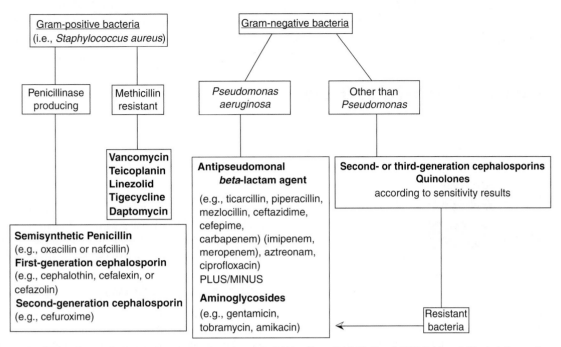

Figure 80-6 Antimicrobial treatment in pyogenic spontaneous spondylodiskitis. *(From Skaf GS, Domloj NT, Fehlings MG, et al: Pyogenic spondylodiscitis: an overview,* J Infect Public Health *3[1]:5–16, 2010.)*

TABLE 80-1

Algorithm for Spinal Cord Compression Resulting From Diskitis

- Immediately obtain blood and urine cultures.
- Immediately start high-dose antibiotics that cover *Staphylococcus aureus.*
- Immediately obtain the most readily available spinal imaging technique that can confirm the presence of spinal cord compression, such as abscess, tumor, and others:
  - Computed tomography
  - Magnetic resonance imaging
  - Myelography
- Simultaneously obtain emergency consultation from a spinal surgeon.
- Continuously and carefully monitor the patient's neurologic status.
- If any of the foregoing are unavailable, arrange emergency transfer of the patient to a tertiary care center by the most rapidly available transportation.
- Repeat imaging and obtain a repeat surgical consultation if the any deterioration is noted in the patient's neurologic status.

Clinical Pearls

Delay in diagnosis and treatment puts the patient and clinician at tremendous risk for a poor outcome. The clinician should assume that all patients who present with fever and back pain have diskitis until proved otherwise and should treat these patients accordingly. Overreliance on a single negative or equivocal imaging test result is a mistake. Serial CT or MRI testing is indicated should any deterioration occur in the patient's neurologic status.

SUGGESTED READINGS

Cottle L, Riordan T: Infectious spondylodiscitis, *J Infect* 56(6):402–412, 2008.

Luzzati R, Giacomazzi D, Danzi MC, et al: Diagnosis, management and outcome of clinically suspected spinal infection, *J Infect* 58(4):259–265, 2009.

Mylona E, Samarkos M, Kakalou E, et al: Pyogenic vertebral osteomyelitis: a systematic review of clinical characteristics, *Semin Arthritis Rheum* 39(1):10–17, 2009.

Sharma SK, Jones JO, Zeballos PP, et al: The prevention of discitis during discography, *Spine J* 9(11):936–943, 2009.

Skaf GS, Domloj NT, Fehlings MG, et al: Pyogenic spondylodiscitis: an overview, *J Infect Public Health* 3(1):5–16, 2010.

Chapter 81

SACROILIAC JOINT PAIN

ICD-9 CODE `724.6`

ICD-10 CODE `M53.3`

THE CLINICAL SYNDROME

Pain from the sacroiliac joint commonly occurs when lifting in an awkward position that puts strain on the joint, its supporting ligaments, and soft tissues. The sacroiliac joint is also susceptible to the development of arthritis from various conditions that can damage the joint cartilage. Osteoarthritis is the most common form of arthritis that results in sacroiliac joint pain; rheumatoid arthritis and posttraumatic arthritis are also common causes of sacroiliac joint pain. Less common causes include the collagen vascular diseases such as ankylosing spondylitis, infection, and Lyme disease. Collagen vascular disease generally manifests as polyarthropathy rather than as monarthropathy limited to the sacroiliac joint, although sacroiliac pain secondary to ankylosing spondylitis responds exceedingly well to the intraarticular injection technique described later. Occasionally, patients present with iatrogenically induced sacroiliac joint dysfunction resulting from overaggressive bone graft harvesting for spinal fusion.

SIGNS AND SYMPTOMS

Most patients presenting with sacroiliac joint pain secondary to strain or arthritis complain of pain localized around the sacroiliac joint and upper leg that radiates into the posterior buttocks and backs of the legs (Fig. 81-1); the pain does not radiate below the knees. Activity makes the pain worse, whereas rest and heat provide some relief. The pain is constant and is characterized as aching; it may interfere with sleep. On physical examination, the affected sacroiliac joint is tender to palpation. The patient often favors the affected leg and lists toward the unaffected side. Spasm of the lumbar paraspinal musculature is often present, as is limited range of motion of the lumbar

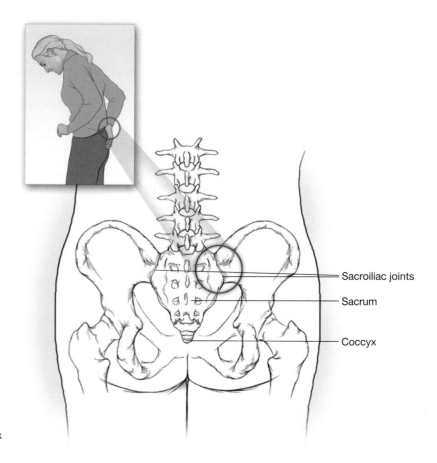

Figure 81-1 Sacroiliac joint pain radiates into the buttock and upper leg.

Sacroiliac joints

Sacrum

Coccyx

spine in the erect position; range of motion improves in the sitting position owing to relaxation of the hamstring muscles.

Patients with pain emanating from the sacroiliac joint exhibit a positive pelvic rock test result. This test is performed by placing the examiner's hands on the iliac crests and the thumbs on the anterior superior iliac spines and then forcibly compressing the patient's pelvis toward the midline. A positive test result is indicated by the production of pain around the sacroiliac joint.

TESTING

Plain radiography is indicated in all patients who present with sacroiliac joint pain (Fig. 81-2). Because the sacrum is susceptible to stress fractures and to the development of both primary and secondary tumors, magnetic resonance imaging of the distal lumbar spine and sacrum is indicated if the cause of the patient's pain is in question (Fig. 81-3). Radionuclide bone scanning should also

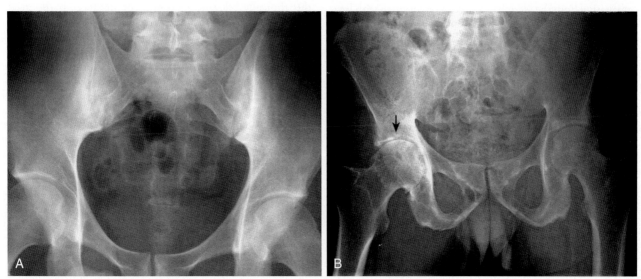

Figure 81-2 Sacroiliitis. **A,** Conventional radiograph of the pelvis of a 32-year-old man with stage II/III ankylosing spondylitis shows bilateral sacroiliitis. **B,** In another patient, a 50-year-old man with advanced disease, both sacroiliac joints are fused. Inflammatory arthritis affects also the right hip joint *(arrow). (From Mansour M, Cheema GS, Naguwa SM, et al: Ankylosing spondylitis: a contemporary perspective on diagnosis and treatment,* Semin Arthritis Rheum *36[4]:210-223, 2007.)*

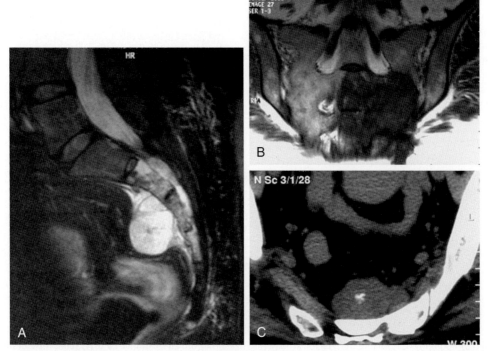

Figure 81-3 Sacral chordoma. Sagittal, fast spin-echo, T2-weighted **(A)** and axial T1-weighted **(B)** magnetic resonance images show a large soft tissue mass arising from the sacrum, with bony destruction. The bulk of the tumor is presacral. Axial computed tomography scan **(C)** demonstrates bony involvement of the left half of the sacrum by a large, midline, presacral mass with calcification. *(From Edelman RR, Hesselink JR, Zlatkin MB, Crues JV, editors:* Clinical magnetic resonance imaging, *ed 3, Philadelphia, 2006, Saunders, p 2333.)*

be considered in such patients to rule out tumor and insufficiency fractures that may be missed on conventional radiographs. Based on the patient's clinical presentation, additional testing may be warranted, including a complete blood count, erythrocyte sedimentation rate, human leukocyte antigen (HLA)-B27 screening, antinuclear antibody testing, and automated blood chemistry.

DIFFERENTIAL DIAGNOSIS

Pain emanating from the sacroiliac joint can be confused with low back strain, lumbar bursitis, lumbar fibromyositis, piriformis syndrome, ankylosing spondylitis, inflammatory arthritis, and disorders of the lumbar spinal cord, roots, plexus, and nerves.

TREATMENT

Initial treatment of the pain and functional disability of sacroiliac joint pain includes a combination of nonsteroidal antiinflammatory drugs or cyclooxygenase-2 inhibitors and physical therapy. The local application of heat and cold may also be beneficial. For patients who do not respond to these treatment modalities, injection with local anesthetic and steroid is a reasonable next step.

Injection of the sacroiliac joint is carried out by placing the patient in the supine position and preparing the skin overlying the affected sacroiliac joint space with antiseptic solution. A sterile syringe containing 4 mL of 0.25% preservative-free bupivacaine and 40 mg methylprednisolone is attached to a 25-gauge needle by using strict aseptic technique. The posterior superior spine of the ilium is identified. At this point, the needle is carefully advanced through the skin and subcutaneous tissues at a 45-degree angle toward the affected sacroiliac joint (Fig. 81-4). If bone is encountered, the needle is withdrawn into the subcutaneous tissues and is redirected superiorly and slightly more laterally. After the joint space is entered, the contents of the syringe are gently injected. Little resistance to injection should be felt. If resistance is encountered, the needle is probably in a ligament and should be advanced slightly into the joint space until the injection can proceed without significant resistance. The needle is then removed, and a sterile pressure dressing and ice pack are applied to the injection site. The use of fluoroscopy, computed tomography, and ultrasound guidance may be required in patients in whom the anatomic landmarks are difficult to identify (Fig. 81-5).

Physical modalities, including local heat and gentle range-of-motion exercises, should be introduced several days after the patient undergoes injection for sacroiliac pain. Vigorous exercises should be avoided, because they will exacerbate the patient's symptoms.

COMPLICATIONS AND PITFALLS

The injection technique is safe if careful attention is paid to the clinically relevant anatomy. For instance, if the needle is inserted too laterally, it may traumatize the sciatic nerve. The major complication of intraarticular injection of the sacroiliac joint is infection, although it should be exceedingly rare if strict aseptic technique is followed, as well as universal precautions to minimize any risk to the operator. The incidence of ecchymosis and hematoma formation can be decreased if pressure is applied to the injection site immediately after injection. Approximately 25% of patients complain of a transient increase in pain after intraarticular injection, and patients should be warned of this possibility.

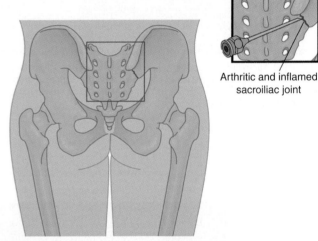

Arthritic and inflamed
sacroiliac joint

Figure 81-4 Correct needle placement for injection of the sacroiliac joint. *(From Waldman SD: Atlas of pain management injection techniques, Philadelphia, 2000, Saunders.)*

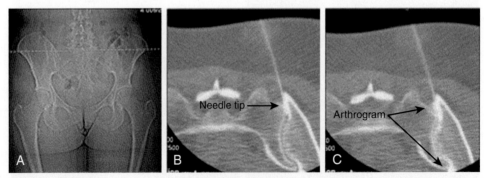

Figure 81-5 Computed tomography (CT) images from sacroiliac joint (SIJ) injection from an illustrative case. **A,** Scout tomogram for planed injection. **B,** Needle (22-gauge) directly inserted into the SIJ. **C,** CT image after injection of 1 mL Omnipaque 300. *(From Block BM, Hobelmann G, Murphy KJ, Grabow TS: An imaging review of sacroiliac joint injection under computed tomography guidance, Reg Anesth Pain Med 30[3]:295–298, 2005.)*

Clinical Pearls

Disorders of the sacroiliac joint can be distinguished from those of the lumbar spine by having the patient bend forward while seated. Patients with sacroiliac pain can bend forward with relative ease because of relaxation of the hamstring muscles in this position. In contrast, patients with lumbar spine pain experience an exacerbation of symptoms when they bend forward while seated.

The injection technique described is extremely effective in the treatment of sacroiliac joint pain. Coexistent bursitis and tendinitis may contribute to sacroiliac pain, thus necessitating additional treatment with more localized injection of local anesthetic and methylprednisolone.

SUGGESTED READINGS

Block BM, Hobelmann G, Murphy KJ, et al: An imaging review of sacroiliac joint injection under computed tomography guidance, *Reg Anesth Pain Med* 30(3):295–298, 2005.

Clemence ML: Ankylosing spondylitis and the seronegative spondyloarthropathies. In Dziedzic K, Hammond A, editors: *Rheumatology*, New York, 2010, Elsevier, pp. 273–287.

McGrath M: Clinical considerations of sacroiliac joint anatomy: a review of function, motion and pain, *J Osteopath Med* 7(1):16–24, 2004.

Slipman CW, Jackson HB, Lipetz JS, et al: Sacroiliac joint pain referral zones, *Arch Phys Med Rehabil* 81(3):334–338, 2000.

Waldman SD: Sacroiliac joint injection. In *Pain review*, Philadelphia, 2009, Saunders, pp 544–545.

Chapter 82

OSTEITIS PUBIS

ICD-9 CODE **733.5**

ICD-10 CODE **M85.30**

THE CLINICAL SYNDROME

Osteitis pubis causes localized tenderness over the symphysis pubis, pain radiating into the inner thigh, and a waddling gait. Radiographic changes consisting of erosion, sclerosis, and widening of the symphysis pubis are pathognomonic for osteitis pubis (Fig. 82-1). This is a disease of the second through fourth decades, and girls and women are affected more frequently than are boys and men. Osteitis pubis occurs most commonly after bladder, inguinal, or prostate surgery and is thought to result from the hematogenous spread of infection to the relatively avascular symphysis pubis. Osteitis pubis can also occur without an obvious inciting factor or infection.

SIGNS AND SYMPTOMS

On physical examination, patients exhibit point tenderness over the symphysis pubis, and the pain may radiate into the inner thigh with palpation of the symphysis pubis. Patients may also have tenderness over the anterior pelvis. Patients often adopt a waddling gait to avoid movement of the symphysis pubis (Fig. 82-2). This dysfunctional gait may result in lower extremity bursitis and tendinitis, which can confuse the clinical picture and add to the patient's pain and disability.

TESTING

Plain radiography is indicated in all patients who present with pain thought to be emanating from the symphysis pubis, to rule out occult bony disorders and tumor. Based on the patient's clinical presentation, additional testing may be warranted, including a complete blood count, prostate-specific antigen level, erythrocyte sedimentation rate, serum protein electrophoresis, and antinuclear antibody testing. Magnetic resonance imaging of the pelvis is indicated if occult mass or tumor is suspected (Fig. 82-3). Radionuclide bone scanning may be useful to exclude stress fractures not visible

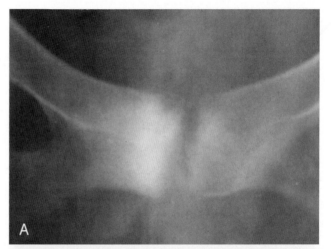

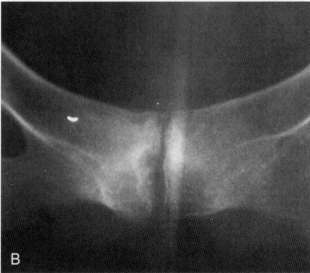

Figure 82-1 This 26-year-old woman developed pain and tenderness about the symphysis pubis during the third trimester of pregnancy. Radiographs obtained 2 years apart (**A** and **B**) reveal partial resolution of the abnormalities of osteitis pubis. *(From Resnick D:* Diagnosis of bone and joint disorders, *ed 4, Philadelphia, 2002, Saunders, p 2133.)*

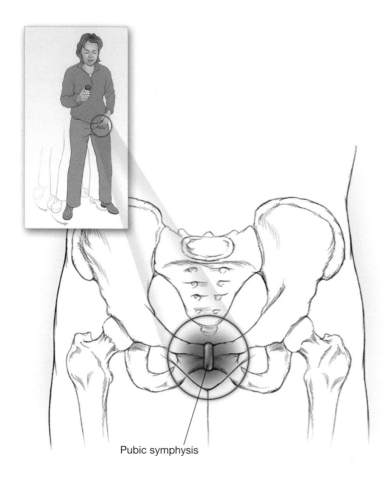

Pubic symphysis

Figure 82-2 Patients with osteitis pubis often develop a waddling gait.

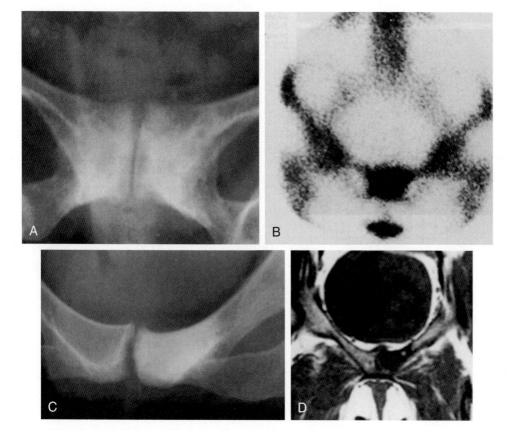

Figure 82-3 **A** and **B,** In this 61-year-old woman with osteitis pubis, local pain and tenderness about the symphysis pubis were the major clinical abnormalities. The radiograph **(A)** reveals considerable bone sclerosis on both sides of the symphysis, with narrowing of the joint space. A marked increase in the accumulation of a bone-seeking radiopharmaceutical agent is observed **(B)**. **C** and **D,** In this 34-year-old woman, a routine radiograph **(C)** shows unilateral osteitis pubis. A coronal T1-weighted spin-echo magnetic resonance image **(D)** shows low signal intensity in the involved bone. *(From Resnick D:* Diagnosis of bone and joint disorders, *ed 4, Philadelphia, 2002, Saunders, p 2132.)*

on plain radiographs. The injection technique described later serves as both a diagnostic and a therapeutic maneuver.

DIFFERENTIAL DIAGNOSIS

A pain syndrome that is clinically similar to osteitis pubis may occur in patients with rheumatoid arthritis or ankylosing spondylitis; however, the characteristic radiographic changes of osteitis pubis are lacking. Multiple myeloma and metastatic tumor may also mimic the pain and radiographic changes of osteitis pubis. Insufficiency fractures of the pubic rami should be considered if generalized osteoporosis is present.

TREATMENT

Initial treatment of the pain and functional disability associated with osteitis pubis includes a combination of nonsteroidal anti-inflammatory drugs (NSAIDs) or cyclooxygenase-2 inhibitors and physical therapy. The local application of heat and cold may also be beneficial. For patients who do not respond to these treatment modalities, injection with local anesthetic and steroid is a reasonable next step.

Injection for osteitis pubis is carried out by placing the patient in the supine position. The midpoints of the pubic bones and the symphysis pubis are identified by palpation, and the overlying skin is prepared with antiseptic solution. A syringe containing 2 mL of 0.25% preservative-free bupivacaine and 40 mg methylprednisolone is attached to a 3½-inch, 25-gauge needle. The needle is advanced very slowly through the previously identified point at a right angle to the skin, directly toward the center of the symphysis pubis. Once the needle impinges on the fibroelastic cartilage of the joint, it is withdrawn slightly out of the joint. After careful aspiration for blood, and if no paresthesia is present, the contents of the syringe are gently injected. Resistance to injection should be minimal.

Physical modalities, including local heat and gentle stretching exercises, should be introduced several days after the patient undergoes injection. Vigorous exercises should be avoided, because they will exacerbate the patient's symptoms. Simple analgesics, NSAIDs, and antimyotonic agents such as tizanidine may be used concurrently with this injection technique.

COMPLICATIONS AND PITFALLS

The injection technique is safe if careful attention is paid to the clinically relevant anatomy. The proximity to the pelvic contents makes it imperative that injection for osteitis pubis be performed only by those familiar with the regional anatomy and experienced in such techniques. Reactivation of latent infection, although rare, can occur; therefore, strict attention to sterile technique is mandatory, along with universal precautions to minimize any risk to the operator. Most complications of the injection technique are related to needle-induced trauma at the injection site and in underlying tissues. The incidence of ecchymosis and hematoma formation can be decreased if pressure is applied to the injection site immediately after injection. Many patients complain of a transient increase in pain after injection, and patients should be warned of this possibility.

Clinical Pearls

Osteitis pubis should be suspected in patients presenting with pain over the symphysis pubis in the absence of trauma. The injection technique described is an extremely effective treatment.

SUGGESTED READINGS

Kai B, Lee KD, Andrews G, et al: Puck to pubalgia: imaging of groin pain in professional hockey players, *Can Assoc Radiol J* 61(2):74–79, 2010.

Waldman SD: Osteitis pubis. In *Atlas of pain management injection techniques,* ed 2, Philadelphia, 2007, Saunders, pp 400–403.

Waldman SD: Osteitis pubis. In *Pain review,* Philadelphia, 2009, Saunders, p 309.

Wollin M, Lovell G: Osteitis pubis in four young football players: a case series demonstrating successful rehabilitation, *Phys Ther Sport* 7(4):173–174, 2006.

Chapter 83

GLUTEUS MAXIMUS SYNDROME

ICD-9 CODE `729.1`

ICD-10 CODE `M79.7`

THE CLINICAL SYNDROME

The gluteus maximus muscle's primary function is hip extension. It originates at the posterior aspect of the dorsal ilium, the posterior superior iliac crest, the posterior inferior aspect of the sacrum and coccyx, and the sacrotuberous ligament. The muscle inserts on the fascia lata at the iliotibial band and the gluteal tuberosity on the femur. The muscle is innervated by the inferior gluteal nerve.

The gluteus maximus muscle is susceptible to trauma and to wear and tear from overuse and misuse and to the development of myofascial pain syndrome, which may also be associated with gluteal bursitis. Such pain is usually the result of repetitive microtrauma to the muscle during such activities as running on soft surfaces, overuse of exercise equipment, or other repetitive activities that require hip extension (Fig. 83-1). Blunt trauma to the muscle may also incite gluteus maximus myofascial pain syndrome.

Myofascial pain syndrome is a chronic pain syndrome that affects a focal or regional portion of the body. The sine qua non of myofascial pain syndrome is the finding of myofascial trigger points on physical examination. Although these trigger points are generally localized to the part of the body affected, the pain is often referred to other areas. This referred pain may be misdiagnosed or attributed to other organ systems, thus leading to extensive evaluation and ineffective treatment. Patients with myofascial pain syndrome involving the gluteus maximus have primary pain in the medial and lower aspects of the muscle that is referred across the buttocks and into the coccygeal area (Fig. 83-2).

The trigger point is pathognomonic lesion of myofascial pain syndrome and is characterized by a local point of exquisite tenderness in the affected muscle. Mechanical stimulation

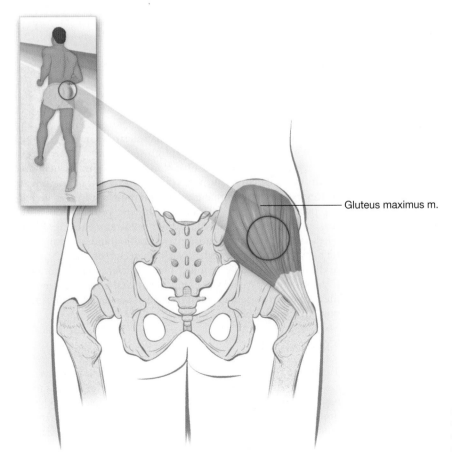

Gluteus maximus m.

Figure 83-1 Gluteus maximus syndrome usually results from repetitive microtrauma to the muscle during such activities as running on soft surfaces, overuse of exercise equipment, or other repetitive activities that require hip extension.

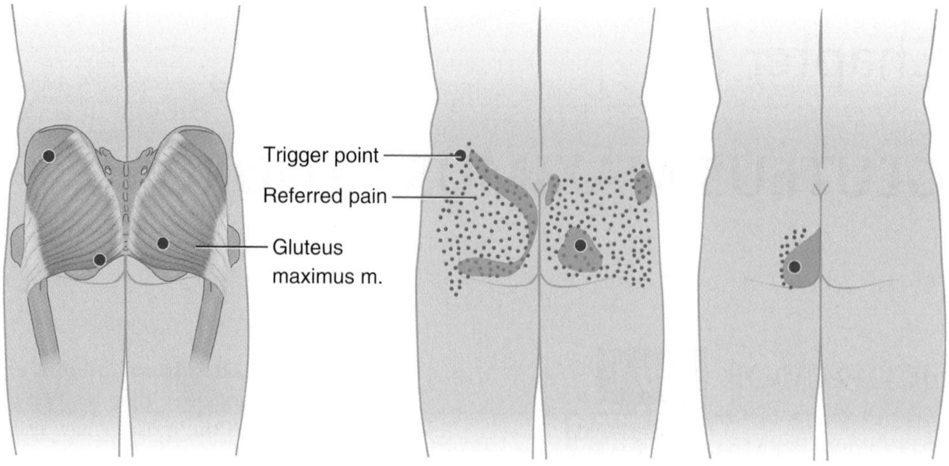

Figure 83-2 Patients with myofascial pain syndrome involving the gluteus maximus have primary pain in the medial and lower aspects of the muscle that is referred across the buttocks and into the coccygeal area. *(From Waldman SD: Gluteus maximus syndrome. In* Atlas of pain management injection techniques, *Philadelphia, 2007, Saunders, p 379.)*

Trigger point
Referred pain
Gluteus maximus m.

of the trigger point by palpation or stretching produces not only intense local pain but also referred pain. In addition, involuntary withdrawal of the stimulated muscle, called a jump sign, often occurs and is characteristic of myofascial pain syndrome. Patients with gluteus maximus syndrome have a trigger point over the upper, medial, and lower aspects of the muscle (see Fig. 83-1).

Taut bands of muscle fibers are often identified when myofascial trigger points are palpated. In spite of this consistent physical finding, the pathophysiology of the myofascial trigger point remains elusive, although trigger points are believed to be caused by microtrauma to the affected muscle. This trauma may result from a single injury, repetitive microtrauma, or chronic deconditioning of the agonist and antagonist muscle unit.

In addition to muscle trauma, various other factors seem to predispose patients to develop myofascial pain syndrome. For instance, a weekend athlete who subjects his or her body to unaccustomed physical activity may develop myofascial pain syndrome. Poor posture while sitting at a computer or while watching television has also been implicated as a predisposing factor. Previous injuries may result in abnormal muscle function and lead to the development of myofascial pain syndrome. All these predisposing factors may be intensified if the patient also suffers from poor nutritional status or coexisting psychological or behavioral abnormalities, including chronic stress and depression. The gluteus maximus muscle seems to be particularly susceptible to stress-induced myofascial pain syndrome.

Stiffness and fatigue often coexist with pain, and they increase the functional disability associated with this disease and complicate its treatment. Myofascial pain syndrome may occur as a primary disease state or in conjunction with other painful conditions, including radiculopathy and chronic regional pain syndromes. Psychological or behavioral abnormalities, including depression, frequently coexist with the muscle abnormalities, and management of these psychological disorders is an integral part of any successful treatment plan.

SIGNS AND SYMPTOMS

The trigger point is the pathognomonic lesion of gluteus maximus syndrome, and it is characterized by a local point of exquisite tenderness in the gluteus maximus muscle. Mechanical stimulation of the trigger point by palpation or stretching produces both intense local pain in the medial and lower aspects of the muscle

and referred pain across the buttocks and into the coccygeal area (see Fig. 83-2). In addition, the jump sign is often present.

TESTING

Biopsies of clinically identified trigger points have not revealed consistently abnormal histologic features. The muscle hosting the trigger points has been described either as "moth-eaten" or as containing "waxy degeneration." Increased plasma myoglobin has been reported in some patients with gluteus maximus syndrome, but this finding has not been corroborated by other investigators. Electrodiagnostic testing has revealed an increase in muscle tension in some patients, but again, this finding has not been reproducible. Because of the lack of objective diagnostic testing, the clinician must rule out other coexisting disease processes that may mimic gluteus maximus syndrome (see "Differential Diagnosis").

DIFFERENTIAL DIAGNOSIS

The diagnosis of gluteus maximus syndrome is based on clinical findings rather than specific laboratory, electrodiagnostic, or radiographic testing. For this reason, a targeted history and physical examination, with a systematic search for trigger points and identification of a positive jump sign, must be carried out in every patient suspected of suffering from gluteus maximus syndrome. The clinician must rule out other coexisting disease processes that may mimic gluteus maximus syndrome, including primary inflammatory muscle disease, primary hip disorders, gluteal bursitis, and gluteal nerve entrapment (Fig. 83-3). The use of electrodiagnostic and radiographic testing can identify coexisting disorders such as rectal or pelvic tumors or lumbosacral nerve lesions. The clinician must also identify coexisting psychological and behavioral abnormalities that may mask or exacerbate the symptoms associated with gluteus maximus syndrome.

TREATMENT

Treatment is focused on eliminating the myofascial trigger and achieving relaxation of the affected muscle. It is hoped that interrupting the pain cycle in this way will allow the patient to obtain prolonged pain relief. The mechanism of action of the treatment modalities used is poorly understood, so an element of trial and error is involved in developing a treatment plan.

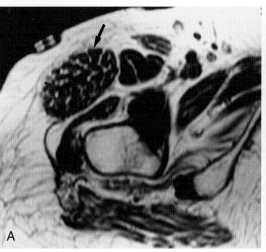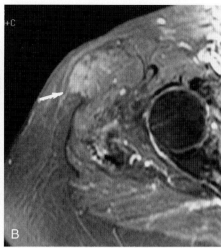

Figure 83-3 Possible entrapment of the superior gluteal nerve. **A,** Transverse, T1-weighted, spin-echo magnetic resonance imaging (MRI) shows denervation hypertrophy of the tensor fasciae latae muscle *(arrow).* **B,** Similar hypertrophy and high signal intensity are seen in the muscle *(arrow)* on transverse, fat-suppressed, T1-weighted, spin-echo MRI obtained after intravenous gadolinium administration. *(From Resnick D: Diagnosis of bone and joint disorders, ed 4, Philadelphia, 2002, Saunders, p 3551.)*

Conservative therapy consisting of trigger point injection with local anesthetic or saline solution is the initial treatment of gluteus maximus syndrome. Because underlying depression and anxiety are present in many patients, antidepressants are an integral part of most treatment plans. Other methods, including physical therapy, therapeutic heat and cold, transcutaneous nerve stimulation, and electrical stimulation, may be helpful on a case-by-case basis. For patients who do not respond to these traditional measures, consideration should be given to the use of botulinum toxin type A; although not currently approved by the Food and Drug Administration for this indication, the injection of minute quantities of botulinum toxin type A directly into trigger points has been successful in the treatment of persistent gluteus maximus syndrome.

COMPLICATIONS AND PITFALLS

Trigger point injections are extremely safe if careful attention is paid to the clinically relevant anatomy. Sterile technique must be used to avoid infection, along with universal precautions to minimize any risk to the operator. Most complications of trigger point injection are related to needle-induced trauma at the injection site and in underlying tissues. The incidence of ecchymosis and hematoma formation can be decreased if pressure is applied to the injection site immediately after injection. The avoidance of overly long needles can decrease the incidence of trauma to underlying structures. Special care must be taken to avoid trauma to the sciatic nerve.

Clinical Pearls

Although gluteus maximus syndrome is a common disorder, it is often misdiagnosed. Therefore, in patients suspected of suffering from gluteus maximus syndrome, a careful evaluation to identify underlying disease processes is mandatory. Gluteus maximus syndrome often coexists with various somatic and psychological disorders.

SUGGESTED READINGS

Arnold LM: The pathophysiology, diagnosis and treatment of fibromyalgia, *Psychiatr Clin North Am* 33(2):375–408, 2010.

Bradley LA: Pathophysiology of fibromyalgia, *Am J Med* 122(12 Suppl 1): S22–S30, 2009.

Imamura M, Cassius DA, Fregni F: Fibromyalgia: from treatment to rehabilitation, *Eur J Pain Suppl* 3(2):117–122, 2009.

Waldman SD: Gluteus maximus syndrome. In *Atlas of pain management injection techniques,* Philadelphia, 2007, Saunders, pp 378–380.

Chapter 84

PIRIFORMIS SYNDROME

ICD-9 CODE **355.0**

ICD-10 CODE **G57.00**

THE CLINICAL SYNDROME

Piriformis syndrome is an entrapment neuropathy that presents as pain, numbness, paresthesias, and weakness in the distribution of the sciatic nerve. It is caused by compression of the sciatic nerve by the piriformis muscle as it passes through the sciatic notch (Fig. 84-1). The piriformis muscle's primary function is to rotate the femur externally at the hip joint; this muscle is innervated by the sacral plexus. With internal rotation of the femur, the tendinous insertion and belly of the muscle can compress the sciatic nerve; if this compression persists, it can cause entrapment of the nerve.

The symptoms of piriformis syndrome usually begin after direct trauma to the sacroiliac and gluteal region. Occasionally, the syndrome is the result of repetitive hip and lower extremity motions or repeated pressure on the piriformis muscle and underlying sciatic nerve.

SIGNS AND SYMPTOMS

Initial symptoms include severe pain in the buttocks that may radiate into the lower extremity and foot. Patients suffering from piriformis syndrome may develop an altered gait, leading to coexistent sacroiliac, back, and hip pain that confuses the clinical picture. Physical findings include tenderness over the sciatic notch. Palpation of the piriformis muscle reveals tenderness and a swollen, indurated muscle belly. A positive Tinel sign over the sciatic nerve as it passes beneath the piriformis muscle is often present. A positive straight leg raising test result suggests sciatic nerve entrapment. Lifting or bending at the waist and hips increases the pain in most patients suffering from piriformis syndrome (Fig. 84-2). Weakness of the affected gluteal muscles and lower extremity and, ultimately, muscle wasting are seen in patients with advanced, untreated cases of piriformis syndrome.

TESTING

Electromyography (EMG) can distinguish lumbar radiculopathy from piriformis syndrome. Plain radiographs of the back, hip, and pelvis are indicated in all patients who present with

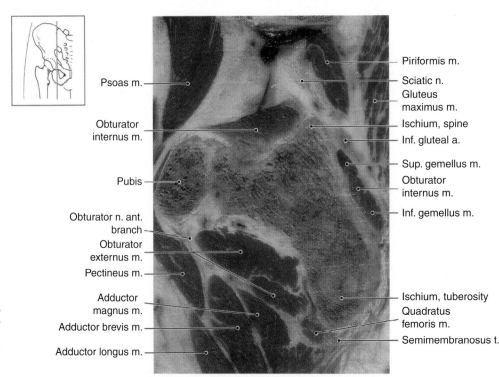

Figure 84-1 Anatomic relationship between the piriformis muscle and the sciatic nerve. *(From Kang HS, Ahn JM, Resnick D:* MRI of the extremities: an anatomic atlas, *ed 2, Philadelphia, 2002, Saunders, p 251.)*

Psoas m.
Obturator internus m.
Pubis
Obturator n. ant. branch
Obturator externus m.
Pectineus m.
Adductor magnus m.
Adductor brevis m.
Adductor longus m.

Piriformis m.
Sciatic n.
Gluteus maximus m.
Ischium, spine
Inf. gluteal a.
Sup. gemellus m.
Obturator internus m.
Inf. gemellus m.
Ischium, tuberosity
Quadratus femoris m.
Semimembranosus t.

piriformis syndrome, to rule out occult bony disorders. Based on the patient's clinical presentation, additional testing may be warranted, including a complete blood count, uric acid level, erythrocyte sedimentation rate, and antinuclear antibody testing. Magnetic resonance imaging (MRI) of the back is indicated if herniated disk, spinal stenosis, or space-occupying lesion is suspected. MRI of the hip may elucidate the cause of compression of the sciatic nerve (Figs. 84-3 and 84-4). Injection in the region of the sciatic nerve at this level serves as both a diagnostic and a therapeutic maneuver.

DIFFERENTIAL DIAGNOSIS

Piriformis syndrome is often misdiagnosed as lumbar radiculopathy or primary hip disease; radiographs of the hip and EMG can make the distinction. In addition, most patients with lumbar radiculopathy have back pain associated with reflex, motor, and sensory changes, whereas patients with piriformis syndrome have only secondary back pain and no reflex changes. The motor and sensory changes of piriformis syndrome are limited to the distribution of the sciatic nerve below the sciatic notch.

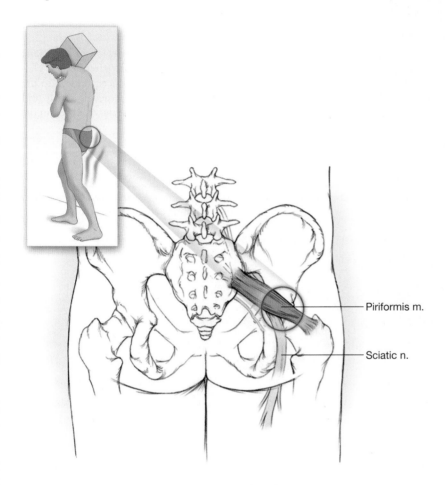

Piriformis m.

Sciatic n.

Figure 84-2 The pain of piriformis syndrome can be exacerbated by lifting.

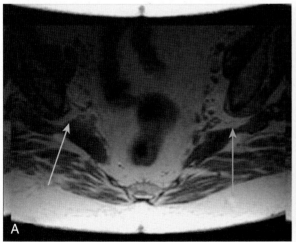

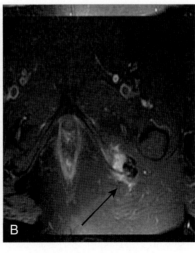

Figure 84-3 **A,** Axial T1-weighted pelvic magnetic resonance neurography (MRN) showing left piriformis muscle asymmetry and atrophy. **B,** Axial postcontrast fat-saturated T1-weighted pelvic MRN showing left ischial bone marrow edema and hamstring tendinopathy. The *left arrow* in **A** shows an atrophic and asymmetric piriformis muscle, and the *arrow* in **B** shows bone marrow edema and tendinopathy. *(From Kulcu DG, Naderi S: Differential diagnosis of intraspinal and extraspinal nondiscogenic sciatica,* J Clin Neurosci *15[11]:1246–1252, 2008.)*

Lumbar radiculopathy and sciatic nerve entrapment may coexist as the double-crush syndrome.

TREATMENT

Initial treatment of the pain and functional disability associated with piriformis syndrome includes a combination of non-steroidal antiinflammatory drugs or cyclooxygenase-2 inhibitors

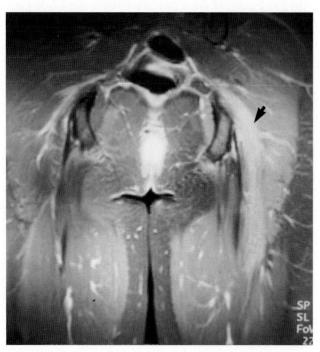

Figure 84-4 Coronal, fat-suppressed, T1-weighted, spin-echo magnetic resonance image obtained after intravenous gadolinium administration shows gross enlargement of and enhancement of signal intensity in the left sciatic nerve *(arrow)*. Transverse magnetic resonance images (not shown) suggested the presence of a fibrolipomatous hamartoma, although a plexiform neurofibroma was also considered. *(From Resnick D: Diagnosis of bone and joint disorders, ed 4, Philadelphia, 2002, Saunders, p 3550.)*

and physical therapy. The local application of heat and cold may also be beneficial. Any repetitive activity that may exacerbate the patient's symptoms should be avoided. If the patient sleeps on his or her side, placing a pillow between the legs may be helpful. If the patient is suffering from significant paresthesias, gabapentin may be added. For patients who do not respond to these treatment modalities, injection of local anesthetic and methylprednisolone in the region of the sciatic nerve at the level of the piriformis muscle is a reasonable next step. Rarely, surgical release of the entrapment is required to obtain relief.

COMPLICATIONS AND PITFALLS

The main complications of injection in the region of the sciatic nerve are ecchymosis and hematoma. Because paresthesia is elicited with the injection technique, needle-induced trauma to the sciatic nerve is a possibility. By advancing the needle slowly and withdrawing the needle slightly away from the nerve, injury to the sciatic nerve can be avoided.

Clinical Pearls

> Because patients suffering from piriformis syndrome may develop an altered gait, resulting in coexistent sacroiliac, back, and hip pain, careful physical examination and appropriate testing are required to sort out the diagnostic possibilities.

SUGGESTED READINGS

Filler AG: Piriformis and related entrapment syndromes: diagnosis and management, *Neurosurg Clin N Am* 19(4):609–622, 2008.

Tibor LM, Sekiya JK: Differential diagnosis of pain around the hip joint, *Arthroscopy* 24(12):1407–1421, 2008.

Tiel RL: Piriformis and related entrapment syndromes: myth and fallacy, *Neurosurg Clin N Am* 19(4):623–627, 2008.

Waldman SD: Injection technique for piriformis syndrome. In *Pain review*, Philadelphia, 2009, Saunders, pp 558–559.

Waldman SD: Piriformis syndrome. In *Pain review*, Philadelphia, 2009, Saunders, p 310.

Chapter 85

ISCHIOGLUTEAL BURSITIS

ICD-9 CODE 726.5

ICD-10 CODE M70.70

THE CLINICAL SYNDROME

The ischial bursa lies between the gluteus maximus muscle and the bone of the ischial tuberosity. It may exist as a single bursal sac or, in some patients, as a multisegmented series of loculated sacs. The ischial bursa is vulnerable to injury from both acute trauma and repeated microtrauma. Acute injuries are often caused by direct trauma to the bursa from falls onto the buttocks or by overuse, such as prolonged riding of horses or bicycles. Running on uneven or soft surfaces such as sand may also cause ischiogluteal bursitis (Fig. 85-1). If inflammation of the ischial bursa becomes chronic, calcification may occur.

SIGNS AND SYMPTOMS

Patients suffering from ischiogluteal bursitis frequently complain of pain at the base of the buttock with resisted extension of the lower extremity. The pain is localized to the area over the ischial tuberosity; referred pain is noted in the hamstring muscle, which may develop coexistent tendinitis. Patients are often unable to sleep on the affected hip and may complain of a sharp, catching sensation when they extend and flex the hip, especially on first awakening. Physical examination may reveal point tenderness over the ischial tuberosity. Passive straight leg raising and active

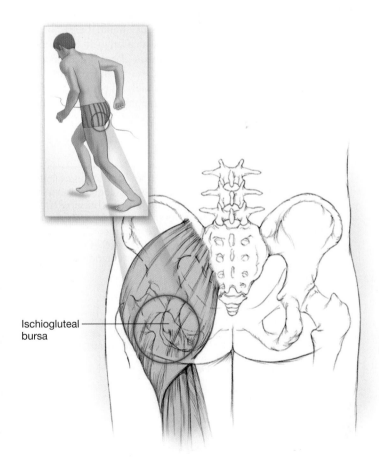

Ischiogluteal
bursa

Figure 85-1 Ischiogluteal bursitis can be caused by running on soft, uneven surfaces. It manifests clinically as point tenderness over the ischial tuberosity.

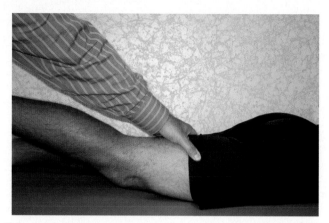

Figure 85-2 Resisted hip extension test for ischiogluteal bursitis. *(From Waldman SD: Physical diagnosis of pain: an atlas of signs and symptoms, Philadelphia, 2006, Saunders, p 309.)*

resisted extension of the affected lower extremity reproduce the pain (Fig. 85-2). Sudden release of resistance during this maneuver causes a marked increase in pain.

TESTING

Plain radiographs of the hip may reveal calcification of the bursa and associated structures, consistent with chronic inflammation. Magnetic resonance imaging is indicated if disruption of the hamstring musculotendinous unit is suspected. The injection technique described later serves as both a diagnostic and a therapeutic maneuver and is also used to treat hamstring tendinitis. Laboratory tests, including a complete blood count, erythrocyte sedimentation rate, and antinuclear antibody testing, are indicated if collagen vascular disease is suspected. Plain radiography and radionuclide bone scanning are indicated in the presence of trauma or if tumor is a possibility.

DIFFERENTIAL DIAGNOSIS

Although the diagnosis of ischiogluteal bursitis is usually straightforward, this painful condition is occasionally confused with sciatica, primary disease of the hip, insufficiency fractures of the pelvis, and tendinitis of the hamstrings. Tumors of the hip and pelvis should also be considered in the differential diagnosis of ischiogluteal bursitis.

TREATMENT

Initial treatment of the pain and functional disability associated with ischiogluteal bursitis includes a combination of nonsteroidal antiinflammatory drugs (NSAIDs) or cyclooxygenase-2 inhibitors and physical therapy. The local application of heat and cold may also be beneficial. Any repetitive activity that may exacerbate the patient's symptoms should be avoided. For patients who do not respond to these treatment modalities, injection with local anesthetic and steroid is a reasonable next step.

To inject the ischiogluteal bursa, the patient is placed in the lateral position with the affected side upward and the affected leg flexed at the knee. The skin overlying the ischial tuberosity is prepared with antiseptic solution. A syringe containing 4 mL of 0.25% preservative-free bupivacaine and 40 mg methylprednisolone is attached to a 1½-inch, 25-gauge needle. The ischial tuberosity is identified with a sterilely gloved finger. Before needle placement, the patient should be instructed to say "There!" immediately if he or she feels paresthesia in the lower extremity, indicating that the needle has impinged on the sciatic nerve. Should paresthesia occur, the needle is immediately withdrawn and is repositioned more medially. The needle is then carefully advanced at that point through the skin, subcutaneous tissues, muscle, and tendon until it impinges on the bone of the ischial tuberosity. Care must be taken to keep the needle in the midline and not to advance it laterally, to avoid contacting the sciatic nerve. After careful aspiration, and if no paresthesia is present, the contents of the syringe are gently injected into the bursa.

Physical modalities, including local heat and gentle stretching exercises, should be introduced several days after the patient undergoes injection. Vigorous exercises should be avoided, because they will exacerbate the patient's symptoms. Simple analgesics, NSAIDs, and antimyotonic agents such as tizanidine may be used concurrently with this injection technique.

COMPLICATIONS AND PITFALLS

The injection technique is safe if careful attention is paid to the clinically relevant anatomy. Because of the proximity to the sciatic nerve, injection for ischiogluteal bursitis should be performed only by those familiar with the regional anatomy and experienced in the technique. Many patients complain of a transient increase in pain after injection of the affected bursa and tendons, and patients should be warned of this possibility. If patients continue to engage in the repetitive activities responsible for ischiogluteal bursitis, improvement will be limited.

Clinical Pearls

To distinguish ischiogluteal bursitis from hamstring tendinitis, the clinician should remember that ischiogluteal bursitis manifests with point tenderness over the ischial bursa, whereas the tenderness of hamstring tendinitis is more diffuse over the upper muscle and tendons. The treatment is the same, however. Injection is extremely effective in relieving the pain of both ischiogluteal bursitis and hamstring tendinitis.

SUGGESTED READINGS

Hodnett PA, Shelly MJ, MacMahon PJ, et al: MR imaging of overuse injuries of the hip, *Magn Reson Imaging Clin N Am* 17(4):667–679, 2009.

Tibor LM, Sekiya JK: Differential diagnosis of pain around the hip joint, *Arthroscopy* 24(12):1407–1421, 2008.

Waldman SD: Injection technique for gluteal bursitis. In *Pain review,* Philadelphia, 2009, Saunders, pp 549–551.

Chapter 86

LEVATOR ANI SYNDROME

ICD-9 CODE   729.1

ICD-10 CODE   M79.7

THE CLINICAL SYNDROME

The levator ani muscle is susceptible to the development of myofascial pain syndrome. Such pain is often the result of repetitive microtrauma to the muscle during such activities as mountain biking and horseback riding (Fig. 86-1). Injury to the muscle during childbirth or blunt trauma to the muscle may also incite levator ani myofascial pain syndrome (Fig. 86-2).

Myofascial pain syndrome is a chronic pain syndrome that affects a focal or regional portion of the body. The sine qua non of myofascial pain syndrome is the finding of myofascial trigger points on physical examination. Although these trigger points are generally localized to the part of the body affected, the pain is often referred to other areas. This referred pain may be misdiagnosed or attributed to other organ systems, thus leading to extensive evaluation and ineffective treatment. Patients with myofascial pain syndrome involving the levator ani have primary pain in the pelvic floor that may be referred to the posterior buttocks and posterior lower extremity (Fig. 86-3).

The trigger point is pathognomonic lesion of myofascial pain syndrome and is characterized by a local point of exquisite tenderness in the affected muscle. Mechanical stimulation of the trigger point by palpation or stretching produces not only intense local pain but also referred pain. In addition, involuntary withdrawal of the stimulated muscle, called a jump sign, often occurs and is characteristic of myofascial pain syndrome. Patients with levator ani syndrome have a trigger point along the rectum or perineum.

Taut bands of muscle fibers are often identified when myofascial trigger points are palpated. In spite of this consistent physical finding, the pathophysiology of the myofascial trigger point remains elusive, although trigger points are believed to be caused by microtrauma to the affected muscle. This trauma may result from a single injury, repetitive microtrauma, or chronic deconditioning of the agonist and antagonist muscle unit.

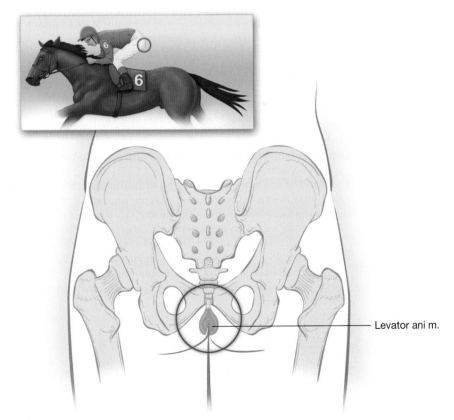

Levator ani m.

Figure 86-1 Levator ani syndrome may be caused by repetitive microtrauma to the muscle during such activities as mountain biking and horseback riding.

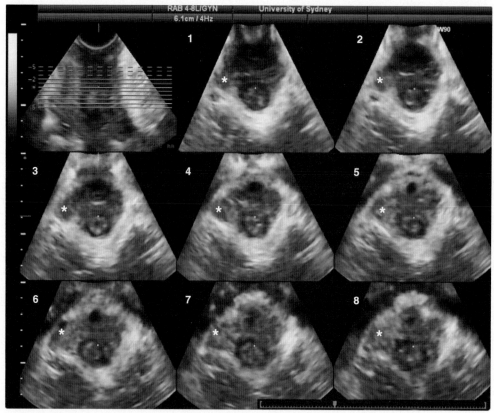

Figure 86-2 Tomographic ultrasound imaging showing right-sided avulsion. The *asterisks* indicate a right-sided levator avulsion. *(From Shek KL, Dietz HP: Can levator avulsion be predicted antenatally? Am J Obstet Gynecol 202[6]:586, 2010.)*

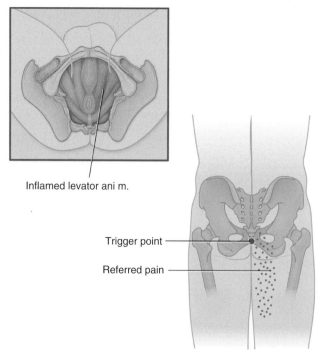

Inflamed levator ani m.

Trigger point

Referred pain

Figure 86-3 Patients with myofascial pain syndrome involving the levator ani have primary pain in the pelvic floor that may be referred to the posterior buttocks and posterior lower extremity. *(From Waldman SD: Atlas of pain management injection techniques, ed 2, Philadelphia, 2007, Saunders, p 385.)*

In addition to muscle trauma, various other factors seem to predispose patients to develop myofascial pain syndrome. For instance, a weekend athlete who subjects his or her body to unaccustomed physical activity may develop myofascial pain syndrome. Poor posture while sitting at a computer or while watching television has also been implicated as a predisposing factor. Previous injuries may result in abnormal muscle function and lead to the development of myofascial pain syndrome. All these predisposing factors may be intensified if the patient also suffers from poor nutritional status or coexisting psychological or behavioral abnormalities, including chronic stress and depression. The levator ani muscle seems to be particularly susceptible to stress-induced myofascial pain syndrome.

Stiffness and fatigue often coexist with pain, and they increase the functional disability associated with this disease and complicate its treatment. Myofascial pain syndrome may occur as a primary disease state or in conjunction with other painful conditions, including radiculopathy and chronic regional pain syndromes. Psychological or behavioral abnormalities, including depression, frequently coexist with the muscle abnormalities, and management of these psychological disorders is an integral part of any successful treatment plan.

SIGNS AND SYMPTOMS

The trigger point is the pathognomonic lesion of levator ani syndrome, and it is characterized by a local point of exquisite tenderness in the levator ani muscle. Mechanical stimulation of

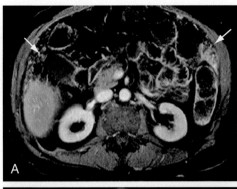

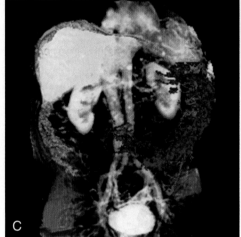

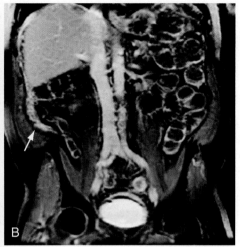

Figure 86-4 Recurrent rectal cancer with carcinomatosis. Axial **(A)** and coronal **(B)** gadolinium-enhanced spoiled gradient-echo magnetic resonance images show heterogeneously enhancing peritoneal and omental metastases *(arrows)* from recurrent rectal cancer. **C,** Three-dimensional color model generated from the coronal gadolinium-enhanced images shows the distribution of the peritoneal and omental tumor in purple. *(From Edelman RR, Hesselink JR, Zlatkin MB, Crues JV, editors:* Clinical magnetic resonance imaging, *ed 3, Philadelphia, 2006, Saunders, p 2780.)*

the trigger point by palpation or stretching produces primary pain in the pelvic floor and referred pain in the posterior buttocks and posterior lower extremity (see Fig. 86-3). In addition, the jump sign is often present.

TESTING

Biopsies of clinically identified trigger points have not revealed consistently abnormal histologic features. The muscle hosting the trigger points has been described either as "moth-eaten" or as containing "waxy degeneration." Increased plasma myoglobin has been reported in some patients with levator ani syndrome, but this finding has not been corroborated by other investigators. Electrodiagnostic testing has revealed an increase in muscle tension in some patients, but again, this finding has not been reproducible. Because of the lack of objective diagnostic testing, the clinician must rule out other coexisting disease processes that may mimic levator ani syndrome (see "Differential Diagnosis"). Imaging modalities including computed tomography, magnetic resonance imaging, and ultrasound should be considered if the diagnosis of levator ani syndrome is in question (see Fig. 86-2).

DIFFERENTIAL DIAGNOSIS

The diagnosis of levator ani syndrome is based on clinical findings rather than specific laboratory, electrodiagnostic, or radiographic testing. For this reason, a targeted history and physical examination, with a systematic search for trigger points and identification of

a positive jump sign, must be carried out in every patient suspected of suffering from levator ani syndrome. The clinician must rule out other coexisting disease processes that may mimic levator ani syndrome, including primary inflammatory muscle disease, primary hip disorders, rectal and pelvic tumors, gluteal bursitis, and gluteal nerve entrapment (Fig. 86-4). The use of electrodiagnostic and radiographic testing can identify coexisting disorders such as rectal and pelvic tumors and lumbosacral nerve lesions. The clinician must also identify coexisting psychological and behavioral abnormalities that may mask or exacerbate the symptoms of levator ani syndrome.

TREATMENT

Treatment is focused on eliminating the myofascial trigger and achieving relaxation of the affected muscle. It is hoped that interrupting the pain cycle in this way will allow the patient to obtain prolonged pain relief. The mechanism of action of the treatment modalities used is poorly understood, so an element of trial and error is involved in developing a treatment plan.

Conservative therapy consisting of trigger point injection with local anesthetic or saline solution is the initial treatment of levator ani syndrome. Because underlying depression and anxiety are present in many patients, antidepressants are an integral part of most treatment plans. Other methods, including physical therapy, therapeutic heat and cold, transcutaneous nerve stimulation, and electrical stimulation, may be helpful on a case-by-case basis. For patients who do not respond to these traditional measures, consideration should be given to the use of botulinum toxin type A; although not currently approved by the Food and Drug Administration for this indication, the injection of minute quantities of botulinum toxin type A directly into trigger points has been successful in the treatment of persistent levator ani syndrome.

COMPLICATIONS AND PITFALLS

Trigger point injections are extremely safe if careful attention is paid to the clinically relevant anatomy. Sterile technique must be used to avoid infection, along with universal precautions to minimize any risk to the operator. Most complications of trigger point injection are related to needle-induced trauma at the injection site and in underlying tissues. The incidence of ecchymosis and hematoma formation can be decreased if pressure is applied to the injection site immediately after injection. The avoidance of overly long needles can decrease the incidence of trauma to underlying structures. Special care must be taken to avoid trauma to the sciatic nerve.

Clinical Pearls

Although levator ani syndrome is a common disorder, it is often misdiagnosed. Therefore, in patients suspected of suffering from levator ani syndrome, a careful evaluation to identify underlying disease processes is mandatory. Levator ani syndrome often coexists with various somatic and psychological disorders.

SUGGESTED READINGS

Arnold LM: The pathophysiology, diagnosis and treatment of fibromyalgia, *Psychiatr Clin North Am* 33(2):375–408, 2010.

Bradley LA: Pathophysiology of fibromyalgia, *Am J Med* 122(12 Suppl 1): S22–S30, 2009.

Corton MM: Anatomy of pelvic floor dysfunction, *Obstet Gynecol Clin North Am* 36(3):401–419, 2009.

Imamura M, Cassius DA, Fregni F: Fibromyalgia: from treatment to rehabilitation, *Eur J Pain Suppl* 3(2):117–122, 2009.

Waldman SD: Levator ani syndrome. In *Atlas of pain management injection techniques,* Philadelphia, 2007, Saunders, pp 384–386.

Chapter 87

COCCYDYNIA

ICD-9 CODE 724.79

ICD-10 CODE M53.3

THE CLINICAL SYNDROME

Coccydynia is a common syndrome characterized by pain localized to the tailbone that radiates into the lower sacrum and perineum. Coccydynia affects female patients more frequently than male patients. It occurs most commonly after direct trauma from a kick or a fall directly onto the coccyx. Coccydynia can also occur after a difficult vaginal delivery. The pain of coccydynia is thought to be the result of strain of the sacrococcygeal ligament or, occasionally, fracture of the coccyx. Less commonly, arthritis of the sacrococcygeal joint can cause coccydynia.

SIGNS AND SYMPTOMS

On physical examination, patients exhibit point tenderness over the coccyx; the pain increases with movement of the coccyx. Movement of the coccyx may also cause sharp paresthesias into the rectum, which patients find quite distressing. On rectal examination, the levator ani, piriformis, and coccygeus muscles may feel indurated, and palpation of these muscles may induce severe spasm. Sitting exacerbates the pain of coccydynia, and patients often attempt to sit on one buttock to avoid pressure on the coccyx (Fig. 87-1).

TESTING

Plain radiography is indicated in all patients who present with pain thought to be emanating from the coccyx, to rule out occult bony disease and tumor. Based on the patient's clinical presentation, additional testing may be warranted, including a complete blood count, prostate-specific antigen level, erythrocyte sedimentation rate, and antinuclear antibody testing. Magnetic resonance imaging of the pelvis is indicated if occult mass or tumor is suspected. Radionuclide bone scanning may be useful to exclude stress fractures not visible on plain radiographs. The injection technique described later serves as both a diagnostic and a therapeutic maneuver.

DIFFERENTIAL DIAGNOSIS

Primary disease of the rectum and anus is occasionally confused with the pain of coccydynia. Primary tumors or metastatic lesions of the sacrum or coccyx may also manifest as coccydynia (Fig. 87-2). Proctalgia fugax can be distinguished from coccydynia because movement of the coccyx does not reproduce the pain.

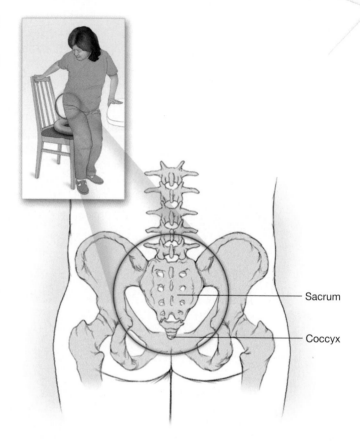

Sacrum

Coccyx

Figure 87-1 The pain of coccydynia is localized to the coccyx and is made worse by sitting.

Insufficiency fractures of the pelvis or sacrum and disorders of the sacroiliac joints may on occasion mimic coccydynia.

TREATMENT

A short course of conservative therapy consisting of simple analgesics, nonsteroidal antiinflammatory drugs (NSAIDs) or cyclooxygenase-2 inhibitors, and a foam donut to prevent further irritation to the sacrococcygeal ligament is a reasonable first step in the treatment of coccydynia. If the patient does not experience rapid improvement, injection is a reasonable next step.

To treat the pain of coccydynia, the patient is placed in the prone position. The legs and heels are abducted to prevent tightening of the gluteal muscles, which can make identification of the sacrococcygeal joint difficult. A wide area of skin is prepared with antiseptic solution so that all the landmarks can be palpated aseptically. A fenestrated sterile drape is placed to avoid

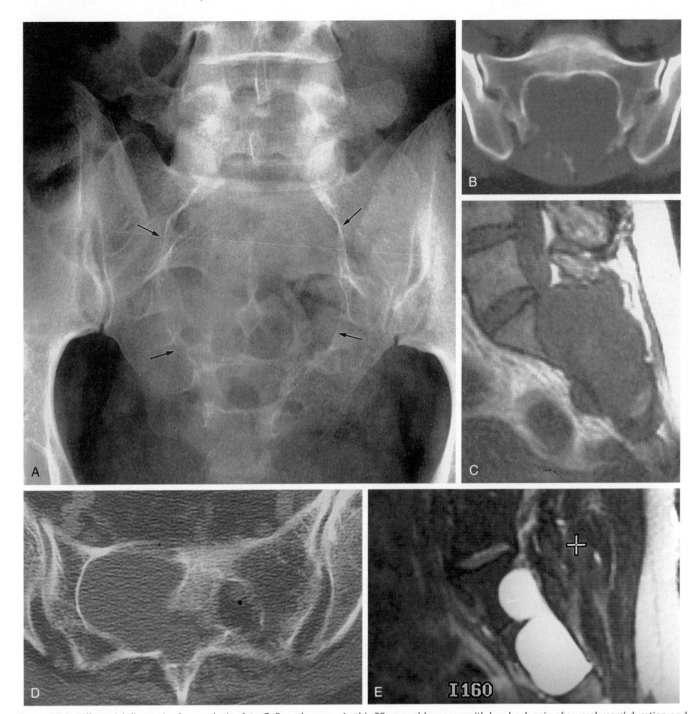

Figure 87-2 Differential diagnosis of coccydynia. **A** to **C**, Ependymoma. In this 28-year-old woman with low back pain of several years' duration and a normal neurologic examination, routine radiography **(A)** reveals an osteolytic lesion *(arrows)* in the sacrum. Transaxial computed tomography (CT) scan **(B)** confirms its central location and posterior extension. Sagittal, T1-weighted, spin-echo magnetic resonance imaging (MRI) **(C)** shows its large size, posterior extension, and low signal intensity. The tumor was of high signal intensity on T2-weighted spin-echo MRI (not shown). Histologic analysis confirmed a myxopapillary ependymoma that did not communicate with the dural sac. **D** and **E**, Meningocele. Transaxial CT scan **(D)** shows a right-sided sacral lesion distorting the neural foramen. It is sharply delineated, with a sclerotic margin. Sagittal fast spin-echo MRI **(E)** reveals a lesion of high signal intensity with bone erosion. *(From Resnick D:* Diagnosis of bone and joint disorders, *ed 4, Philadelphia, 2002, Saunders, p 4018.)*

contamination of the palpating finger. The middle finger of the operator's nondominant hand is placed over the sterile drape into the natal cleft, with the fingertip palpating the sacrococcygeal joint at the base of the sacrum. After locating the sacrococcygeal joint, a 1½-inch, 25-gauge needle is inserted through the skin at a 45-degree angle into the region of the sacrococcygeal joint and ligament. If the ligament is penetrated, a "pop" will be felt, and the needle should be withdrawn through the ligament. If contact with the bony wall of the sacrum occurs, the needle should be withdrawn slightly to disengage the needle tip from the periosteum. When the needle is satisfactorily positioned, a syringe containing 5 mL of 1% preservative-free lidocaine and 40 mg methylprednisolone is attached to the needle. Gentle aspiration is carried out to identify cerebrospinal fluid or blood. If the

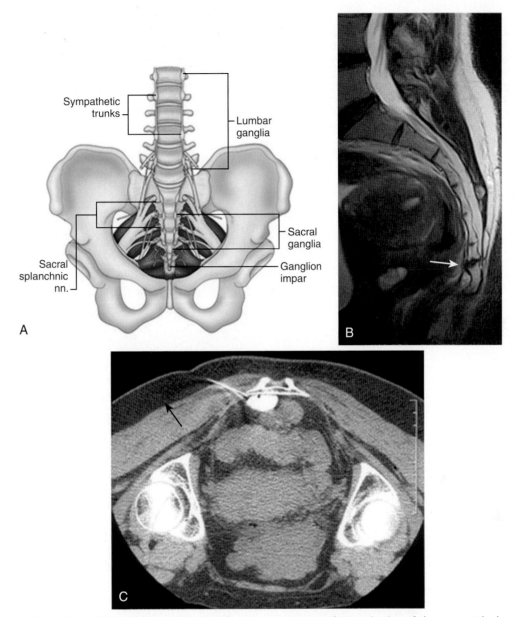

Figure 87-3 **A,** Anatomic location of the ganglion impar. Ganglion impar represents the termination of the paravertebral sympathetic chains, converging at the sacrococcygeal level. **B,** Sagittal, T2-weighted magnetic resonance imaging showing the ganglion impar as a small, isointense signal structure anterior to the sacrococcygeal level *(white arrow)*. **C,** Contrast medium outlining the ganglion impar, seen as filling defect *(black arrow)* in the pool of contrast. *(From Datir A, Connell D: CT-guided injection for ganglion impar blockade: a radiological approach to the management of coccydynia,* Clin Radiol 65[1]:21–25, 2010.)

aspiration test result is negative, the contents of the syringe are slowly injected. Little resistance to injection should be felt. Any significant pain or sudden increase in resistance during injection suggests incorrect needle placement, and the clinician should stop injecting immediately and reassess the needle position. After injection, the needle is removed, and a sterile pressure dressing and ice pack are applied to the injection site. If prolonged pain relief is not obtained with the technique, blockade of the ganglion impar should be considered (Fig. 87-3).

Physical modalities, including local heat, gentle range-of-motion exercises, and rectal massage of the affected muscles, should be introduced several days after the patient undergoes injection for coccygeal pain. Vigorous exercises should be avoided, because they will exacerbate the patient's symptoms. Simple analgesics and NSAIDs can be used concurrently with the injection technique.

COMPLICATIONS AND PITFALLS

Coccydynia should be considered a diagnosis of exclusion in the absence of trauma to the coccyx and its ligaments, because failure to diagnose underlying tumor can have disastrous consequences. The injection technique is safe if careful attention is paid to clinically relevant anatomy. The major complication of injection is infection, given the proximity to the rectum. This complication should be exceedingly rare if strict aseptic technique is followed, as well as universal precautions to minimize any risk to the operator. The incidence of ecchymosis and hematoma formation can be decreased if pressure is applied to the injection site immediately after injection. Approximately 25% of patients complain of a transient increase in pain after injection, and patients should be warned of this possibility.

Clinical Pearls

The use of a foam donut when sitting, along with the other treatment modalities discussed, may provide symptomatic relief and allow the sacrococcygeal ligament to heal. The injection technique described is extremely effective in the treatment of coccydynia. Coexistent sacroiliitis may contribute to coccygeal pain, thus necessitating additional treatment with more localized injection of local anesthetic and methylprednisolone.

SUGGESTED READINGS

De Andrés J, Chaves S: Coccygodynia: a proposal for an algorithm for treatment, *J Pain* 4(5):257–266, 2003.

Hodges SD, Eck JC, Humphreys SC: A treatment and outcomes analysis of patients with coccydynia, *Spine J* 4(2):138–140, 2004.

Waldman SD: Coccydynia. In *Atlas of pain management injection techniques,* Philadelphia, 2007, Saunders, pp 412–416.

Waldman SD: Coccydynia. In *Pain review,* Philadelphia, 2009, Saunders, pp 252–253.

Chapter **88**

ARTHRITIS PAIN OF THE HIP

ICD-9 CODE `715.95`

ICD-10 CODE `M16.9`

THE CLINICAL SYNDROME

Arthritis of the hip is commonly encountered in clinical practice. The hip joint is susceptible to the development of arthritis from various conditions that have the ability to damage the joint cartilage. Osteoarthritis is the most common form of arthritis that results in hip joint pain; rheumatoid arthritis and posttraumatic arthritis are also common causes of hip pain. Less frequent causes of arthritis-induced hip pain include the collagen vascular diseases, infection, villonodular synovitis, and Lyme disease. Acute infectious arthritis is usually accompanied by significant systemic symptoms, including fever and malaise, and should be easily recognized; it is treated with culture and antibiotics rather than injection therapy. Collagen vascular disease generally manifests as polyarthropathy rather than as monarthropathy limited to the hip joint, although hip pain secondary to collagen vascular disease responds exceedingly well to the treatment modalities described here.

SIGNS AND SYMPTOMS

Most patients presenting with hip pain secondary to arthritis complain of pain localized around the hip and upper leg (Fig. 88-1). Most patients with intrinsic hip disorders have a positive Patrick-FABERE (flexion, abduction, external rotation, extension) test result (Fig. 88-2). Patients may initially present with ill-defined pain in the groin; occasionally, the pain is localized to the buttocks. Activity makes the pain worse, whereas rest and heat provide some relief. The pain is constant and is characterized as aching; it may interfere with sleep. Some patients complain of a grating or popping sensation with use of the joint, and crepitus may be noted on physical examination.

In addition to pain, patients often experience a gradual decrease in functional ability caused by reduced hip range of motion that makes simple everyday tasks such as walking, climbing stairs,

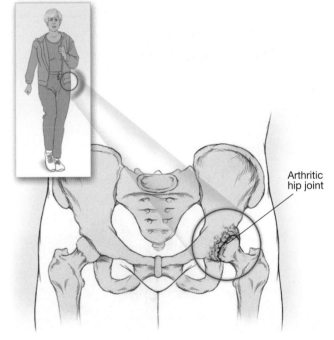

Figure 88-1 The pain of arthritis of the hip is localized to the hip, groin, and upper leg; it is made worse by weight-bearing exercise.

and getting into and out of a car quite difficult. With continued disuse, muscle wasting may occur, and a frozen hip secondary to adhesive capsulitis may develop.

TESTING

Plain radiography is indicated in all patients who present with hip pain. Based on the patient's clinical presentation, additional testing may be warranted, including a complete blood count, erythrocyte sedimentation rate, and antinuclear antibody testing. Magnetic resonance imaging of the hip is indicated if aseptic necrosis or an occult mass or tumor is suspected or if the diagnosis is in question (Fig. 88-3).

279

DIFFERENTIAL DIAGNOSIS

Many diseases can cause hip pain (Table 88-1). Lumbar radiculopathy may mimic the pain and disability associated with arthritis of the hip; however, in such patients, hip examination results should be negative. Entrapment neuropathies, such as meralgia paresthetica, and trochanteric bursitis may confuse the diagnosis; both these conditions can coexist with arthritis of the hip. Primary and metastatic tumors of the hip and spine may also manifest similarly to arthritis of the hip.

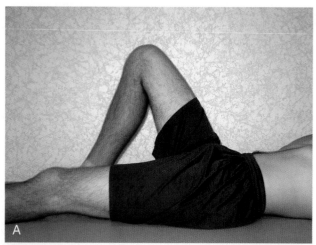

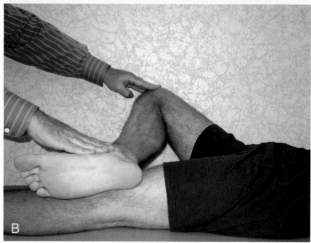

Figure 88-2 **A** and **B,** Performing the Patrick-FABERE test. *(From Waldman SD: Physical diagnosis of pain: an atlas of signs and symptoms, Philadelphia, 2006, Saunders, p 304.)*

TREATMENT

Initial treatment of the pain and functional disability of arthritis of the hip includes a combination of nonsteroidal antiinflammatory drugs or cyclooxygenase-2 inhibitors and physical therapy. The local application of heat and cold may also be beneficial. For patients who do not respond to these treatment modalities, intraarticular injection of local anesthetic and steroid is a reasonable next step.

Intraarticular injection of the hip is performed by placing the patient in the supine position. The skin overlying the hip, subacromial region, and joint space is prepared with antiseptic solution. A sterile syringe containing 4 mL of 0.25% preservative-free bupivacaine and 40 mg methylprednisolone is attached to a 2-inch, 25-gauge needle by using strict aseptic technique. The femoral artery is identified; then, at a point approximately 2 inches lateral to the femoral artery, just below the inguinal ligament, the hip joint space is identified. The needle is carefully advanced through the skin and subcutaneous tissues through the joint capsule into the joint. If bone is encountered, the needle is withdrawn into the subcutaneous tissues and is redirected superiorly and slightly more medially. After the joint space is entered, the contents of the syringe are gently injected. Little resistance to injection should be felt. If resistance is encountered, the needle is probably in a ligament or tendon and should be advanced slightly into the joint space until the injection can proceed without significant resistance. The needle is removed, and a sterile pressure dressing and ice pack are applied to the injection site.

Physical modalities, including local heat and gentle range-of-motion exercises, should be introduced several days after the patient undergoes injection for hip pain. Vigorous exercises should be avoided, because they will exacerbate the patient's symptoms.

COMPLICATIONS AND PITFALLS

Failure to identify a primary or metastatic tumor of the hip or spine that is causing the patient's pain can be disastrous. The injection technique is safe if careful attention is paid to the clinically relevant anatomy. The major complication of intraarticular injection of the hip is infection; however, it should be exceedingly rare if strict aseptic technique is followed, along with universal precautions to minimize any risk to the operator. The incidence of ecchymosis and hematoma formation can be decreased if pressure is applied to the injection site immediately after injection. Approximately 25% of patients complain of a transient increase in pain after intraarticular injection of the hip joint, and patients should be warned of this possibility.

Figure 88-3 Monoarticular left hip pain of 6 months' duration in a 29-year-old man. **A,** Radiograph of the pelvis shows mild axial narrowing of the hip without erosions *(large arrow).* **B,** Coronal T1-weighted magnetic resonance image shows soft tissue thickening (synovitis) of intermediate density about the hip *(small arrowhead)* and acetabular erosion *(large arrowheads). (From Haaga JR, Lanzieri CF, Gilkeson RC, editors: CT and MR imaging of the whole body, ed 4, Philadelphia, 2003, Mosby, 2003, p 1913.)*

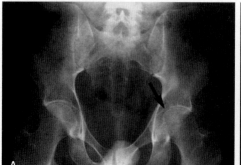

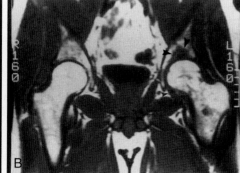

TABLE 88-1

Causes of Hip Pain and Dysfunction

Localized Bony or Joint Space Pathology	Periarticular Pathology	Systemic Disease	Sympathetically Mediated Pain	Referred From Other Body Areas	Vascular Disease
Fracture	Bursitis	Rheumatoid arthritis	Causalgia	Lumbar plexopathy	Aortoiliac atherosclerosis
Primary bone tumor	Tendinitis	Collagen vascular disease	Reflex sympathetic dystrophy	Lumbar radiculopathy	Internal iliac artery occlusion
Primary synovial tissue tumor	Adhesive capsulitis	Reiter's syndrome		Lumbar spondylosis	
Joint instability	Joint instability	Gout		Fibromyalgia	
Localized arthritis	Muscle strain	Other crystal arthropathies		Myofascial pain syndromes	
Osteophyte formation	Muscle sprain	Charcot's neuropathic arthritis		Inguinal hernia	
Osteonecrosis of femoral head	Periarticular infection not involving joint space			Entrapment neuropathies	
Joint space infection				Intrapelvic tumors	
Hemarthrosis				Retroperitoneal tumors	
Villonodular synovitis					
Intraarticular foreign body					
Slipped capital femoral epiphysis (Legg's disease)					
Chronic hip dislocation					

From Waldman SD: *Physical diagnosis of pain: an atlas of signs and symptoms,* Philadelphia, 2006, Saunders, 2006.

Clinical Pearls

> Coexistent bursitis and tendinitis may contribute to hip pain, thus necessitating additional treatment with more localized injection of local anesthetic and methylprednisolone. The injection technique described is extremely effective in the treatment of pain secondary to arthritis of the hip joint.

SUGGESTED READINGS

Mamisch TC, Zilkens C, Siebenrock KA, et al: MRI of hip osteoarthritis and implications for surgery, *Magn Reson Imaging Clin N Am* 18(1):111–120, 2010.

McAlindon TE, Bannuru RR: OARSI recommendations for the management of hip and knee osteoarthritis: the semantics of differences and changes, *Osteoarthritis Cartilage* 18(4):473–475, 2010.

Waldman SD: Arthritis pain of the hip. In *Pain review,* Philadelphia, 2009, Saunders, pp 311–312.

Waldman SD: Functional anatomy of the hip. In *Pain review,* Philadelphia, 2009, Saunders, pp 135–138.

Zhang W, Nuki G, Moskowitz RW, et al: OARSI recommendations for the management of hip and knee osteoarthritis. Part III. Changes in evidence following systematic cumulative update of research published through January 2009, *Osteoarthritis Cartilage* 18(4):476–499, 2010.

Chapter **89**

SNAPPING HIP SYNDROME

ICD-9 CODE **727.09**

ICD-10 CODE **M65.80**

THE CLINICAL SYNDROME

Patients with snapping hip syndrome experience a snapping sensation in the lateral hip associated with sudden, sharp pain in the area of the greater trochanter. The snapping sensation and pain are the result of the iliopsoas tendon subluxating over the greater trochanter or iliopectineal eminence (Fig. 89-1). The trochanteric bursa lies between the greater trochanter and the tendon of the gluteus medius and the iliotibial tract. The gluteus medius muscle originates from the outer surface of the ilium, and its fibers pass downward and laterally to attach on the lateral surface of the greater trochanter. The gluteus medius muscle locks the pelvis in place during walking and running; this muscle is innervated by the superior gluteal nerve. The iliopectineal eminence is the point at which the ilium and the pubis bone merge. The psoas and iliacus muscles join at the lateral side of the psoas, and the combined fibers are referred to as the iliopsoas muscle. Like the psoas muscle, the iliacus flexes the thigh on the trunk or, if the thigh is fixed, flexes the trunk on the thigh, such as when moving from a supine to a sitting position.

The symptoms of snapping hip syndrome occur most commonly when rising from a sitting to a standing position or when walking briskly (Fig. 89-2). Often, trochanteric bursitis coexists with snapping hip syndrome and increases the patient's pain and disability.

SIGNS AND SYMPTOMS

Physical examination reveals that patients can recreate the snapping and pain by moving from a sitting to a standing position and adducting the hip. This positive snap sign is considered diagnostic for snapping hip syndrome (Fig. 89-3). Point tenderness over the trochanteric bursa, indicative of trochanteric bursitis, is often present.

TESTING

Plain radiographs are indicated in all patients who present with pain thought to be emanating from the hip, to rule out occult bony disorders and tumor. Based on the patient's clinical presentation, additional testing may be warranted, including a complete blood count, prostate-specific antigen level, erythrocyte sedimentation rate, and antinuclear antibody testing. Magnetic resonance imaging of the affected hip is indicated if an occult mass or aseptic necrosis is suspected and to aid in confirmation of the diagnosis

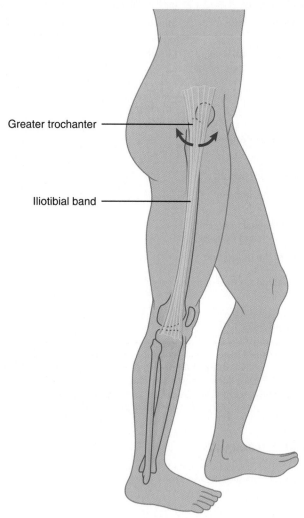

Greater trochanter

Iliotibial band

Figure 89-1 The snapping sensation and pain are the result of the iliopsoas tendon subluxating over the greater trochanter or iliopectineal eminence. *(From Waldman SD: Snapping hip syndrome. In* Atlas of pain management injection techniques, *ed 2, Philadelphia, 2007, Saunders, p 368.)*

(Fig. 89-4). Electrodiagnostic and radiographic testing can identify coexisting disease such as internal derangement of the hip joint and lumbosacral nerve lesions. The injection technique described later serves as both a diagnostic and a therapeutic maneuver.

DIFFERENTIAL DIAGNOSIS

The diagnosis of snapping hip syndrome is based on clinical findings rather than specific laboratory, electrodiagnostic, or radiographic testing. For this reason, a targeted history and physical

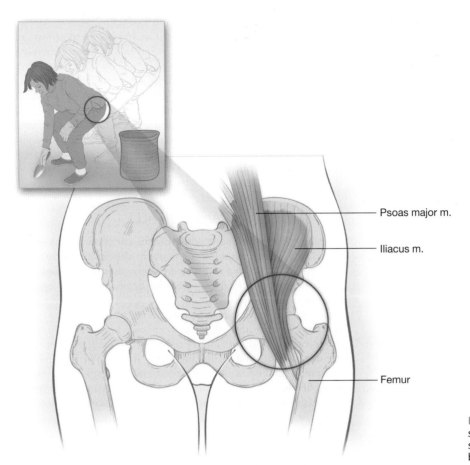

Psoas major m.

Iliacus m.

Femur

Figure 89-2 The symptoms of snapping hip syndrome commonly occur when rising from a sitting to a standing position or when walking briskly.

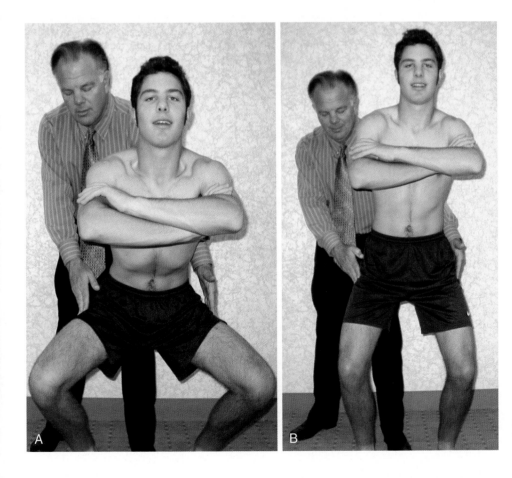

Figure 89-3 A and **B,** Eliciting the snap sign. *(From Waldman SD: Physical diagnosis of pain: an atlas of signs and symptoms, Philadelphia, 2006, Saunders, 2006, p 320.)*

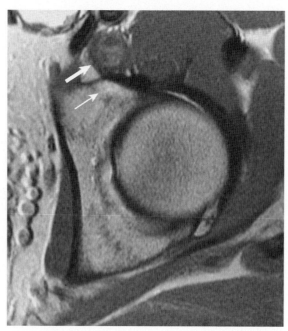

Figure 89-4 Magnetic resonance axial T1-weighted imaging showing osseous protuberance anteriorly *(thin arrow)* resulting in intratendinous high signal intensity (tendinosis) within the iliopsoas tendon *(thick arrow)*, also referred to as internal snapping hip syndrome. *(From Hodnett PA, Shelly MJ, MacMahon PJ, et al: MR imaging of overuse injuries of the hip, Magn Reson Imaging Clin N Am 17[4]:667–679, 2009.)*

examination, with a systematic search for other causes of hip pain, should be performed. The clinician must rule out other coexisting disease processes that may mimic snapping hip syndrome, including primary inflammatory muscle disease, primary hip disorders, and rectal and pelvic tumors.

TREATMENT

Initial treatment of the pain and functional disability associated with snapping hip syndrome includes a combination of nonsteroidal antiinflammatory drugs or cyclooxygenase-2 inhibitors and physical therapy. The local application of heat and cold may also be beneficial. For patients who do not respond to these treatment modalities, injection with local anesthetic and steroid is a reasonable next step.

To perform the injection, the patient is placed in the lateral decubitus position with the affected side upward. The midpoint of the greater trochanter is identified, and the skin overlying this point is prepared with antiseptic solution. A syringe containing 2 mL of 0.25% preservative-free bupivacaine and 40 mg

methylprednisolone is attached to a 3½-inch, 25-gauge needle. Before needle placement, the patient should be instructed to say "There!" as soon as a paresthesia is felt in the lower extremity, thus indicating that the needle has impinged on the sciatic nerve. Should a paresthesia occur, the needle is immediately withdrawn and is repositioned more laterally. The needle is slowly advanced through the previously identified point at a right angle to the skin, directly toward the center of the greater trochanter, until the needle hits bone; the needle is then withdrawn out of the periosteum. After careful aspiration for blood, and if no paresthesia is present, the contents of the syringe are gently injected. Resistance to injection should be minimal.

COMPLICATIONS AND PITFALLS

The injection technique is safe if careful attention is paid to the clinically relevant anatomy, particularly the sciatic nerve. The proximity to the sciatic nerve makes it imperative that this procedure be performed only by those familiar with the regional anatomy and experienced in the technique. Although infection is rare, sterile technique must be used, along with universal precautions to minimize any risk to the operator. Most complications of the injection technique are related to needle-induced trauma at the injection site and in the underlying tissues. The incidence of ecchymosis and hematoma formation can be decreased if pressure is applied to the injection site immediately after injection. Many patients complain of a transient increase in pain after injection, and patients should be warned of this possibility.

Clinical Pearls

Snapping hip syndrome is a common disorder that often coexists with trochanteric bursitis. Because snapping hip syndrome is often misdiagnosed, a careful evaluation to identify underlying disease processes is mandatory. The injection technique described is extremely effective in the treatment of snapping hip syndrome.

SUGGESTED READINGS

Byrd TWT: Snapping hip, *Oper Tech Sports Med* 13(1):46–54, 2005.

Hodnett PA, Shelly MJ, MacMahon PJ, et al: MR imaging of overuse injuries of the hip, *Magn Reson Imaging Clin N Am* 17(4):667–679, 2009.

Tibor LM, Sekiya JK: Differential diagnosis of pain around the hip joint, *Arthroscopy* 24(12):1407–1421, 2008.

Waldman SD: Snapping hip syndrome. In *Atlas of pain management injection techniques*, ed 2, Philadelphia, 2007, Saunders, pp 367–370.

Waldman SD: Functional anatomy of the hip. In *Pain review*, Philadelphia, 2009, Saunders, pp 135–138.

Chapter 90

ILIOPECTINEAL BURSITIS

ICD-9 CODE **726.5**

ICD-10 CODE **M70.70**

THE CLINICAL SYNDROME

Bursae are formed from synovial sacs, whose purpose is to allow the easy sliding of muscles and tendons across one another at areas of repetitive movement. Lining these synovial sacs is a synovial membrane invested with a network of blood vessels that secrete synovial fluid. With overuse or misuse, the bursa may become inflamed or, rarely, infected; inflammation of the bursa results in an increase in the production of synovial fluid that causes swelling of the bursal sac. Although significant interpatient variability exists in the number, size, and location of bursae, the iliopectineal bursa generally lies between the psoas and iliacus muscles and the iliopectineal eminence. This bursa may exist as a single bursal sac or, in some patients, as a multisegmented series of loculated sacs.

The iliopectineal bursa, which is also known as the limbo dancer's bursa, is vulnerable to injury from both acute trauma and repeated microtrauma. Acute injuries often involve direct trauma to the bursa through hip injuries (Fig. 90-1); overuse injuries may also occur, such as the use of exercise equipment for lower extremity strengthening. If inflammation of the iliopectineal bursa becomes chronic, calcification may occur.

SIGNS AND SYMPTOMS

Patients with iliopectineal bursitis frequently complain of pain in the anterior hip and groin. The pain is localized to the area just below the crease of the groin anteriorly, with referred pain noted in the hip joint and anterior pelvis. Often, patients are unable to sleep on the affected hip and may complain of a sharp "catching" sensation with range of motion of the hip. Iliopectineal bursitis often coexists with arthritis of the hip joint.

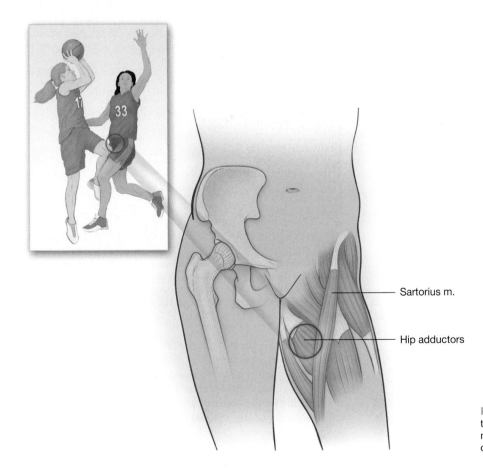

Sartorius m.

Hip adductors

Figure 90-1 The iliopectineal bursa is vulnerable to injury from both acute trauma and repeated microtrauma. Acute injuries may be caused by direct trauma to the bursa through hip injuries.

Figure 90-2 Pubic insufficiency fracture simulating a neoplasm in a 61-year-old woman. **A,** Pelvic radiograph shows changes in the symphysis on the left with sclerosis that suggest a chondroid- or osteoid-producing lesion *(arrows).* **B,** Computed tomography reveals a linear fracture plane and surrounding callus *(arrowheads)* resulting from a healing fracture; no evidence of a soft tissue mass is present. *(From Haaga JR, Lanzieri CF, Gilkeson RC, editors: CT and MR imaging of the whole body, ed 4, Philadelphia, 2003, Mosby, p 1924.)*

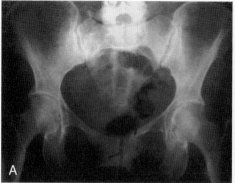
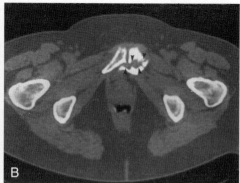

Physical examination may reveal point tenderness in the upper thigh just below the crease of the groin. Passive flexion, adduction, and abduction, as well as active resisted flexion and adduction of the affected lower extremity, can reproduce the pain. Sudden release of resistance during this maneuver causes a marked increase in pain.

TESTING

Plain radiographs or computed tomography scanning may reveal calcification of the bursa and associated structures that is consistent with chronic inflammation (Fig. 90-2). Magnetic resonance imaging of the hip and pelvis is indicated if tendinitis, partial disruption of the ligaments, stress fracture, internal derangement of the hip, or pelvic mass is suspected. Ultrasonography may confirm the cystic nature of the structures (Fig. 90-3). Radionuclide bone scanning is indicated if occult fracture, metastatic disease, or primary tumor involving the hip or pelvis is being considered. Based on the patient's clinical presentation, additional testing may be warranted, including a complete blood count, erythrocyte sedimentation rate, and antinuclear antibody testing. The injection technique described later serves as both a diagnostic and a therapeutic maneuver.

DIFFERENTIAL DIAGNOSIS

Iliopectineal bursitis is a common cause of hip and groin pain. Osteoarthritis, rheumatoid arthritis, posttraumatic arthritis, and, less frequently, aseptic necrosis of the femoral head are also common causes of hip and groin pain that may coexist with iliopectineal bursitis. Less common causes of arthritis-induced pain include the collagen vascular diseases, infection, villonodular synovitis, and Lyme disease. Acute infectious arthritis is usually accompanied by significant systemic symptoms, including fever and malaise, and should be easily recognized; it is treated with culture and antibiotics rather than injection therapy. Collagen vascular disease generally manifests as polyarthropathy rather than as monarthropathy limited to the hip joint, although pain secondary to collagen vascular disease responds exceedingly well to the injection technique described here.

TREATMENT

Initial treatment of the pain and functional disability associated with iliopectineal bursitis includes a combination of nonsteroidal antiinflammatory drugs (NSAIDs) or cyclooxygenase-2 inhibitors and physical therapy. The local application of heat and cold may

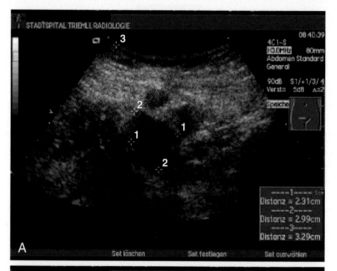

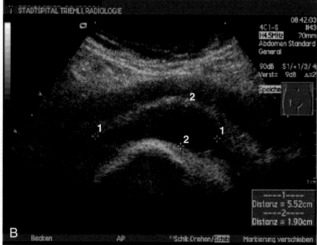

Figure 90-3 **A** and **B,** Sonography of the right groin with extensive iliopectineal bursitis. *(From Weber M, Prim P, Lüthy R: Inguinal pain with limping: iliopectineal bursitis as first sign of polymyalgia rheumatica,* Joint Bone Spine *75[3]:332–333, 2008.)*

also be beneficial. For patients who do not respond to these treatment modalities, injection of local anesthetic and steroid into the iliopectineal bursa is a reasonable next step.

Injection into the iliopectineal bursa is performed with the patient in the supine position. The pulsation of the femoral artery at the midpoint of the inguinal ligament is identified. At a point 2½ inches below and 3½ inches lateral to this pulsation lies the entry point of the needle; this point should be at the lateral edge

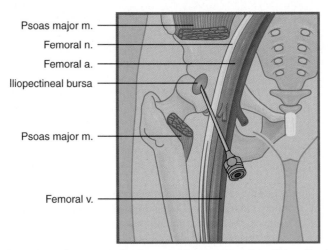

Psoas major m.
Femoral n.
Femoral a.
Iliopectineal bursa

Psoas major m.

Femoral v.

Figure 90-4 Correct needle placement for injection of the iliopectineal bursa. *(From Waldman SD:* Atlas of pain management injection techniques, *ed 2, Philadelphia, 2007, Saunders, p 359.)*

Physical modalities, including local heat and gentle stretching exercises, should be introduced several days after the patient undergoes injection. Vigorous exercises should be avoided, because they will exacerbate the patient's symptoms. Simple analgesics and NSAIDs can be used concurrently with this injection technique.

COMPLICATIONS AND PITFALLS

The injection technique is safe if careful attention is paid to the clinically relevant anatomy. Specifically, care must be taken to avoid trauma to the femoral nerve. The major complication of injection of the iliopectineal bursa is infection, although it should be exceedingly rare if strict aseptic technique is followed, along with universal precautions to minimize any risk to the operator. Other complications are related to needle-induced trauma at the injection site and in the underlying tissues. The incidence of ecchymosis and hematoma formation can be decreased if pressure is applied to the injection site immediately after injection. Approximately 25% of patients complain of a transient increase in pain after injection, and patients should be warned of this possibility.

Clinical Pearls

The injection technique described is extremely effective in the treatment of iliopectineal bursitis. Iliopectineal bursitis frequently coexists with arthritis of the hip, which may require specific treatment to achieve pain relief and return of function.

of the sartorius muscle. The skin overlying this point is prepared with antiseptic solution. A syringe containing 9 mL of 0.25% preservative-free bupivacaine and 40 mg methylprednisolone is attached to a 3½-inch, 25-gauge needle. Before needle placement, the patient should be instructed to say "There!" as soon as a paresthesia is felt in the lower extremity, thus indicating that the needle has impinged on the femoral nerve. Should a paresthesia occur, the needle is immediately withdrawn and is repositioned more laterally. The needle is then carefully advanced through the previously identified point at a 45-degree angle cephalad, to allow the needle to pass safely beneath the femoral artery, vein, and nerve. The needle is advanced very slowly to avoid trauma to the femoral nerve until the needle hits bone at the point where the ilium and pubic bones merge (Fig. 90-4); the needle is then withdrawn out of the periosteum. After careful aspiration for blood, and if no paresthesia is present, the contents of the syringe are gently injected into the bursa. Resistance to injection should be minimal.

SUGGESTED READINGS

Ramakrishnan R, Krieves MA, Lavelle WF, et al: Hip pain. In *Current therapy in pain,* New York, 2009, Elsevier, pp 177–181.

Tibor LM, Sekiya JK: Differential diagnosis of pain around the hip joint, *Arthroscopy* 24(12):1407–1421, 2008.

Waldman SD: Iliopectinate bursitis. In *Atlas of pain management injection techniques,* ed 2, Philadelphia, 2007, Saunders, pp 358–360.

Waldman SD: Injection technique for iliopectineal bursitis. In *Pain review,* Philadelphia, 2009, Saunders, pp 553–554.

Chapter 91

ISCHIAL BURSITIS

ICD-9 CODE 726.5

ICD-10 CODE M70.70

The Clinical Syndrome

Bursae are formed from synovial sacs, whose purpose is to allow the easy sliding of muscles and tendons across one another at areas of repetitive movement. Lining these synovial sacs is a synovial membrane invested with a network of blood vessels that secrete synovial fluid. With overuse or misuse, the bursa may become inflamed or, rarely, infected; inflammation of the bursa results in an increase in the production of synovial fluid that causes swelling of the bursal sac. Although significant interpatient variability exists in the number, size, and location of bursae, the ischial bursa generally lies between the gluteus maximus muscle and the bone of the ischial tuberosity. It may exist as a single bursal sac or, in some patients, as a multisegmented series of loculated sacs.

The ischial bursa is vulnerable to injury from both acute trauma and repeated microtrauma. Acute injuries are often caused by direct trauma to the bursa from falls onto the buttocks and from overuse, such as prolonged riding of horses or bicycles (Fig. 91-1). Running on uneven or soft surfaces such as sand also may cause ischial bursitis. If inflammation of the ischial bursa becomes chronic, calcification may occur.

Signs and Symptoms

Patients suffering from ischial bursitis frequently complain of pain at the base of the buttock with resisted extension of the lower extremity. The pain is localized to the area over the ischial tuberosity; referred pain is noted in the hamstring muscle, which may develop coexistent tendinitis. Often, patients are unable to sleep on the affected hip and may complain of a sharp "catching" sensation when extending and flexing the hip, especially on first awakening. Physical examination may reveal point tenderness over the ischial tuberosity. Passive straight leg raising and active

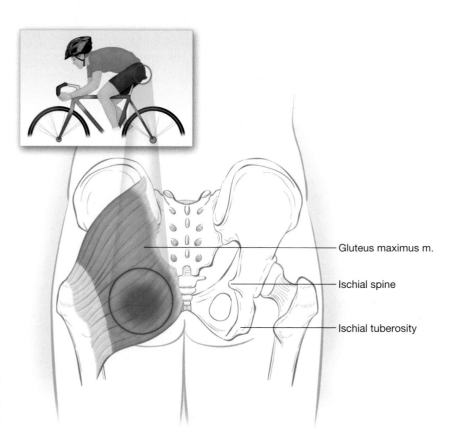

Figure 91-1 The ischial bursa is vulnerable to injury from both acute trauma and repeated microtrauma. Acute injuries are caused by direct trauma to the bursa from falls onto the buttocks and from overuse, such as prolonged riding of horses or bicycles.

Gluteus maximus m.

Ischial spine

Ischial tuberosity

resisted extension of the affected lower extremity reproduce the pain. Sudden release of resistance during this maneuver causes a marked increase in pain; this increase in pain is considered a positive resisted hip extension test, a finding supporting the diagnosis of ischial bursitis (Fig. 91-2).

TESTING

Plain radiographs may reveal calcification of the bursa and associated structures that is consistent with chronic inflammation. Magnetic resonance imaging of the hip and pelvis is indicated if tendinitis, partial disruption of the ligaments, stress fracture, internal derangement of the hip, or hip or pelvic mass is suspected (Fig. 91-3). Radionuclide bone scanning is indicated if occult fracture, metastatic disease, or primary tumor involving the hip or pelvis is being considered. Based on the patient's clinical presentation, additional testing may be warranted, including a complete blood count, erythrocyte sedimentation rate, and antinuclear antibody testing. The injection technique described later serves as both a diagnostic and a therapeutic maneuver.

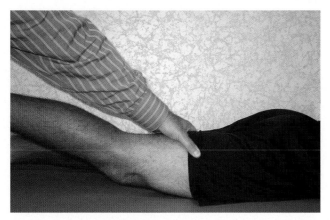

Figure 91-2 The resisted hip extension test for ischial bursitis. *(From Waldman SD: Physical diagnosis of pain: an atlas of signs and symptoms, Philadelphia, 2006, Saunders, p 309.)*

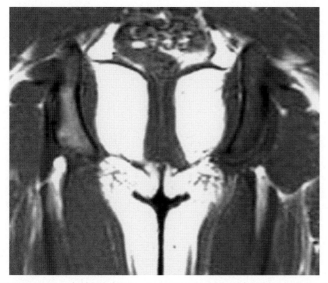

Figure 91-3 Ischial stress injury in a 16-year-old female athlete. Coronal T1-weighted magnetic resonance imaging shows asymmetrical decreased marrow signal intensity involving the left ischium. *(From Edelman RR, Hesselink JR, Zlatkin MB, Crues JV, editors:* Clinical magnetic resonance imaging, *ed 3, Philadelphia, 2006, Saunders, p 3385.)*

DIFFERENTIAL DIAGNOSIS

Ischial bursitis is a common cause of hip and groin pain. Osteoarthritis, rheumatoid arthritis, posttraumatic arthritis, and, less frequently, aseptic necrosis of the femoral head are also common causes of hip and groin pain that may coexist with ischial bursitis. Hamstring tendinitis or tears of the hamstring muscles may also be present. Less common causes of arthritis-induced pain include the collagen vascular diseases, infection, villonodular synovitis, and Lyme disease. Acute infectious arthritis is usually accompanied by significant systemic symptoms, including fever and malaise, and should be easily recognized; it is treated with culture and antibiotics rather than injection therapy. Collagen vascular disease generally manifests as polyarthropathy rather than as monarthropathy limited to the hip joint, although pain secondary to collagen vascular disease responds exceedingly well to the injection technique described here.

TREATMENT

Initial treatment of the pain and functional disability associated with ischial bursitis includes a combination of nonsteroidal antiinflammatory drugs (NSAIDs) or cyclooxygenase-2 inhibitors and physical therapy. The local application of heat and cold may also be beneficial. For patients who do not respond to these treatment modalities, injection of local anesthetic and steroid into the ischial bursa is a reasonable next step.

To inject the ischial bursa, the patient is placed in the lateral position with the affected side upward and the affected leg flexed at the knee. The skin overlying the ischial tuberosity is prepared with antiseptic solution. A syringe containing 4 mL of 0.25% preservative-free bupivacaine and 40 mg methylprednisolone is attached to a 1½-inch, 25-gauge needle. The ischial tuberosity is identified with a sterilely gloved finger. Before needle placement, the patient should be instructed to say "There!" as soon as a paresthesia is felt in the lower extremity, thus indicating that the needle has impinged on the sciatic nerve. Should a paresthesia occur, the needle is immediately withdrawn and is repositioned more medially. The needle is then carefully advanced through the skin, subcutaneous tissues, muscle, and tendon until it impinges on the bone of the ischial tuberosity (Fig. 91-4). Care must be taken to keep the needle in the midline and not to advance it laterally,

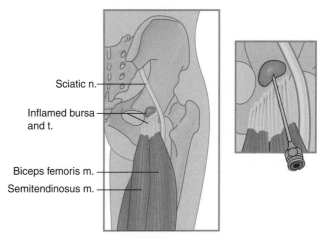

Sciatic n.

Inflamed bursa and t.

Biceps femoris m.

Semitendinosus m.

Figure 91-4 Correct needle placement for injection of the ischial bursa. *(From Waldman SD:* Atlas of pain management injection techniques, *ed 2, Philadelphia, 2007, Saunders.)*

or it could contact the sciatic nerve. After careful aspiration, and if no paresthesia is present, the contents of the syringe are gently injected into the bursa.

Physical modalities, including local heat and gentle stretching exercises, should be introduced several days after the patient undergoes injection. Vigorous exercises should be avoided, because they will exacerbate the patient's symptoms. Simple analgesics and NSAIDs can be used concurrently with this injection technique.

COMPLICATIONS AND PITFALLS

The injection technique is safe if careful attention is paid to the clinically relevant anatomy. Special care must be taken to avoid trauma to the sciatic nerve. The major complication of injection of the ischial bursa is infection, although it should be exceedingly rare if strict aseptic technique is followed, along with universal precautions to minimize any risk to the operator. Other complications are related to needle-induced trauma at the injection site and in the underlying tissues. The incidence of ecchymosis and hematoma formation can be decreased if pressure is applied to the injection site immediately after injection. Approximately 25% of patients complain of a transient increase in pain after injection, and patients should be warned of this possibility.

Clinical Pearls

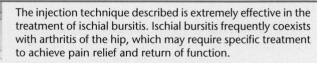

The injection technique described is extremely effective in the treatment of ischial bursitis. Ischial bursitis frequently coexists with arthritis of the hip, which may require specific treatment to achieve pain relief and return of function.

SUGGESTED READINGS

Hodnett PA, Shelly MJ, MacMahon PJ, et al: MR imaging of overuse injuries of the hip, *Magn Reson Imaging Clin N Am* 17(4):667–679, 2009.

Waldman SD: Ischial bursitis. In *Atlas of pain management injection techniques,* ed 2, Philadelphia, 2007, Saunders, pp 345–348.

Waldman SD: Injection technique for ischial bursitis. In *Pain review,* Philadelphia, 2009, Saunders, pp 547–549.

Zacher J, Gursche A: "Hip" pain, *Best Pract Res Clin Rheumatol* 17(1):71–85, 2003.

Chapter 92

MERALGIA PARESTHETICA

ICD-9 CODE `355.1`

ICD-10 CODE `G57.10`

THE CLINICAL SYNDROME

Meralgia paresthetica is caused by compression of the lateral femoral cutaneous nerve by the inguinal ligament. This entrapment neuropathy manifests as pain, numbness, and dysesthesias in the distribution of the lateral femoral cutaneous nerve. The symptoms often begin as a burning pain in the lateral thigh, with associated cutaneous sensitivity. Patients suffering from meralgia paresthetica note that sitting, squatting, or wearing wide belts causes the symptoms to worsen (Fig. 92-1). Although traumatic lesions to the lateral femoral cutaneous nerve have been implicated in meralgia paresthetica, in most patients, no obvious antecedent trauma can be identified.

SIGNS AND SYMPTOMS

Physical findings include tenderness over the lateral femoral cutaneous nerve at the origin of the inguinal ligament at the anterior superior iliac spine. A positive Tinel sign over the lateral femoral cutaneous nerve as it passes beneath the inguinal ligament may be present. Patients may complain of burning dysesthesias in the nerve's distribution (Fig. 92-2). Careful sensory examination of the lateral thigh reveals a sensory deficit in the distribution of the lateral femoral cutaneous nerve; no motor deficit should be present. Sitting or the wearing of tight waistbands or wide belts can compress the nerve and exacerbate the symptoms of meralgia paresthetica.

TESTING

Electromyography (EMG) can distinguish lumbar radiculopathy and diabetic femoral neuropathy from meralgia paresthetica. Plain radiographs of the back, hip, and pelvis are indicated in all patients

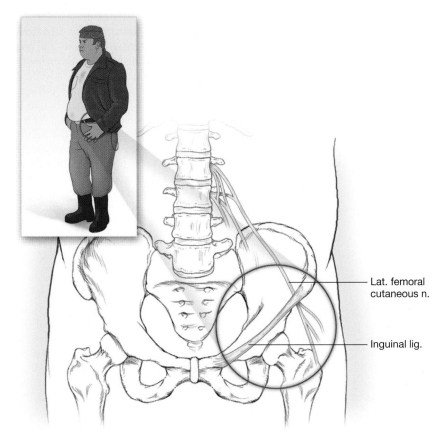

Lat. femoral cutaneous n.

Inguinal lig.

Figure 92-1 Obesity and the wearing of wide belts may compress the lateral femoral cutaneous nerve, thus resulting in meralgia paresthetica.

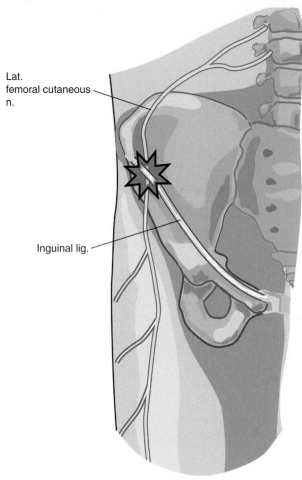

Figure 92-2 Burning pain in the lateral thigh is indicative of meralgia paresthetica. *(From Waldman SD: Physical diagnosis of pain: an atlas of signs and symptoms, Philadelphia, 2006, Saunders, p 279.)*

who present with meralgia paresthetica, to rule out occult bony disease. Based on the patient's clinical presentation, additional testing may be warranted, including a complete blood count, uric acid level, erythrocyte sedimentation rate, and antinuclear antibody testing. Magnetic resonance imaging (MRI) of the back is indicated if a herniated disk, spinal stenosis, or space-occupying lesion is suspected. The injection technique described later serves as both a diagnostic and a therapeutic maneuver.

DIFFERENTIAL DIAGNOSIS

Meralgia paresthetica is often misdiagnosed as lumbar radiculopathy, trochanteric bursitis, or primary hip disease. Radiographs of the hip and EMG can distinguish meralgia paresthetica from radiculopathy or pain emanating from the hip. In addition, most patients suffering from lumbar radiculopathy have back pain associated with reflex, motor, and sensory changes, whereas patients with meralgia paresthetica have no back pain and no motor or reflex changes; the sensory changes of meralgia paresthetica are limited to the distribution of the lateral femoral cutaneous nerve and should not extend below the knee. Lumbar radiculopathy and lateral femoral cutaneous nerve entrapment may coexist as the double-crush syndrome. Occasionally, diabetic femoral neuropathy produces anterior thigh pain, which may confuse the diagnosis.

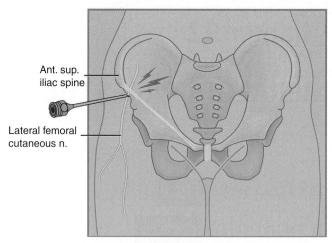

Figure 92-3 Correct needle placement for injection of the lateral femoral cutaneous nerve to treat meralgia paresthetica. *(From Waldman SD: Atlas of pain management injection techniques, Philadelphia, 2000, Saunders, 2000.)*

TREATMENT

Patients suffering from meralgia paresthetica should be instructed in avoidance techniques to reduce the symptoms and pain associated with this entrapment neuropathy. A short course of conservative therapy consisting of simple analgesics, nonsteroidal antiinflammatory drugs, or cyclooxygenase-2 inhibitors is a reasonable first step in the treatment of meralgia paresthetica. If patients do not experience rapid improvement, injection is the next step.

To treat the pain of meralgia paresthetica, the patient is placed in the supine position with a pillow under the knees if lying with the legs extended increases the pain because of traction on the nerve. The anterior superior iliac spine is identified by palpation. A point 1 inch medial to the anterior superior iliac spine and just inferior to the inguinal ligament is identified and is prepared with antiseptic solution. A 1½-inch, 25-gauge needle is slowly advanced perpendicular to the skin until the needle is felt to pop through the fascia. A paresthesia is often elicited. After careful aspiration, a solution of 5 to 7 mL of 1% preservative-free lidocaine and 40 mg methylprednisolone is injected in a fanlike pattern as the needle pierces the fascia of the external oblique muscle. Care must be taken not to place the needle deep enough to enter the peritoneal cavity and perforate the abdominal viscera (Fig. 92-3). After injection of the solution, pressure is applied to the injection site to decrease the incidence of ecchymosis and hematoma formation, which can be quite dramatic, especially in anticoagulated patients. If anatomic landmarks are difficult to identify, the use of fluoroscopic or ultrasound guidance should be considered (Fig. 92-4).

COMPLICATIONS AND PITFALLS

Care must be taken to rule out other conditions that may mimic the pain of meralgia paresthetica. The main complications of the injection technique are ecchymosis and hematoma. If the needle is placed too deep and it enters the peritoneal cavity, perforation of the colon may result in the formation of an intraabdominal abscess and fistula. Early detection of infection is crucial to avoid potentially life-threatening sequelae. If the needle is placed too medially, blockade of the femoral nerve may occur, thus making ambulation difficult.

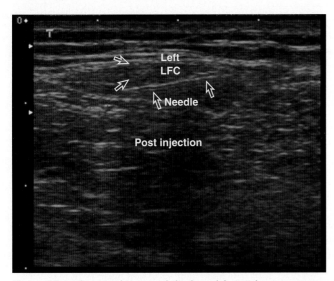

Figure 92-4 Ultrasound image of the lateral femoral cutaneous nerve (LFC) following the injection of 2 mL of local anesthetic. Perineural spread of the local anesthetic can be visualized. The needle is visualized as a linear hyperechoic structure deep to the nerve. *(From Hurdle MF, Weingarten TN, Crisostomo RA, et al: Ultrasound-guided blockade of the lateral femoral cutaneous nerve: technical description and review of 10 cases, Arch Phys Med Rehabil 88[10]:1362–1364, 2007.)*

Clinical Pearls

Meralgia paresthetica is a common complaint that is often misdiagnosed as lumbar radiculopathy. The injection technique described can produce dramatic pain relief. If a patient presents with pain suggestive of meralgia paresthetica but does not respond to lateral femoral cutaneous nerve block, however, a lesion more proximal in the lumbar plexus or an L2-3 radiculopathy should be considered. Such patients often respond to epidural block with steroid. EMG and MRI of the lumbar plexus are indicated in this patient population to rule out other causes of their pain, including malignant disease invading the lumbar plexus or epidural or vertebral metastatic disease at L2-3.

SUGGESTED READINGS

Moucharafieh R, Wehbe J, Maalouf G: Meralgia paresthetica: a result of tight new trendy low cut trousers ("taille basse"), *Int J Surg* 6(2):164–168, 2008.

Trummer M, Flaschka G, Under F, et al: Lumbar disc herniation mimicking meralgia paresthetica: case report, *Surg Neurol* 54(1):80–81, 2000.

Waldman SD: Injection technique for meralgia paresthetica. In *Pain review*, Philadelphia, 2009, Saunders, pp 556–557.

Waldman SD: Meralgia paresthetica. In *Pain review*, Philadelphia, 2009, Saunders, p 301.

Chapter 93

PHANTOM LIMB PAIN

ICD-9 CODE `353.6`

ICD-10 CODE `M54.6`

THE CLINICAL SYNDROME

Almost all patients who undergo amputation experience the often painful and distressing sensation that the absent body part is still present (Fig. 93-1). The cause of this phenomenon is not fully understood, but it is thought to be mediated in large part at the spinal cord level. Congenitally absent limbs do not seem to be subject to the same phenomenon. Patients may be able to describe the limb in vivid detail, although it is often distorted or in an abnormal position. In many patients, the sensation of the phantom limb fades with time, but in some patients, phantom pain remains a distressing part of daily life. Phantom limb pain is often described as a constant, unpleasant, dysesthetic pain that may be exacerbated by movement or stimulation of the affected cutaneous regions; a sharp, shooting neuritic pain may be superimposed on the constant dysesthetic symptoms, and some patients also note a burning component reminiscent of reflex sympathetic dystrophy. Some investigators reported that severe limb pain before amputation increases the incidence of phantom limb pain, but other investigators failed to find this correlation.

SIGNS AND SYMPTOMS

Phantom limb pain can take multiple forms, but it usually consists of dysesthetic pain. Additionally, patients may experience abnormal kinesthetic sensations (i.e., that the limb is in an abnormal position) or abnormal kinetic sensations (i.e., that the limb is moving). Investigators have reported that many patients with phantom limb pain experience a telescoping phenomenon; for example, a patient may report that the phantom foot feels like it is attached directly to the proximal thigh. Phantom limb pain may fade over time, and younger patients are more likely to experience this diminution in symptoms. Because of the unusual nature of phantom limb pain, a behavioral component is invariably present.

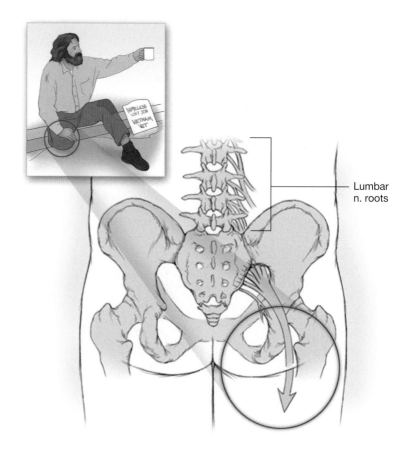

Lumbar n. roots

Figure 93-1 Phantom limb pain occurs with varying degrees of intensity in almost all patients who undergo amputation.

Testing

In most cases, the diagnosis of phantom limb pain is easily made on clinical grounds. Testing is generally used to identify other treatable coexisting diseases, such as radiculopathy. Such testing includes the following: basic laboratory tests; examination of the stump for neuroma, tumor, or occult infection; and plain radiographs and radionuclide bone scanning if fracture or osteomyelitis is suspected.

Differential Diagnosis

A careful initial evaluation, including a thorough history and physical examination, is indicated in all patients suffering from phantom limb pain if infection or fracture is a possibility. If the amputation was necessitated by malignant disease, occult tumor must be excluded. Other causes of pain in the distribution of the innervation of the affected limb, including radiculopathy and peripheral neuropathy, should be considered.

Treatment

The first step is to reassure patients that phantom pain is normal after the loss of a limb and that these sensations are real, not imagined; this knowledge alone can reduce patients' anxiety and suffering. Many pain specialists agree that preemptive analgesia early in the natural course of a disease that may lead to amputation, such as peripheral vascular insufficiency, can reduce the likelihood that patients will develop phantom limb pain. The following treatments may be useful to relieve phantom limb pain.

Analgesics

The anticonvulsant gabapentin is a first-line treatment in the palliation of phantom limb pain. It should be administered early in the course of the pain syndrome and can be used concurrently with neural blockade, opioid analgesics, and other adjuvant analgesics, including antidepressants, if care is taken to avoid central nervous system side effects. Gabapentin is started at a bedtime dose of 300 mg and is titrated upward in 300-mg increments to a maximum of 3600 mg/day given in divided doses, as side effects allow. Pregabalin represents a reasonable alternative to gabapentin and is better tolerated in some patients. Pregabalin is started at 50 mg three times a day and may be titrated upward to 100 mg three times a day as side effects allow. Because pregabalin is excreted primarily by the kidneys, the dosage should be decreased in patients with compromised renal function.

Carbamazepine should be considered in patients with severe neuritic pain who do not respond to nerve block and gabapentin. If this drug is used, rigid monitoring of hematologic parameters is indicated, especially in patients receiving chemotherapy or radiation therapy. Phenytoin may also be beneficial in the treatment of neuritic pain, but it should not be used in patients with lymphoma; the drug may induce a pseudolymphoma-like state that is difficult to distinguish from the actual lymphoma.

Antidepressants

Antidepressants may be useful adjuncts in the initial treatment of phantom limb pain. On a short-term basis, these drugs can alleviate the significant sleep disturbance that is common in this setting. In addition, antidepressants may be valuable in ameliorating the neuritic component of the pain, which is treated less effectively with opioid analgesics. After several weeks of treatment, antidepressants may exert a mood-elevating effect, which may be desirable in some patients. Care must be taken to observe closely for central nervous system side effects in this patient population, and these drugs may cause urinary retention and constipation.

Nerve Block

Neural blockade with local anesthetic and steroid by either epidural nerve block or blockade of the sympathetic nerves subserving the painful area is a reasonable next step if the aforementioned pharmacologic modalities fail to control phantom limb pain. The exact mechanism by which neural blockade relieves phantom limb pain is unknown, but it may be related to the modulation of pain transmission at the spinal cord level. In general, neurodestructive procedures have a very low success rate and should be used only after all other treatments have failed, if at all.

Opioid Analgesics

Opioid analgesics have a limited role in the management of phantom limb pain, and they frequently do more harm than good. Careful administration of potent, long-acting opioid analgesics (e.g., oral morphine elixir, methadone) on a time-contingent rather than as-needed basis may be a beneficial adjunct to sympathetic neural blockade. Because many patients suffering from phantom limb pain are older or have severe multisystem disease, close monitoring for the potential side effects of opioid analgesics (e.g., confusion or dizziness, which may cause a patient to fall) is warranted. Daily dietary fiber supplementation and Milk of Magnesia should be started along with opioid analgesics to prevent constipation.

Adjunctive Treatments

The application of ice packs to the stump may provide relief in some patients with phantom limb pain. The application of heat increases pain in most patients, presumably because of increased conduction of small fibers, but it may be worth trying if the application of cold is ineffective. Transcutaneous electrical nerve stimulation and vibration may also be effective in a limited number of patients. The favorable risk-to-benefit ratio of these modalities makes them reasonable alternatives for patients who cannot or will not undergo sympathetic neural blockade or who cannot tolerate pharmacologic treatment. A trial of spinal cord stimulation is also a reasonable option. The topical application of capsaicin may be beneficial in some patients suffering from phantom limb pain; however, the burning associated with application of this drug often limits its usefulness.

Complications and Pitfalls

Although no complications are associated with phantom limb pain itself, the consequences of unremitting pain can be devastating. Failure to treat phantom limb pain and the associated symptoms of sleep disturbance and depression aggressively can result in suicide.

Clinical Pearls

> Because phantom limb pain can be so severe and have such devastating consequences, the clinician must treat it rapidly and aggressively. Special attention must be paid to the insidious onset of severe depression, which mandates hospitalization with suicide precautions.

SUGGESTED READINGS

Anderson-Barnes VC, McAuliffe C, Swanberg KM, et al: Phantom limb pain: a phenomenon of proprioceptive memory? *Med Hypotheses* 73(4):555–558, 2009.

Giummarra MJ, Gibson SJ, Georgiou-Karistianis N, et al: Central mechanisms in phantom limb perception: the past, present, and future, *Brain Res Rev* 54(1):219–232, 2007.

Ketz AK: The experience of phantom limb pain in patients with combat-related traumatic amputations, *Arch Phys Med Rehabil* 89(6):1127–1132, 2008.

Wade NJ: Beyond body experiences: phantom limbs, pain and the locus of sensation, *Cortex* 45(2):243–255, 2009.

Waldman SD: Phantom limb pain. In *Pain review,* Philadelphia, 2009, Saunders, pp 313–314.

Chapter 94

TROCHANTERIC BURSITIS

ICD-9 CODE **726.5**

ICD-10 CODE **M70.60**

THE CLINICAL SYNDROME

Trochanteric bursitis is commonly encountered in clinical practice. Patients suffering from trochanteric bursitis frequently complain of pain in the lateral hip that radiates down the leg and mimics sciatica (Fig. 94-1). The pain is localized to the area over the trochanter. Often, patients are unable to sleep on the affected hip and may complain of a sharp "catching" sensation with range of motion of the hip, especially on first arising. Patients may note that walking upstairs is becoming increasingly difficult. Trochanteric bursitis often coexists with arthritis of the hip, back and sacroiliac joint disease, and gait disturbance.

The trochanteric bursa lies between the greater trochanter and the tendon of the gluteus medius and the iliotibial tract.

This bursa may exist as a single bursal sac or, in some patients, as a multisegmented series of loculated sacs. The trochanteric bursa is vulnerable to injury from both acute trauma and repeated microtrauma. Acute injuries may be caused by direct trauma to the bursa from falls onto the greater trochanter or previous hip surgery, as well as by overuse injuries, including running on soft or uneven surfaces. If inflammation of the trochanteric bursa becomes chronic, calcification may occur.

SIGNS AND SYMPTOMS

Physical examination reveals point tenderness in the lateral thigh just over the greater trochanter. Passive adduction and abduction, as well as active resisted abduction, of the affected lower extremity reproduce the pain. Sudden release of resistance during this maneuver causes a marked increase in pain (Fig. 94-2). No sensory deficit should be noted in the distribution of the lateral femoral cutaneous nerve; this feature distinguishes trochanteric bursitis from meralgia paresthetica.

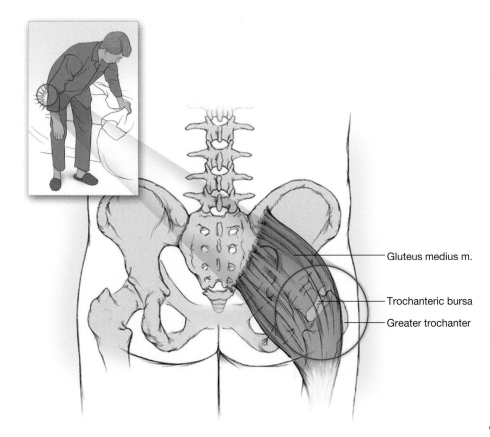

Gluteus medius m.

Trochanteric bursa

Greater trochanter

Figure 94-1 The pain of trochanteric bursitis often mimics that of sciatica.

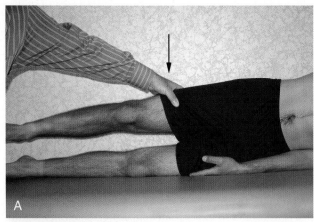

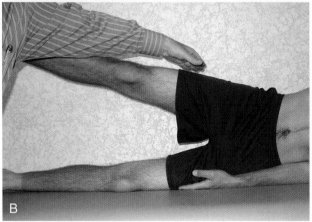

Figure 94-2 **A** and **B,** The resisted abduction release test. *(From Waldman SD: Physical diagnosis of pain: an atlas of signs and symptoms, Philadelphia, 2006, Saunders, p 316.)*

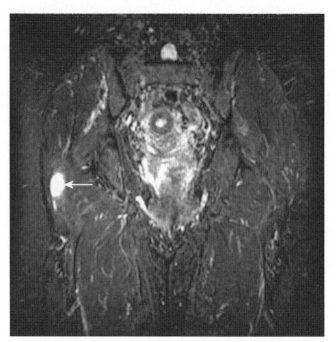

Figure 94-3 Magnetic resonance T2 short tau inversion recovery (STIR)–weighted coronal imaging showing signal hyperintensity within a distended trochanteric bursal complex *(arrow),* historically referred to as trochanteric bursitis. *(From Hodnett PA, Shelly MJ, MacMahon PJ, et al: MR imaging of overuse injuries of the hip,* Magn Reson Imaging Clin N Am *17[4]:667–679, 2009.)*

TESTING

Plain radiographs of the hip may reveal calcification of the bursa and associated structures, findings consistent with chronic inflammation. Magnetic resonance imaging is indicated if an occult mass or tumor of the hip or groin is suspected or to confirm the diagnosis (Figs. 94-3 and 94-4). A complete blood count and erythrocyte sedimentation rate are useful if infection is suspected. Electromyography (EMG) can distinguish trochanteric bursitis from meralgia paresthetica and sciatica. The injection technique described later serves as both a diagnostic and a therapeutic maneuver.

DIFFERENTIAL DIAGNOSIS

Trochanteric bursitis frequently coexists with arthritis of the hip. Occasionally, trochanteric bursitis can be confused with meralgia paresthetica, because both manifest with pain in the lateral thigh. In patients with meralgia paresthetica, however, palpation over the greater trochanter does not elicit pain. EMG can help sort out confusing clinical presentations. Primary or secondary tumors of the hip must also be considered in the differential diagnosis of trochanteric bursitis.

TREATMENT

A short course of conservative therapy consisting of simple analgesics, nonsteroidal antiinflammatory drugs (NSAIDs), or cyclooxygenase-2 inhibitors is a reasonable first step in the treatment of trochanteric

bursitis. Patients should be instructed to avoid repetitive activities that may be responsible for the development of trochanteric bursitis, such as running on sand. If patients do not experience rapid improvement, injection is a reasonable next step.

Injection of the trochanteric bursa is carried out by placing the patient in the lateral decubitus position with the affected side upward. The midpoint of the greater trochanter is identified, and the skin overlying this point is prepared with antiseptic solution. A syringe containing 2 mL of 0.25% preservative-free bupivacaine and 40 mg methylprednisolone is attached to a 3½-inch, 25-gauge needle. Before needle placement, the patient should be instructed to say "There!" as soon as a paresthesia is felt in the lower extremity, thus indicating that the needle has impinged on the sciatic nerve. If a paresthesia occurs, the needle is immediately withdrawn and is repositioned more laterally. The needle is then slowly advanced through the previously identified point at a right angle to the skin, directly toward the center of the greater trochanter (Fig. 94-5), until it hits bone; the needle is then withdrawn out of the periosteum. After careful aspiration for blood, and if no paresthesia is present, the contents of the syringe are gently injected into the bursa. Resistance to injection should be minimal.

Physical modalities, including local heat and gentle stretching exercises, should be introduced several days after the patient undergoes injection. Vigorous exercises should be avoided, because they will exacerbate the patient's symptoms. Simple analgesics, NSAIDs, and antimyotonic agents can be used concurrently with this injection technique.

COMPLICATIONS AND PITFALLS

Other conditions that may mimic the pain of trochanteric bursitis must be excluded. The injection technique is safe if careful attention is paid to the clinically relevant anatomy. Special care

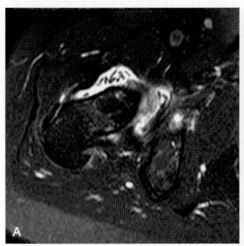

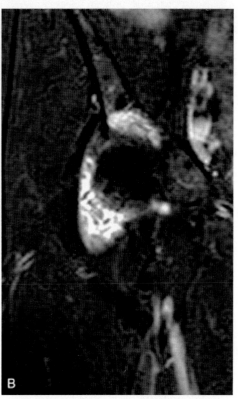

Figure 94-4 Synovial osteochondromatosis or chondromatosis. **A,** Axial, fat-saturated, T2-weighted magnetic resonance imaging (MRI). **B,** Coronal, fat-saturated, T2-weighted MRI. *(From Edelman RR, Hesselink JR, Zlatkin MB, Crues JV, editors: Clinical magnetic resonance imaging, ed 3, Philadelphia, 2006, Saunders, p 3392.)*

must be taken to avoid trauma to the sciatic nerve, which makes it imperative that this procedure be performed only by those familiar with the regional anatomy and experienced in the technique. Most complications of the injection technique are related to needle-induced trauma at the injection site and in the underlying tissues. Infection, although rare, can occur, and this possibility makes careful attention to sterile technique mandatory. Many patients complain of a transient increase in pain after injection, and patients should be warned of this possibility.

Clinical Pearls

Trochanteric bursitis frequently coexists with arthritis of the hip, which may require specific treatment to achieve pain relief and return of function. The injection technique described is extremely effective in the treatment of trochanteric bursitis.

SUGGESTED READINGS

Hodnett PA, Shelly MJ, MacMahon PJ, et al: MR imaging of overuse injuries of the hip, *Magn Reson Imaging Clin N Am* 17(4):667–679, 2009.

Segal NA, Felson DT, Torner JC, et al: Greater trochanteric pain syndrome: epidemiology and associated factors, *Arch Phys Med Rehabil* 88(8):988–992, 2007.

Waldman SD: Injection technique for trochanteric bursitis. In *Pain review,* Philadelphia, 2009, Saunders, pp 554–555.

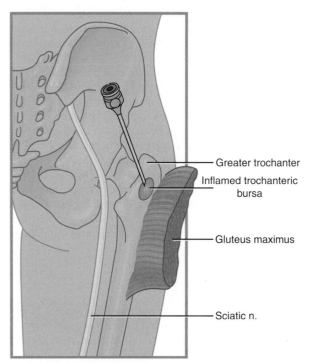

Greater trochanter

Inflamed trochanteric bursa

Gluteus maximus

Sciatic n.

Figure 94-5 Correct needle placement for injection of the trochanteric bursa. *(From Waldman SD: Atlas of pain management injection techniques, Philadelphia, 2000, Saunders.)*

Chapter 95

ARTHRITIS PAIN OF THE KNEE

ICD-9 CODE 715.96

ICD-10 CODE M17.9

THE CLINICAL SYNDROME

Arthritis of the knee is a common painful condition. The knee joint is susceptible to the development of arthritis from various conditions that have the ability to damage the joint cartilage. Osteoarthritis is the most common form of arthritis that results in knee pain; rheumatoid arthritis and posttraumatic arthritis are also common causes of knee pain. Less frequent causes of arthritis-induced knee pain include the collagen vascular diseases, infection, villonodular synovitis, and Lyme disease. Acute infectious arthritis is usually accompanied by significant systemic symptoms, including fever and malaise, and should be easily recognized; it is treated with culture and antibiotics rather than injection therapy. Collagen vascular disease generally manifests as polyarthropathy rather than as monarthropathy limited to the knee joint, although knee pain secondary to collagen vascular disease responds exceedingly well to the treatment modalities described here.

SIGNS AND SYMPTOMS

Most patients with osteoarthritis or posttraumatic arthritis of the knee complain of pain localized around the knee and distal femur. Activity makes the pain worse, whereas rest and heat provide some relief. The pain is constant and is characterized as aching; it may interfere with sleep. Some patients complain of a grating or popping sensation with use of the joint, and crepitus may be present on the physical examination.

In addition to pain, patients often experience a gradual reduction in functional ability because of decreasing knee range of motion that makes simple everyday tasks such as walking, climbing stairs, and getting in and out of a car quite difficult (Fig. 95-1). With continued disuse, muscle wasting may occur, and a frozen knee resulting from adhesive capsulitis may develop.

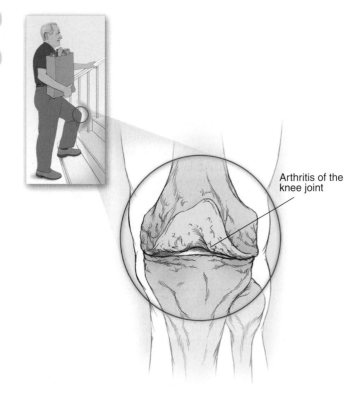

Arthritis of the knee joint

Figure 95-1 The pain of arthritis of the knee is made worse with weight-bearing activities.

TESTING

Plain radiographs or magnetic resonance imaging (MRI) is indicated in all patients who present with knee pain (Fig. 95-2). Based on the patient's clinical presentation, additional testing may be warranted, including a complete blood count, erythrocyte sedimentation rate, and antinuclear antibody testing. MRI of the knee is also indicated if the diagnosis is in question, if an occult mass or tumor is suspected, or in the presence of trauma.

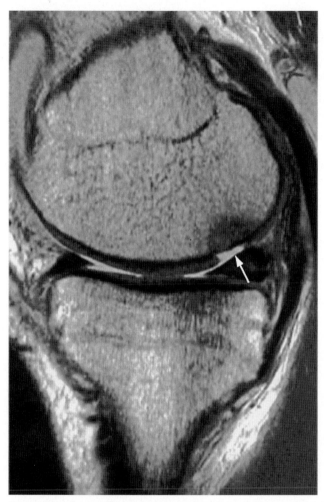

Figure 95-2 Sagittal fast spin-echo image through the medial joint line demonstrates focal full-thickness chondral injury with associated subchondral osseous changes *(arrow)*. *(From Edelman RR, Hesselink JR, Zlatkin MB, Crues JV, editors:* Clinical magnetic resonance imaging, *ed 3, Philadelphia, 2006, Saunders, p 3425.)*

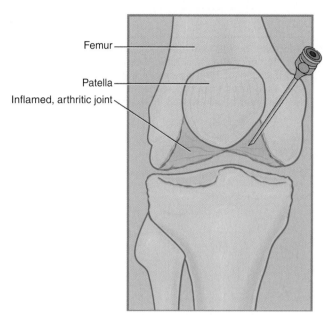

Figure 95-3 Proper needle placement for intraarticular injection of the knee. *(From Waldman SD:* Atlas of pain management injection techniques, *Philadelphia, 2000, Saunders.)*

DIFFERENTIAL DIAGNOSIS

Lumbar radiculopathy may mimic the pain and disability associated with arthritis of the knee. In such patients, results of the knee examination should be negative. Bursitis of the knee and entrapment neuropathies such as meralgia paresthetica may also confuse the diagnosis; both these conditions may coexist with arthritis of the knee. Primary and metastatic tumors of the femur and spine may also manifest in a manner similar to arthritis of the knee.

TREATMENT

Initial treatment of the pain and functional disability associated with arthritis of the knee includes a combination of nonsteroidal antiinflammatory drugs or cyclooxygenase-2 inhibitors and physical therapy. The local application of heat and cold may also be beneficial. For patients who do not respond to these treatment modalities, intraarticular injection of local anesthetic and steroid is a reasonable next step.

For intraarticular injection of the knee, the patient is placed in the supine position with a rolled blanket underneath the knee to flex the joint gently. The skin overlying the medial joint is prepared with antiseptic solution. A sterile syringe containing

5 mL of 0.25% preservative-free bupivacaine and 40 mg methylprednisolone is attached to a 1½-inch, 25-gauge needle by using strict aseptic technique. The joint space is identified, and the clinician places his or her thumb on the lateral margin of the patella and pushes it medially. At a point in the middle of the medial edge of the patella, the needle is inserted between the patella and the femoral condyles. The needle is then carefully advanced through the skin and subcutaneous tissues through the joint capsule and into the joint (Fig. 95-3). If bone is encountered, the needle is withdrawn into the subcutaneous tissues and is redirected superiorly. After the joint space is entered, the contents of the syringe are gently injected. Little resistance to injection should be felt. If resistance is encountered, the needle is probably in a ligament or tendon and should be advanced slightly into the joint space until the injection can proceed without significant resistance. The needle is then removed, and a sterile pressure dressing and ice pack are applied to the injection site.

Physical modalities, including local heat and gentle range-of-motion exercises, should be introduced several days after the patient undergoes injection. Vigorous exercises should be avoided, because they will exacerbate the patient's symptoms.

COMPLICATIONS AND PITFALLS

Failure to identify primary or metastatic tumor of the knee or spine that is causing the patient's pain can have disastrous results. The injection technique is safe if careful attention is paid to the clinically relevant anatomy. The major complication of intraarticular injection of the knee is infection, although it should be exceedingly rare if strict aseptic technique is followed, along with universal precautions to minimize any risk to the operator. The incidence of ecchymosis and hematoma formation can be decreased if pressure is applied to the injection site immediately after the injection. Approximately 25% of patients complain of a transient increase in pain after injection, and patients should be warned of this possibility.

Clinical Pearls

Coexistent bursitis and tendinitis may contribute to knee pain, thus necessitating additional treatment with more localized injection of local anesthetic and methylprednisolone. The injection technique described is extremely effective in the treatment of pain secondary to arthritis of the knee.

SUGGESTED READINGS

Blagojevic M, Jinks C, Jeffery A, et al: Risk factors for onset of osteoarthritis of the knee in older adults: a systematic review and meta-analysis, *Osteoarthritis Cartilage* 18(1):24–33, 2010.

Javaid MK, Lynch JA, Tolstykh I, et al: Pre-radiographic MRI findings are associated with onset of knee symptoms: the most study, *Osteoarthritis Cartilage* 18(3):323–328, 2010.

Rannou F, Poiraudeau S: Non-pharmacological approaches for the treatment of osteoarthritis, *Best Pract Res Clin Rheumatol* 24(1):93–106, 2010.

Teichtahl AJ, Wluka AE, Wang Y, et al: Occupational activity is associated with knee cartilage morphology in females, *Maturitas* 66(1):72–76, 2010.

Waldman SD: Intra-articular injection of the knee. In *Atlas of pain management injection techniques,* Philadelphia, 2007, Saunders, pp 417–421.

Waldman SD: Arthritis pain of the knee. In *Pain review,* Philadelphia, 2009, Saunders, pp 311–312.

Chapter 96

AVASCULAR NECROSIS OF THE KNEE JOINT

ICD-9 CODE **733.43**

ICD-10 CODE **M87.059**

THE CLINICAL SYNDROME

Avascular necrosis of the knee joint is an often missed diagnosis. Like the scaphoid, the knee joint is extremely susceptible to this disease because of the tenuous blood supply of the articular cartilage. This blood supply is easily disrupted, often leaving the proximal portion of the bone without nutrition leading to osteonecrosis (Fig. 96-1). A disease of the fourth and fifth decades, with exception of patients suffering from avascular necrosis of the knee joint secondary to collagen vascular disease, avascular necrosis of the knee joint is more common in men (Fig. 96-2). The disease is bilateral in 45% to 50% of cases.

Predisposing factors to avascular necrosis of the knee joint are listed in Table 96-1. They include trauma to the joint, corticosteroid use, Cushing's disease, alcohol abuse, connective tissue diseases especially systemic lupus erythematosus, osteomyelitis, human immunodeficiency virus infection, organ transplantation, hemoglobinopathies including sickle cell disease, hyperlipidemia, gout, renal failure, pregnancy, and radiation therapy involving the femoral head.

The patient with avascular necrosis of the knee joint complains of pain over the affected knee joint or knee joints that may radiate into the proximal lower extremity. The pain is deep and aching, and the patient often complains of a "catching" sensation with range of motion of the affect knee joint or knee joints. Range of motion decreases as the disease progresses.

SIGNS AND SYMPTOMS

Physical examination of patients suffering from avascular necrosis of the knee joint reveals pain to deep palpation of the knee joint. The pain can worsened by passive and active range of motion. A click or crepitus may also be appreciated by the examiner when the knee joint is put through range of motion. The range of motion is invariably decreased.

TESTING

Plain radiographs are indicated in all patients who present with avascular necrosis of the knee joint, to rule out underlying occult bony disease and to identify sclerosis and fragmentation of the osseous support of the articular surface. Early in the course of the disease, however, plain radiographs can be notoriously unreliable, and magnetic resonance imaging (MRI) reveals articular changes before significant changes are evident

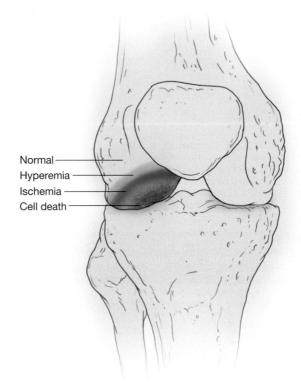

Normal
Hyperemia
Ischemia
Cell death

Figure 96-1 The pain of avascular necrosis of the knee joint is worsened by passive and active range of motion.

on plain radiographs (Fig. 96-3). Based on the patient's clinical presentation, additional testing including complete blood cell count, uric acid, sedimentation rate, and antinuclear antibody testing may also be indicated. MRI of the knee joint is indicated in all patients suspected of suffering from avascular necrosis of the knee joint or if other causes of joint instability, infection, or tumor is suspected, or if the plain radiographs are nondiagnostic (Fig. 96-4). Administration of gadolinium followed by post-contrast imaging may help delineate the adequacy of blood supply; contrast enhancement of the knee joint is a good prognostic sign. Electromyography is indicated if coexistent cervical radiculopathy or brachial plexopathy is suspected. A very gentle intraarticular injection of the knee joint with small volumes local anesthetic provides immediate improvement of the pain and helps demonstrate that the nidus of the patient's pain is in fact the knee joint. Ultimately, total joint replacement is required in most patients suffering from avascular necrosis of the knee joint, although newer joint preservation techniques are becoming more popular in younger, more active patients, given the short life expectancy of total knee prosthesis.

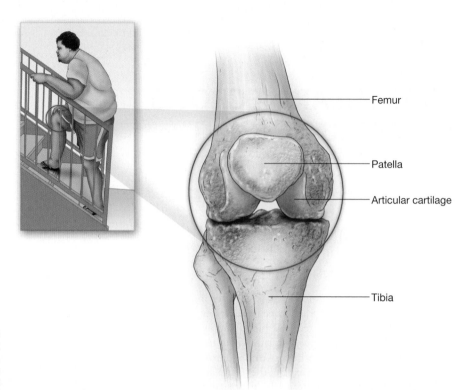

Femur

Patella

Articular cartilage

Tibia

Figure 96-2 Physical examination of patients suffering from avascular necrosis of the knee joint reveals pain to deep palpation of the knee joint. The pain is worsened by passive and active range of motion, and a click or crepitus, as well as decreased range of motion, may also be present.

TABLE 96-1

Predisposing Factors for Avascular Necrosis of the Knee Joint

- Trauma to the knee joint
- Steroids
- Cushing's disease
- Alcohol abuse
- Connective tissue diseases, especially systemic lupus erythematosus
- Osteomyelitis
- Human immunodeficiency virus infection
- Organ transplantation
- Hemoglobinopathies including sickle cell disease
- Hyperlipidemia
- Gout
- Renal failure
- Pregnancy
- Radiation therapy

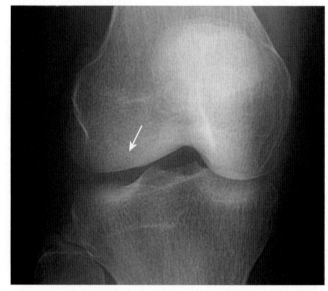

Figure 96-3 Anteroposterior radiograph revealing a subchondral lucency of the lateral femoral condyle *(arrow)* consistent with early avascular necrosis. *(From Zywiel MG, Armocida FM, McGrath MS, et al: Bicondylar spontaneous osteonecrosis of the knee: a case report,* Knee *17[2]:167–171, 2010.)*

DIFFERENTIAL DIAGNOSIS

Coexistent arthritis and gout of the knee joints, bursitis, and tendinitis may also coexist with avascular necrosis of the knee joints and exacerbate the pain and disability of the patient. Tears of the ligaments, bone cysts, bone contusions, and fractures may also mimic the pain of avascular necrosis of the knee joint, as can occult metastatic disease.

TREATMENT

Initial treatment of the pain and functional disability associated with avascular necrosis of the knee joint should include a combination of the nonsteroidal antiinflammatory agents (NSAIDs) or

cyclooxygenase-2 inhibitors and decreased weight bearing of the affect knee joint or knee joints. The local application of heat and cold may also be beneficial. For patients who do not respond to these treatment modalities, an injection of a local anesthetic into the knee joint may be a reasonable next step to provide palliation of acute pain. Vigorous exercises should be avoided, because they will exacerbate the patient's symptoms. Ultimately, surgical repair in the form of total joint arthroplasty is the treatment of choice.

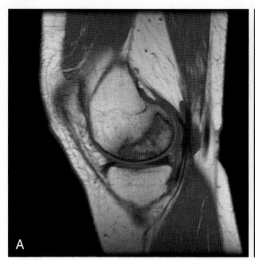 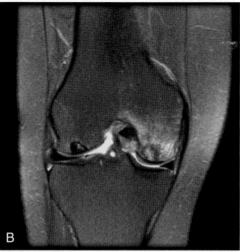

Figure 96-4 T1-weighted **(A)** and T2-weighted **(B)** magnetic resonance images taken 3 months before the plain radiograph in Figure 96-3 show subchondral lesions in both the medial and lateral femoral condyle. *(From Zywiel MG, Armocida FM, McGrath MS, et al: Bicondylar spontaneous osteonecrosis of the knee: a case report,* Knee *17[2]:167–171, 2010.)*

COMPLICATIONS AND PITFALLS

Failure to treat significant avascular necrosis of the knee joint surgically usually results in continued pain and disability and usually leads to ongoing damage to the knee joint (see Fig. 96-3). Injection of the joint with local anesthetic is a relatively safe technique if the clinician is attentive to detail, specifically uses small amounts of local anesthetic and avoids high injection pressures that may further damage the joint. Another complication of this injection technique is infection. This complication should be exceedingly rare if strict aseptic technique is followed. Approximately 25% of patients complain of a transient increase in pain after this injection technique, and patients should be warned of this possibility.

Clinical Pearls

Avascular necrosis of the knee joint is a diagnosis that is often missed, thus leading to much unnecessary pain and disability. The clinician should include avascular necrosis of the knee joint in the differential diagnosis in all patients complaining of knee joint pain, especially if any of the predisposing factors listed in Table 96-1 are present. Coexistent arthritis, tendinitis, and gout may also contribute to the pain and may require additional treatment. The use of physical modalities, including local heat and cold, as well as decreased weight bearing, may provide symptomatic relief. Vigorous exercises should be avoided, because they will exacerbate the patient's symptoms and may cause further damage to the knee. Simple analgesics and NSAIDs may be used concurrently with this injection technique.

SUGGESTED READINGS

Kattapuram TM, Kattapuram SV: Spontaneous osteonecrosis of the knee, *Clin Imaging* 32(6):495, 2008.

Pape D, Seil R, Kohn D, et al: Imaging of early stages of osteonecrosis of the knee, *Orthop Clin North Am* 35(3):293–303, 2004.

Savini CJ, James CW: HIV infection and avascular necrosis, *J Assoc Nurses AIDS Care* 12(5):83–85, 2001.

Yates PY, Calder JD, Stranks GJ, et al: Early MRI diagnosis and non-surgical management of spontaneous osteonecrosis of the knee, *Knee* 14(2):112–116, 2007.

Zywiel MG, McGrath MS, Seyler TM, et al: Osteonecrosis of the knee: a review of three disorders, *Orthop Clin North Am* 40(2):193–211, 2009.

Chapter 97

MEDIAL COLLATERAL LIGAMENT SYNDROME

ICD-9 CODE `717.82`

ICD-10 CODE `M23.50`

THE CLINICAL SYNDROME

Medial collateral ligament syndrome is characterized by pain at the medial aspect of the knee joint. This syndrome is usually the result of trauma to the medial collateral ligament from falls with the leg in valgus and externally rotated, typically during snow skiing accidents or football clipping injuries (Fig. 97-1). The medial collateral ligament, which is also known as the tibial collateral ligament, is a broad, flat, bandlike ligament that runs from the medial condyle of the femur to the medial aspect of the shaft of the tibia, where it attaches just above the groove where the semimembranosus muscle attaches (Fig. 97-2). It also attaches to the edge of the medial semilunar cartilage. The ligament is susceptible to strain at the joint line or avulsion at its origin or insertion.

SIGNS AND SYMPTOMS

Patients with medial collateral ligament syndrome present with pain over the medial joint and increased pain on passive valgus and external rotation of the knee. Activity, especially flexion and external rotation of the knee, makes the pain worse, whereas rest and heat provide some relief. The pain is constant and is characterized as aching; it may interfere with sleep. Patients with injury to the medial collateral ligament may complain of locking or popping with flexion of the affected knee. Coexistent bursitis, tendinitis, arthritis, or internal derangement of the knee may confuse the clinical picture after trauma to the knee joint.

On physical examination, patients with injury to the medial collateral ligament exhibit tenderness along the course of the ligament from the medial femoral condyle to its tibial insertion. If the ligament is avulsed from its bony insertions, tenderness may be localized to the proximal or distal ligament, whereas patients suffering from strain of the ligament have more diffuse tenderness. Patients with severe injury to the ligament may exhibit joint laxity when valgus and varus stress is placed on the affected knee (Fig. 97-3). Because pain may produce muscle guarding, magnetic resonance imaging (MRI) of the knee may be necessary to confirm the clinical impression. Joint effusion and swelling may be present with injury to the medial collateral ligament, but these findings are also suggestive of intraarticular damage. Again, MRI can confirm the diagnosis.

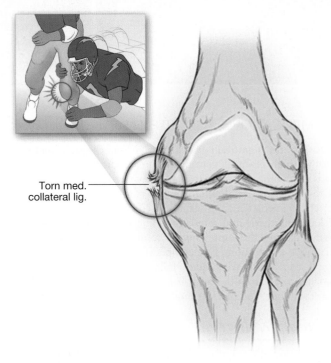

Torn med. collateral lig.

Figure 97-1 Medial collateral ligament syndrome is characterized by medial joint pain that is made worse with flexion or external rotation of the knee.

TESTING

MRI is indicated in all patients who present with medial collateral ligament pain, particularly if internal derangement or an occult mass or tumor is suspected (Fig. 97-4). In addition, MRI should be performed in all patients with injury to the medial collateral ligament who fail to respond to conservative therapy or who exhibit joint instability on clinical examination. Bone scan may be useful to identify occult stress fractures involving the joint, especially if trauma has occurred. Based on the patient's clinical presentation, additional testing may be warranted, including a complete blood count, erythrocyte sedimentation rate, and antinuclear antibody testing.

DIFFERENTIAL DIAGNOSIS

Any condition affecting the medial compartment of the knee joint may mimic the pain of medial collateral ligament syndrome. Bursitis, arthritis, and entrapment neuropathies may also confuse the diagnosis, as may primary tumors of the knee and spine.

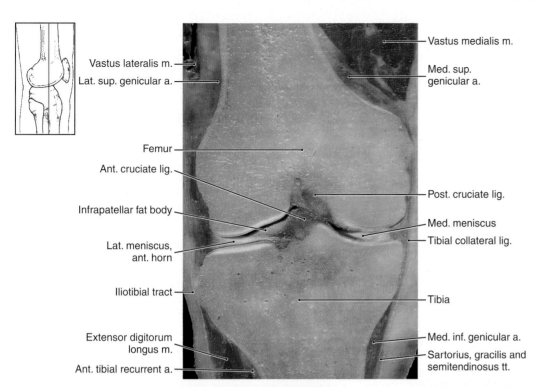

Vastus lateralis m.
Lat. sup. genicular a.
Femur
Ant. cruciate lig.
Infrapatellar fat body
Lat. meniscus, ant. horn
Iliotibial tract
Extensor digitorum longus m.
Ant. tibial recurrent a.

Vastus medialis m.
Med. sup. genicular a.
Post. cruciate lig.
Med. meniscus
Tibial collateral lig.
Tibia
Med. inf. genicular a.
Sartorius, gracilis and semitendinosus tt.

Figure 97-2 The medial collateral ligament is also known as the tibial collateral ligament. *(From Kang HS, Ahn JM, Resnick D: MRI of the extremities: an anatomic atlas, ed 2, Philadelphia, 2002, Saunders, 2002.)*

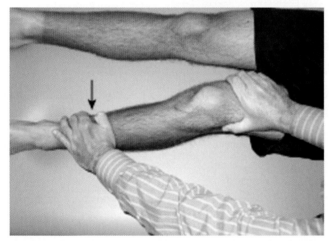

Figure 97-3 The valgus stress test for medial collateral ligament integrity. *(From Waldman SD: Physical diagnosis of pain: an atlas of signs and symptoms, ed 2, Philadelphia, 2010, Saunders, p 291.)*

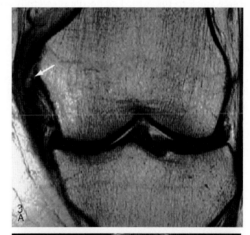

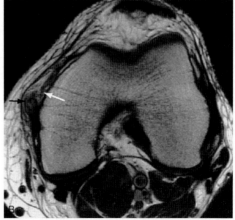

Figure 97-4 A, Coronal fast spin-echo magnetic resonance imaging (MRI) demonstrates a high-grade proximal medial collateral ligament tear *(arrow).* **B,** Axial fast spin-echo MRI in the same patient demonstrates a tear *(arrow)* of the medial collateral ligament from the femur. *(From Edelman RR, Hesselink JR, Zlatkin MB, Crues JV, editors:* Clinical magnetic resonance imaging, *ed 3, Philadelphia, 2006, Saunders, p 3407.)*

TREATMENT

Initial treatment of the pain and functional disability associated with injury to the medial collateral ligament includes a combination of nonsteroidal anti-inflammatory drugs or cyclooxygenase-2 inhibitors and physical therapy. The local application of heat and cold may also be beneficial. Any repetitive activity that exacerbates the patient's symptoms should be avoided. For patients who do not respond to these treatment modalities and who do not have lesions that require surgical repair, injection is a reasonable next step.

Injection of the medial collateral ligament is carried out with the patient in the supine position with a rolled blanket underneath the knee to flex the joint gently. The skin overlying the lateral aspect of the knee joint is prepared with antiseptic solution. A sterile

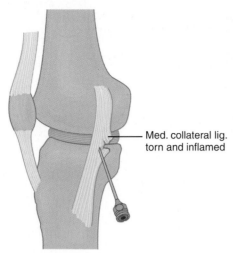

Med. collateral lig.
torn and inflamed

Figure 97-5 Injection technique for medial collateral ligament syndrome. *(From Waldman SD: Atlas of pain management injection techniques, ed 2, Philadelphia, 2007, Saunders, p 435.)*

syringe containing 2 mL of 0.25% preservative-free bupivacaine and 40 mg methylprednisolone is attached to a 1½-inch, 25-gauge needle by using strict aseptic technique. The tenderest portion of the ligament is identified, and the needle is inserted at this point at a 45-degree angle to the skin. The needle is carefully advanced through the skin and subcutaneous tissues into proximity with the medial collateral ligament (Fig. 97-5). If bone is encountered, the needle is withdrawn into the subcutaneous tissues and is redirected superiorly. The contents of the syringe are then gently injected. Little resistance to injection should be felt. If resistance is encountered, the needle is probably in a ligament or tendon and should be advanced or withdrawn slightly until the injection can proceed without significant resistance. The needle is then removed, and a sterile pressure dressing and ice pack are applied to the injection site.

COMPLICATIONS AND PITFALLS

The major complication of injection is infection, although this should be exceedingly rare if strict aseptic technique is followed. Approximately 25% of patients complain of a transient increase in pain after injection of the medial collateral ligament, and patients should be warned of this possibility.

Clinical Pearls

Patients with injury to the medial collateral ligament are best examined with the knee in the slightly flexed position. The clinician may want to examine the nonpainful knee first to reduce the patient's anxiety and to ascertain the findings of a normal examination. The injection technique described is extremely effective in the treatment of pain secondary to medial collateral ligament syndrome. Coexistent bursitis, tendinitis, arthritis, and internal derangement of the knee may contribute to the patient's pain, thus necessitating additional treatment with more localized injection of local anesthetic and methylprednisolone.

SUGGESTED READINGS

Beall DP, Googe JD, Moss JT, et al: Magnetic resonance imaging of the collateral ligaments and the anatomic quadrants of the knee, *Radiol Clin North Am* 45(6):983–1002, 2007.

Jones L, Bismil Q, Alvas F, et al: Persistent symptoms following nonoperative management in low grade MCL injury of the knee: the role of the deep MCL, *Knee* 16(1):64–68, 2009.

Kastelein M, Wagemakers HP, Luijsterburg PA, et al: Assessing medial collateral ligament knee lesions in general practice, *Am J Med* 121(11):982–988, 2008.

Malone WJ, Verde F, Weiss D, et al: MR imaging of knee instability, *Magn Reson Imaging Clin N Am* 17(4):697–724, 2009.

Waldman SD: Medial collateral ligament syndrome. In *Atlas of pain management injection techniques,* ed 2, Philadelphia, 2007, Saunders, pp 434–436.

Chapter 98

MEDIAL MENISCAL TEAR

ICD-9 CODE 717.1

ICD-10 CODE M23.219

THE CLINICAL SYNDROME

The meniscus is a unique anatomic structure that fulfills various functions to allow ambulation in the upright position (Table 98-1). The meniscus is susceptible to both acute injury from trauma and degenerative tears, which are more chronic. Tears of the medial meniscus are classified by their orientation and shape (Table 98-2).

Acute medial meniscal injury is the most commonly encountered cause of significant knee pain secondary to trauma in clinical practice. The incidence of acute tear is approximately 60 cases per 100,000 individuals. Acute tears often result from sudden twisting or squatting with weight bearing (Fig. 98-1). The male predominance is more than 2:1. Medial meniscal tear is a disease of the third and fourth decades in men and the second decade in girls and women. In older patients, the incidence of degenerative medial meniscal tears approaches 60%, although not all these tears cause significant pain and functional disability for the patient.

The pain of medial meniscal tear is characterized by pain at the medial aspect of the knee joint line. The medial meniscus is a triangular structure on cross section that is approximately 3.5 cm in length from anterior to posterior (Fig. 98-2). This structure is wider posteriorly and is attached to the tibia by the coronary ligaments,

TABLE 98-1
Functions of the Medial Meniscus

- Load bearing
- Conversion of compressive forces to tensile forces
- Load distribution
- Stabilization of the joint
- Lubrication of the joint
- Proprioception

TABLE 98-2
Classification of Tears of the Medial Meniscus

- Longitudinal tears
- Bucket handle tears
- Parrot beak–shaped oblique tears
- Horizontal tears
- Radial tears
- Complex combination tears

which are also susceptible to trauma, as are the fibrous connections from the joint capsule and medial collateral ligament.

SIGNS AND SYMPTOMS

Patients with medial meniscal tear present with pain over the medial joint space and increased pain on the McMurray, squat, and Apley grinding tests (Fig. 98-3). Activity, especially flexion and external rotation of the knee, makes the pain worse, whereas rest and heat provide some relief. The pain is constant and is characterized as aching; it may interfere with sleep. Patients with injury to the medial meniscus may complain of locking or popping with flexion of the affected knee. An effusion is often present and can be quite pronounced in some patients. Coexistent bursitis, tendinitis, arthritis, or other internal derangement of the knee may confuse the clinical picture after trauma to the knee joint.

On physical examination, patients with injury to the medial collateral ligament exhibit tenderness along the medial joint line. Patients with tear of the medial meniscus may exhibit a positive McMurray, squat, and Apley test result. Because pain may produce muscle guarding that makes accurate joint examination difficult, magnetic resonance imaging (MRI) of the knee may be necessary to confirm the clinical impression.

TESTING

Plain radiographs and MRI are indicated in all patients who present with knee pain, particularly if internal derangement or an occult mass or tumor is suspected (Fig. 98-4). In addition, MRI should be performed in all patients with injury to the medial meniscus who fail to respond to conservative therapy or who exhibit joint instability on clinical examination. Bone scan may be useful to identify occult stress fractures involving the joint, especially if trauma has occurred. Based on the patient's clinical presentation, additional testing may be warranted, including a complete blood count, erythrocyte sedimentation rate, and antinuclear antibody testing. Arthroscopy of the affected joint may serve as both a diagnostic and therapeutic maneuver.

DIFFERENTIAL DIAGNOSIS

Any condition affecting the medial compartment of the knee joint may mimic the pain of medial meniscal tear. Bursitis, arthritis, and entrapment neuropathies may also confuse the diagnosis, as may primary tumors of the knee and spine.

TREATMENT

Initial treatment of the pain and functional disability associated with injury to the medial collateral ligament includes a combination of nonsteroidal antiinflammatory drugs or cyclooxygenase-2 inhibitors and physical therapy. The local application of heat and

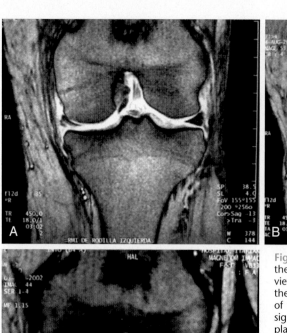

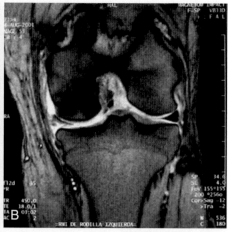

Figure 98-1 A 63-year-old man with pain over the medial joint line of the knee. **A,** Coronal view magnetic resonance imaging (MRI) shows the presence of a lesion of the posterior horn of the medial meniscus. The osseous marrow signal in the medial femoral condyle and tibial plateau appears with normal intensity. **B,** Six weeks after the first MRI, a T2-weighted coronal image shows diffuse low signal intensity area in the subchondral region of the medial femoral condyle. **C,** One year after the first MRI, a frontal image shows a subchondral area of low signal with a surrounding zone of intermediate low signal, diagnosed as osteonecrosis of the medial femoral condyle. *(From Muscolo DL, Costa-Paz M, Ayerza M, Makino A: Medial meniscal tears and spontaneous osteonecrosis of the knee,* Arthroscopy *22[4]:457–460, 2006.)*

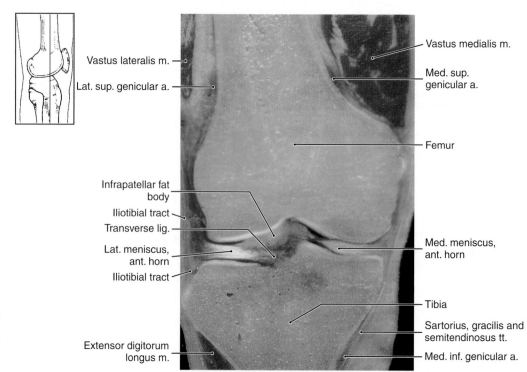

Figure 98-2 The medial meniscus is subject to degenerative changes, as well as tearing secondary to acute trauma. *(From Kang HS, Ahn JM, Resnick D: MRI of the extremities: an anatomic atlas, ed 2, Philadelphia, 2002, Saunders, p 305.)*

Vastus lateralis m.
Lat. sup. genicular a.
Vastus medialis m.
Med. sup. genicular a.
Femur
Infrapatellar fat body
Iliotibial tract
Transverse lig.
Lat. meniscus, ant. horn
Iliotibial tract
Med. meniscus, ant. horn
Tibia
Sartorius, gracilis and semitendinosus tt.
Extensor digitorum longus m.
Med. inf. genicular a.

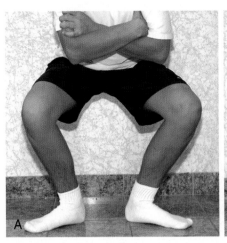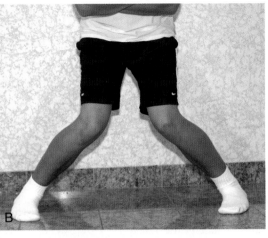

Figure 98-3 The squat test for meniscal tear. **A,** The patient is asked first to perform a full squat with the feet and legs fully externally rotated. **B,** The patient is then asked to perform a full squat with the feet and legs fully internally rotated. *(From Waldman SD: Physical diagnosis of pain: an atlas of signs and symptoms, ed 2, Philadelphia, 2010, Saunders, 2010, p 308.)*

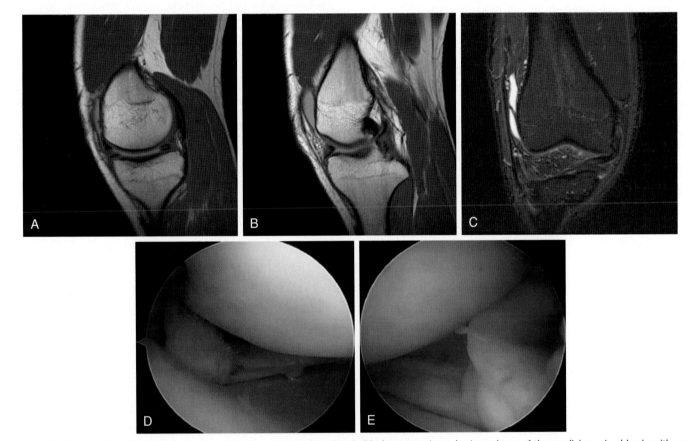

Figure 98-4 **A** to **C,** Sagittal proton density magnetic resonance imaging (MRI) demonstrating a horizontal tear of the medial meniscal body with an anterior horn fragment displaced anterior to the medial femoral condyle **(A)** and a posterior horn fragment displaced into the intercondylar notch adjacent to the posterior cruciate ligament **(B)**. Both displaced fragments were missed on MRI. **C,** Coronal short tau inversion recovery (STIR) MRI also demonstrating the displaced anterior horn meniscal fragment mentioned in **A**. This fragment was palpable to the patient, who brought it to the attention of the surgeon before arthroscopy. **D** and **E,** Arthroscopic images of the same case demonstrating the horizontal tear of the meniscal body and the displaced posterior horn **(D)** and anterior horn fragments **(E)**. *(From Sampson MJ, Jackson MP, Moran CJ, et al: Three Tesla MRI for the diagnosis of meniscal and anterior cruciate ligament pathology: a comparison to arthroscopic findings,* Clin Radiol *63[10]:1106–1111, 2008.)*

cold may also be beneficial. Any repetitive activity that exacerbates the patient's symptoms should be avoided. For patients who do not respond to these treatment modalities and who do not have lesions that require surgical repair, injection is a reasonable next step.

Injection of the medial meniscus is carried out by injecting the intraarticular space of the affected knee with local anesthetic and

steroid. To perform intraarticular injection of the knee, the patient is placed in the supine position with a rolled blanket underneath the knee to flex the joint gently. The skin overlying the medial joint is prepared with antiseptic solution. A sterile syringe containing 5 mL of 0.25% preservative-free bupivacaine and 40 mg methylprednisolone is attached to a 1½-inch, 25-gauge needle by using strict aseptic technique. The joint space is identified, and the clinician places his or her thumb on the lateral margin of the patella and pushes it medially. At a point in the middle of the medial edge of the patella, the needle is inserted between the patella and the femoral condyles. The needle is then carefully advanced through the skin and subcutaneous tissues through the joint capsule and into the joint (see Fig. 95-3). If bone is encountered, the needle is withdrawn into the subcutaneous tissues and is redirected superiorly. After the joint space is entered, the contents of the syringe are gently injected. Little resistance to injection should be felt. If resistance is encountered, the needle is probably in a ligament or tendon and should be advanced slightly into the joint space until the injection can proceed without significant resistance. The needle is then removed, and a sterile pressure dressing and ice pack are applied to the injection site.

Physical modalities, including local heat and gentle range-of-motion exercises, should be introduced several days after the patient undergoes injection. Vigorous exercises should be avoided, because they will exacerbate the patient's symptoms.

COMPLICATIONS AND PITFALLS

The major complication of injection is infection, although this should be exceedingly rare if strict aseptic technique is followed. Approximately 25% of patients complain of a transient increase in pain after injection of the medial collateral ligament, and patients should be warned of this possibility.

Clinical Pearls

Patients with injury to the medial collateral ligament are best examined with the knee in the slightly flexed position. The clinician may want to examine the nonpainful knee first to reduce the patient's anxiety and to ascertain the findings of a normal examination. The injection technique described is extremely effective in the treatment of pain secondary to medial meniscal tear. Coexistent bursitis, tendinitis, arthritis, and internal derangement of the knee may contribute to the patient's pain, thus necessitating additional treatment with more localized injection of local anesthetic and methylprednisolone.

SUGGESTED READINGS

Malone WJ, Verde F, Weiss D, et al: MR imaging of knee instability, *Magn Reson Imaging Clin N Am* 17(4):698–724, 2009.

Muscolo DL, Costa-Paz M, Ayerza M, et al: Medial meniscal tears and spontaneous osteonecrosis of the knee, *Arthroscopy* 22(4):457–460, 2006.

Sampson MJ, Jackson MP, Moran CJ, et al: Three Tesla MRI for the diagnosis of meniscal and anterior cruciate ligament pathology: a comparison to arthroscopic findings, *Clin Radiol* 63(10):1106–1111, 2008.

Waldman SD: An overview of painful conditions of the knee. In *Physical diagnosis of pain: an atlas of signs and symptoms,* ed 2, Philadelphia, 2010, Saunders, p 309.

Waldman SD: The Apley grinding test for meniscal tear. In *Physical diagnosis of pain: an atlas of signs and symptoms,* ed 2, Philadelphia, 2010, Saunders, p 307.

Waldman SD: The McMurray test for torn meniscus. In *Physical diagnosis of pain: an atlas of signs and symptoms,* ed 2, Philadelphia, 2010, Saunders, p 306.

Waldman SD: The squat test for meniscal tear. In *Physical diagnosis of pain: an atlas of signs and symptoms,* ed 2, Philadelphia, 2010, Saunders, p 308.

Chapter 99

ANTERIOR CRUCIATE LIGAMENT SYNDROME

ICD-9 CODE **844.2**

ICD-10 CODE **S83.509A**

THE CLINICAL SYNDROME

Anterior cruciate ligament syndrome is characterized by pain in the anterior aspect of the knee joint. It is usually the result of trauma to the anterior cruciate ligament from sudden deceleration secondary to planting of the affected lower extremity while extreme twisting or hyperextension forces are placed on the knee, typically during snow skiing accidents, football, and basketball injuries (Fig. 99-1). Unlike many other painful knee syndromes, anterior cruciate ligament syndrome occurs significantly more frequently in female patients.

The anterior cruciate ligament controls the amount of anterior movement or translation of the tibia relative to the femur, as well as providing important proprioceptive information regarding the position of the knee. This ligament is made up of dense fibroelastic fibers that run from the posteromedial surface of the lateral condyle of the distal femur through the intercondylar notch to the anterior surface of the tibia (Fig. 99-2). The anterior cruciate ligament is innervated by the posterior branch of the posterior tibial nerve. The ligament is susceptible to sprain or partial or complete tear.

SIGNS AND SYMPTOMS

Patients with anterior cruciate ligament syndrome present with pain over the anterior knee joint and increased pain on passive valgus stress and range of motion of the knee. Activity makes the pain worse, whereas rest and heat provide some relief. The pain is constant and is characterized as aching; it may interfere with sleep. Patients with injury to the anterior cruciate ligament may complain of a sudden popping of the affected knee at the time

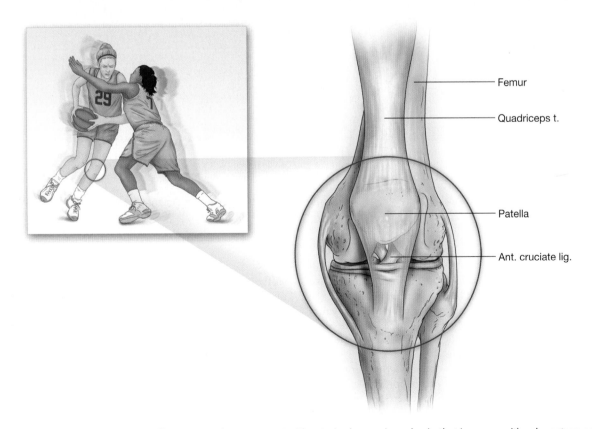

— Femur

— Quadriceps t.

— Patella

— Ant. cruciate lig.

Figure 99-1 Patients with anterior cruciate ligament syndrome present with anterior knee pain and pain that increases with valgus stress applied to the knee.

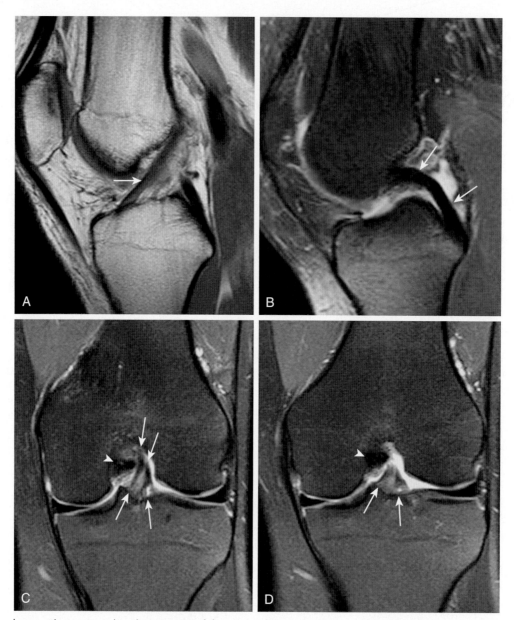

Figure 99-2 Normal magnetic resonance imaging anatomy of the cruciate ligaments. **A,** Sagittal fast spin-echo proton density (FSE PD)–weighted image shows streaky areas of isointense signal within a normal anterior cruciate ligament (ACL). Note the straight anterior border of the ACL *(arrow)*, which is parallel to Blumensaat's line. **B,** Sagittal fat-saturated FSE PD–weighted image shows the dark signal intensity of the posterior cruciate ligament (PCL), which has a posterior convex configuration *(arrows)*. **C** and **D,** Contiguous coronal fat-saturated FSE PD–weighted images of a normal ACL and PCL. Note the dark signal intensity of the PCL *(arrowhead)* and relatively high signal intensity of the ACL near its tibial insertion. The anteromedial and posterolateral bundles of the ACL are visualized *(arrows)*. *(From Kam CK, Chee DW, Peh WC: Magnetic resonance imaging of cruciate ligament injuries of the knee, Can Assoc Radiol J 61[2]:80–89, 2010.)*

of acute injury, as well as a sensation that the knee wants to give way or slip backward. Coexistent bursitis, tendinitis, arthritis, or internal derangement of the knee may confuse the clinical picture after trauma to the knee joint. The menisci of the knee are often injured when the patient sustains knee trauma severe enough to disrupt the anterior cruciate ligament.

On physical examination, patients with injury to the anterior cruciate ligament exhibit tenderness to palpation of the anterior knee. If the ligament is avulsed from its bony insertions, tenderness may be localized to the site of insertion, whereas patients suffering from strain of the ligament have more diffuse tenderness. Patients with severe injury to the ligament may exhibit joint laxity when anterior stress is placed on the affected knee. This maneuver is best accomplished by performing an anterior drawer test for anterior cruciate ligament integrity (Fig. 99-3). Other tests to assess the integrity of the anterior cruciate ligament include the flexion-rotation anterior drawer test and the Lachman test.

Because pain may produce muscle guarding, magnetic resonance imaging (MRI) of the knee may be necessary to confirm

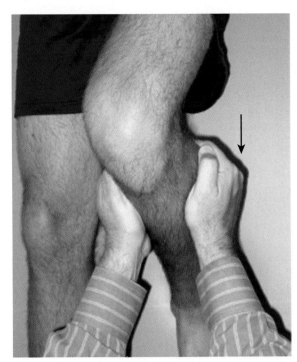

Figure 99-3 The anterior drawer test for anterior cruciate ligament integrity. *(From Waldman SD: Physical diagnosis of pain: an atlas of signs and symptoms, ed 2, Philadelphia, 2010, Saunders, p 293.)*

the clinical impression. Joint effusion and swelling may be present with injury to the ligament, but these findings can also suggest meniscal damage. Again, MRI can confirm the diagnosis.

TESTING

MRI is indicated in all patients who present with anterior cruciate ligament injury, both to rule out coexistent internal derangement, occult mass, or tumor and to confirm the diagnosis (Fig. 99-4). In addition, MRI should be performed in all patients with injury to the anterior cruciate ligament who fail to respond to conservative therapy or who exhibit joint instability on clinical examination. Bone scan may be useful to identify occult stress fractures involving the joint, especially if trauma has occurred. Based on the patient's clinical presentation, additional testing may be warranted, including a complete blood count, erythrocyte sedimentation rate, and antinuclear antibody testing.

DIFFERENTIAL DIAGNOSIS

Any condition affecting the medial compartment of the knee joint may mimic the pain of anterior cruciate ligament syndrome. Bursitis, arthritis, and entrapment neuropathies may also confuse the diagnosis, as may primary tumors of the knee and spine.

TREATMENT

Initial treatment of the pain and functional disability associated with injury to the anterior cruciate ligament includes a combination of nonsteroidal antiinflammatory drugs or cyclooxygenase-2

inhibitors and physical therapy. The local application of heat and cold may also be beneficial. Any repetitive activity that exacerbates the patient's symptoms should be avoided. For patients who do not respond to these treatment modalities and do not have lesions that require surgical repair, injection is a reasonable next step.

Injection to treat anterior cruciate ligament syndrome is carried out by injecting the interarticular space of the affected knee with local anesthetic and steroid. To perform intraarticular injection of the knee, the patient is placed in the supine position with a rolled blanket underneath the knee to flex the joint gently. The skin overlying the medial joint is prepared with antiseptic solution. A sterile syringe containing 5 mL of 0.25% preservative-free bupivacaine and 40 mg methylprednisolone is attached to a 1½-inch, 25-gauge needle using strict aseptic technique. The joint space is identified, and the clinician places his or her thumb on the lateral margin of the patella and pushes it medially. At a point in the middle of the medial edge of the patella, the needle is inserted between the patella and the femoral condyles. The needle is then carefully advanced through the skin and subcutaneous tissues through the joint capsule and into the joint (see Fig. 95-3). If bone is encountered, the needle is withdrawn into the subcutaneous tissues and is redirected superiorly. After the joint space is entered, the contents of the syringe are gently injected. Little resistance to injection should be felt. If resistance is encountered, the needle is probably in a ligament or tendon and should be advanced slightly into the joint space until the injection can proceed without significant resistance. The needle is then removed, and a sterile pressure dressing and ice pack are applied to the injection site.

Physical modalities, including local heat and gentle range-of-motion exercises, should be introduced several days after the patient undergoes injection. Vigorous exercises should be avoided, because they will exacerbate the patient's symptoms. Orthotic devices to stabilize the knee may also help improve the patient's functional ability as well as relieve pain.

COMPLICATIONS AND PITFALLS

The major complication of injection is infection, although this should be exceedingly rare if strict aseptic technique is followed. Approximately 25% of patients complain of a transient increase in pain after injection of the medial collateral ligament, and patients should be warned of this possibility.

Clinical Pearls

Patients with injury to the anterior cruciate ligament are best examined with the knee in the slightly flexed position. The clinician may want to examine the nonpainful knee first to reduce the patient's anxiety and to ascertain the findings of a normal examination. The injection technique described is extremely effective in the treatment of pain secondary to anterior cruciate ligament syndrome. Coexistent bursitis, tendinitis, arthritis, and internal derangement of the knee may contribute to the patient's pain, thus necessitating additional treatment with more localized injection of local anesthetic and methylprednisolone.

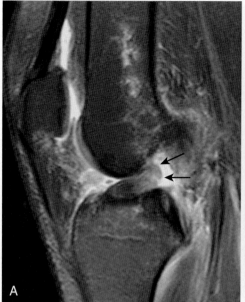
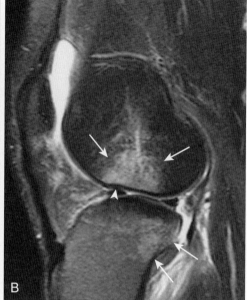
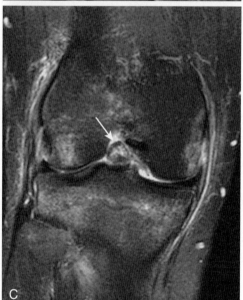

Figure 99-4 Acute complete anterior cruciate ligament (ACL) tear. **A,** Midsagittal fat-saturated fast spin-echo (FSE) T2-weighted image shows the distal portion of the ruptured ACL, which is thickened, hyperintense, and horizontally oriented *(arrows)*. Its axis is abnormally flattened (away from the Blumensaat's line). **B,** Lateral parasagittal fat-saturated FSE T2-weighted image shows bone contusions *(arrows)* in the lateral femoral condyle and posterolateral tibial plateau. A deepened lateral femoral sulcus *(arrowhead)* and anterior tibial translation are present. **C,** Coronal fat-saturated FSE T2-weighted image shows the thickened ACL, with increased signal intensity within its fibers *(arrow). (From Kam CK, Chee DW, Peh WC: Magnetic resonance imaging of cruciate ligament injuries of the knee,* Can Assoc Radiol J *61[2]:80–89, 2010.)*

SUGGESTED READINGS

Giugliano DN, Solomon JL: ACL tears in female athletes, *Phys Med Rehabil Clin N Am* 18(3):417–438, 2007.

Kam CK, Chee DW, Peh WC: Magnetic resonance imaging of cruciate ligament injuries of the knee, *Can Assoc Radiol J* 61(2):80–89, 2010.

Malone WJ, Verde F, Weiss D, et al: MR imaging of knee instability, *Magn Reson Imaging Clin N Am* 17(4):698–724, 2009.

Shelbourne KD, Urch SE: Treatment approach to anterior cruciate ligament injuries, *Oper Tech Sports Med* 17(1):24–31, 2009.

Waldman SD: An overview of painful conditions of the knee. In *Physical diagnosis of pain: an atlas of signs and symptoms,* ed 2, Philadelphia, 2010, Saunders, p 309.

Waldman SD: The anterior drawer test for anterior cruciate ligament instability. In *Physical diagnosis of pain: an atlas of signs and symptoms,* ed 2, Philadelphia, 2010, Saunders, p 293.

Waldman SD: The flexion-rotation anterior drawer test for anterior cruciate ligament instability. In *Physical diagnosis of pain: an atlas of signs and symptoms,* ed 2, Philadelphia, 2010, Saunders, p 294.

Chapter 100

JUMPER'S KNEE

ICD-9 CODE **726.90**

ICD-10 CODE **M77.9**

THE CLINICAL SYNDROME

Jumper's knee is characterized by pain at the inferior or superior pole of the patella. It occurs in up to 20% of jumping athletes at some point in their careers. It may affect one or both knees; boys and men are affected twice as commonly as are girls and women when just one knee is involved. Jumper's knee is usually the result of overuse or misuse of the knee joint caused by running, jumping, or overtraining on hard surfaces or direct trauma to the quadriceps or patellar tendon, such as from kicks or head butts during football or kickboxing (Fig. 100-1).

The quadriceps tendon is made up of fibers from the four muscles that constitute the quadriceps muscle: vastus lateralis, vastus intermedius, vastus medialis, and rectus femoris. These muscles are the primary extensors of the lower extremity at the knee. The tendons of these muscles converge and unite to form a single, exceedingly strong tendon (Fig. 100-2). The patella functions as a sesamoid bone within the quadriceps tendon, with fibers of the tendon expanding around the patella and forming the medial and lateral patella retinacula, which strengthen the knee joint. The patellar tendon extends from the patella to the tibial tuberosity. Weak or poor quadriceps and hamstring muscle flexibility, congenital variants in knee anatomy (e.g., patella alta or baja), and limb length discrepancies have been implicated as risk factors for the development of jumper's knee. Investigators have postulated that the strong eccentric contraction of the quadriceps muscle to strengthen the knee joint during landing is the inciting factor rather than the jump itself.

SIGNS AND SYMPTOMS

Patients with jumper's knee present with pain over the superior or inferior pole (or both) of the sesamoid. Jumper's knee can affect both the medial and lateral sides of both the quadriceps and the

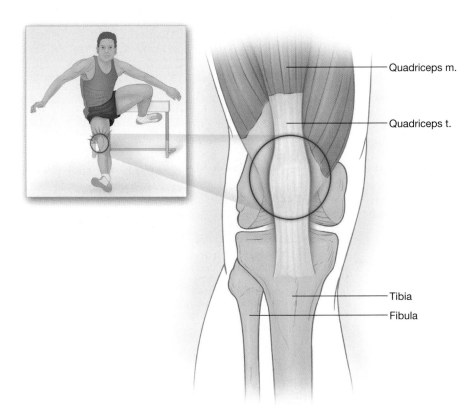

Quadriceps m.

Quadriceps t.

Tibia

Fibula

Figure 100-1 Jumper's knee—characterized by pain at the inferior or superior pole of the patella—occurs in up to 20% of jumping athletes at some point in their careers.

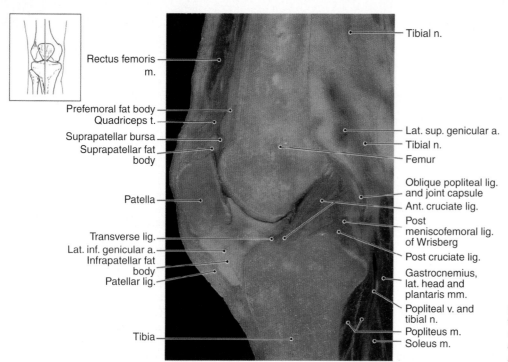

Rectus femoris m.

Prefemoral fat body
Quadriceps t.
Suprapatellar bursa
Suprapatellar fat body
Patella
Transverse lig.
Lat. inf. genicular a.
Infrapatellar fat body
Patellar lig.
Tibia

Tibial n.

Lat. sup. genicular a.
Tibial n.
Femur
Oblique popliteal lig. and joint capsule
Ant. cruciate lig.
Post meniscofemoral lig. of Wrisberg
Post cruciate lig.
Gastrocnemius, lat. head and plantaris mm.
Popliteal v. and tibial n.
Popliteus m.
Soleus m.

Figure 100-2 Sagittal view of the knee. (From Kang HS, Ahn JM, Resnick D: MRI of the extremities: an anatomic atlas, ed 2, Philadelphia, 2002, Saunders, 2002, p 341.)

patellar tendons. Patients note increased pain on walking down slopes or down stairs. Activity using the knee, especially jumping, makes the pain worse, whereas rest and heat provide some relief. The pain is constant and is characterized as aching; it may interfere with sleep. On physical examination, the patient notes tenderness of the quadriceps or patellar tendon (or both), and joint effusion may be present. Active resisted extension of the knee reproduces the pain. Coexistent suprapatellar and infrapatellar bursitis, tendinitis, arthritis, or internal derangement of the knee may confuse the clinical picture after trauma to the knee.

TESTING

Plain radiographs are indicated in all patients who present with knee pain. Magnetic resonance imaging of the knee is indicated if jumper's knee is suspected, because this imaging modality readily demonstrates tendinosis of the quadriceps or patellar tendon (Fig. 100-3). Ultrasound imaging may also provide beneficial information regarding the vascularity and integrity of the patellar and quadriceps tendons. Bone scan may be useful to identify occult stress fractures involving the joint, especially if trauma has occurred. Based on the patient's clinical presentation, additional testing may be indicated, including a complete blood count, erythrocyte sedimentation rate, and antinuclear antibody testing.

DIFFERENTIAL DIAGNOSIS

Jumper's knee is a repetitive stress disorder that causes tendinosis of the quadriceps and patellar tendons and is a distinct clinical entity from tendinitis of those tendons or quadriceps expansion syndrome, which may coexist with jumper's knee and confuse the clinical picture. Quadriceps expansion syndrome has a predilection for the medial side of the superior pole of the patella. The quadriceps tendon is also subject to acute calcific tendinitis, which may coexist with acute strain injuries and the more chronic changes of jumper's

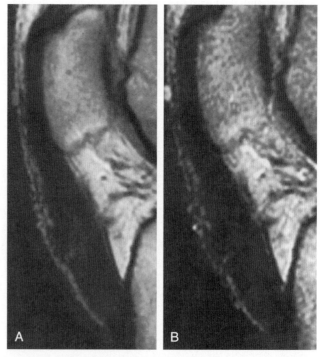

Figure 100-3 Chronic patellar tendinosis. Sagittal intermediate-weighted (A) and T2-weighted (B) spin echo magnetic resonance images show marked thickening of the entire patellar tendon that is more pronounced in the middle and distal segments. The anterior margin of the tendon is indistinct. There is no increase in signal intensity within the patellar tendon in B. (From Resnick D: Diagnosis of bone and joint disorders, ed 4, Philadelphia, 2002, Saunders, p 3236.)

knee. Calcific tendinitis of the quadriceps has a characteristic radiographic appearance of whiskers on the anterosuperior patella. The suprapatellar, infrapatellar, and prepatellar bursae also may become inflamed with dysfunction of the quadriceps tendon.

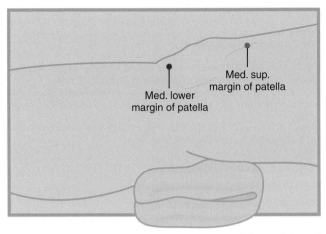

Figure 100-4 Identification of the superior margin of the medial patella (blue) and of the medial lower margin of the patella (red). *(From Waldman SD: Atlas of pain management injection techniques, Philadelphia, 2000, Saunders, pp 269, 278.)*

TREATMENT

Initial treatment of the pain and functional disability associated with jumper's knee includes a combination of nonsteroidal anti-inflammatory drugs (NSAIDs) or cyclooxygenase-2 inhibitors and physical therapy. A nighttime splint to protect the knee may also help relieve the symptoms. For patients who do not respond to these treatment modalities, injection with local anesthetic and steroid is a reasonable next step.

To perform the injection, the patient is placed in the supine position with a rolled blanket underneath the knee to flex the joint gently. If only the quadriceps tendon is affected, the skin overlying the medial aspect of the knee joint is prepared with antiseptic solution. A sterile syringe containing 2 mL of 0.25% preservative-free bupivacaine and 40 mg methylprednisolone is attached to a 1½-inch, 25-gauge needle by using strict aseptic technique. The superior margin of the medial patella is identified (Fig. 100-4). Just above this point, the needle is inserted horizontally to slide just beneath the quadriceps tendon (Fig. 100-5). If the needle strikes the femur, it is withdrawn slightly and is redirected with a more anterior trajectory. When the needle is in position just below the quadriceps tendon, the contents of the syringe are gently injected. Little resistance to injection should be felt. If resistance is encountered, the needle is probably in a ligament or tendon and should be advanced or withdrawn slightly until the injection can proceed without significant resistance. The needle is removed, and a sterile pressure dressing and ice pack are applied to the injection site.

If only the patellar tendon is affected, the skin overlying the medial portion of the lower margin of the patella is prepared with antiseptic solution. A sterile syringe containing 2 mL of 0.25% preservative-free bupivacaine and 40 mg methylprednisolone is attached to a 1½-inch, 25-gauge needle by using strict aseptic technique. The medial lower margin of the patella is identified (see Fig. 100-4). Just below this point, the needle is inserted at a right angle to the patella to slide beneath the patellar ligament into the deep infrapatellar bursa (Fig. 100-6). If the needle strikes the patella, it is withdrawn slightly and is redirected with a more inferior trajectory. When the needle is in position in proximity to the deep infrapatellar bursa, the contents of the syringe are gently injected. Little resistance to injection should be felt. If resistance is encountered, the needle is probably in a ligament or tendon and should be advanced or withdrawn slightly until the injection can

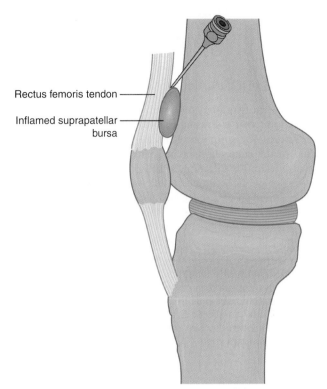

Figure 100-5 Correct needle placement for injection of the suprapatellar bursa. *(From Waldman SD: Atlas of pain management injection techniques, Philadelphia, 2000, Saunders, p 269.)*

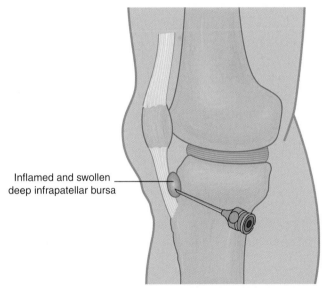

Figure 100-6 Correct needle placement for injection of the deep infrapatellar bursa. *(From Waldman SD: Atlas of pain management injection techniques, Philadelphia, 2000, Saunders, p 278.)*

proceed without significant resistance. The needle is removed, and a sterile pressure dressing and ice pack are applied to the injection site. If both the quadriceps and patellar tendons are affected, both injections should be performed.

Physical modalities, including local heat and gentle range-of-motion exercises, should be introduced several days after the patient undergoes injection. Vigorous exercises should be avoided, because they will exacerbate the patient's symptoms. Simple analgesics and NSAIDs can be used concurrently with this injection technique. Reports suggest that the injection of platelet-rich plasma may aid in the healing of the tendinopathy associated with jumper's knee.

COMPLICATIONS AND PITFALLS

Failure to identify primary or metastatic tumor of the distal femur or knee joint that is causing the patient's pain can have disastrous results. The injection technique is safe if careful attention is paid to the clinically relevant anatomy. The major complication of injection is infection, although it should be exceedingly rare if strict aseptic technique is followed. Approximately 25% of patients complain of a transient increase in pain after injection, and patients should be warned of this possibility.

Clinical Pearls

Coexistent bursitis, tendinitis, arthritis, and internal derangement of the knee may contribute to the patient's pain, thus necessitating additional treatment with more localized injection of local anesthetic and methylprednisolone. The injection technique described is extremely effective in treating the pain of jumper's knee.

SUGGESTED READINGS

Benjamin M, Kumai T, Milz S, et al: The skeletal attachment of tendons: tendon "entheses, *Comp Biochem Physiol A Mol Integr Physiol* 133(4):931–945, 2002.

Draghi F, Danesino GM, Coscia D, et al: Overload syndromes of the knee in adolescents: sonographic findings, *J Ultrasound* 11(4):151–157, 2008.

Kon E, Filardo G, Delcogliano M, et al: Platelet-rich plasma: new clinical application. A pilot study for treatment of jumper's knee, *Injury* 40(6):598–603, 2009.

Waldman SD: Jumper's knee. In *Atlas of pain management injection techniques*, ed 2, Philadelphia, 2007, Saunders, p 443–449.

Chapter 101

RUNNER'S KNEE

ICD-9 CODE **726.61**

ICD-10 CODE **M76.899**

THE CLINICAL SYNDROME

Runner's knee, also known as iliotibial band friction syndrome, is a common cause of lateral knee pain. The iliotibial band is an extension of the fascia lata, which inserts at the lateral condyle of the tibia. The iliotibial band bursa lies between the iliotibial band and the lateral condyle of the femur. Runner's knee is an overuse syndrome caused by friction injury to the iliotibial band as it rubs back and forth across the lateral epicondyle of the femur during running (Fig. 101-1); this rubbing can also irritate the iliotibial bursa beneath it. If inflammation of the iliotibial band becomes chronic, calcification may occur.

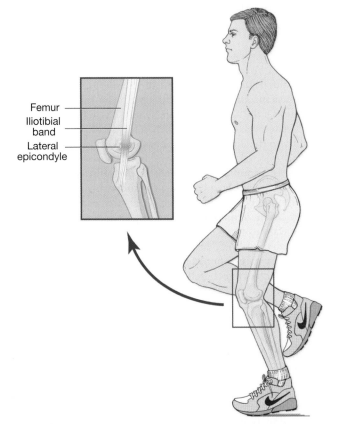

Figure 101-1 Runner's knee is an overuse syndrome caused by friction injury to the iliotibial band as it rubs back and forth across the lateral epicondyle of the femur. (From Waldman SD: Atlas of pain management injection techniques, ed 2, Philadelphia, 2000, Saunders, p 476.)

Runner's knee is a distinct clinical entity from iliotibial bursitis, although these two painful conditions frequently coexist. Runner's knee occurs more commonly in patients with genu varum and planus feet, although worn-out jogging shoes have also been implicated in the development of this syndrome.

SIGNS AND SYMPTOMS

Patients with runner's knee present with pain over the lateral side of the distal femur just over the lateral femoral epicondyle. Compared with iliotibial bursitis, the pain tends to be a little less localized, and effusion is rare. The onset of runner's knee frequently occurs after long-distance biking or jogging in worn-out shoes that lack proper cushioning (Fig. 101-2). Activity, especially that involving resisted abduction and passive adduction of the lower extremity, makes the pain worse, whereas rest and heat provide some relief. Flexion of the affected knee reproduces the pain in many patients with runner's knee. Often, patients are unable to kneel or walk down stairs. The pain is constant and is characterized as aching; it may interfere with sleep. Coexistent bursitis, tendinitis, arthritis, or internal derangement of the knee may confuse the clinical picture after trauma to the knee.

Physical examination may reveal point tenderness over the lateral epicondyle of the femur just above the tendinous insertion of the iliotibial band (see Fig. 101-1). If iliotibial bursitis is also present, the patient may have swelling and fluid accumulation around the bursa. Palpation of this area while the patient flexes and extends the knee may result in a creaking or "catching" sensation. Active resisted abduction of the lower extremity reproduces the pain, as does passive adduction. Sudden release of resistance during this maneuver causes a marked increase in pain. Pain is exacerbated when the patient stands with all his or her weight on the affected extremity and then flexes the affected knee 30 to 40 degrees.

TESTING

Plain radiographs of the knee may reveal calcification of the bursa and associated structures, including the iliotibial band tendon, findings consistent with chronic inflammation. Magnetic resonance imaging is indicated if runner's knee, iliotibial band bursitis, internal derangement, an occult mass, or a tumor of the knee is suspected (Figs. 101-3 and 101-4). Ultrasound imaging may also help clarify the diagnosis (Fig. 101-5). Electromyography can distinguish iliotibial band bursitis from neuropathy, lumbar radiculopathy, and plexopathy. Bone scan may be useful to identify occult stress fractures involving the joint, especially if trauma has occurred.

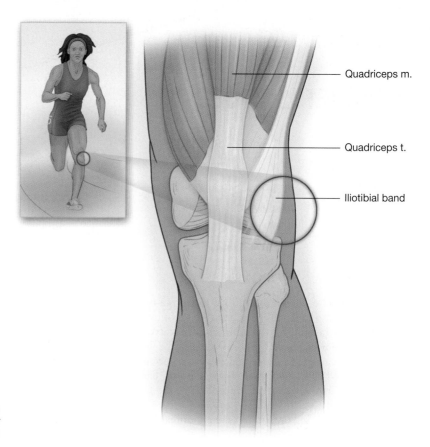

Quadriceps m.

Quadriceps t.

Iliotibial band

Figure 101-2 Patients with runner's knee present with pain over the lateral side of the distal femur, just over the lateral femoral epicondyle. The condition is often associated with running or jogging in worn-out shoes.

DIFFERENTIAL DIAGNOSIS

The iliotibial, suprapatellar, infrapatellar, and prepatellar bursae may become inflamed with dysfunction of the iliotibial band. The patellar tendon, which extends from the patella to the tibial tuberosity, is also subject to tendinitis, which may confuse the clinical picture. Internal derangement of the knee joint may coexist with iliotibial band bursitis.

TREATMENT

Initial treatment of the pain and functional disability associated with runner's knee includes a combination of nonsteroidal anti-inflammatory drugs (NSAIDs) or cyclooxygenase-2 inhibitors and physical therapy. A nighttime splint to protect the knee may also relieve the symptoms. For patients who fail to respond to these treatment modalities, injection with local anesthetic and steroid is a reasonable next step.

To perform the injection, the patient is placed in the supine position with a rolled blanket underneath the knee to flex the joint gently. The skin over the lateral epicondyle of the femur is prepared with antiseptic solution. A sterile syringe containing 2 mL of 0.25% preservative-free bupivacaine and 40 mg methylprednisolone is attached to a 1½-inch, 25-gauge needle by using strict aseptic technique. The iliotibial band bursa is identified by locating the point of maximal tenderness over the lateral condyle

of the femur. At this point, the needle is inserted at a 45-degree angle to the femoral condyle, and the needle passes through the skin, subcutaneous tissues, and iliotibial band into the iliotibial band bursa. If the needle strikes the femur, it is withdrawn slightly into the substance of the bursa. When the needle is positioned in proximity to the iliotibial band bursa, the contents of the syringe are gently injected. Little resistance to injection should be felt. If resistance is encountered, the needle is probably in a ligament or tendon and should be advanced or withdrawn slightly until the injection can proceed without significant resistance. The needle is removed, and a sterile pressure dressing and ice pack are applied to the injection site.

Physical modalities, including local heat and gentle range-of-motion exercises, should be introduced several days after the patient undergoes injection. Vigorous exercises should be avoided, because they will exacerbate the patient's symptoms. Simple analgesics and NSAIDs can be used concurrently with this injection technique.

COMPLICATIONS AND PITFALLS

Failure to identify primary or metastatic tumor of the distal femur or knee joint that is causing the patient's pain can have disastrous results. The injection technique is safe if careful attention is paid to the clinically relevant anatomy. The major complication of injection is infection, although this

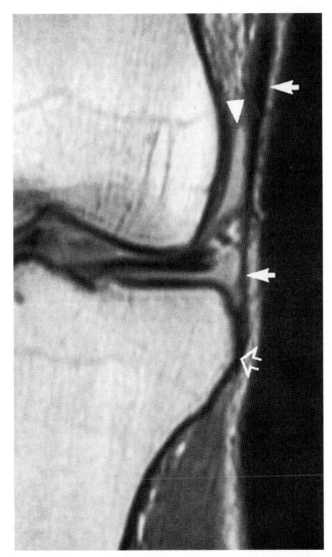

Figure 101-3 Normal iliotibial tract. Coronal, intermediate-weighted, spin-echo magnetic resonance image shows the iliotibial tract *(solid arrows)* attaching to Gerdy's tubercle *(open arrow)* in the tibia. A small joint effusion is evident just medial to the iliotibial tract *(arrowhead).* *(From Resnick D: Diagnosis of bone and joint disorders, ed 4, Philadelphia, 2002, Saunders, p 3231.)*

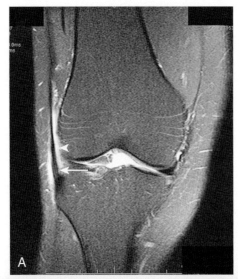

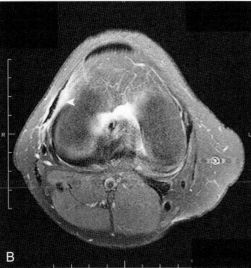

Figure 101-4 Iliotibial band friction syndrome. **A,** Coronal T2-weighted fat-saturated magnetic resonance imaging (MRI) demonstrates high signal intensity in the fatty tissue deep to the iliotibial band *(arrowhead)* with loss of definition of the normally low-signal-intensity band *(arrow).* **B,** Axial T2-weighted fat-saturated MRI demonstrates high signal intensity in the fatty tissue deep to the iliotibial band consistent with replacement by inflammatory tissue *(arrowhead). (From O'Keeffe SA, Hogan BA, Eustace SJ, Kavanaugh EC: Overuse injuries of the knee,* Magn Reson Imaging Clin N Am *17[4]:725–739, 2009.)*

should be exceedingly rare if strict aseptic technique is followed. Approximately 25% of patients complain of a transient increase in pain after injection, and patients should be warned of this possibility.

Clinical Pearls

Coexistent bursitis, tendinitis, arthritis, and internal derangement of the knee may contribute to the patient's pain, thus necessitating additional treatment with more localized injection of local anesthetic and methylprednisolone. The injection technique described is extremely effective in treating the pain of runner's knee.

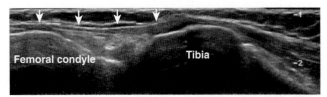

Figure 101-5 Iliotibial band syndrome. Wide longitudinal ultrasound scan along the iliotibial band *(arrows):* edematous swelling of the soft tissues deep to the iliotibial band, whose fibers do not show any alteration. *(From Draghi F, Danesino GM, Coscia D, et al: Overload syndromes of the knee in adolescents: sonographic findings,* J Ultrasound *11[4]:151–157, 2008.)*

SUGGESTED READINGS

Draghi F, Danesino GM, Coscia D, et al: Overload syndromes of the knee in adolescents: sonographic findings, *J Ultrasound* 11(4):151–157, 2008.

Ellis R, Hing W, Reid D: Iliotibial band friction syndrome: a systematic review, *Man Ther* 12(3):200–208, 2007.

Fairclough J, Hayashi K, Toumi H, et al: Is iliotibial band syndrome really a friction syndrome? *J Sci Med Sport* 10(2):74–76, 2007.

Hamill J, Miller R, Noehren B, et al: A prospective study of iliotibial band strain in runners, *Clin Biomech* 23(8):1018–1025, 2008.

Waldman SD: Runner's knee. In *Atlas of pain management injection techniques,* ed 2, Philadelphia, 2007, Saunders, pp 475–480.

Waldman SD: The iliotibial band bursa. In *Pain review,* Philadelphia, 2009, Saunders, pp 154–155.

Chapter **102**

SUPRAPATELLAR BURSITIS

ICD-9 CODE **726.60**

ICD-10 CODE **M70.50**

THE CLINICAL SYNDROME

The suprapatellar bursa extends superiorly from beneath the patella under the quadriceps femoris muscle and its tendon. The bursa is held in place by a small portion of the vastus intermedius muscle called the articularis genus muscle. The suprapatellar bursa may exist as a single bursal sac or, in some patients, as a multisegmented series of loculated sacs. The suprapatellar bursa is vulnerable to injury from both acute trauma and repeated microtrauma. Acute injuries may be caused by direct trauma to the bursa during falls onto the knee or patellar fractures. Overuse injuries may result from running on soft or uneven surfaces or from jobs that require crawling on the knees, such as carpet laying. If inflammation of the suprapatellar bursa becomes chronic, calcification may occur.

SIGNS AND SYMPTOMS

Patients suffering from suprapatellar bursitis complain of pain in the anterior knee above the patella that may radiate superiorly into the distal anterior thigh. Often, patients are unable to kneel or walk down stairs (Fig. 102-1). Patients may also complain of a sharp "catching" sensation with range of motion of the knee, especially on first arising. Suprapatellar bursitis often coexists with arthritis and tendinitis of the knee, thus confusing the clinical picture.

Physical examination may reveal point tenderness in the anterior knee just above the patella. Passive flexion and active resisted extension of the knee reproduce the pain. Sudden release of resistance during this maneuver causes a marked increase in pain. The patient may have swelling in the suprapatellar region, with a boggy feeling on palpation. Occasionally, the suprapatellar bursa becomes infected, with systemic symptoms such as fever and malaise, as well as local symptoms such as rubor, color, and dolor.

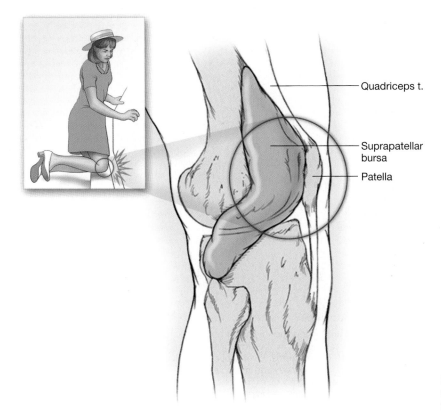

Quadriceps t.

Suprapatellar bursa

Patella

Figure 102-1 Suprapatellar bursitis is usually the result of direct trauma from either acute injury or repeated microtrauma, such as prolonged kneeling.

TESTING

Plain radiographs and magnetic resonance imaging (MRI) of the knee may reveal calcification of the bursa and associated structures, including the quadriceps tendon, findings consistent with chronic inflammation (Fig. 102-2). MRI is indicated if internal derangement, an occult mass, or a tumor of the knee is suspected. Electromyography can distinguish suprapatellar bursitis from femoral neuropathy, lumbar radiculopathy, and plexopathy. The injection technique described later serves as both a diagnostic and a therapeutic maneuver. A complete blood count, automated chemistry profile including uric acid level, erythrocyte sedimentation rate, and antinuclear antibody testing are indicated if collagen vascular disease is suspected. If infection is a possibility, aspiration, Gram stain, and culture of bursal fluid should be performed on an emergency basis.

DIFFERENTIAL DIAGNOSIS

Because of the anatomy of the region, the associated tendons and other bursae of the knee can become inflamed along with the suprapatellar bursa, thus confusing the diagnosis. Both the quadriceps tendon and the suprapatellar bursa are subject to inflammation from overuse, misuse, or direct trauma. The tendon fibers, called expansions, are vulnerable to strain, and the tendon

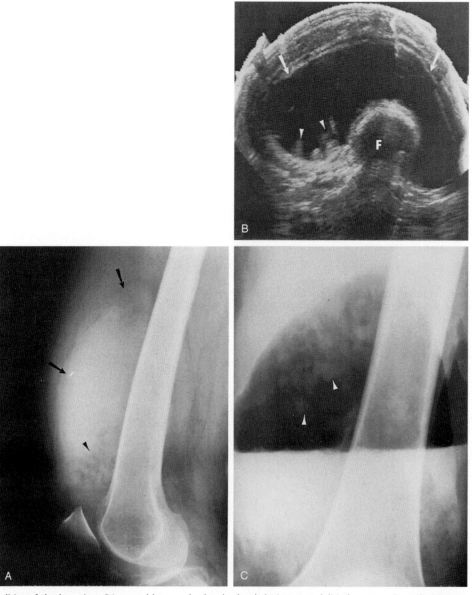

Figure 102-2 Abnormalities of the knee in a 54-year-old man who has had ankylosing spondylitis for approximately 25 years. Multiple episodes of painless swelling of the suprapatellar region were followed by spontaneous resolution. At the time of these imaging studies, aspiration of fluid in the distended suprapatellar pouch produced 3000 cells/mm³ and no growth of organisms. Over a period of several weeks, the swelling resolved. **A,** Lateral radiograph demonstrates massive distention of the suprapatellar pouch *(arrows)* and multiple nodular radiolucent shadows *(arrowhead)*. **B,** On a transverse sonogram, note the distended bursa *(arrows)* containing nodular synovial excrescences *(arrowheads)*. F, femur. **C,** Upright frontal image during double-contrast arthrography documents nodular synovial hyperplasia *(arrowheads)* in the distended suprapatellar pouch. *(From Resnick D: Diagnosis of bone and joint disorders, ed 4, Philadelphia, 2002, Saunders, p 1058.)*

proper is subject to the development of tendinitis. The suprapatellar, infrapatellar, and prepatellar bursae may also become inflamed with dysfunction of the quadriceps tendon. Anything that alters the normal biomechanics of the knee can result in inflammation of the suprapatellar bursa.

TREATMENT

A short course of conservative therapy consisting of simple analgesics, nonsteroidal antiinflammatory drugs (NSAIDs), or cyclooxygenase-2 inhibitors and a knee brace to prevent further trauma is the first step in the treatment of suprapatellar bursitis. If patients do not experience rapid improvement, injection is a reasonable next step.

To perform the injection, the patient is placed in the supine position with a rolled blanket underneath the knee to flex the joint gently. The skin overlying the medial aspect of the knee joint is prepared with antiseptic solution. A sterile syringe containing 2 mL of 0.25% preservative-free bupivacaine and 40 mg methylprednisolone is attached to a 1½-inch, 25-gauge needle by using strict aseptic technique. The superior margin of the medial patella is identified. Just above this point, the needle is inserted horizontally to slide beneath the quadriceps tendon. If the needle strikes the femur, it is withdrawn slightly and is redirected with a more anterior trajectory. When the needle is in position just below the quadriceps tendon, the contents of the syringe are gently injected. Little resistance to injection should be felt. If resistance is encountered, the needle is probably in a ligament or tendon and should be advanced or withdrawn slightly until the injection can proceed without significant resistance. The needle is removed, and a sterile pressure dressing and ice pack are applied to the injection site.

Physical modalities, including local heat and gentle range-of-motion exercises, should be introduced several days after the patient undergoes injection. Vigorous exercises should be avoided, because they will exacerbate the patient's symptoms. Simple analgesics and NSAIDs can be used concurrently with this injection technique.

COMPLICATIONS AND PITFALLS

Failure to identify primary or metastatic tumor of the distal femur or knee joint that is causing the patient's pain can have disastrous results. The injection technique is safe if careful attention is paid to the clinically relevant anatomy. The major complication of injection is infection, although this should be exceedingly rare if strict aseptic technique is followed. Approximately 25% of patients complain of a transient increase in pain after injection, and patients should be warned of this possibility.

Clinical Pearls

Coexistent bursitis, tendinitis, arthritis, and internal derangement of the knee may contribute to the patient's pain, thus necessitating additional treatment with more localized injection of local anesthetic and methylprednisolone. The injection technique described is extremely effective in treating the pain of suprapatellar bursitis.

SUGGESTED READINGS

O'Keeffe SA, Hogan BA, Eustace SJ, et al: Overuse injuries of the knee, *Magn Reson Imaging Clin N Am* 17(4):725–739, 2009.

Waldman SD: Bursitis syndromes of the knee. In *Pain review,* Philadelphia, 2009, Saunders, pp 318–322.

Waldman SD: Injection technique for suprapatellar bursitis. In *Pain review,* Philadelphia, 2009, Saunders, pp 584–585.

Chapter **103**

PREPATELLAR BURSITIS

ICD-9 CODE **726.65**

ICD-10 CODE **M70.40**

THE CLINICAL SYNDROME

The prepatellar bursa lies between the subcutaneous tissues and the patella. This bursa is held in place by the patellar ligament. The prepatellar bursa may exist as a single bursal sac or, in some patients, as a multisegmented series of loculated sacs. The prepatellar bursa is vulnerable to injury from both acute trauma and repeated microtrauma. Acute injuries are caused by direct trauma to the bursa during falls onto the knee or patellar fracture. Overuse injuries may be caused by running on soft or uneven surfaces or jobs that require crawling or kneeling, such as carpet laying or scrubbing floors, hence the other name for prepatellar bursitis: housemaid's knee (Fig. 103-1). If inflammation of the prepatellar bursa becomes chronic, calcification may occur.

SIGNS AND SYMPTOMS

Patients suffering from prepatellar bursitis complain of pain and swelling in the anterior knee over the patella that can radiate superiorly and inferiorly into the surrounding area. Often, patients are unable to kneel or walk down stairs. Patients may also complain of a sharp "catching" sensation with range of motion of the knee, especially on first arising. Prepatellar bursitis often coexists with arthritis and tendinitis of the knee, which can confuse the clinical picture.

TESTING

Plain radiographs and magnetic resonance imaging (MRI) of the knee may reveal calcification of the bursa and associated structures, including the quadriceps tendon, consistent with chronic inflammation. MRI is indicated if internal derangement, an occult mass, infection, or a tumor of the knee is suspected (Fig. 103-2). Ultrasound imaging can also help clarify the diagnosis (Fig. 103-3). Electromyography can distinguish prepatellar bursitis from femoral neuropathy, lumbar radiculopathy, and plexopathy.

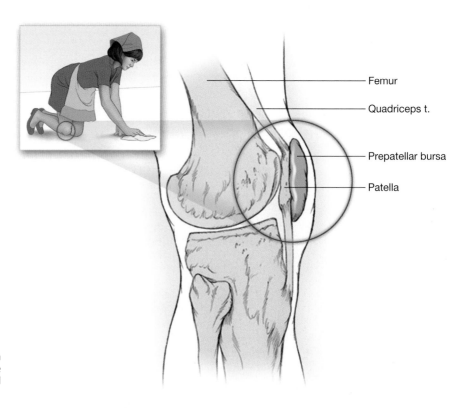

Femur

Quadriceps t.

Prepatellar bursa

Patella

Figure 103-1 Prepatellar bursitis is also known as housemaid's knee because of its prevalence among people whose work requires prolonged crawling or kneeling.

The injection technique described later serves as both a diagnostic and a therapeutic maneuver. Antinuclear antibody testing is indicated if collagen vascular disease is suspected. If infection is a possibility, aspiration, Gram stain, and culture of bursal fluid should be performed on an emergency basis.

DIFFERENTIAL DIAGNOSIS

Because of the anatomy of the region, the associated tendons and other bursae of the knee can become inflamed along with the prepatellar bursa, thus confusing the diagnosis. Both the quadriceps tendon and the prepatellar bursa are subject to inflammation from overuse, misuse, or direct trauma. The tendon fibers, called expansions, are vulnerable to strain, and the tendon proper is subject to the development of tendinitis. The suprapatellar, infrapatellar, and prepatellar bursae may also become inflamed with dysfunction of the quadriceps tendon. Anything that alters the normal biomechanics of the knee can result in inflammation of the prepatellar bursa.

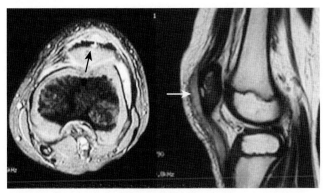

Figure 103-2 Axial and sagittal magnetic resonance imaging views demonstrate inflammatory thickening of the prepatellar bursa. A mild defect on the anterior cortex of the patella *(arrows)* is evident. *(From Choi H-R: Patellar osteomyelitis presenting as prepatellar bursitis,* Knee *14[4]:333–335, 2007.)*

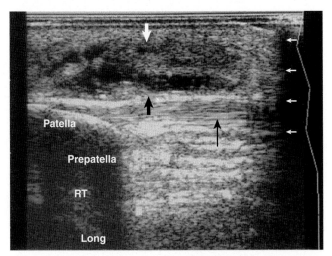

Figure 103-3 Prepatellar bursitis. Longitudinal midline scan over the inferior pole of patella in a 42-year-old garden paver presenting with chronic anterior knee pain. The prepatellar bursa *(between heavy arrows)* is markedly thickened and distended by a combination of synovial proliferation, a finding indicating chronic irritation and fluid. The bursa lies superficial to the patella and the normal fibrillary pattern of the patella tendon *(thin arrow). (From Ptasznik R: Ultrasound in acute and chronic knee injury,* Radiol Clin North Am *37[4]:797–830, 1999.)*

TREATMENT

A short course of conservative therapy consisting of simple analgesics, nonsteroidal antiinflammatory drugs (NSAIDs), or cyclooxygenase-2 inhibitors and a knee brace to prevent further trauma is the first step in the treatment of prepatellar bursitis. If patients do not experience rapid improvement, injection is a reasonable next step.

To perform the injection, the patient is placed in the supine position with a rolled blanket underneath the knee to flex the joint gently. The skin overlying the patella is prepared with antiseptic solution. A sterile syringe containing 2 mL of 0.25% preservative-free bupivacaine and 40 mg methylprednisolone is attached to a 1½-inch, 25-gauge needle by using strict aseptic technique. The center of the medial patella is identified. Just above this point, the needle is inserted horizontally to slide subcutaneously into the prepatellar bursa (Fig. 103-4). If the needle strikes the patella, it is withdrawn slightly and is redirected with a more anterior trajectory. When the needle is positioned in proximity to the prepatellar bursa, the contents of the syringe are gently injected. Little resistance to injection should be felt. If resistance is encountered, the needle is probably in a ligament or tendon and should be advanced or withdrawn slightly until the injection can proceed without significant resistance. The needle is removed, and a sterile pressure dressing and ice pack are applied to the injection site.

Physical modalities, including local heat and gentle range-of-motion exercises, should be introduced several days after the patient undergoes injection. Vigorous exercises should be avoided, because they will exacerbate the patient's symptoms. Simple analgesics and NSAIDs can be used concurrently with this injection technique.

COMPLICATIONS AND PITFALLS

Failure to identify primary or metastatic tumor of the distal femur or knee joint that is causing the patient's pain can have disastrous results. The injection technique is safe if careful attention is paid to the clinically relevant anatomy. The major complication

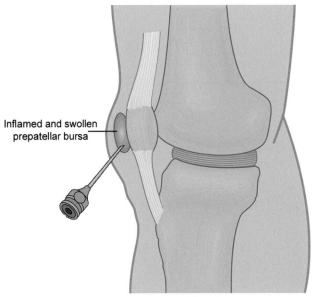

Inflamed and swollen prepatellar bursa

Figure 103-4 Correct needle placement for injection of the prepatellar bursa. *(From Waldman SD: Atlas of pain management injection techniques, Philadelphia, 2000, Saunders.)*

of injection is infection, although this should be exceedingly rare if strict aseptic technique is followed. Approximately 25% of patients complain of a transient increase in pain after injection, and patients should be warned of this possibility.

Clinical Pearls

Coexistent bursitis, tendinitis, arthritis, and internal derangement of the knee may contribute to the patient's pain, thus necessitating additional treatment with more localized injection of local anesthetic and methylprednisolone. The injection technique described is extremely effective in treating the pain of prepatellar bursitis.

SUGGESTED READINGS

Choi H-R: Patellar osteomyelitis presenting as prepatellar bursitis, *Knee* 14(4): 333–335, 2007.

O'Keeffe SA, Hogan BA, Eustace SJ, et al: Overuse injuries of the knee, *Magn Reson Imaging Clin N Am* 17(4):725–739, 2009.

Waldman SD: Prepatellar bursitis pain. In *Atlas of pain management injection techniques,* ed 2, Philadelphia, 2007, Saunders, pp 454–457.

Waldman SD: Prepatellar bursitis. In *Pain review,* Philadelphia, 2009, Saunders, pp 586–587.

Waldman SD: Bursitis syndromes of the knee. In *Pain review,* Philadelphia, 2009, Saunders, pp 318–322.

Chapter 104

SUPERFICIAL INFRAPATELLAR BURSITIS

ICD-9 CODE 726.69

ICD-10 CODE M76.899

THE CLINICAL SYNDROME

The superficial infrapatellar bursa lies between the subcutaneous tissues and the upper part of the patellar ligament. This bursa may exist as a single bursal sac or, in some patients, as a multisegmented series of loculated sacs. The superficial infrapatellar bursa is vulnerable to injury from both acute trauma and repeated microtrauma. Acute injuries are caused by direct trauma to the bursa during falls onto the knee or patellar fracture. Overuse injuries are caused by running on soft or uneven surfaces or doing jobs that require crawling or kneeling, such as carpet laying or scrubbing floors (Fig. 104-1). If inflammation of the superficial infrapatellar bursa becomes chronic, calcification may occur.

SIGNS AND SYMPTOMS

Patients with superficial infrapatellar bursitis complain of pain and swelling in the anterior knee over the patella that can radiate superiorly and inferiorly into the surrounding area. Often, patients are unable to kneel or walk down stairs. Patients may also complain of a sharp "catching" sensation with range of motion of the knee, especially on first arising. Superficial infrapatellar bursitis often coexists with arthritis and tendinitis of the knee, which can confuse the clinical picture.

TESTING

Plain radiographs and magnetic resonance imaging (MRI) of the knee may reveal calcification of the bursa and associated structures, including the quadriceps and patellar tendons, findings consistent with chronic inflammation (Fig. 104-2). Other occult abnormalities may also be identified that may mimic the pain of

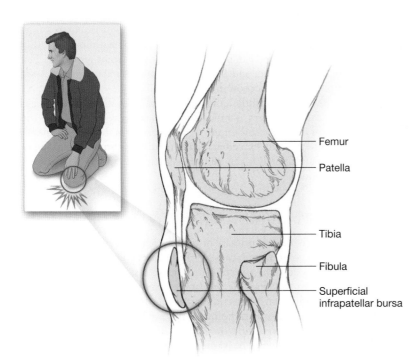

Femur
Patella
Tibia
Fibula
Superficial infrapatellar bursa

Figure 104-1 Infrapatellar bursitis is a common cause of inferior knee pain.

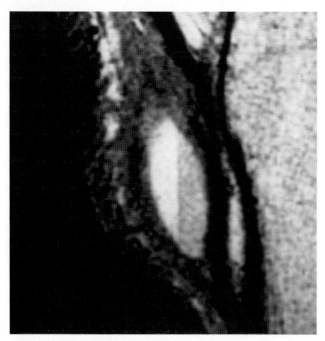

Figure 104-2 Superficial infrapatellar bursitis. A fluid level within the bursa is evident on this sagittal fast spin-echo magnetic resonance image. *(From Resnick D: Diagnosis of bone and joint disorders, ed 4, Philadelphia, 2002, Saunders, p 4257.)*

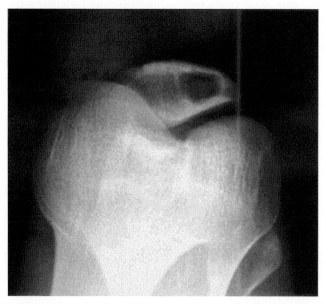

Figure 104-3 Skyline view of the knee showing a well-defined contained osteolytic lesion in the patella with a sequestrum consistent with a diagnosis of tuberculosis of the patella. *(From Mittal R, Trikha V, Rastogi S: Tuberculosis of patella,* Knee *13[1]:54–56, 2006.)*

infrapatellar bursitis (Fig. 104-3). MRI is indicated if internal derangement, an occult mass, or a tumor of the knee is suspected. Electromyography can distinguish superficial infrapatellar bursitis from femoral neuropathy, lumbar radiculopathy, and plexopathy. The injection technique described later serves as both a diagnostic and a therapeutic maneuver. Antinuclear antibody testing is indicated if collagen vascular disease is suspected. If infection is a possibility, aspiration, Gram stain, and culture of bursal fluid should be performed on an emergency basis.

DIFFERENTIAL DIAGNOSIS

Because of the anatomy of the region, the associated tendons and other bursae of the knee can become inflamed along with the superficial infrapatellar bursa, thus confusing the diagnosis. Both the quadriceps tendon and the superficial infrapatellar bursa are subject to inflammation from overuse, misuse, or direct trauma. The tendon fibers, called expansions, are vulnerable to strain, and the tendon proper is subject to the development of tendinitis. The infrapatellar fat pad is also subject to various abnormalities including Hoffa's disease, which can mimic the pain of superficial infrapatellar bursitis. The suprapatellar, infrapatellar, and prepatellar bursae may also become inflamed with dysfunction of the quadriceps tendon. Anything that alters the normal biomechanics of the knee can result in inflammation of the superficial infrapatellar bursa.

TREATMENT

A short course of conservative therapy consisting of simple analgesics, nonsteroidal antiinflammatory drugs (NSAIDs), or cyclooxygenase-2 inhibitors, and a knee brace to prevent further trauma is the first step in the treatment of superficial infrapatellar bursitis. If patients do not experience rapid improvement, injection is a reasonable next step.

To inject the superficial infrapatellar bursa, the patient is placed in the supine position with a rolled blanket underneath the knee to flex the joint gently. The skin overlying the patella is prepared with antiseptic solution. A sterile syringe containing 2 mL of 0.25% preservative-free bupivacaine and 40 mg methylprednisolone is attached to a 1½-inch, 25-gauge needle by using strict aseptic technique. The center of the lower pole of the patella is identified. Just below this point, the needle is inserted at a 45-degree angle to slide subcutaneously into the superficial infrapatellar bursa. If the needle strikes the patella, it is withdrawn slightly and is redirected with a more inferior trajectory. When the needle is positioned in proximity to the superficial infrapatellar bursa, the contents of the syringe are gently injected. Little resistance to injection should be felt. If resistance is encountered, the needle is probably in a ligament or tendon and should be advanced or withdrawn slightly until the injection can proceed without significant resistance. The needle is removed, and a sterile pressure dressing and ice pack are applied to the injection site.

Physical modalities, including local heat and gentle range-of-motion exercises, should be introduced several days after the patient undergoes injection. Vigorous exercises should be avoided, because they will exacerbate the patient's symptoms. Simple analgesics and NSAIDs can be used concurrently with this injection technique.

COMPLICATIONS AND PITFALLS

Failure to identify primary or metastatic tumor of the distal femur or knee joint that is causing the patient's pain can have disastrous results. The injection technique is safe if careful attention is paid to the clinically relevant anatomy. The major complication of injection is infection, although this should be exceedingly rare if strict aseptic technique is followed. Approximately 25% of patients complain of a transient increase in pain after injection, and patients should be warned of this possibility.

Clinical Pearls

Coexistent bursitis, tendinitis, arthritis, and internal derangement of the knee may contribute to the patient's pain, thus necessitating additional treatment with more localized injection of local anesthetic and methylprednisolone. The injection technique described is extremely effective in treating the pain of superficial infrapatellar bursitis.

SUGGESTED READINGS

O'Keeffe SA, Hogan BA, Eustace SJ, et al: Overuse injuries of the knee, *Magn Reson Imaging Clin N Am* 17(4):725–739, 2009.

Waldman SD: Bursitis syndromes of the knee. In *Pain review*, Philadelphia, 2009, Saunders, pp 318–322.

Waldman SD: Injection technique for superficial infrapatellar bursitis. In *Pain review*, Philadelphia, 2009, Saunders, pp 587–588.

Waldman SD: The superficial infrapatellar bursa. In *Pain review*, Philadelphia, 2009, Saunders, pp 151–152.

Chapter **105**

DEEP INFRAPATELLAR BURSITIS

ICD-9 CODE `726.69`

ICD-10 CODE `M76.899`

THE CLINICAL SYNDROME

The deep infrapatellar bursa lies between the patellar ligament and the tibia. This bursa may exist as a single bursal sac or, in some patients, as a multisegmented series of loculated sacs. The deep infrapatellar bursa is vulnerable to injury from both acute trauma and repeated microtrauma. Acute injuries are caused by direct trauma to the bursa during falls onto the knee (Fig. 105-1) or patellar fracture. Overuse injuries are caused by running on soft or uneven surfaces or jobs that require crawling and kneeling, such as carpet laying or scrubbing floors. If inflammation of the deep infrapatellar bursa becomes chronic, calcification may occur.

SIGNS AND SYMPTOMS

Patients with deep infrapatellar bursitis complain of pain and swelling in the anterior knee below the patella that can radiate inferiorly into the surrounding area. Often, patients are unable to kneel or walk down stairs. They may also complain of a sharp "catching" sensation with range of motion of the knee, especially on first arising. Infrapatellar bursitis often coexists with arthritis and tendinitis of the knee, which can confuse the clinical picture.

Physical examination may reveal point tenderness in the anterior knee just below the patella. Swelling and fluid accumulation surrounding the lower patella are often present. Passive flexion and active resisted extension of the knee reproduce the pain. Sudden release of resistance during this maneuver causes a marked increase in pain. The deep infrapatellar bursa is not as susceptible to infection as is the superficial infrapatellar bursa.

TESTING

Plain radiographs, ultrasound, and magnetic resonance imaging (MRI) of the knee may reveal calcification of the bursa and associated structures, including the quadriceps tendon, findings consistent with chronic inflammation (Figs. 105-2 and 105-3). MRI is indicated if internal derangement, an occult mass, or a tumor of the knee is suspected. Electromyography can distinguish deep infrapatellar bursitis from femoral neuropathy, lumbar radiculopathy, and plexopathy. The injection technique described later serves as both a diagnostic and a therapeutic maneuver. Antinuclear

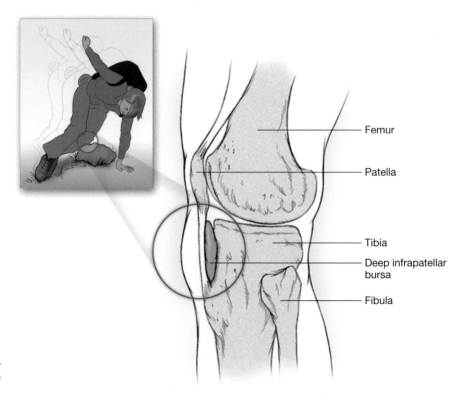

Femur

Patella

Tibia

Deep infrapatellar bursa

Fibula

Figure 105-1 Deep infrapatellar bursitis may result from direct trauma, such as falling on the knee.

antibody testing is indicated if collagen vascular disease is suspected. If infection is a possibility, aspiration, Gram stain, and culture of bursal fluid should be performed on an emergency basis.

DIFFERENTIAL DIAGNOSIS

Because of the anatomy of the region, the associated tendons and other bursae of the knee can become inflamed along with the deep infrapatellar bursa, thus confusing the diagnosis. Both the quadriceps tendon and the deep infrapatellar bursa are subject to inflammation from overuse, misuse, or direct trauma. The tendon fibers, called expansions, are vulnerable to strain, and the tendon proper is subject to the development of tendinitis. The suprapatellar, infrapatellar, and prepatellar bursae may also become inflamed with dysfunction of the quadriceps tendon. Anything that alters the normal biomechanics of the knee can result in inflammation of the deep infrapatellar bursa.

TREATMENT

A short course of conservative therapy consisting of simple analgesics, nonsteroidal antiinflammatory drugs (NSAIDs), or cyclooxygenase-2 inhibitors, and a knee brace to prevent further trauma is the first step in the treatment of deep infrapatellar bursitis. If patients do not experience rapid improvement, injection is a reasonable next step.

To inject the deep infrapatellar bursa, the patient is placed in the supine position with a rolled blanket underneath the knee to flex the joint gently. The skin overlying the medial portion of the lower margin of the patella is prepared with antiseptic solution. A sterile syringe containing 2 mL of 0.25% preservative-free bupivacaine and 40 mg methylprednisolone is attached to a 1½-inch, 25-gauge needle by using strict aseptic technique. The medial lower margin of the patella is identified. Just below this point, the needle is inserted at a right angle to the patella to slide beneath the patellar ligament into the deep infrapatellar bursa. If the needle strikes the patella, it is withdrawn slightly and is redirected with a more inferior trajectory. When the needle is positioned in proximity to the deep infrapatellar bursa, the contents of the syringe are gently injected. Little resistance to injection should be felt. If resistance is encountered, the needle is probably in a ligament or tendon and should be advanced or withdrawn slightly until the injection can proceed without significant resistance. The needle is

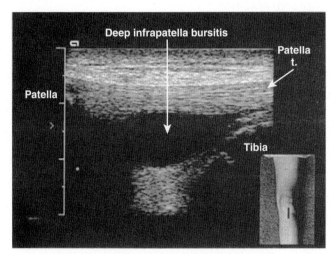

Figure 105-2 Deep infrapatellar bursitis. Longitudinal midline scan over the distal patella in a 24-year-old middle-distance runner presenting with the recent onset of pain over the distal patella tendon. The clinical diagnosis was distal patella tendinopathy. A 2.5 × 1-cm oval sonolucent fluid collection (arrow) can be seen between the normal-appearing patella tendon and the proximal anterior tibial cortex. (From Ptasznik R: Ultrasound in acute and chronic knee injury, Radiol Clin North Am 37[4]:797–830, 1999.)

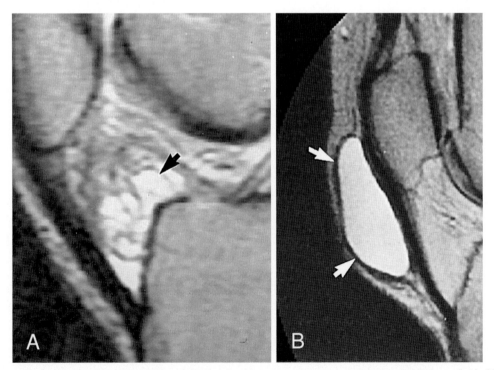

Figure 105-3 **A,** Deep infrapatellar bursitis. Sagittal, T2-weighted, spin-echo magnetic resonance imaging (MRI) shows fluid of high signal intensity (arrow) in the deep infrapatellar bursa. **B,** Prepatellar bursitis. Sagittal, T2-weighted, spin-echo MRI shows fluid of high signal intensity (arrows) in the prepatellar bursa. (From Resnick D: Diagnosis of bone and joint disorders, ed 4, Philadelphia, 2002, Saunders, p 3285.)

removed, and a sterile pressure dressing and ice pack are applied to the injection site.

Physical modalities, including local heat and gentle range-of-motion exercises, should be introduced several days after the patient undergoes injection. Vigorous exercises should be avoided, because they will exacerbate the patient's symptoms. Simple analgesics and NSAIDs can be used concurrently with this injection technique.

COMPLICATIONS AND PITFALLS

Failure to identify primary or metastatic tumor of the distal femur or knee joint that is causing the patient's pain can have disastrous results. The injection technique is safe if careful attention is paid to the clinically relevant anatomy. The major complication of injection is infection, although this should be exceedingly rare if strict aseptic technique is followed. Approximately 25% of patients complain of a transient increase in pain after injection, and patients should be warned of this possibility.

Clinical Pearls

Coexistent bursitis, tendinitis, arthritis, and internal derangement of the knee may contribute to the patient's pain, thus necessitating additional treatment with more localized injection of local anesthetic and methylprednisolone. The injection technique described is extremely effective in treating the pain of deep infrapatellar bursitis.

SUGGESTED READINGS

O'Keeffe SA, Hogan BA, Eustace SJ, et al: Overuse injuries of the knee, *Magn Reson Imaging Clin N Am* 17(4):725–739, 2009.

Ptasznik R: Ultrasound in acute and chronic knee injury, *Radiol Clin North Am* 37(4):797–830, 1999.

Waldman SD: Bursitis syndromes of the knee. In *Pain review,* Philadelphia, 2009, Saunders, pp 318–322.

Waldman SD: Injection technique for deep infrapatellar bursitis. In *Pain review,* Philadelphia, 2009, Saunders, pp 589–590.

Chapter 106

OSGOOD-SCHLATTER DISEASE

ICD-9 CODE 732.4

ICD-10 CODE M92.50

THE CLINICAL SYNDROME

Osgood-Schlatter disease is characterized by anterior knee pain that is exacerbated by stress on the quadriceps mechanism and by direct pressure on the tibial tuberosity. Although the disease can affect all ages, most cases occur in adolescents, with a peak incidence at approximately 13 years of age. Boys and men are affected two to three times more often than are girls and women, although some investigators believe that the number of female cases is on the rise as a result of increased female participation in competitive sports. The pain and functional disability associated with Osgood-Schlatter disease are bilateral in 25% to 30% of patients, and one side often has more severe symptoms. Osgood-Schlatter disease is usually the result of overuse or misuse of the knee joint caused by running, jumping, or overtraining on hard surfaces, as well as any other activities that require repetitive quadriceps contraction (Fig. 106-1). Competitive sports most often implicated in the development of Osgood-Schlatter disease include soccer, gymnastics, basketball, ballet, track, hockey, baseball, and Irish and Scottish Highland–style dancing (Table 106-1).

The quadriceps tendon is made of fibers from the four muscles that constitute the quadriceps muscle: vastus lateralis, vastus intermedius, vastus medialis, and rectus femoris. These muscles are the primary extensors of the lower extremity at the knee. The tendons of these muscles converge and unite to form a single, exceedingly strong tendon. The patella functions as a sesamoid bone within the quadriceps tendon, with fibers of the tendon expanding around the patella and forming the medial and lateral patella retinacula, which strengthen the knee joint. The patellar tendon extends from the patella to the tibial tuberosity (see Fig. 100-2). The tibial tuberosity is the nidus of the pain and functional disability associated with Osgood-Schlatter disease because the repetitive stresses applied to the tibial tuberosity by contraction of the quadriceps mechanism result in apophysitis and heterotopic bone growth. These responses to the damage induced by repetitive stress are most often seen during the period of rapid skeletal growth associated with adolescence, although as mentioned earlier, this disease has been reported in all age groups.

SIGNS AND SYMPTOMS

Patients with Osgood-Schlatter disease present with pain over the anterior knee and with pressure on the tibial tuberosity. Patients note increased pain on walking down slopes or up and down stairs, as well as during any activity that involves contraction of

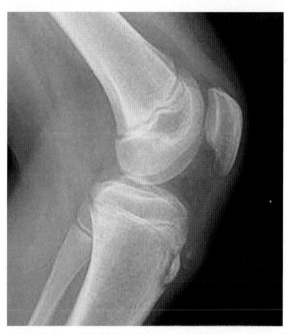

Figure 106-1 Osgood-Schlatter disease of the tibial apophysis. *(From DeLee JC, Drez DD, Miller M, editors:* Orthopaedic sports medicine: principles and practice, *ed 3, Philadelphia, 2010, Saunders, p 1526.)*

TABLE 106-1
Sports Commonly Associated With Osgood-Schlatter Disease
• Soccer
• Gymnastics
• Basketball
• Baseball
• Track
• Hockey
• Ballet
• Irish-style line dancing
• Scottish Highland–style dancing

the quadriceps mechanism. Activity using the knee makes the pain worse, whereas rest and heat provide some relief. The pain is constant and is characterized as aching; it may interfere with sleep. On physical examination, the patient notes significant pain on palpation of the tibial tuberosity, as well as tenderness to palpation of the patellar tendon. Enlargement of the tibial tuberosity is often readily apparent, and this cosmetic defect can cause significant anxiety in the patient and parents. Generalized swelling

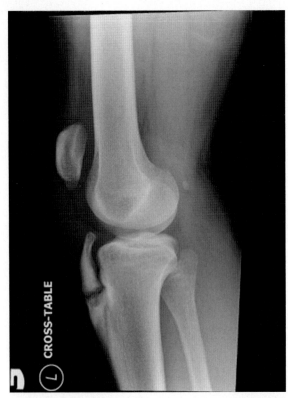

Figure 106-2 Radiograph of the left knee on initial presentation. A large ossicle, 4 cm in length, seen at the tibial tubercle, separated from the tubercle. The ossicle is seen indenting into the joint space. *(From Talawadekar GD, Mostofi B, Housden P: Unusually large sized bony ossicle in Osgood Schlatter disease, Eur J Radiol Extra 69[1]:e37–e39, 2009.)*

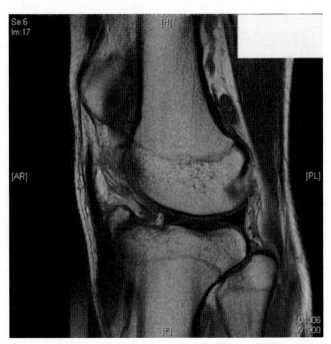

Figure 106-3 Magnetic resonance imaging of the left knee shows a large accessory apophysis indenting into Hoffa's fat pad with high signal changes between the tibia and the accessory apophysis and the patellar tendon, findings signifying inflammation. *(From Talawadekar GD, Mostofi B, Housden P: Unusually large sized bony ossicle in Osgood-Schlatter disease, Eur J Radiol Extra 69[1]:e37–e39, 2009.)*

of the joint may be present, and thickening of the patellar tendon may be appreciated on careful physical examination. Active resisted extension of the knee reproduces the pain, as does pressure on the tibial tuberosity. Coexistent suprapatellar and infrapatellar bursitis, tendinitis, arthritis, or internal derangement of the knee may confuse the clinical picture after trauma to the knee.

TESTING

Plain radiographs are indicated in all patients who present with knee pain who are suspected of suffering from Osgood-Schlatter disease (Fig. 106-2). Magnetic resonance imaging of the knee is indicated if Osgood-Schlatter disease is suspected, because it readily detects any disorder of the patellar tendon, as well as the condition of the tibial tuberosity (Fig. 106-3). Ultrasound imaging may also provide beneficial information regarding the vascularity and integrity of the patellar tendons and the presence of tibial tuberosity abnormalities (Fig. 106-4). Bone scan may be useful to identify occult stress fractures involving the joint, especially if trauma has occurred. Based on the patient's clinical presentation, additional testing may be indicated, including a complete blood count, erythrocyte sedimentation rate, and antinuclear antibody testing.

DIFFERENTIAL DIAGNOSIS

Osgood-Schlatter disease is a repetitive stress disorder that is a distinct clinical entity from tendinitis of the patellar tendons or quadriceps expansion syndrome. However, such tendinitis, bursitis, and other painful conditions that affect the anterior knee may coexist with Osgood-Schlatter disease and may confuse the clinical picture. Quadriceps expansion syndrome has a predilection for the medial side of the superior pole of the patella. The quadriceps tendon is also subject to acute calcific tendinitis, which may coexist with acute strain injuries and the more chronic changes of Osgood-Schlatter disease. Calcific tendinitis of the quadriceps has a characteristic radiographic appearance of whiskers on the anterosuperior patella. The suprapatellar, infrapatellar, and prepatellar bursae also may become inflamed with dysfunction of the quadriceps tendon. Hoffa's syndrome, which is a disease affecting the infrapatellar fat pad, may also coexist with Osgood-Schlatter disease.

TREATMENT

Initial treatment of the pain and functional disability associated with Osgood-Schlatter disease includes a combination of nonsteroidal antiinflammatory drugs or cyclooxygenase-2 inhibitors and rest, with the patient avoiding activities that involve contraction of the quadriceps mechanism. The use of therapeutic cold may also provide symptom relief. Gentle physical therapy consisting of stretching of the quadriceps mechanism and the opposing hamstring muscles should be implemented as the patient's symptoms allow. A nighttime splint and knee pads to protect the knee, as well as the use of an infrapatellar strap during activity, may also help relieve symptoms. For patients who do not respond to these treatment modalities, injection of the tibial tuberosity with local anesthetic and steroid is a reasonable next step.

To perform the injection, the patient is placed in the supine position with a rolled blanket underneath the knee to flex the

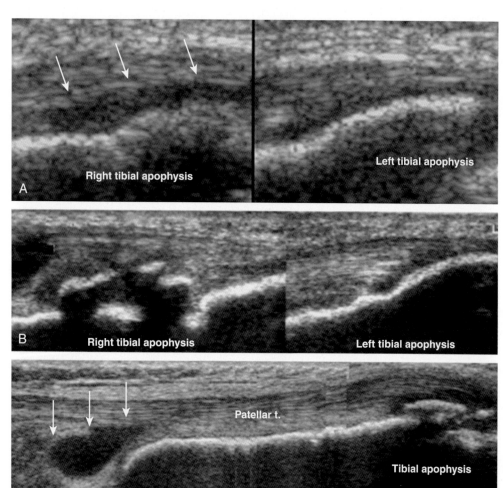

Figure 106-4 Osgood-Schlatter disease. **A,** Comparative sagittal ultrasound scans: cartilage swelling can be seen in the right tibial apophysis *(arrows)*. **B,** Comparative sagittal ultrasound scans: fragmentation of the right tibial tubercle ossification center. **C,** The sagittal ultrasound scan shows reactive bursitis of the deep tibial patellar bursa *(arrows)*, besides fragmentation of the tibial tubercle ossification center. *(From Draghi F, Danesino GM, Coscia D, et al: Overload syndromes of the knee in adolescents: sonographic findings,* J Ultrasound *11[4]:151–157, 2008.)*

joint gently. The patellar tendon is identified, and the skin overlying the medial portion of the lower margin of the patella is prepared with antiseptic solution. A sterile syringe containing 2 mL of 0.25% preservative-free bupivacaine and 40 mg methylprednisolone is attached to a 1½-inch, 25-gauge needle by using strict aseptic technique. The medial lower margin of the patella is identified. Just below this point, the needle is inserted at a right angle to the patella to slide beneath the patellar ligament into the region of the deep infrapatellar bursa. If the needle strikes the patella, it is withdrawn slightly and is redirected with a more inferior trajectory. When the needle is in position in proximity to the region beneath the patellar tendon, the contents of the syringe are gently injected. Little resistance to injection should be felt. If resistance is encountered, the needle is probably in a ligament or tendon and should be advanced or withdrawn slightly until the injection can proceed without significant resistance. The needle is removed, and a sterile pressure dressing and ice pack are applied to the injection site.

If the foregoing modalities fail to relieve the patient's symptoms, some experts recommend complete rest of the affected knee by application of a cast for a 4- to 6-week period. In recalcitrant cases, excision of the tibial tuberosity and associated ossicles may be required.

COMPLICATIONS AND PITFALLS

Failure to identify primary or metastatic tumor of the distal femur or knee joint that is causing the patient's pain can have disastrous results. The injection technique is safe if careful attention is paid to the clinically relevant anatomy. The major complication of injection is infection, although it should be exceedingly rare if strict aseptic technique is followed. Approximately 25% of patients complain of a transient increase in pain after injection, and patients should be warned of this possibility.

Clinical Pearls

Coexistent bursitis, tendinitis, arthritis, and internal derangement of the knee may contribute to the patient's pain, thus necessitating additional treatment with more localized injection of local anesthetic and methylprednisolone. The injection technique described is extremely effective in treating the pain of Osgood-Schlatter disease. Patients and their families often require repeated reassurance regarding the enlargement of the tibial tuberosity and clear statements that such enlargement is definitely not cancer. Such reassurance is the only thing that will lessen their anxiety regarding the common cause of anterior knee pain.

SUGGESTED READINGS

Benjamin M, Kumai T, Milz S, et al: The skeletal attachment of tendons: tendon "entheses", *Comp Biochem Physiol A Mol Integr Physiol* 133(4):931–945, 2002.

Draghi F, Danesino GM, Coscia D, et al: Overload syndromes of the knee in adolescents: sonographic findings, *J Ultrasound* 11(4):151–157, 2008.

Nicholas JA: Osgood-Schlatter disease. In Garfunkel LC, Kaczorowski J, Christy C, editors: *Pediatric clinical advisor,* ed 2, St Louis, 2007, Mosby, p 411.

Smith AD: Osgood-Schlatter disorder and related extensor mechanism problems. In Micheli LJ, Kocher M, editors: *The pediatric and adolescent knee,* Philadelphia, 2006, Saunders, pp 198–214.

Talawadekar GD, Mostofi B, Housden P: Unusually large sized bony ossicle in Osgood-Schlatter disease, *Eur J Radiol Extra* 69(1):e37–e39, 2009.

Chapter 107

BAKER'S CYST OF THE KNEE

ICD-9 CODE `727.51`

ICD-10 CODE `M70.20`

THE CLINICAL SYNDROME

When bursae become inflamed, they may overproduce synovial fluid, which can become trapped in a saclike cyst. Because of a one-way valve effect, this cyst gradually expands. Baker's cyst is the result of an abnormal accumulation of synovial fluid in the medial aspect of the popliteal fossa. Often, a tear of the medial meniscus or tendinitis of the medial hamstring is responsible for the development of Baker's cyst. Patients suffering from rheumatoid arthritis are especially susceptible to the development of Baker's cysts.

SIGNS AND SYMPTOMS

Patients with Baker's cysts complain of a feeling of fullness behind the knee. They may notice a lump behind the knee that becomes more apparent when they flex the knee. The cyst may continue to enlarge and dissect inferiorly into the calf (Fig. 107-1).

Patients suffering from rheumatoid arthritis are prone to this phenomenon, and the pain associated with dissection into the calf may be confused with thrombophlebitis, thus leading to inappropriate treatment with anticoagulants. Occasionally, Baker's cyst spontaneously ruptures, usually after frequent squatting. In this case, rubor and calor may be evident in the calf, again mimicking thrombophlebitis; however, Homans' sign is negative, and no cords are palpable.

On physical examination, patients with Baker's cysts have a cystic swelling in the medial aspect of the popliteal fossa that may be quite large. Activity that includes squatting or walking makes the pain worse, whereas rest and heat provide some relief. The pain is constant and is characterized as aching; it may interfere with sleep.

TESTING

Plain radiographs and magnetic resonance imaging (MRI) of the knee are indicated for all patients who present with Baker's cyst (Fig. 107-2). MRI can also detect internal derangement or an occult mass or tumor. Based on the patient's clinical presentation, additional testing may be warranted, including a complete blood count, erythrocyte sedimentation rate, and antinuclear antibody testing.

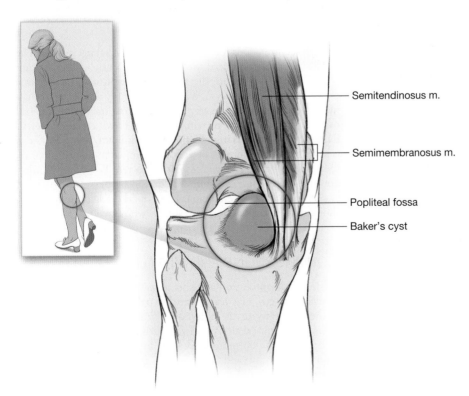

Semitendinosus m.

Semimembranosus m.

Popliteal fossa

Baker's cyst

Figure 107-1 Patients with Baker's cyst often complain of a sensation of fullness or a lump behind the knee.

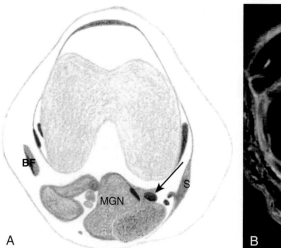

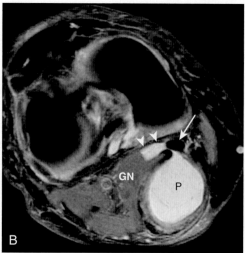

Figure 107-2 **A,** Drawing illustrating a popliteal cyst. This axial view shows a popliteal cyst (blue) located between the semimembranosus tendon *(arrow)* and the medial gastrocnemius muscle (MGN). BF, biceps femoris muscle and tendon; S, sartorius muscle. **B,** Axial proton density (PD) –weighted magnetic resonance image with fat suppression showing a large popliteal cyst (P) extending posteriorly between the medial gastrocnemius muscle (GN) and the semimembranosus tendon *(arrow)*. Note the communication between the popliteal cyst and the subgastrocnemius bursa *(arrowheads)*. *(From Marra MD, Crema MD, Chung M, et al: MRI features of cystic lesions around the knee,* Knee *15[6]:423–438, 2008.)*

Figure 107-3 Treatment of Baker's cyst. **A,** A needle *(arrows)* is introduced into the cyst under sonographic guidance. **B,** Once the cyst is empty, 40 mg triamcinolone acetate is injected. The injected substance appears as a fluid with echogenic dots filling the cyst *(open arrows)*. The *solid arrow* points to the needle.

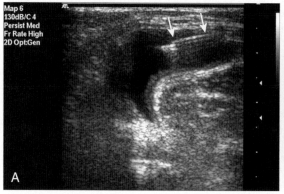

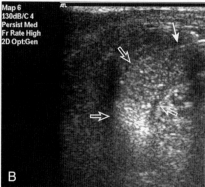

DIFFERENTIAL DIAGNOSIS

As mentioned, Baker's cysts may rupture spontaneously, thus leading to a misdiagnosis of thrombophlebitis. Occasionally, tendinitis of the medial hamstring or injury to the medial meniscus is confused with Baker's cyst. Primary or metastatic tumors in the region, although rare, must also be considered in the differential diagnosis. Care must be taken not to mistake a popliteal artery aneurysm for Baker's cyst. Careful palpation of the popliteal fossa should reveal a pulsatile mass if the artery is involved.

TREATMENT

Although surgery is often required to treat Baker's cyst, a short trial of conservative therapy consisting of an elastic bandage and nonsteroidal antiinflammatory drugs or cyclooxygenase-2 inhibitors is warranted. If these conservative measures fail, injection is a reasonable next step.

To inject Baker's cyst, the patient is placed in the prone position with the anterior ankle resting on a folded towel to flex the knee slightly. The middle of the popliteal fossa is identified, and at a point two finger breadths medial to and two finger breadths below the popliteal crease, the skin is prepared with antiseptic solution. A syringe containing 2 mL of 0.25% preservative-free bupivacaine and 40 mg

methylprednisolone is attached to a 2-inch, 22-gauge needle. The needle is carefully advanced through the previously identified point at a 45-degree angle from the medial border of the popliteal fossa directly toward Baker's cyst. While continuously aspirating, the clinician advances the needle very slowly, to avoid trauma to the tibial nerve or popliteal artery or vein. When the cyst is entered, synovial fluid suddenly appears in the syringe. At this point, if no paresthesia is noted in the distribution of the common peroneal or tibial nerve, the contents of the syringe are gently injected. Resistance to injection should be minimal. A pressure dressing is placed over the cyst to prevent fluid reaccumulation. Ultrasound guidance may aid the clinician in needle placement in patients whose anatomic landmarks are difficult to identify (Fig. 107-3).

COMPLICATIONS AND PITFALLS

Failure to diagnose primary knee disorders, such as tears of the medial meniscus, may lead to further pain and disability. Because of the proximity to the common peroneal and tibial nerves, as well as the popliteal artery and vein, it is imperative that injection of Baker's cysts be performed only by those familiar with the regional anatomy and experienced in the technique. Many patients complain of a transient increase in pain after injection, and infection, although rare, may occur.

Clinical Pearls

The injection technique described is extremely effective in treating the pain and swelling of Baker's cysts. Coexistent semimembranosus bursitis, medial hamstring tendinitis, and internal derangement of the knee may contribute to the patient's pain, thus necessitating additional treatment with more localized injection of local anesthetic and methylprednisolone.

SUGGESTED READINGS

Drescher MJ, Smally AJ: Thrombophlebitis and pseudothrombophlebitis in the ED, *Am J Emerg Med* 15(7):683–685, 1997.

Marra MD, Crema MD, Chung M, et al: MRI features of cystic lesions around the knee, *Knee* 15(6):423–438, 2008.

Torreggiani WC, Al-Ismail K, Munk PL, et al: The imaging spectrum of Baker's (popliteal) cysts, *Clin Radiol* 57(8):681–691, 2002.

Waldman SD: Baker's cyst of the knee. In *Atlas of pain management injection techniques*, ed 2, Philadelphia, 2007, Saunders, pp 484–486.

Waldman SD: Baker's cyst of the knee. In *Pain review*, Philadelphia, 2009, Saunders, p 317.

Chapter 108

PES ANSERINE BURSITIS

ICD-9 CODE `726.61`

ICD-10 CODE `M76.899`

THE CLINICAL SYNDROME

The pes anserine bursa lies beneath the pes anserine tendon, which is the insertional tendon of the sartorius, gracilis, and semitendinous muscles on the medial side of the tibia. This bursa may exist as a single bursal sac or, in some patients, as a multisegmented series of loculated sacs. The pes anserine bursa is prone to the development of inflammation from overuse, misuse, or direct trauma. If inflammation of the pes anserine bursa becomes chronic, calcification may occur. Rarely, the pes anserine bursa becomes infected.

With trauma to the medial knee, the medial collateral ligament is often involved, along with the pes anserine bursa. This broad, flat, bandlike ligament runs from the medial condyle of the femur to the medial aspect of the shaft of the tibia, where it attaches just above the groove of the semimembranosus muscle; it also attaches to the edge of the medial semilunar cartilage. The medial collateral ligament is crossed at its lower part by the tendons of the sartorius, gracilis, and semitendinosus muscles.

SIGNS AND SYMPTOMS

Patients with pes anserine bursitis present with pain over the medial knee joint and increased pain on passive valgus and external rotation of the knee. Activity, especially that involving flexion and external rotation of the knee, makes the pain worse, whereas rest and heat provide some relief. Often, patients are unable to kneel or walk down stairs (Fig. 108-1). The pain of pes anserine bursitis is constant and is characterized as aching; it may interfere with sleep. Coexistent bursitis, tendinitis, arthritis, or internal derangement of the knee may confuse the clinical picture after trauma to the knee.

Physical examination may reveal point tenderness in the anterior knee just below the medial knee joint at the tendinous insertion of the pes anserine. Swelling and fluid accumulation surrounding the bursa are often present. Active resisted flexion of the knee reproduces the pain. Sudden release of resistance during this maneuver causes a marked increase in pain.

TESTING

Plain radiographs of the knee may reveal calcification of the bursa and associated structures, including the pes anserine tendon, findings consistent with chronic inflammation. Magnetic resonance

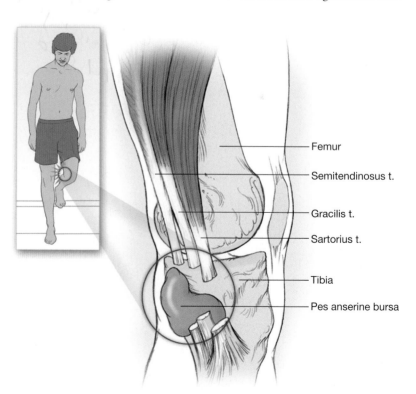

Figure 108-1 Patients with pes anserine bursitis complain of medial knee pain that is made worse with kneeling or walking down stairs.

imaging (MRI) is indicated if internal derangement, an occult mass, or a tumor of the knee is suspected. Electromyography can distinguish pes anserine bursitis from neuropathy, lumbar radiculopathy, and plexopathy. The injection technique described later serves as both a diagnostic and a therapeutic maneuver.

DIFFERENTIAL DIAGNOSIS

Pes anserine spurs may coexist with pes anserine bursitis, thus confusing the clinical picture (Fig. 108-2). Because of the unique anatomic relationships present in the medial knee, it is often difficult to make an accurate clinical diagnosis that identifies the structure responsible for the patient's pain. MRI can rule out lesions that may require surgical intervention, such as tears of the medial meniscus. Anything that alters the normal biomechanics of the knee can result in inflammation of the pes anserine bursa.

TREATMENT

A short course of conservative therapy consisting of simple analgesics, nonsteroidal antiinflammatory drugs (NSAIDs) or cyclooxygenase-2 inhibitors, and a knee brace to prevent further trauma is the first step in the treatment of pes anserine bursitis. If patients do not experience rapid improvement, injection is a reasonable next step.

To inject the pes anserine bursa, the patient is placed in the supine position with a rolled blanket underneath the knee to flex the joint gently. The skin just below the medial knee joint is prepared with antiseptic solution. A sterile syringe containing 2 mL of 0.25% preservative-free bupivacaine and 40 mg methylprednisolone is attached to a 1½-inch, 25-gauge needle by using strict aseptic technique. The pes anserine tendon is identified by having the patient strongly flex his or her leg against resistance. The pes anserine bursa is located at a point distal to the medial joint space where the pes anserine tendon attaches to the tibia. The bursa can usually be identified by point tenderness. At that point, the needle is inserted at a 45-degree angle to the tibia and passes through the skin and subcutaneous tissues into the pes anserine bursa. If the needle strikes the tibia, the needle is withdrawn slightly into the substance of the bursa. When the needle is positioned in proximity to the pes anserine bursa, the contents of the syringe are gently injected. Little resistance to injection should be felt. If resistance is encountered, the needle is probably in a ligament or tendon and should be advanced or withdrawn slightly until the injection can proceed without significant resistance. The needle is removed, and a sterile pressure dressing and ice pack are applied to the injection site.

Physical modalities, including local heat and gentle range-of-motion exercises, should be introduced several days after the patient undergoes injection. Vigorous exercises should be avoided, because they will exacerbate the patient's symptoms. Simple analgesics and NSAIDs can be used concurrently with this injection technique.

COMPLICATIONS AND PITFALLS

Failure to identify primary or metastatic tumor of the distal femur or knee joint that is causing the patient's pain can have disastrous results. The injection technique is safe if careful attention is paid to the clinically relevant anatomy. The major complication of injection is infection, although this should be exceedingly rare if strict aseptic technique is followed. Approximately 25% of patients complain of a transient increase in pain after injection, and patients should be warned of this possibility.

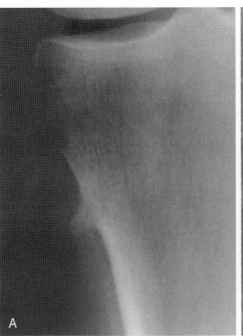 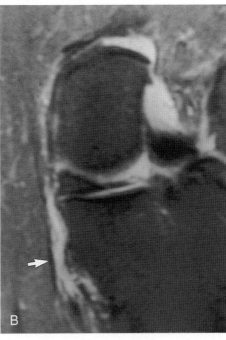

Figure 108-2 Pes anserine spurs. In this 65-year-old woman with a history of pes anserine bursitis, a conventional radiograph **(A)** reveals a small excrescence in the medial portion of the tibia. On a coronal, fat-suppressed, fast spin-echo magnetic resonance image **(B)**, fluid of high signal intensity *(arrow)* is seen about the bone outgrowth. *(From Resnick D: Diagnosis of bone and joint disorders, ed 4, Philadelphia, 2002, Saunders, p 3898.)*

Clinical Pearls

Coexistent bursitis, tendinitis, arthritis, and internal derangement of the knee may contribute to the patient's pain, thus necessitating additional treatment with more localized injection of local anesthetic and methylprednisolone. The injection technique described is extremely effective in treating the pain of pes anserine bursitis.

SUGGESTED READINGS

Maheshwari AV, Muro-Cacho CA, Pitcher JD Jr: Pigmented villonodular bursitis/diffuse giant cell tumor of the pes anserine bursa: a report of two cases and review of literature, *Knee* 14(5):402–407, 2007.

Waldman SD: Bursitis syndromes of the knee. In *Pain review,* Philadelphia, 2009, Saunders, pp 318–322.

Waldman SD: Functional anatomy of the knee. In *Pain review,* Philadelphia, 2009, Saunders, pp 144–149.

Wood LR, Peat G, Thomas E, et al: The contribution of selected non-articular conditions to knee pain severity and associated disability in older adults, *Osteoarthritis Cartilage* 16(6):647–653, 2008.

Chapter 109

TENNIS LEG

ICD-9 CODE **844.9**

ICD-10 CODE **S86.919A**

THE CLINICAL SYNDROME

Tennis leg is the term applied to acute injury of the musculo-tendinous unit of the gastrocnemius muscle. This injury occurs most commonly following an acute, forceful push-off with the foot of the affected leg. Although this injury has been given the name tennis leg because of its common occurrence in tennis players, tennis leg can also be seen in divers, jumpers, hill runners, and basketball players. Occurring most commonly in men in the fourth to sixth decade, tennis leg is usually the result of an acute traumatic event secondary to a sudden push-off or lunge with the back leg while the knee is extended and the foot dorsi-flexed, thus placing maximal eccentric tension on the lengthened gastrocnemius muscle (Fig. 109-1).

The main functions of the gastrocnemius muscle are to plantar flex the ankle and to provide stability to the posterior knee. The medial head of the muscle finds it origin at the posterior aspect of the medial femoral condyle, and, coursing inferiorly, it merges with the musculotendinous unit of the soleus muscle to form the Achilles tendon. Several tendinous insertions are spread through-out the belly of the gastrocnemius muscle, and strain or complete rupture is most likely to occur at these points.

SIGNS AND SYMPTOMS

In most patients, the pain of tennis leg occurs acutely, is often quite severe, and is accompanied by an audible pop or snapping sound. The pain is constant and severe and is localized to the medal calf. The patient often complains that it felt like a knife was sud-denly stuck into the medial calf. Patients with complete rupture of the gastrocnemius musculotendinous unit experience significant swelling, ecchymosis, and hematoma formation that may extend from the medial thigh to the ankle. If this swelling is not too severe, the clinician may identify a palpable defect in the medial calf, as well as obvious asymmetry when compared with the unin-jured side. The clinician can elicit pain by passively dorsiflexing the ankle of the patient's affected lower extremity and by having the patient plantar flex the ankle against active resistance.

TESTING

Magnetic resonance imaging of the calf is indicated if tennis leg is suspected, as well as to rule out other disorders that which may mimic this condition (Fig. 109-2). Ultrasound imaging may also aid in diagnosis; the common finding of fluid between the gastrocnemius and soleus muscles is highly suggestive of

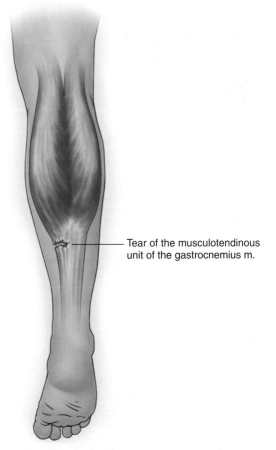

Tear of the musculotendinous unit of the gastrocnemius m.

Figure 109-1 The pain of tennis leg occurs acutely and is accompanied by an audible snap or pop that emanates from the tearing of the musculotendinous unit of the gastrocnemius muscle.

the diagnosis of tennis leg (Figs. 109-3 and 109-4). Ultrasound imaging can also identify defects in the musculotendinous unit. Based on the patient's clinical presentation, additional testing may be indicated, including a complete blood count, erythrocyte sedimentation rate, and antinuclear antibody testing.

DIFFERENTIAL DIAGNOSIS

Tennis leg is usually a straightforward clinical diagnosis that can be made on the basis of history and clinical findings. However, coexisting bursitis or tendinitis of the knee and distal lower extremity from over-use or misuse may confuse the diagnosis. In some clinical situations, consideration should be given to primary or secondary tumors involv-ing the affected region. Nerve entrapments of the lower extremity secondary to compression by massive hematoma formation (especially in anticoagulated patients) can also confuse the diagnosis.

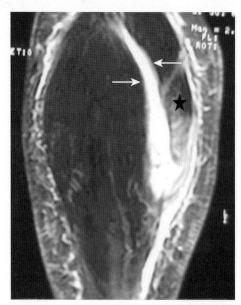

Figure 109-2 A 53-year-old woman reported a sudden pop and sharp pain in the back of her leg during arising from sajdah (the placing of the forehead on the prayer mat covered floor during prayer. A T2-weighted coronal magnetic resonance image reveals fluid *(arrows)* between the gastrocnemius and soleus muscles. Also noted is an increased signal *(star)* within the medial gastrocnemius head near the midtarsal joint that indicates muscle injury. *(From Yilmaz C, Orgenc Y, Ergenc R, Erkan N: Rupture of the medial gastrocnemius muscle during namaz praying: an unusual cause of tennis leg, Comput Med Imaging Graph 32[8]:728–731, 2008.)*

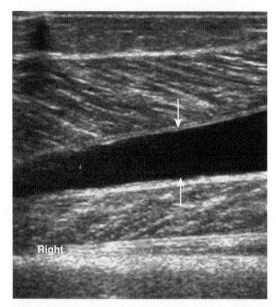

Figure 109-3 Ultrasound image of an intermuscular fluid collection between the medial gastrocnemius and soleus muscles on ultrasound *(arrows)* in a patient with tennis leg. *(From Armfield DR, Kim DH, Towers JD, et al: Sports-related muscle injury in the lower extremity, Clin Sports Med 25[4]:803–842, 2006.)*

TREATMENT

Initial treatment of the pain and functional disability associated with tennis leg includes rest, elevation, use of elastic compressive wraps, and application of ice to the affected extremity to reduce swelling and pain. The use of acetaminophen or cyclooxygenase-2 inhibitors, with or without the addition of a short-acting opioid

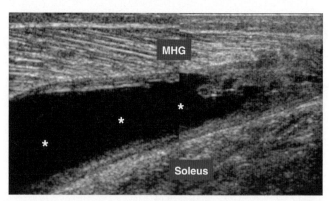

Figure 109-4 Ultrasound image of a patient with complete rupture *(asterisks)* of the medial head of the gastrocnemius (MHG); the soleus muscle is also visible. *(From Flecca D, Tomei A, Ravazzolo N, et al: US evaluation and diagnosis of rupture of the medial head of the gastrocnemius (tennis leg), J Ultrasound 10[4]:194–198, 2007.)*

such as hydrocodone, is indicated for pain. Aspirin should be avoided because of its effects on platelets, given the sometimes significant bleeding associated with the injury in tennis leg. Gentle physical therapy to normalize gait and to maintain range of motion should be implemented in a few days, as the swelling subsides.

Vigorous exercises should be avoided, because they will exacerbate the patient's symptoms. Occasionally, surgical repair of the tendon is undertaken if the patient is experiencing significant functional disability or is unhappy with the cosmetic defect resulting from the retracted tendon and muscle.

COMPLICATIONS AND PITFALLS

Careful observation for the development of lower extremity compartment syndrome during the early phase of this condition is important if bleeding is significant, especially in anticoagulated patients.

Given the overlap of symptoms of tennis leg with deep venous thrombosis, the clinician must have a high index of suspicion for the development of deep venous thrombosis, especially during the rest phase of recovery or if anticoagulants have been discontinued. As the damage to the musculotendinous unit heals, scar formation can occur and can lead to chronic pain and functional disability. If this occurs, surgical excision and reconstruction of the musculotendinous unit may be required.

Clinical Pearls

The amount of swelling and bruising associated with the acute injury causing tennis leg may be impressive and may cause extreme anxiety for the injured patient and his or her family. Reassurance should be given early and often. A high index of suspicion for the insidious onset of lower extremity compartment syndrome or deep venous thrombosis is important, to avoid disaster.

SUGGESTED READINGS

Armfield DR, Kim DH, Towers JD, et al: Sports-related muscle injury in the lower extremity, *Clin Sports Med* 25(4):803–842, 2006.
Flecca D, Tomei A, Ravazzolo N, et al: US evaluation and diagnosis of rupture of the medial head of the gastrocnemius (tennis leg), *J Ultrasound* 10(4):194–198, 2007.
Kwak H-S, Lee K-B, Han Y-M: Ruptures of the medial head of the gastrocnemius ("tennis leg"): clinical outcome and compression effect, *Clin Imaging* 30(1):48–53, 2006.
Pai V, Pai V: Acute compartment syndrome after rupture of the medial head of gastrocnemius in a child, *J Foot Ankle Surg* 46(4):288–290, 2007.

Chapter 110

ARTHRITIS PAIN OF THE ANKLE

ICD-9 CODE `715.97`

ICD-10 CODE `M19.90`

THE CLINICAL SYNDROME

Arthritis of the ankle is a common condition. The ankle joint is susceptible to the development of arthritis from various conditions that have the ability to damage the joint cartilage. Osteoarthritis is the most common form of arthritis that results in ankle pain; rheumatoid arthritis and post-traumatic arthritis are also frequent causes of ankle pain. Less common causes include the collagen vascular diseases, infection, villonodular synovitis, and Lyme disease. Acute infectious arthritis is usually accompanied by significant systemic symptoms, including fever and malaise, and should be easily recognized; it is treated with culture and antibiotics rather than injection therapy. Collagen vascular disease generally manifests as polyarthropathy rather than as monarthropathy limited to the ankle joint, although ankle pain secondary to collagen vascular disease responds exceedingly well to the treatment modalities described here.

SIGNS AND SYMPTOMS

Most patients complain of pain localized around the ankle and distal lower extremity. Activity makes the pain worse, whereas rest and heat provide some relief. The pain is constant and is characterized as aching; it may interfere with sleep. Some patients complain of a grating or popping sensation with use of the joint, and crepitus may be present on physical examination.

In addition to pain, patients with arthritis of the ankle often experience a gradual decrease in functional ability because of reduced ankle range of motion that makes simple everyday tasks such as walking and climbing stairs and ladders quite difficult (Fig. 110-1). With continued disuse, muscle wasting may occur, and a frozen ankle secondary to adhesive capsulitis may develop.

TESTING

Plain radiographs are indicated in all patients who present with ankle pain. Magnetic resonance imaging of the ankle is indicated in the case of trauma, if the diagnosis is in question, or if an occult mass or tumor is suspected. Based on the patient's clinical presentation, additional testing may be warranted, including a complete blood count, erythrocyte sedimentation rate, and antinuclear antibody testing.

DIFFERENTIAL DIAGNOSIS

Lumbar radiculopathy may mimic the pain and disability of arthritis of the ankle; however, results of the ankle examination are negative. Bursitis of the ankle and entrapment neuropathies such as tarsal tunnel syndrome may also confuse the diagnosis; both these conditions may coexist with arthritis of the ankle. Primary and metastatic tumors of the distal tibia and fibula and spine, as well as occult fractures, may also manifest in a manner similar to arthritis of the ankle.

TREATMENT

Initial treatment of the pain and functional disability associated with arthritis of the ankle includes a combination of nonsteroidal antiinflammatory drugs or cyclooxygenase-2 inhibitors and physical therapy. The local application of heat and cold may also be beneficial. Avoidance of repetitive activities that aggravate the patient's symptoms, as well as short-term immobilization of the ankle joint, may provide relief. For patients who do not respond to these treatment modalities, intraarticular injection of local anesthetic and steroid is a reasonable next step.

To perform intraarticular injection of the ankle, the patient is placed in the supine position, and the skin overlying the ankle joint is prepared with antiseptic solution. A sterile syringe containing 2 mL of 0.25% preservative-free bupivacaine and 40 mg methyl-prednisolone is attached to a 1½-inch, 25-gauge needle by using strict aseptic technique. With the patient's foot in the neutral position, the junction of the tibia and fibula just above the talus

349

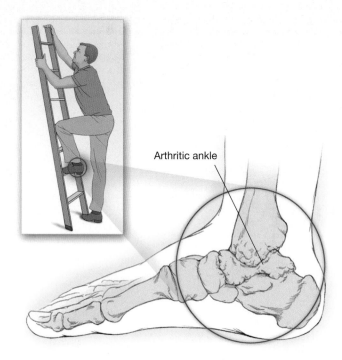

Figure 110-1 Arthritis of the ankle is often made worse with activity.

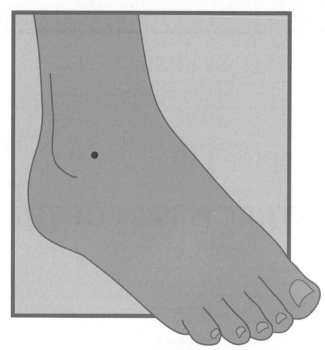

Figure 110-2 With the foot in the neutral position, the junction of the tibia and fibula just above the talus can be identified. At this point, a triangular indentation indicating the joint space is easily palpable. *(From Waldman SD:* Atlas of pain management injection techniques, *Philadelphia, 2000, Saunders, p 301.)*

is identified. At this point, a triangular indentation indicating the joint space is easily palpable (Fig. 110-2). The needle is carefully advanced through the skin, subcutaneous tissues, and joint capsule and into the joint. If bone is encountered, the needle is withdrawn into the subcutaneous tissues and is redirected superiorly and slightly more medially. After the joint space is entered, the contents of the syringe are gently injected. Little resistance to injection should be felt. If resistance is encountered, the needle is probably in a ligament or tendon and should be advanced slightly into the joint space until the injection can proceed without significant resistance. The needle is removed, and a sterile pressure dressing and ice pack are applied to the injection site.

Physical modalities, including local heat and gentle range-of-motion exercises, should be introduced several days after the patient undergoes injection. Vigorous exercises should be avoided, because they will exacerbate the patient's symptoms.

COMPLICATIONS AND PITFALLS

Failure to identify primary or metastatic tumor of the ankle that is causing the patient's pain can have disastrous results. The injection technique is safe if careful attention is paid to the clinically relevant anatomy. The major complication of intraarticular injection of the ankle is infection, although this should be exceedingly rare

if strict aseptic technique is followed. Approximately 25% of patients complain of a transient increase in pain after injection, and patients should be warned of this possibility.

Clinical Pearls

Coexistent bursitis and tendinitis may contribute to the patient's ankle pain, thus necessitating additional treatment with more localized injection of local anesthetic and methylprednisolone. The injection technique described is extremely effective in treating the pain of arthritis of the ankle joint.

SUGGESTED READINGS

Alcaraz MJ, Megías J, García-Arnandis I, et al: New molecular targets for the treatment of osteoarthritis, *Biochem Pharmacol* 80(1):13–21, 2010.

Collins MS: Imaging evaluation of chronic ankle and hindfoot pain in athletes, *Magn Reson Imaging Clin N Am* 16(1):39–58, 2008.

Waldman SD: Intraarticular injection of the ankle and foot. In *Atlas of pain management injection techniques,* ed 2, Philadelphia, 2007, Saunders, pp 497–500.

Waldman SD: Functional anatomy of the ankle and foot. In *Pain review,* Philadelphia, 2009, Saunders, pp 155–156.

Chapter 111

ARTHRITIS OF THE MIDTARSAL JOINTS

ICD-9 CODE 715.97

ICD-10 CODE M19.90

THE CLINICAL SYNDROME

Arthritis of the midtarsal joints is a common condition. The midtarsal joints are susceptible to the development of arthritis from various conditions that have the ability to damage the joint cartilage. Osteoarthritis is the most common form of arthritis that results in midtarsal joint pain; rheumatoid arthritis and posttraumatic arthritis are also frequent causes of midtarsal pain. Less common causes include the collagen vascular diseases, infection, and Lyme disease. Acute infectious arthritis is usually accompanied by significant systemic symptoms, including fever and malaise, and should be easily recognized; it is treated with culture and antibiotics rather than injection therapy. Collagen vascular disease generally manifests as polyarthropathy rather than as monarthropathy limited to the midtarsal joint, although midtarsal pain secondary to collagen vascular disease responds exceedingly well to the treatment modalities described here.

SIGNS AND SYMPTOMS

Most patients present with pain localized to the dorsum of the foot. Activity, especially that involving inversion and adduction of the midtarsal joint, makes the pain worse (Fig. 111-1), whereas rest and heat provide some relief. The pain is constant and is characterized as aching; it may interfere with sleep. Some patients complain of a grating or popping sensation with use of the joints, and crepitus may be present on physical examination. In addition to pain, patients with arthritis of the midtarsal joint often experience a gradual decrease in functional ability because of reduced midtarsal range of motion that makes simple everyday tasks such as walking and climbing stairs quite difficult.

TESTING

Plain radiographs are indicated for all patients who present with midtarsal pain (Fig. 111-2). Magnetic resonance imaging of the midtarsal joint is indicated if aseptic necrosis, an occult mass, or a tumor is suspected. Based on the patient's clinical presentation, additional testing may be warranted, including a complete blood count, erythrocyte sedimentation rate, and antinuclear antibody testing.

DIFFERENTIAL DIAGNOSIS

Primary disorders of the foot, including gout and occult fractures, may mimic the pain and disability of arthritis of the midtarsal joint. Bursitis and plantar fasciitis of the foot, as well as entrapment

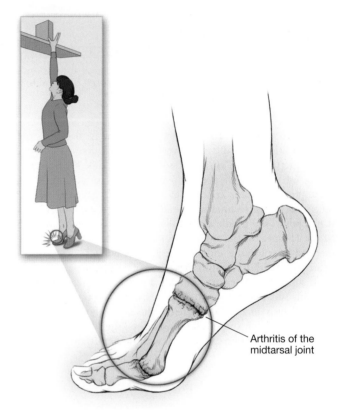

Figure 111-1 Arthritis of the midtarsal joint manifests as pain in the dorsum of the foot that is made worse with inversion and adduction of the affected joint.

neuropathies such as tarsal tunnel syndrome, may also confuse the diagnosis; these conditions may coexist with arthritis of the midtarsal joint. Primary and metastatic tumors of the foot may also manifest in a manner similar to arthritis of the midtarsal joint.

TREATMENT

Initial treatment of the pain and functional disability associated with arthritis of the midtarsal joint includes a combination of nonsteroidal antiinflammatory drugs or cyclooxygenase-2 inhibitors and physical therapy. The local application of heat and cold may also be beneficial. Avoidance of repetitive activities that aggravate the patient's symptoms, as well as short-term immobilization of the midtarsal joint, may provide relief. For patients who do not respond to these treatment modalities, intra-articular injection of local anesthetic and steroid is a reasonable next step.

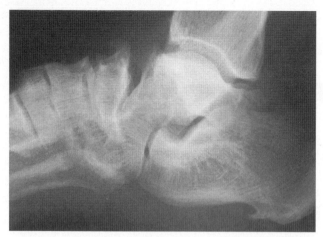

Figure 111-2 Lateral view of the tarsal bones shows osteoarthritis secondary to a vertical talus. *(From Brower AC, Flemming DJ:* Arthritis in black and white, *ed 2, Philadelphia, 1997, Saunders.)*

To perform midtarsal injection, the patient is placed in the supine position, and the skin overlying the tenderest midtarsal joint is prepared with antiseptic solution. A sterile syringe containing 2 mL of 0.25% preservative-free bupivacaine and 40 mg methylprednisolone is attached to a ⅝-inch, 25-gauge needle by using strict aseptic technique. The affected joint space is identified. At this point, the needle is carefully advanced at a right angle to the dorsal aspect of the ankle through the skin, subcutaneous tissues, and joint capsule and into the joint. If bone is encountered, the needle is withdrawn into the subcutaneous tissues and is redirected superiorly. After the joint space is entered, the contents of the syringe are gently injected. Little resistance to injection should be felt. If resistance is encountered, the needle is probably in a ligament or tendon and should be advanced slightly into the joint space until the injection can proceed without significant resistance.

The needle is removed, and a sterile pressure dressing and ice pack are applied to the injection site.

Physical modalities, including local heat and gentle range-of-motion exercises, should be introduced several days after the patient undergoes injection. Vigorous exercises should be avoided, because they will exacerbate the patient's symptoms.

COMPLICATIONS AND PITFALLS

Failure to identify primary or metastatic tumor of the midtarsal joint that is causing the patient's pain can have disastrous results. The injection technique is safe if careful attention is paid to the clinically relevant anatomy. The major complication of intra-articular injection of the midtarsal joint is infection, although this should be exceedingly rare if strict aseptic technique is followed. Approximately 25% of patients complain of a transient increase in pain after injection, and patients should be warned of this possibility.

Clinical Pearls

> Coexistent bursitis and tendinitis may contribute to the patient's pain, thus necessitating additional treatment with more localized injection of local anesthetic and methylprednisolone. The injection technique described is extremely effective in treating the pain of arthritis of the midtarsal joint.

SUGGESTED READINGS

Alcaraz MJ, Megías J, García-Arnandis I, et al: New molecular targets for the treatment of osteoarthritis, *Biochem Pharmacol* 80(1):13–21, 2010.

Collins MS: Imaging evaluation of chronic ankle and hindfoot pain in athletes, *Magn Reson Imaging Clin N Am* 16(1):39–58, 2008.

Waldman SD: Intra-articular injection of the ankle and foot. In *Atlas of pain management injection techniques,* ed 2, Philadelphia, 2007, Saunders, pp 497–500.

Waldman SD: Functional anatomy of the ankle and foot. In *Pain review,* Philadelphia, 2009, Saunders, pp 155–156.

Chapter 112

DELTOID LIGAMENT STRAIN

ICD-9 CODE **845.01**

ICD-10 CODES **S93.429A**

THE CLINICAL SYNDROME

The deltoid ligament is exceptionally strong and is not as easily strained as is the anterior talofibular ligament. However, the deltoid ligament is susceptible to strain from acute injury resulting from sudden overpronation of the ankle or repetitive microtrauma to the ligament from overuse or misuse, such as long-distance running on soft or uneven surfaces. The deltoid ligament has two layers, both of which attach to the medial malleolus above it (Fig. 112-1). The deep layer attaches below to the medial body of the talus, and the superficial fibers attach to the medial talus, the sustentaculum tali of the calcaneus, and the navicular tuberosity.

SIGNS AND SYMPTOMS

Patients with deltoid ligament strain complain of pain just below the medial malleolus. Plantar flexion and eversion of the ankle joint exacerbate the pain. Often, patients with injury to the deltoid ligament note a pop, followed by significant swelling and the inability to walk (Fig. 112-2).

On physical examination, patients have point tenderness over the medial malleolus. With acute trauma, ecchymosis over the ligament may be noted. Patients with deltoid ligament strain have a positive result of the eversion test, which is performed by passively everting and plantar flexing the affected ankle joint (Fig. 112-3). Coexistent bursitis and arthritis of the ankle and subtalar joint may also be present and may confuse the clinical picture.

TESTING

Plain radiographs are indicated for all patients who present with ankle pain. Magnetic resonance imaging (MRI) of the ankle is indicated if disruption of the deltoid ligament, joint instability, an occult mass, or a tumor is suspected. Radionuclide bone scanning should be performed if occult fracture is suspected. Based on the patient's clinical presentation, additional testing may be warranted, including a complete blood count, erythrocyte sedimentation rate, and antinuclear antibody testing.

DIFFERENTIAL DIAGNOSIS

Avulsion fracture of the calcaneus, talus, medial malleolus, or base of the fifth metatarsal can mimic deltoid ligament pain. Bursitis, tendinitis, and gout of the midtarsal joints may coexist with deltoid ligament strain, thus confusing the diagnosis. Tarsal tunnel

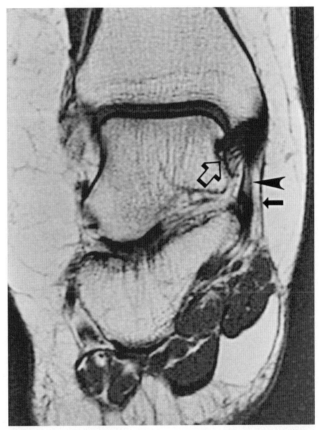

Figure 112-1 Normal medial ankle ligaments on a coronal, T1-weighted magnetic resonance image. The two layers of the deltoid (medial) ligament are seen. The deep tibiotalar ligament is striated *(open arrow)*. The more superficial tibiocalcaneal ligament *(arrowhead)* may have vertical striations as well. The thin, vertical, low-signal structure superficial to the tibiocalcaneal ligament is the flexor retinaculum *(solid arrow)*. *(From Kaplan PA, Helms CA, Dussault R, et al:* Musculoskeletal MRI, *Philadelphia, 2001, Saunders, p 835.)*

syndrome may occur after ankle trauma and further complicate the clinical picture.

TREATMENT

Initial treatment of the pain and functional disability associated with deltoid ligament strain includes a combination of nonsteroidal antiinflammatory drugs (NSAIDs) or cyclooxygenase-2 inhibitors and physical therapy. The local application of heat and cold may also be beneficial. Avoidance of repetitive activities that aggravate the patient's symptoms, as well as short-term immobilization of the ankle joint, may provide relief. For patients who do not respond to these treatment modalities, injection is a reasonable next step.

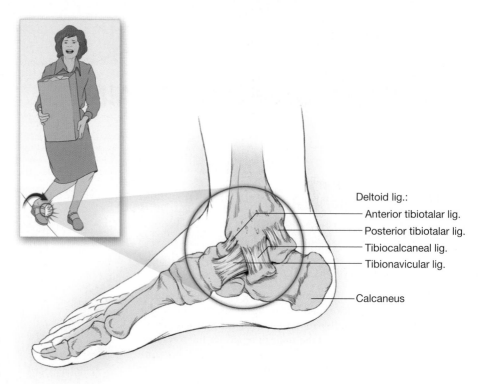

Figure 112-2 With deltoid ligament strain, patients may notice a pop, followed by significant swelling.

Deltoid lig.:
- Anterior tibiotalar lig.
- Posterior tibiotalar lig.
- Tibiocalcaneal lig.
- Tibionavicular lig.

Calcaneus

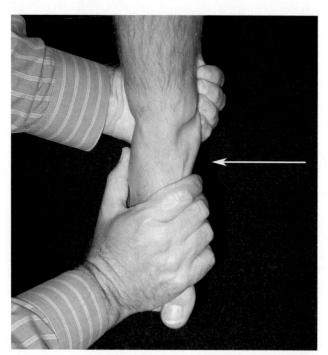

Figure 112-3 Eversion test for deltoid ligament insufficiency. *(From Waldman SD: Physical diagnosis of pain: an atlas of signs and symptoms, Philadelphia, 2006, Saunders, p 369.)*

To perform deltoid ligament injection, the patient is placed in the supine position, and the skin overlying the area of the medial malleolus is prepared with antiseptic solution. A sterile syringe containing 2 mL of 0.25% preservative-free bupivacaine and 40 mg methylprednisolone is attached to a 1½-inch, 25-gauge needle by using strict aseptic technique. With the lower extremity slightly abducted, the lower margin of the medial malleolus is identified. At this point, the needle is carefully advanced at a 30-degree angle to the ankle through the skin and subcutaneous tissues to impinge on the lower margin of the medial malleolus. The needle is then withdrawn slightly, and the contents of the syringe are gently injected. Resistance to injection should be slight. If significant resistance is encountered, the needle is probably in the ligament and should be withdrawn slightly until the injection can proceed without significant resistance. The needle is removed, and a sterile pressure dressing and ice pack are applied to the injection site.

Physical modalities, including local heat and gentle range-of-motion exercises, should be introduced several days after the patient undergoes injection. Vigorous exercises should be avoided, because they will exacerbate the patient's symptoms. Simple analgesics and NSAIDs can be used concurrently with this injection technique.

COMPLICATIONS AND PITFALLS

Failure to identify occult fractures of the ankle and foot may result in significant morbidity; therefore, radionuclide bone scanning and MRI should be performed in all patients with unexplained ankle and foot pain, especially if trauma is present. The major complication of injection is infection, although this should be exceedingly rare if strict aseptic technique is followed. Approximately 25% of patients complain of a transient increase in pain after injection, and patients should be warned of this possibility. A gentle technique should always be used when injecting around strained ligaments, to avoid further damage to the already compromised ligament.

Clinical Pearls

Approximately 25,000 people are estimated to sprain an ankle every day. Although the public generally views this injury as minor, ankle sprains can result in significant permanent pain and disability. The injection technique described is extremely effective in treating the pain of deltoid ligament strain. Coexistent arthritis, bursitis, and tendinitis may contribute to medial ankle pain, thus necessitating additional treatment with more localized injection of local anesthetic and methylprednisolone.

SUGGESTED READINGS

Collins MS: Imaging evaluation of chronic ankle and hindfoot pain in athletes, *Magn Reson Imaging Clin N Am* 16(1):39–58, 2008.

Hintermann B, Knupp M, Pagenstert GI: Deltoid ligament injuries: diagnosis and management, *Foot Ankle Clin* 11(3):625–637, 2006.

Waldman SD: Intra-articular injection of the ankle and foot. In *Atlas of pain management injection techniques,* ed 2, Philadelphia, 2007, Saunders, pp 497–500.

Waldman SD: The deltoid ligament. In *Pain review,* Philadelphia, 2009, Saunders, p 157.

Chapter 113

ANTERIOR TARSAL TUNNEL SYNDROME

ICD-9 CODE **355.5**

ICD-10 CODE **G57.50**

THE CLINICAL SYNDROME

Anterior tarsal tunnel syndrome is caused by compression of the deep peroneal nerve as it passes beneath the superficial fascia of the ankle (Fig. 113-1). The most common cause of this compression is trauma to the dorsum of the foot. Severe, acute plantar flexion of the foot has been implicated in anterior tarsal tunnel syndrome, as has wearing tight shoes or squatting and bending forward, such as when planting flowers (Fig. 113-2). Anterior tarsal tunnel syndrome is much less common than is posterior tarsal tunnel syndrome.

SIGNS AND SYMPTOMS

This entrapment neuropathy manifests primarily as pain, numbness, and paresthesias in the dorsum of the foot that radiate into the first dorsal web space; these symptoms may also radiate proximal to the entrapment, into the anterior ankle. No motor involvement occurs unless the distal lateral division of the deep peroneal nerve

is affected. Nighttime foot pain analogous to that of carpal tunnel syndrome is often present. Patients may report that holding the foot in the everted position decreases the pain and paresthesias.

Physical findings include tenderness over the deep peroneal nerve at the dorsum of the foot. A positive Tinel sign just medial to the dorsalis pedis pulse over the deep peroneal nerve as it passes beneath the fascia is usually present (Fig. 113-3). Active plantar flexion often reproduces the symptoms of anterior tarsal tunnel syndrome. Weakness of the extensor digitorum brevis may be present if the lateral branch of the deep peroneal nerve is affected.

TESTING

Electromyography (EMG) can distinguish lumbar radiculopathy and diabetic polyneuropathy from anterior tarsal tunnel syndrome. Plain radiographs are indicated in all patients who present with foot or ankle pain, to rule out occult bony disease. Magnetic resonance imaging (MRI) of the ankle and foot is indicated if joint instability or a space-occupying lesion is suspected. Based on the patient's clinical presentation, additional testing may be warranted, including a complete blood count, uric acid level, erythrocyte sedimentation rate, and antinuclear antibody testing. The injection technique described later serves as both a diagnostic and a therapeutic maneuver.

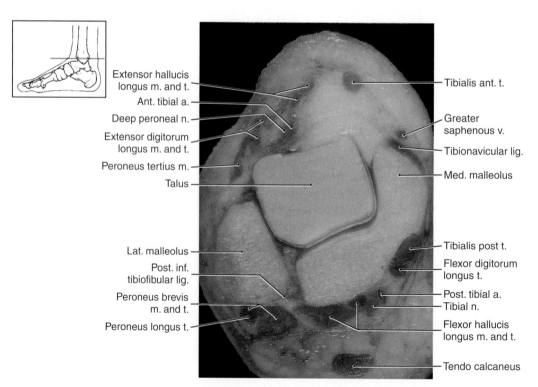

Extensor hallucis longus m. and t.
Ant. tibial a.
Deep peroneal n.
Extensor digitorum longus m. and t.
Peroneus tertius m.
Talus

Tibialis ant. t.
Greater saphenous v.
Tibionavicular lig.
Med. malleolus

Lat. malleolus
Post. inf. tibiofibular lig.
Peroneus brevis m. and t.
Peroneus longus t.

Tibialis post t.
Flexor digitorum longus t.
Post. tibial a.
Tibial n.
Flexor hallucis longus m. and t.
Tendo calcaneus

Figure 113-1 The relationships among the medial malleolus, the tibial artery and nerve, and the flexor tendons of the ankle. *(From Kang HS, Ahn JM, Resnick D: MRI of the extremities: an anatomic atlas, ed 2, Philadelphia, 2002, Saunders, p 415.)*

DIFFERENTIAL DIAGNOSIS

Anterior tarsal tunnel syndrome is often misdiagnosed as arthritis of the ankle joint, lumbar radiculopathy, or diabetic polyneuropathy. Patients with arthritis of the ankle, however, have radiographic evidence of arthritis. Most patients suffering from lumbar radiculopathy have reflex, motor, and sensory changes associated with back pain, whereas patients with anterior tarsal tunnel syndrome have no reflex changes or motor deficits, and sensory changes are limited to the distribution of the distal deep peroneal nerve. However, lumbar radiculopathy and deep peroneal nerve entrapment may coexist as the double-crush syndrome. Diabetic polyneuropathy generally manifests as a symmetrical sensory deficit involving the entire foot, rather than a disorder limited to the distribution of the deep peroneal nerve. When anterior tarsal tunnel syndrome occurs in diabetic patients, diabetic polyneuropathy is usually also present.

TREATMENT

Mild cases of tarsal tunnel syndrome usually respond to conservative therapy; surgery should be reserved for severe cases. Initial treatment of tarsal tunnel syndrome consists of simple analgesics, nonsteroidal antiinflammatory drugs, or cyclooxygenase-2 inhibitors and splinting of the ankle. At a minimum, the splint should be worn at night, but wearing it for 24 hours a day is ideal. Avoidance of repetitive activities that may be responsible for the development of tarsal tunnel syndrome, such as prolonged squatting or wearing shoes that are too tight, can also ameliorate the symptoms. If patients fail to respond to these conservative measures, injection of the tarsal tunnel with local anesthetic and steroid is a reasonable next step.

Tarsal tunnel injection is performed by placing the patient in the supine position with the leg extended. The extensor hallucis longus tendon is identified by having the patient extend his or her big toe against resistance. A point just medial to the tendon at the skin crease of the ankle is identified and prepared with antiseptic solution. A 1½-inch, 25-gauge needle is advanced through this point very slowly toward the tibia until a paresthesia is elicited in the web space between the first and second toes, usually at a needle depth of ¼ to ½ inch. The patient should be warned to expect this paresthesia and instructed to say "There!" as soon as it is felt. If no paresthesia is elicited, the needle is withdrawn and is redirected slightly more posteriorly until a paresthesia is induced. The needle is then withdrawn 1 mm, and the patient is observed to ensure that he or she is not experiencing any persistent paresthesia. After careful aspiration, a total of 6 mL of 1% preservative-free lidocaine and 40 mg ethylprednisolone is slowly injected. Care must be taken not to advance the needle into the substance of the nerve and inadvertently inject the solution intraneurally. After injection, pressure is applied to the injection site to decrease the incidence of ecchymosis and hematoma formation.

COMPLICATIONS AND PITFALLS

Failure to treat tarsal tunnel syndrome adequately can result in permanent pain, numbness, and functional disability; these problems can be exacerbated if coexistent reflex sympathetic dystrophy is not treated aggressively with sympathetic neural blockade. The main complications of deep peroneal nerve block are ecchymosis and hematoma, which can be avoided by applying pressure to the injection site. Because a paresthesia is elicited with this technique, needle-induced trauma to the common peroneal nerve is a possibility. By advancing the needle slowly and then withdrawing it slightly away from the nerve, needle-induced trauma can be avoided.

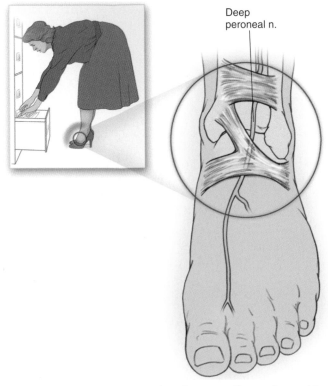

Figure 113-2 Anterior tarsal tunnel syndrome manifests as deep, aching pain in the dorsum of the foot, weakness of the extensor digitorum brevis, and numbness in the distribution of the deep peroneal nerve.

Deep peroneal n.

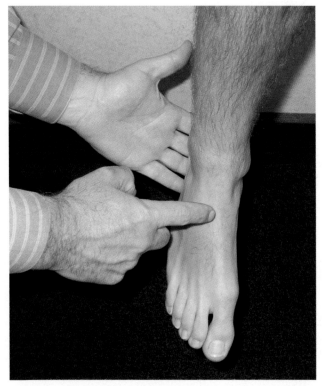

Figure 113-3 Eliciting Tinel's sign for anterior tarsal tunnel syndrome. *(From Waldman SD: Physical diagnosis of pain: an atlas of signs and symptoms, Philadelphia, 2006, Saunders, p 373.)*

Clinical Pearls

The most common cause of pain radiating into the lower extremity is herniated lumbar disk or nerve impingement secondary to degenerative arthritis of the spine, not disorders involving the common or deep peroneal nerve. Lesions above the origin of the common peroneal nerve, such as lesions of the sciatic nerve, or lesions at the point where the common peroneal nerve winds around the head of the fibula, may be confused with deep peroneal nerve entrapment. EMG and MRI of the lumbar spine, combined with the clinical history and physical examination, can determine the cause of distal lower extremity and foot pain. Diabetic patients and other patients with vulnerable nerve syndrome may be more susceptible to the development of anterior tarsal tunnel syndrome.

The injection technique described is useful in the treatment of anterior tarsal tunnel syndrome. Careful preinjection neurologic assessment is important to identify preexisting neurologic deficits that could later be attributed to the deep peroneal nerve block. These assessments are especially important in patients who have sustained trauma to the ankle or foot and in those suffering from diabetic neuropathy in whom deep peroneal nerve block is being used for acute pain control.

SUGGESTED READINGS

DiDomenico LA, Masternick EB: Anterior tarsal tunnel syndrome, *Clin Podiatr Med Surg* 23(3):611–620, 2006.

Kennedy JG, Baxter DE: Nerve disorders in dancers, *Clin Sports Med* 27(2):329–334, 2008.

Waldman SD: Anterior tarsal tunnel syndrome. In *Pain review*, Philadelphia, 2009, Saunders, pp 322–323.

Waldman SD: The anterior tarsal tunnel. In *Pain review*, Philadelphia, 2009, Saunders, p 159.

Chapter 114

POSTERIOR TARSAL TUNNEL SYNDROME

ICD-9 CODE   355.5

ICD-10 CODE   G57.50

THE CLINICAL SYNDROME

Posterior tarsal tunnel syndrome is caused by compression of the posterior tibial nerve as it passes through the posterior tarsal tunnel. The posterior tarsal tunnel is made up of the flexor retinaculum, the bones of the ankle, and the lacunate ligament. In addition to the posterior tibial nerve, the tunnel contains the posterior tibial artery and certain flexor tendons that are subject to tenosynovitis. The most common cause of compression of the posterior tibial nerve at this location is trauma to the ankle, including fracture, dislocation, and crush injury. Thrombophlebitis involving the posterior tibial artery has also been implicated in the development of posterior tarsal tunnel syndrome. Patients with rheumatoid arthritis have a higher incidence of posterior tarsal tunnel syndrome than does the general population. Posterior tarsal tunnel syndrome is much more common than anterior tarsal tunnel syndrome.

SIGNS AND SYMPTOMS

Posterior tarsal tunnel syndrome manifests in a manner analogous to carpal tunnel syndrome. Patients complain of pain, numbness, and paresthesias in the sole of the foot; these symptoms may also radiate proximal to the entrapment, into the medial ankle (Fig. 114-1). Patients may note weakness of the toe flexors and instability of the foot resulting from weakness of the lumbrical muscles. Nighttime foot pain analogous to that of carpal tunnel syndrome is often present.

Physical findings include tenderness over the posterior tibial nerve at the medial malleolus. A positive Tinel sign just below and behind the medial malleolus over the posterior tibial nerve is usually present. Active inversion of the ankle often reproduces the symptoms of posterior tarsal tunnel syndromes. Medial and lateral plantar divisions of the posterior tibial nerve provide motor innervation to the intrinsic muscles of the foot; thus, weakness of the flexor digitorum brevis and the lumbrical muscles may be present if these branches of the nerve are affected.

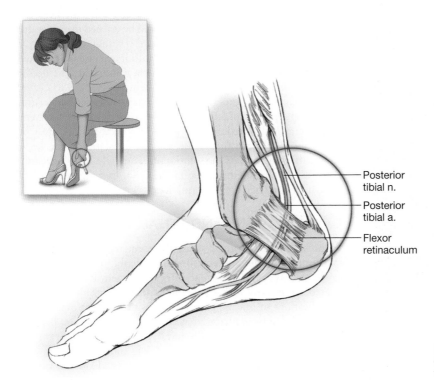

Posterior tibial n.

Posterior tibial a.

Flexor retinaculum

Figure 114-1 Posterior tarsal tunnel syndrome is characterized by pain, numbness, and paresthesias of the sole of the foot.

TESTING

Electromyography (EMG) can distinguish lumbar radiculopathy and diabetic polyneuropathy from posterior tarsal tunnel syndrome. Plain radiographs and magnetic resonance imaging (MRI) are indicated for all patients who present with posterior tarsal tunnel syndrome, to rule out occult bony disease (Fig. 114-2). MRI of the ankle and foot is also indicated if joint instability or a space-occupying lesion is suspected. Based on the patient's clinical presentation, additional testing may be warranted, including a complete blood count, uric acid level, erythrocyte sedimentation rate, and antinuclear antibody testing. The injection technique described later serves as both a diagnostic and a therapeutic maneuver.

DIFFERENTIAL DIAGNOSIS

Posterior tarsal tunnel syndrome is often misdiagnosed as arthritis of the ankle joint, lumbar radiculopathy, or diabetic polyneuropathy. Patients with arthritis of the ankle, however, have radiographic evidence of arthritis. Most patients suffering from lumbar radiculopathy have reflex, motor, and sensory changes associated with back pain, whereas those with posterior tarsal tunnel syndrome have no reflex changes, and motor and sensory changes are limited to the distribution of distal posterior tibial nerve. However, lumbar radiculopathy and posterior tibial nerve entrapment may coexist as the double-crush syndrome. Diabetic polyneuropathy generally manifests as a symmetrical sensory deficit involving the entire foot, rather than a condition limited to the distribution of the posterior tibial nerve. When posterior tarsal tunnel syndrome occurs in diabetic patients, diabetic polyneuropathy is usually also present.

TREATMENT

Mild cases of tarsal tunnel syndrome usually respond to conservative therapy; surgery should be reserved for severe cases. Initial treatment of tarsal tunnel syndrome consists of simple analgesics, nonsteroidal antiinflammatory drugs, or cyclooxygenase-2 inhibitors and splinting of the ankle. At a minimum, the splint should be worn at night, but wearing it for 24 hours a day is ideal. Avoidance of repetitive activities that may be responsible for the development of tarsal tunnel syndrome can also ameliorate the symptoms. If patients fail to respond to these conservative measures, injection of the tarsal tunnel with local anesthetic and steroid is a reasonable next step.

Posterior tarsal tunnel injection is performed with the patient in the lateral position and the affected leg in the dependent position and slightly flexed. The posterior tibial artery is palpated, and the area between the medial malleolus and the Achilles tendon is identified and prepared with antiseptic solution. A 1½-inch, 25-gauge needle is inserted at this level and is directed anteriorly toward the pulsation of the posterior tibial artery. If the arterial pulsation cannot be identified, the needle is directed toward the posterior superior border of the medial malleolus. The needle is advanced slowly toward the tibial nerve, which lies in the posterior groove of the medial malleolus, until a paresthesia is elicited in the distribution of the tibial nerve, usually after the needle is advanced ½ to ¾ inch. The patient should be warned to expect this paresthesia and instructed to say "There!" as soon as it is felt. If no paresthesia is elicited, the needle is withdrawn and is redirected slightly more cephalad until a paresthesia is induced. The needle is then withdrawn 1 mm, and the patient is observed to ensure that he or she is not experiencing any persistent paresthesia. After careful aspiration, a total of 6 mL of 1% preservative-free lidocaine and 40 mg methylprednisolone is slowly injected. Care must be taken not to advance the needle into the substance of the nerve and inadvertently inject the solution intraneurally. After injection, pressure is applied to the injection site to decrease the incidence of ecchymosis and hematoma formation.

COMPLICATIONS AND PITFALLS

Failure to treat tarsal tunnel syndrome adequately can result in permanent pain, numbness, and functional disability; these problems can be exacerbated if coexistent reflex sympathetic dystrophy is not treated aggressively with sympathetic neural blockade. The main complications of injection are ecchymosis and hematoma, which can be avoided by applying pressure to the injection site. Because a paresthesia is elicited, needle-induced trauma to the nerve is a possibility. By advancing the needle slowly and then withdrawing it slightly away from the nerve, needle-induced trauma can be avoided.

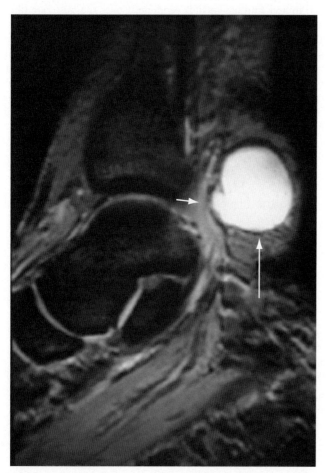

Figure 114-2 Tarsal tunnel syndrome. Sagittal short tau inversion recovery magnetic resonance image shows a ganglion cyst *(long arrow)* compressing the neurovascular bundle in the tarsal tunnel *(short arrow)*. *(From Edelman RR, Hesselink JR, Zlatkin MB, Crues JV, editors: Clinical magnetic resonance imaging, ed 3, Philadelphia, 2006, Saunders, p 3454.)*

Clinical Pearls

The most common cause of pain radiating into the lower extremity is herniated lumbar disk or nerve impingement secondary to degenerative arthritis of the spine, not disorders involving the tibial, common, or deep peroneal nerve. Lesions above the origin of the tibial or common peroneal nerve may be confused with posterior tarsal tunnel syndrome. EMG and MRI of the lumbar spine, combined with the clinical history and physical examination, can determine the cause of distal lower extremity and foot pain.

SUGGESTED READINGS

Cancilleri F, Ippolito M, Amato C, et al: Tarsal tunnel syndrome: four uncommon cases, *Foot Ankle Surg* 13(4):214–217, 2007.

Kennedy JG, Baxter DE: Nerve disorders in dancers, *Clin Sports Med* 27(2):329–334, 2008.

Waldman SD: Posterior tarsal tunnel syndrome. In *Pain review*, Philadelphia, 2009, Saunders, pp 323–324.

Williams TH, Robinson AH: Entrapment neuropathies of the foot and ankle, *Orthop Trauma* 23(6):404–411, 2009.

Allen JM, Greer BJ, Sorge DS, et al: MR Imaging of neuropathies of the leg, ankle, and foot, *Magn Reson Imaging Clin N Am* 16(1):117–131, 2008.

Chapter 115

ACHILLES TENDINITIS

ICD-9 CODE 727.00

ICD-10 CODE M65.879

THE CLINICAL SYNDROME

Achilles tendinitis has become more common as jogging has increased in popularity. The Achilles tendon is susceptible to the development of tendinitis both at its insertion on the calcaneus and at its narrowest part, a point approximately 5 cm above its insertion. The Achilles tendon is subjected to repetitive motion that may result in microtrauma, which heals poorly owing to the tendon's avascular nature. Running is often the inciting factor in acute Achilles tendinitis, which frequently coexists with bursitis and thus causes additional pain and functional disability. Calcium deposition around the tendon may occur if inflammation persists, and this complication makes subsequent treatment more difficult. Continued trauma to the inflamed tendon may ultimately result in tendon rupture.

SIGNS AND SYMPTOMS

The onset of Achilles tendinitis is usually acute, occurring after overuse or misuse of the ankle joint. Inciting activities include running with sudden stops and starts, such as when playing tennis. Improper stretching of the gastrocnemius and Achilles tendon before exercise has also been implicated in Achilles tendinitis, as well as in acute tendon rupture. The pain of Achilles tendinitis is constant and severe and is localized in the posterior ankle (Fig. 115-1). Significant sleep disturbance is often reported. Patients may attempt to splint the inflamed Achilles tendon by adopting a flatfooted gait to avoid plantar flexing the tendon. Pain is induced with resisted plantar flexion of the foot, and a creaking or grating sensation may be palpated when the foot is passively plantar flexed (Fig. 115-2). A chronically inflamed Achilles tendon may suddenly rupture from stress or during injection into the tendon itself.

TESTING

Plain radiographs and magnetic resonance imaging (MRI) are indicated in all patients who present with posterior ankle pain (Fig. 115-3). MRI of the ankle is also indicated if joint instability is suspected. Radionuclide bone scanning is useful to identify stress fractures not seen on plain radiographs. Based on the patient's clinical presentation, additional testing may be warranted, including a complete blood count, erythrocyte sedimentation rate, and antinuclear antibody testing. The injection technique described later serves as both a diagnostic and a therapeutic maneuver.

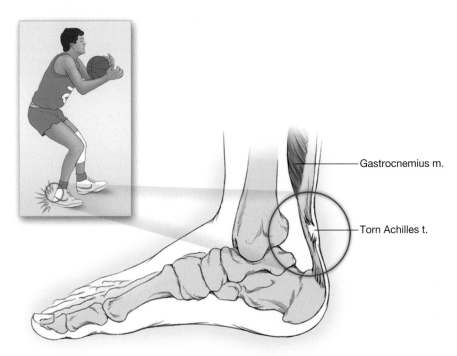

Gastrocnemius m.

Torn Achilles t.

Figure 115-1 The pain of Achilles tendinitis is constant and severe and is localized to the posterior ankle.

DIFFERENTIAL DIAGNOSIS

Achilles tendinitis is usually easily identified on clinical grounds. However, if the bursa located between the Achilles tendon and the base of the tibia and the upper posterior calcaneus is inflamed, coexistent bursitis may confuse the diagnosis. Stress fractures of the ankle may also mimic Achilles tendinitis.

TREATMENT

Initial treatment of the pain and functional disability associated with Achilles tendinitis includes a combination of nonsteroidal antiinflammatory drugs (NSAIDs) or cyclooxygenase-2 inhibitors and physical therapy. The local application of heat and cold may also be beneficial. Repetitive activities thought to be responsible for the development of tendinitis, such as jogging, should be avoided. For patients who do not respond to these treatment modalities, injection with local anesthetic and steroid is a reasonable next step.

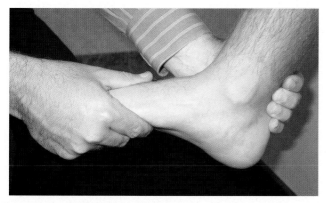

Figure 115-2 Eliciting the creak sign for Achilles tendinitis. *(From Waldman SD: Physical diagnosis of pain: an atlas of signs and symptoms, Philadelphia, 2006, Saunders, p 377.)*

Injection for Achilles tendinitis is carried out by placing the patient in the prone position with the affected foot hanging off the end of the table. The foot is gently dorsiflexed to facilitate identification of the margin of the tendon, because injection directly into the tendon should be avoided. The tender point at the tendinous insertion or at its narrowest part approximately 5 cm above the insertion is identified and marked with a sterile marker. The skin overlying this point is prepared with antiseptic solution. A sterile syringe containing 2 mL of 0.25% preservative-free bupivacaine and 40 mg methylprednisolone is attached to a 1½-inch, 25-gauge needle by using strict aseptic technique. The previously marked point is palpated, and the needle is carefully advanced at this point along the tendon and through the skin and subcutaneous tissues, with care taken not to enter the substance of the tendon. The contents of the syringe are gently injected while the clinician slowly withdraws the needle. Resistance to injection should be minimal. If resistance is significant, the needle tip is probably in the substance of the Achilles tendon and should be withdrawn slightly until the injection can proceed without significant resistance. The needle is removed, and a sterile pressure dressing and ice pack are applied to the injection site.

Physical modalities, including local heat and gentle range-of-motion exercises, should be introduced several days after the patient undergoes injection. Vigorous exercises should be avoided, because they will exacerbate the patient's symptoms. Simple analgesics and NSAIDs can be used concurrently with this injection technique.

COMPLICATIONS AND PITFALLS

Trauma to the Achilles tendon from the injection itself is an ever-present possibility. Tendons that are highly inflamed or previously damaged are subject to rupture if they are injected directly. This complication can be avoided if the clinician uses gentle technique and stops injecting immediately if significant resistance is encountered. Approximately 25% of patients complain of a transient increase in pain after injection, and patients should be warned of this possibility.

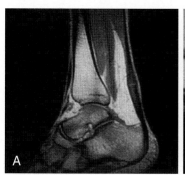
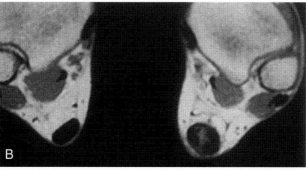

Figure 115-3 Magnetic resonance imaging of chronic, degenerative tendinosis with thickening of the tendon in the sagittal **(A)** and coronal **(B)** planes compared with the opposite Achilles tendon. *(From Lesic A, Bumbasirevic M: Disorders of the Achilles tendon, Curr Orthop 18[1]:63–75, 2004.)*

Clinical Pearls

Although the Achilles tendon is the thickest and strongest tendon in the body, it is susceptible to inflammation or even rupture. It begins at the midcalf and continues downward, narrowing as it goes, to attach to the posterior calcaneus; it becomes narrowest approximately 5 cm above its calcaneal insertion. At these two points, tendinitis is most likely to develop. The injection technique described is extremely effective in treating Achilles tendinitis. Coexistent bursitis and arthritis may contribute to the patient's symptoms, thus necessitating additional treatment with more localized injection of local anesthetic and methylprednisolone.

SUGGESTED READINGS

Grivas TB, Koufopoulos GE, Vasiliadis E, et al: The management of lower extremity soft tissue and tendon trauma, *Clin Podiatr Med Surg* 23(2):257–282, 2006.

Lesic A, Bumbasirevic M: Disorders of the Achilles tendon, *Curr Orthop* 18(1):63–75, 2004.

Stephenson K, Saltzman CL, Brotzman SB: Foot and ankle injuries. In Brotzman SB, Wilk KE, editors: *Handbook of orthopaedic rehabilitation,* ed 2, St Louis, 2007, Mosby, pp 547–646.

Waldman SD: Achilles tendinitis. In *Pain review,* Philadelphia, 2009, Saunders, p 325.

Chapter **116**

ACHILLES TENDON RUPTURE

ICD-9 CODE 727.67

ICD-10 CODE M66.369

THE CLINICAL SYNDROME

Achilles tendon rupture most often occurs following an injury after acute push-off during jumping or sprinting as the result of extreme ankle dorsiflexion, Occurring in otherwise healthy adults, it is a disease of the third to fifth decades and has a male predominance. Rupture of the Achilles tendon most often occurs in the left leg because right-handed individuals usually push off with the left leg when they jump.

The Achilles tendon is most susceptible to rupture at its narrowest part, a point approximately 5 cm above its insertion. The Achilles tendon is subjected to repetitive motion that may result in microtrauma, which heals poorly owing to the tendon's avascular nature. The repeated microtrauma leads to tendinitis and tendinopathy that may predispose the tendon to rupture. Achilles tendinitis frequently coexists with bursitis, which causes additional pain and functional disability.

In addition to traumatic rupture of the Achilles tendon, sudden, nontraumatic rupture may occur. Factors that predispose the patient to traumatic and nontraumatic rupture of the Achilles tendon include steroid use, dialysis, gout, rheumatoid arthritis, systemic lupus erythematosus, diabetes, endocrinopathies, renal transplant, hyperlipidemias, and the use of fluoroquinolones (Table 116-1).

SIGNS AND SYMPTOMS

The onset of Achilles tendon rupture is usually acute, occurring after acute push-off during jumping or sprinting as the result of extreme ankle dorsiflexion. Improper stretching of the gastrocnemius and Achilles tendon before exercise has also been implicated in the development of Achilles tendinitis and acute tendon rupture. The pain of Achilles tendon rupture is constant and severe and is localized in the posterior ankle. The patient often complains of a feeling like being kicked in the ankle. Significant ecchymosis, swelling, and hematoma are frequently present. Palpation of the ruptured Achilles tendon may reveal a lack of tendon continuity. The patient suffering from Achilles tendon rupture exhibit positive results of the toe raise and Thompson squeeze tests (Fig. 116-1).

TABLE 116-1

Factors Associated With Rupture of the Achilles Tendon

- Steroid use
- Dialysis
- Gout
- Rheumatoid arthritis
- Systemic lupus erythematosus
- Diabetes
- Endocrinopathies
- Renal transplantation
- Hyperlipidemias
- Fluoroquinolone use

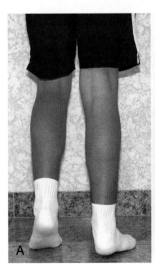 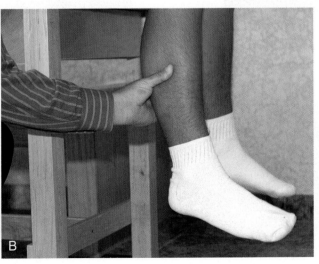

Figure 116-1 **A,** To perform the toe raise test for Achilles tendon rupture, the patient is asked to stand in a comfortable position and then to raise himself or herself on tiptoe. **B,** To perform the Thompson squeeze test for Achilles tendon rupture, the examiner grasps the calf on the patient's affected side just below the point of the calf's maximum girth and firmly squeezes the calf. Absence of plantar flexion on the affected side provides a presumptive diagnosis of rupture of the Achilles tendon. *(From Waldman SD: Physical diagnosis of pain: an atlas of signs and symptoms, ed 2, Philadelphia, 2010, Saunders, pp 344, 346.)*

TESTING

Plain radiographs and magnetic resonance imaging (MRI) are indicated in all patients who present with posterior ankle pain and who are suspected of suffering from Achilles tendon rupture (Fig. 116-2). MRI of the ankle is also indicated if joint instability, bursitis, or occult tumor is suspected. Radionuclide bone scanning is useful to identify stress fractures not seen on plain radiographs. Ultrasound imaging may also help assess the integrity of the Achilles tendon (Fig. 116-3). Based on the patient's clinical presentation, additional testing may be warranted, including a complete blood count, erythrocyte sedimentation rate, and antinuclear antibody testing.

DIFFERENTIAL DIAGNOSIS

Achilles tendon rupture is usually easily identified on clinical grounds. However, if the bursa located between the Achilles tendon and the base of the tibia and the upper posterior calcaneus is inflamed, coexistent bursitis may confuse the diagnosis. Stress fractures of the ankle may also mimic the pain of Achilles tendon rupture.

TREATMENT

Initial treatment of the pain and functional disability associated with Achilles tendon rupture includes elevation, relative rest, and ice. A combination of nonsteroidal antiinflammatory drugs or cyclooxygenase-2 inhibitors and short-acting opioid analgesics such as hydrocodone may be necessary to manage the acute pain associated with this condition. Although some specialists recommend conservative therapy, most believe that surgical repair of the tendon with postoperative immobilization is the best option in otherwise healthy patients (Fig. 116-4).

COMPLICATIONS AND PITFALLS

Repeat rupture of the affected Achilles tendon represents a real risk whether conservative or operative treatment is pursued. Care must be taken to avoid immobilization with casts until the acute swelling associated with tendon rupture is resolved or nerve compression and pressure ulcers may result. Gentle physical therapy during the healing phase is essential if functional ability is to be maintained.

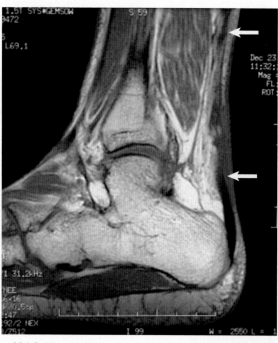

Figure 116-2 A magnetic resonance image with *arrows* pointing to the ends of the Achilles tendon ends. The area between the arrows represents the gap between the tendon ends. *(From Padanilam TG: Chronic Achilles tendon ruptures,* Foot Ankle Clin *14[4]:711–728, 2009.)*

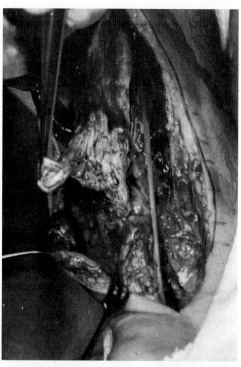

Figure 116-4 The standard method for repair of Achilles tendon ruptures. The frayed ends of the tendon are not routinely débrided. *(From DeLee JC, Drez DD, Miller M, editors:* Orthopaedic sports medicine: principles and practice, *ed 3, Philadelphia, 2010, Saunders, p 2010.)*

Figure 116-3 **A,** Longitudinal ultrasound scan of a ruptured Achilles tendon during plantar flexion shows less than 1 cm of separation between the torn tendon ends. The patient was successfully treated with casting in plantar flexion. **B,** Same patient with longitudinal scanning in dorsiflexion shows increased separation and better delineation of the complete tendon rupture. *(From Fessell DP, Jacobson JA: Ultrasound of the hindfoot and midfoot,* Radiol Clin North Am *46[6]:1027–1043, 2008.)*

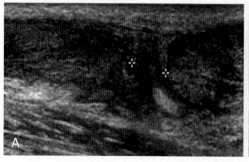
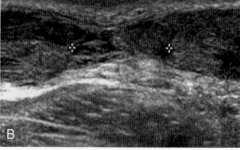

Clinical Pearls

Although the Achilles tendon is the thickest and strongest tendon in the body, it is susceptible to inflammation or even rupture. It begins at the midcalf and continues downward, narrowing as it goes, to attach to the posterior calcaneus; it becomes narrowest approximately 5 cm above its calcaneal insertion. Coexistent bursitis and arthritis may contribute to the patient's symptoms, thus necessitating additional treatment with more localized injection of local anesthetic and methylprednisolone.

SUGGESTED READINGS

Fessell DP, Jacobson JA: Ultrasound of the hindfoot and midfoot, *Radiol Clin North Am* 46(6):1027–1043, 2008.

Grivas TB, Koufopoulos GE, Vasiliadis E, et al: The management of lower extremity soft tissue and tendon trauma, *Clin Podiatr Med Surg* 23(2):257–282, 2006.

Lesic A, Bumbasirevic M: Disorders of the Achilles tendon, *Curr Orthop* 18(1):63–75, 2004.

Stephenson K, Saltzman CL, Brotzman SB: Foot and ankle injuries. In Brotzman SB, Wilk KE, editors: *Handbook of orthopaedic rehabilitation*, ed 2, St Louis, 2007, Mosby, pp 547–646.

Waldman SD: The Achilles tendon. In *Pain review*, Philadelphia, 2009, Saunders, p 161.

Chapter 117

ARTHRITIS PAIN OF THE TOES

ICD-9 CODE 715.97

ICD-10 CODE M19.90

THE CLINICAL SYNDROME

The toe joint is susceptible to the development of arthritis from various conditions that have the ability to damage the joint cartilage. Osteoarthritis is the most common form of arthritis that results in toe joint pain; rheumatoid arthritis and posttraumatic arthritis are also frequent causes of toe pain. Less common causes include the collagen vascular diseases, infection, and Lyme disease. Acute infectious arthritis is usually accompanied by significant systemic symptoms, including fever and malaise, and should be easily recognized; it is treated with culture and antibiotics rather than injection therapy. Collagen vascular disease generally manifests as polyarthropathy rather than as monarthropathy limited to the toe joint, although toe pain secondary to collagen vascular disease responds exceedingly well to the intraarticular injection technique described later.

SIGNS AND SYMPTOMS

Most patients present with pain localized to the affected joint of the foot, most commonly the great toe. Activity, especially flexion of the toe joints, makes the pain worse (Fig. 117-1), whereas rest and heat provide some relief. The pain is constant and is characterized as aching; it may interfere with sleep. Some patients complain of a grating or popping sensation with use of the joint, and crepitus may be present on physical examination. In addition to pain, patients often experience a gradual decrease in functional ability because of reduced toe range of motion that makes simple everyday tasks such as walking, standing on tiptoes, and climbing stairs quite difficult.

TESTING

Plain radiographs are indicated in all patients who present with toe joint pain (Figs. 117-2 and 117-3). Magnetic resonance imaging of the toe is indicated if joint instability, an occult mass, or a tumor is suspected. Based on the patient's clinical presentation, additional

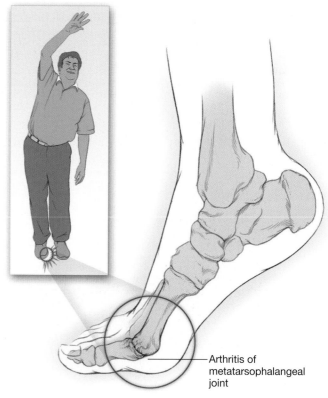

Arthritis of metatarsophalangeal joint

Figure 117-1 Arthritis of the toe manifests as pain that is made worse with weight-bearing activity.

testing may be warranted, including a complete blood count, erythrocyte sedimentation rate, and antinuclear antibody testing.

DIFFERENTIAL DIAGNOSIS

Bursitis and tendinitis of the foot, as well as entrapment neuropathies such as tarsal tunnel syndrome, may confuse the diagnosis; these conditions may coexist with arthritis of the toes. Primary and metastatic tumors of the foot, occult fractures of the tarsals and metatarsals, and fractures of the sesamoid bones of the foot may manifest in a manner similar to arthritis of the toes.

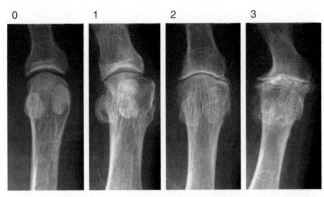

Figure 117-2 Examples of first metatarsophalangeal joint (dorsal) joint space narrowing in osteoarthritis. *(From Menz HB, Munteanu SE, Landorf KB, et al: Radiographic classification of osteoarthritis in commonly affected joints of the foot,* Osteoarthritis Cartilage *15[11]:1333–1338, 2007.)*

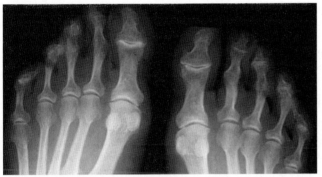

Figure 117-3 Feet radiographs showing joint narrowing, bone proliferation, and ankylosis. *(From Mas AJ, Rotés-Querol J: Erosive osteoarthritis of the feet: description of two patients,* Joint Bone Spine *74[3]:296–298, 2007.)*

TREATMENT

Initial treatment of the pain and functional disability associated with arthritis of the toes includes a combination of nonsteroidal antiinflammatory drugs or cyclooxygenase-2 inhibitors and physical therapy. The local application of heat and cold may also be beneficial. Avoidance of repetitive activities that aggravate the patient's symptoms, as well as short-term immobilization of the toe joints, may provide relief. For patients who do not respond to these treatment modalities, intraarticular injection with local anesthetic and steroid is a reasonable next step.

To perform intraarticular injection of the toes, the patient is placed in the supine position, and the skin overlying the affected toe joint is prepared with antiseptic solution. A sterile syringe containing 1.5 mL of 0.25% preservative-free bupivacaine and 40 mg methylprednisolone is attached to a ⅝-inch, 25-gauge needle by using strict aseptic technique. The affected toe is distracted to open the joint space, which is identified. At this point, the needle is carefully advanced perpendicular to the joint space next to the extensor tendons through the skin, subcutaneous tissues, and joint capsule and into the joint. If bone is encountered, the needle is withdrawn into the subcutaneous tissues and is redirected superiorly. Once the needle is in the joint space, the contents of the syringe are gently injected. Little resistance to injection should be felt. If resistance is encountered, the needle is probably in a ligament or tendon and should be advanced slightly into the joint space until the injection can proceed without significant resistance. The needle is removed, and a sterile pressure dressing and ice pack are applied to the injection site.

Physical modalities, including local heat and gentle range-of-motion exercises, should be introduced several days after the patient undergoes injection. Vigorous exercises should be avoided, because they will exacerbate the patient's symptoms.

COMPLICATIONS AND PITFALLS

Failure to identify primary or metastatic tumor of the foot that is causing the patient's pain can have disastrous results. The injection technique is safe if careful attention is paid to the clinically relevant anatomy. The major complication of injection is infection, although this should be exceedingly rare if strict aseptic technique is followed. Approximately 25% of patients complain of a transient increase in pain after injection, and patients should be warned of this possibility.

Clinical Pearls

Coexistent bursitis and tendinitis may contribute to the patient's pain, thus necessitating additional treatment with more localized injection of local anesthetic and methylprednisolone. The injection technique described is extremely effective in treating the pain of arthritis of the toe joints.

SUGGESTED READINGS

Menz HB, Munteanu SE, Landorf KB, et al: Radiographic classification of osteoarthritis in commonly affected joints of the foot, *Osteoarthritis Cartilage* 15(11):1333–1338, 2007.

Milner S: Common disorders of the foot and ankle, *Surgery* 24(11):382–385, 2006.

Waldman SD: Intraarticular injection of the ankle and foot. In *Atlas of pain management injection techniques,* ed 2, Philadelphia, 2007, Saunders, pp 497–500.

Waldman SD: Functional anatomy of the ankle and foot. In *Pain review,* Philadelphia, 2009, Saunders, pp 155–156.

Chapter 118

BUNION PAIN

ICD-9 CODE `727.1`

ICD-10 CODE `M20.10`

THE CLINICAL SYNDROME

Bunion is one of the most common causes of foot pain. The term *bunion* refers to soft tissue swelling over the first metatarsophalangeal joint associated with abnormal angulation of the joint that results in a prominent first metatarsal head and overlapping of the first and second toes, called the hallux valgus deformity. The first metatarsophalangeal joint may ultimately subluxate and cause the overlapping of the first and second toes to worsen. An inflamed adventitious bursa may accompany bunion formation. The most common cause of bunions is the wearing of narrow-toed shoes, and high heels may exacerbate the problem (Fig. 118-1); thus, bunions are more common in women.

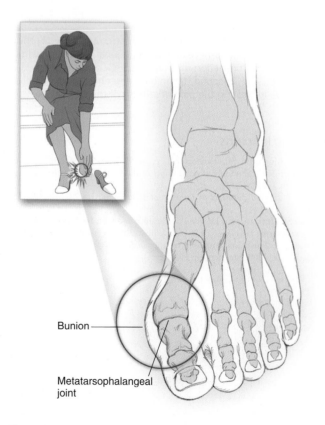

Bunion

Metatarsophalangeal joint

Figure 118-1 Narrow-toed shoes are implicated in the development of bunions.

SIGNS AND SYMPTOMS

Most patients present with pain localized to the affected first metatarsophalangeal joint and complain of being unable to get shoes to fit. Walking makes the pain worse, whereas rest and heat provide some relief. The pain is constant and is characterized as aching; it may interfere with sleep. Some patients complain of a grating or popping sensation with use of the joint, and crepitus may be present on physical examination. In addition to pain, patients with bunions develop the characteristic hallux valgus deformity, with a prominent first metatarsal head, improper angulation of the joint, and overlapping first and second toes.

TESTING

Plain radiographs are indicated in all patients who present with bunion pain (Fig. 118-2). Magnetic resonance imaging of the toe is indicated if joint instability, an occult mass, or a tumor is suspected. Based on the patient's clinical presentation, additional testing may be warranted, including a complete blood count, erythrocyte sedimentation rate, and antinuclear antibody testing.

DIFFERENTIAL DIAGNOSIS

The diagnosis of bunion is usually obvious on clinical grounds alone. Bursitis and tendinitis of the foot and ankle often coexist with bunion pain. In addition, stress fractures of the metatarsals, phalanges, or sesamoid bones may confuse the diagnosis and require specific treatment.

TREATMENT

Initial treatment of the pain and functional disability associated with bunion includes a combination of nonsteroidal antiinflammatory drugs or cyclooxygenase-2 inhibitors and physical therapy. The local application of heat and cold may also be beneficial. Avoidance of repetitive activities that aggravate the patient's symptoms, avoidance of narrow-toed or high-heeled shoes, and short-term immobilization of the affected toes may also provide relief. For patients who do not respond to these treatment modalities, injection with local anesthetic and steroid is a reasonable next step.

To inject the bunion deformity, the patient is placed in the supine position, and the skin overlying the bunion is prepared with antiseptic solution. A sterile syringe containing 1.5 mL of 0.25% preservative-free bupivacaine and 40 mg methylprednisolone is attached to a ⅝-inch, 25-gauge needle by using strict aseptic technique. The bunion is identified, and the needle is carefully advanced against the first metatarsal head. The needle is then withdrawn slightly out of the periosteum, and the contents of the syringe are gently injected. Little resistance to injection should be

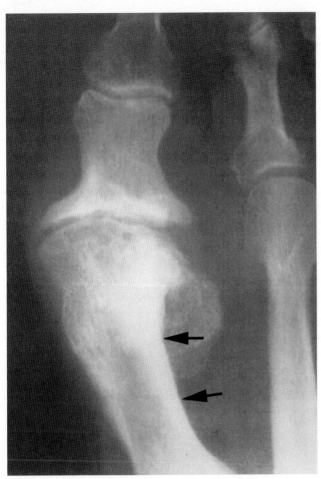

Figure 118-2 Osteoarthritis of the first metatarsophalangeal joint in a patient with hallux valgus deformity. The sesamoids are lateral to the metatarsal head. The radiograph shows narrowing of the joint space, with subchondral bone and osteophyte formation. Marked thickening of the lateral cortex of the metatarsal shaft *(arrows)* is evident. *(From Brower AC, Flemming DJ: Arthritis in black and white, ed 2, Philadelphia, 1997, Saunders.)*

felt. If resistance is encountered, the needle is probably in a ligament or tendon and should be advanced or withdrawn slightly until the injection can proceed without significant resistance. The needle is removed, and a sterile pressure dressing and ice pack are applied to the injection site.

Physical modalities, including local heat and gentle range-of-motion exercises, should be introduced several days after the patient undergoes injection.

COMPLICATIONS AND PITFALLS

Failure to identify primary or metastatic tumor of the foot that is causing the patient's pain can have disastrous results. The injection technique is safe if careful attention is paid to the clinically relevant anatomy. The major complication of injection is infection, although this should be exceedingly rare if strict aseptic technique is followed. Approximately 25% of patients complain of a transient increase in pain after injection, and patients should be warned of this possibility.

Clinical Pearls

Coexistent bursitis and tendinitis may contribute to the patient's foot pain, thus necessitating additional treatment with more localized injection of local anesthetic and methylprednisolone. The injection technique described is extremely effective in treating bunion pain. Narrow-toed and high-heeled shoes should be avoided, because they will exacerbate the patient's symptoms.

SUGGESTED READINGS

Albert A, Leemrijse T: The dorsal bunion: an overview, *Foot Ankle Surg* 11(2):65–68, 2005.
Kennedy JG, Collumbier JA: Bunions in dancers, *Clin Sports Med* 27(2):321–328, 2008.
Lavelle WF, Bellapianta JM, Lavelle ED: Foot pain. In Smith HS, editor: *Current therapy in pain*, 2009, pp 189–194.
Mann R: Bunion deformity in elite athletes. In Porter DA, Schon LC, editors: *Baxter's the foot and ankle in sport*, ed 2, St Louis, 2008, Mosby, pp 435–443.

Chapter 119

MORTON'S NEUROMA

ICD-9 CODE `355.6`

ICD-10 CODE `G57.60`

THE CLINICAL SYNDROME

Morton's neuroma is one of the most common pain syndromes affecting the forefoot. It is characterized by tenderness and burning pain in the plantar surface of the forefoot, with painful paresthesias in the two affected toes. This pain syndrome is thought to be caused by perineural fibrosis of the interdigital nerves. Although the nerves between the third and fourth toes are affected most commonly, the second and third toes and, rarely, the fourth and fifth toes can be affected as well (Fig. 119-1). Patients may feel like they are walking with a stone in the shoe. The pain of Morton's neuroma worsens with prolonged standing or walking for long distances and is exacerbated by poorly fitting or improperly padded shoes. As with bunion and hammer toe deformities, Morton's neuroma is associated with wearing tight, narrow-toed shoes.

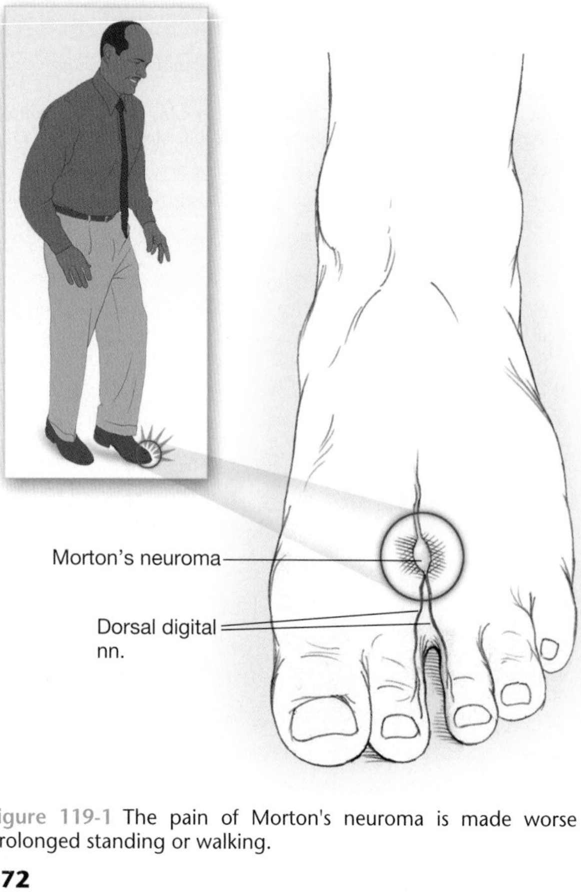

SIGNS AND SYMPTOMS

On physical examination, pain can be reproduced by performing Mulder's maneuver: firmly squeezing the two metatarsal heads together with one hand while placing firm pressure on the interdigital space with the other (Fig. 119-2). In contrast to metatarsalgia, in which the tender area is over the metatarsal heads, with Morton's neuroma, the tender area is localized to only the plantar surface of the affected interspace, with paresthesias radiating into the two affected toes. Patients with Morton's neuroma often exhibit an antalgic gait in an effort to reduce weight bearing during walking.

TESTING

Plain radiographs and magnetic resonance imaging (MRI) are indicated in all patients who present with Morton's neuroma, to rule out fractures and to identify sesamoid bones that may have become inflamed (Fig. 119-3). MRI of the metatarsal bones is also indicated if joint instability, an occult mass, or a tumor is suspected. Ultrasound imaging may also aid in the diagnosis of Morton's neuroma. Radionuclide bone scanning may be useful to identify stress fractures of the metatarsal or sesamoid bones that may be missed on plain radiographs. Based on the patient's clinical presentation, additional testing may be warranted, including a complete blood count, erythrocyte sedimentation rate, and antinuclear antibody testing.

Morton's neuroma —

Dorsal digital nn. —

Figure 119-1 The pain of Morton's neuroma is made worse with prolonged standing or walking.

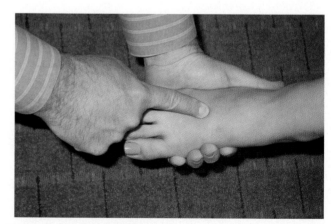

Figure 119-2 Eliciting Mulder's sign for Morton's neuroma. *(From Waldman SD: Physical diagnosis of pain: an atlas of signs and symptoms, Philadelphia, 2006, Saunders, p 381.)*

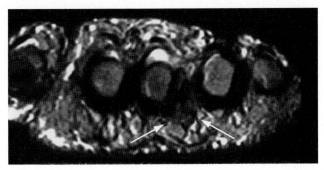

Figure 119-3 Morton's neuroma. Coronal (short axis) T2-weighted magnetic resonance image through the forefoot demonstrates a hypointense lesion located between the third and fourth metatarsal heads *(arrows)*. *(From Edelman RR, Hesselink JR, Zlatkin MB, Crues JV, editors:* Clinical magnetic resonance imaging, *ed 3, Philadelphia, 2006, Saunders, p 4355.)*

DIFFERENTIAL DIAGNOSIS

Fractures of the sesamoid bones of the foot are often confused with Morton's neuroma; although the pain of sesamoid fracture is localized to the plantar surface of the foot, it is less neuritic than is that of Morton's neuroma. Tendinitis, bursitis, and stress fractures of the foot can also mimic the pain of Morton's neuroma.

TREATMENT

Initial treatment of the pain and functional disability associated with Morton's neuroma includes a combination of nonsteroidal antiinflammatory drugs or cyclooxygenase-2 inhibitors and physical therapy. The local application of heat and cold may also be beneficial. Avoidance of repetitive activities that aggravate the patient's symptoms, avoidance of narrow-toed or high-heeled shoes, and short-term immobilization of the affected foot may also provide relief. For patients who do not respond to these treatment modalities, injection with local anesthetic and steroid is a reasonable next step.

To inject Morton's neuroma, the patient is placed in the supine position with a pillow under the knee to slightly flex the leg. A total of 3 mL non-epinephrine-containing local anesthetic and 40 mg methylprednisolone is drawn up in a 12-mL sterile syringe. The affected interdigital space is identified, the dorsal surface of the foot at this point is marked with a sterile marker, and the skin is prepared with antiseptic solution. At a point proximal to the metatarsal head, a 1½-inch, 25-gauge needle is inserted between the two metatarsal bones in the area to be blocked (Fig. 119-4). While the clinician is slowly injecting, the needle is advanced from the dorsal surface of the foot toward the palmar surface. Because the plantar digital nerve is situated on the dorsal side of the flexor retinaculum, the needle must be advanced almost to the palmar surface of the foot. The needle is removed, and pressure is applied to the injection site to avoid hematoma formation.

Physical modalities, including local heat and gentle range-of-motion exercises, should be introduced several days after the patient undergoes injection.

COMPLICATIONS AND PITFALLS

Failure to identify primary or metastatic tumor of the foot that is causing the patient's pain can have disastrous results. The major complication of injection is infection, although this should be

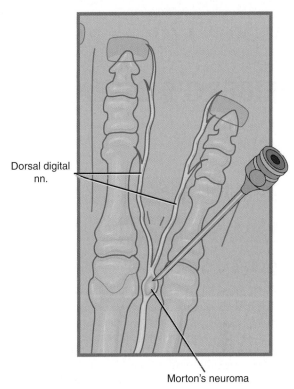

Dorsal digital nn.

Morton's neuroma

Figure 119-4 Proper needle placement for injection of Morton's neuroma. *(From Waldman SD:* Atlas of pain management injection techniques, *Philadelphia, 2000, Saunders.)*

exceedingly rare if strict aseptic technique is followed. Because of the confined space of the soft tissues surrounding the metatarsals and digits, mechanical compression of the blood supply after injection is a possibility. To prevent vascular insufficiency and gangrene from occurring, the clinician must avoid rapidly injecting a large volume of solution into these confined spaces; epinephrine-containing solutions should not be used, for the same reasons. Approximately 25% of patients complain of a transient increase in pain after injection, and patients should be warned of this possibility.

Clinical Pearls

Coexistent bursitis and tendinitis may contribute to the patient's foot pain, thus necessitating additional treatment with more localized injection of local anesthetic and methylprednisolone. The injection technique described is extremely effective in treating the pain of Morton's neuroma; however, patients often require shoe orthoses and shoes with a wider toe box to take pressure off the affected interdigital nerves.

SUGGESTED READINGS

Clinical Practice Guideline Forefoot Disorders Panel, Thomas JL, Blitch EL IV, et al: Diagnosis and treatment of forefoot disorders. Section 3. Morton's intermetatarsal neuroma, *J Foot Ankle Surg* 48(2):251–256, 2009.
George VA, Khan AM, Hutchinson CE, et al: Morton's neuroma: the role of MR scanning in diagnostic assistance, *Foot* 15(1):14–16, 2005.
Williams TH, Robinson AH: Entrapment neuropathies of the foot and ankle, *Orthop Trauma* 23(6):404–411, 2009.
Wu KK: Morton's interdigital neuroma: a clinical review of its etiology, treatment, and results, *J Foot Ankle Surg* 35(2):112–119, 1996.

Chapter 120

FREIBERG'S DISEASE

ICD-9 CODE 732.5

ICD-10 CODE M72.90

The Clinical Syndrome

Freiberg's disease is an often missed clinical diagnosis. The disease may be identified as a result of the characteristic radiographic findings of collapse of the second and, less commonly, third metatarsal head or heads. Like the scaphoid, the second metatarsal joint is extremely susceptible to this disease because of the tenuous blood supply of the articular cartilage. This blood supply is easily disrupted, and this often leaves the proximal portion of the bone without nutrition and leads to osteonecrosis. Although Freiberg's disease can occur at any age, it is a disease of adolescence through the second decade. Freiberg's disease is five times more common in female patients.

Although the exact cause of Freiberg's disease remains elusive, many investigators believe that this condition is the result of repetitive microtrauma to second and third metatarsal heads. Investigators believe that the relative immobility of the second and third metatarsals, combined with the extreme load transmission, makes these bones particularly susceptible to the development of avascular necrosis. High heels, which increase the load on the metatarsal heads, may raise the risk of the development of Freiberg's disease, as well as of any disease that impairs the blood supply to the foot (e.g., diabetes, vasculitis, and human immunodeficiency virus infection).

The patient with Freiberg's disease complains of pain over the affected metatarsal head or heads that may radiate into the adjacent toes (Fig. 120-1). The pain is deep and aching, and the patient often complains of increased pain on weight bearing and a limp when walking. The patient may or may not have a clear history of foot trauma that can be identified as the inciting incident for the disease.

Signs and Symptoms

Physical examination of patients suffering from Freiberg's disease reveals pain on deep palpation of the affected metatarsal joints. The pain can worsened by passive and active range of motion. Subtle swelling over the affected joint or joints may be appreciated on careful physical examination. An antalgic gait is invariably present.

Testing

Plain radiographs are indicated in all patients who present with Freiberg's disease, to confirm the diagnosis, as well as to rule out underlying occult bony disease (Fig. 120-2). Early subtle sclerotic

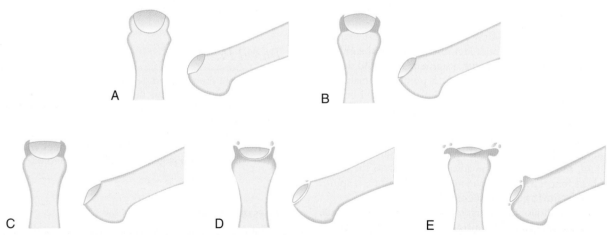

Figure 120-1 Levels of progression of Freiberg's disease. **A,** Early fracture of the subchondral epiphysis. **B,** Early collapse of the dorsal central portion of the metatarsal with flattening of the articular surface. **C,** Further flattening of the metatarsal head with continued collapse of the central portion of the articular surface with medial and lateral projections; the plantar articular cartilage remains intact. **D,** Loose bodies form from fractures of lateral projections and separation of a central articular fragment. **E,** End-stage degenerative arthrosis with marked flattening of the metatarsal head and joint space narrowing. *(Redrawn from Katcherian DA: Treatment of Freiberg's disease, Orthop Clin North Am 25:69–81, 1994, in DeLee JC, Drez DD, Miller M, editors: Orthopaedic sports medicine: principles and practice, ed 3, Philadelphia, 2010, Saunders, p 2167.)*

changes and joint space narrowing are often attributed to degenerative arthritis. Magnetic resonance imaging (MRI) may reveal articular changes before significant changes are evident on plain radiographs (Fig. 120-3). Based on the patient's clinical presentation, additional testing, including complete blood cell count, uric acid, sedimentation rate, and antinuclear antibody testing, may also be indicated. MRI of the foot is indicated in all patients suspected of suffering from Freiberg's disease, as well as when other causes of joint instability, infection, or tumor is suspected, or if the plain radiographs are nondiagnostic (Fig. 120-4). Administration of gadolinium followed by postcontrast imaging may help delineate the adequacy of blood supply; contrast enhancement of the metatarsal joint is a good prognostic sign. Electromyography is indicated if coexistent lumbar radiculopathy or lumbar plexopathy is suspected. A very gentle intraarticular injection of the affected joint with small volumes of local anesthetic provides immediate improvement of the pain and helps demonstrate that the nidus of the patient's pain is, in fact, the metatarsal joint. Ultimately, joint replacement is required in most patients suffering from Freiberg's disease.

DIFFERENTIAL DIAGNOSIS

Coexistent arthritis and gout of the metatarsal joints, bursitis, synovitis, and tendinitis may also coexist with Freiberg's disease and exacerbate the patient's pain and disability. Morton's neuroma can mimic the pain of Freiberg's disease. Tears of the ligaments, bone cysts, bone contusions, and fractures may also mimic the pain of Freiberg's disease, as can occult metastatic disease.

TREATMENT

Initial treatment of the pain and functional disability associated with Freiberg's disease should include a combination of the nonsteroidal antiinflammatory agents (NSAIDs) or

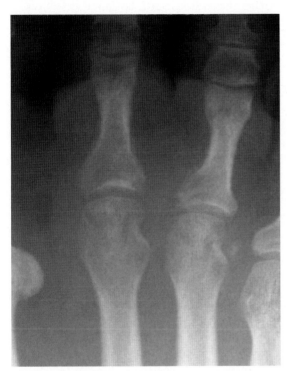

Figure 120-2 Anteroposterior radiograph showing distinct tissue swelling and periostitis of the diaphyses of the second and third proximal phalanges. *(From Dolce M, Osher L, McEneany P, Prins D: The use of surgical core decompression as treatment for avascular necrosis of the second and third metatarsal heads,* Foot *17[3]:162–166, 2007.)*

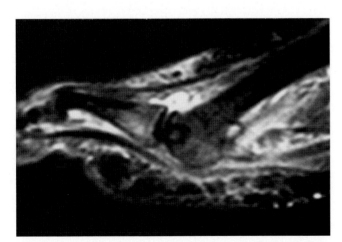

Figure 120-3 Sagittal short tau inversion recovery magnetic resonance image demonstrating higher juxta-articular marrow edema with a well-delineated low-signal defect of the second metatarsal head. *(From Dolce M, Osher L, McEneany P, Prins D: The use of surgical core decompression as treatment for avascular necrosis of the second and third metatarsal heads,* Foot *17[3]:162–166, 2007.)*

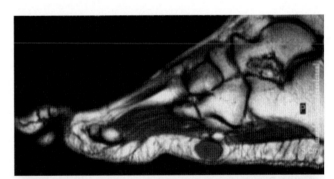

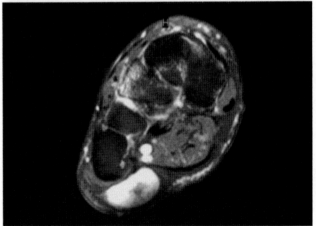

Figure 120-4 Sagittal and axial magnetic resonance images showing a lesion arising from the sole and not involving the deeper structures. This lesion was later shown to be a fibroma of the flexor tendon sheath. *(From Vasconez HC, Nisanci M, Lee EY: Giant cell tumour of the flexor tendon sheath of the foot,* J Plast Reconstr Aesthet Surg *61[7]:815–818, 2008.)*

cyclooxygenase-2 (COX-2) inhibitors and decreased weight bearing of the joint or joints. The local application of heat and cold may also be beneficial. For patients who do not respond to these treatment modalities, an injection of a local anesthetic and steroid into joint may be a reasonable next step to provide palliation of acute pain. Vigorous exercises should be avoided, because they will exacerbate the patient's symptoms. Ultimately, surgical repair in the form of total joint arthroplasty is the treatment of choice.

COMPLICATIONS AND PITFALLS

Failure to treat significant Freiberg's disease surgically usually results in continued pain and disability and, in most patients, leads to ongoing damage to the knee joint (see Fig. 120-2). Injection of the joint with local anesthetic and steroid is a relatively safe technique if the clinician is attentive to detail and specifically uses small amounts of local anesthetic and avoids high injection pressures that may further damage the joint. Another complication of this injection technique is infection. This complication should be exceedingly rare if strict aseptic technique is followed. Approximately 25% of patients will complain of a transient increase in pain after this injection technique, and patients should be warned of this possibility.

Clinical Pearls

Freiberg's disease is a diagnosis that is often missed, thus leading to much unnecessary pain and disability. The clinician should include Freiberg's disease in the differential diagnosis in all patients complaining of forefoot pain. Coexistent arthritis, tendinitis, and gout may also contribute to the pain and may require additional treatment. The use of physical modalities, including local heat and cold, as well as decreased weight bearing, may provide symptomatic relief. Vigorous exercises should be avoided, because they will exacerbate the patient's symptoms and may cause further damage to the foot. Simple analgesics and NSAIDs may be used concurrently with this injection technique.

SUGGESTED READINGS

Blitz NM, Yu JH: Freiberg's infraction in identical twins: a case report, *J Foot Ankle Surg* 44(3):218–221, 2005.

Hay SM, Harris NJ, Duckworth T: Freiberg's disease present in adjacent metatarsals, *Foot* 5(2):95–97, 1995.

Lavelle WF, Bellapianta JM, Lavelle ED: Foot pain. In Smith HS, editor: *Current therapy in pain,* 2009, pp 189–194.

Love JN, O'Mara S: Freiberg's disease in the emergency department, *J Emerg Med* 38(4):e23–e25, 2010.

Savini CJ, James CW: HIV infection and avascular necrosis, *J Assoc Nurses AIDS Care* 12(5):83–85, 2001.

Chapter 121

PLANTAR FASCIITIS

ICD-9 CODE **728.71**

ICD-10 CODE **M72.9**

THE CLINICAL SYNDROME

Plantar fasciitis is characterized by pain and tenderness over the plantar surface of the calcaneus. It is twice as common in women as in men. Plantar fasciitis is thought to be caused by inflammation of the plantar fascia, which can occur alone or as part of a systemic inflammatory condition such as rheumatoid arthritis, Reiter's syndrome, or gout. Obesity seems to predispose patients to the development of plantar fasciitis, as does going barefoot or wearing house slippers for prolonged periods (Fig. 121-1). High-impact aerobic exercise has also been implicated as a causative factor.

SIGNS AND SYMPTOMS

The pain of plantar fasciitis is most severe when first walking after a period of non–weight bearing and is made worse by prolonged standing or walking. On physical examination, patients exhibit a positive calcaneal jump sign, which consists of point tenderness over the plantar medial calcaneal tuberosity (Fig. 121-2). Patients may also have tenderness along the plantar fascia as it moves anteriorly. Pain is increased by dorsiflexing the toes, which pulls the plantar fascia taut, and then palpating along the fascia from the heel to the forefoot.

TESTING

Plain radiographs and magnetic resonance imaging are indicated in all patients who present with pain thought to be caused by plantar fasciitis, to rule out occult bony disorders and tumor (Figs. 121-3 and 121-4). Although characteristic radiographic changes are lacking in plantar fasciitis, radionuclide bone scanning may show increased uptake where the plantar fascia attaches to the medial calcaneal tuberosity; it can also rule out stress fractures not visible on plain radiographs. Based on the patient's clinical presentation, additional testing may be warranted, including a complete blood count, prostate-specific antigen level, erythrocyte sedimentation rate, and antinuclear antibody testing. The injection technique described later serves as both a diagnostic and a therapeutic maneuver.

DIFFERENTIAL DIAGNOSIS

Common causes of heel pain are listed in Table 121-1. The pain of plantar fasciitis may be confused with many diseases including the pain of Sever's disease, Morton's neuroma, or sesamoiditis.

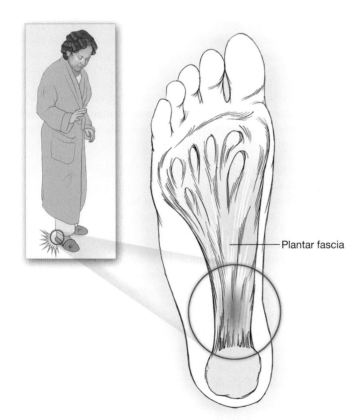

Figure 121-1 The pain of plantar fasciitis is localized to the hindfoot and can cause significant functional disability.

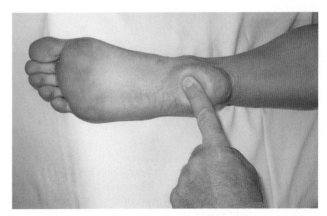

Figure 121-2 Eliciting the calcaneal jump sign for plantar fasciitis. *(From Waldman SD: Physical diagnosis of pain: an atlas of signs and symptoms, Philadelphia, 2006, Saunders, p 379.)*

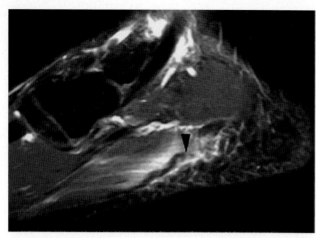

Figure 121-3 Rupture of the central cord of the plantar fascia. This sagittal short tau inversion recovery magnetic resonance image demonstrates discontinuity of the plantar fascia, with extensive edema of the flexor digitorum brevis muscle *(arrowhead)*. *(From Edelman RR, Hesselink JR, Zlatkin MB, Crues JV, editor: Clinical magnetic resonance imaging, ed 3, Philadelphia, 2006, Saunders, p 3456.)*

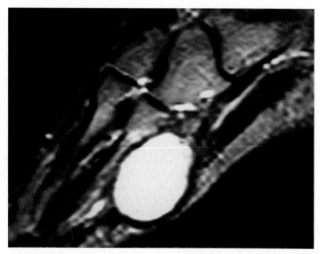

Figure 121-4 Synovial sarcoma. This sagittal T2-weighted magnetic resonance image demonstrates a large soft tissue mass in the plantar aspect of the foot. The mass is homogeneous and exhibits a thick capsule, simulating a fluid collection. *(From Edelman RR, Hesselink JR, Zlatkin MB, Crues JV, editor: Clinical magnetic resonance imaging, ed 3, Philadelphia, 2006, Saunders, p 3456.)*

TABLE 121-1	
Common Causes of Heel Pain	
Skeletal	Calcaneal epiphysitis (Sever's disease)
	Calcaneal stress fracture
	Tarsal stress fractures
	Infections, osteomyelitis
	Inflammatory arthropathies (e.g., Reiter's syndrome, psoriatic arthritis)
	Subtalar arthritis
Soft tissue	Achilles tendinitis
	Achilles tendon rupture
	Fat pad atrophy
	Heel pad contusion
	Plantar fascia rupture
	Posterior tibial tendinitis
	Retrocalcaneal bursitis
Neurologic	Abductor digiti quinti nerve entrapment
	Lumbar spine disorders
	Problems with medial calcaneal branch of the posterior tibial nerve
	Neuropathies
	Tarsal tunnel syndrome
Miscellaneous	Metabolic disorders
	Osteomalacia
	Paget's disease
	Sickle cell disease
	Tumors
	Neuromas
	Vascular insufficiency

Modified from Karabat N, Toros T, Hurel C: Ultrasonographic evaluation in plantar fasciitis, *J Foot Ankle Surg* 46(6):442–446, 2007.

that do not provide good support, and short-term immobilization of the affected foot may provide relief. For patients who do not respond to these treatment modalities, injection with local anesthetic and steroid is a reasonable next step.

To perform an injection for plantar fasciitis, the patient is placed in the supine position. The medial aspect of the heel is identified by palpation, and the skin overlying this point is prepared with antiseptic solution. A syringe containing 2 mL of 0.25% preservative-free bupivacaine and 40 mg methylprednisolone is attached to a 1½-inch, 25-gauge needle. The needle is slowly advanced through the previously identified point at a right angle to the skin, directly toward the center of the medial aspect of the calcaneus, until the needle impinges on bone. The needle is then withdrawn slightly out of the periosteum, and the contents of the syringe are gently injected as the needle is slowly withdrawn. The operator should feel slight resistance to injection, given the closed nature of the heel.

Physical modalities, including local heat and gentle stretching exercises, should be introduced several days after the patient undergoes injection. Vigorous exercises should be avoided, because they will exacerbate the patient's symptoms. Heel pads or molded orthotic devices may also be of value. Simple analgesics, NSAIDs, and antimyotonic agents such as tizanidine can be used concurrently with this injection technique.

COMPLICATIONS AND PITFALLS

Most complications of injection are related to needle-induced trauma at the injection site and in the underlying tissues. Many patients complain of a transient increase in pain after injection,

However, the characteristic pain on dorsiflexion of the toes associated with plantar fasciitis should help distinguish these conditions. Stress fractures of the metatarsal or sesamoid bones, bursitis, and tendinitis may also confuse the clinical picture.

TREATMENT

Initial treatment of the pain and functional disability associated with plantar fasciitis includes a combination of nonsteroidal anti-inflammatory drugs (NSAIDs) or cyclooxygenase-2 inhibitors and physical therapy. The local application of heat and cold may also be beneficial. Avoidance of repetitive activities that aggravate the patient's symptoms, avoidance of walking barefoot or with shoes which can be minimized by injecting gently and slowly. Infection, although rare, may occur if sterile technique is not followed.

Clinical Pearls

The injection technique described is extremely effective in treating the pain of plantar fasciitis. It is a safe procedure if careful attention is paid to the clinically relevant anatomy, sterile technique is used to avoid infection, and universal precautions are implemented to minimize any risk to the operator.

SUGGESTED READINGS

Karabat N, Toros T, Hurel C: Ultrasonographic evaluation in plantar fasciitis, *J Foot Ankle Surg* 46(6):442–446, 2007.

Puttaswamaiah R, Chandran P: Degenerative plantar fasciitis: a review of current concepts, *Foot* 17(1):3–9, 2007.

Rajput B, Abboud RJ: Common ignorance, major problem: the role of footwear in plantar fasciitis, *Foot* 14(4):214–218, 2004.

Waldman SD: Intraarticular injection of the ankle and foot. In *Atlas of pain management injection techniques,* ed 2, Philadelphia, 2007, Saunders, pp 497–500.

Waldman SD: Functional anatomy of the ankle and foot. In *Pain review,* Philadelphia, 2009, Saunders, pp 155–156.

Waldman SD: Plantar fasciitis. In *Pain review,* Philadelphia, 2009, Saunders, p 327.

Chapter 122

CALCANEAL SPUR SYNDROME

ICD-9 CODE **726.73**

ICD-10 CODE **M77.30**

THE CLINICAL SYNDROME

Calcaneal spurs are a common cause of heel pain. They can occur anywhere along the calcaneal tuberosity but are most frequent at the insertion of the plantar fascia (Fig. 122-1). Calcaneal spurs are usually asymptomatic, but when they are painful, the condition is generally the result of inflammation of the insertional fibers of the plantar fascia at the medial tuberosity. Symptomatic calcaneal spurs are often found in association with plantar fasciitis. Like plantar fasciitis, calcaneal spurs can occur alone or may be part of a systemic inflammatory condition such as rheumatoid arthritis, Reiter's syndrome, or gout. In some patients, the cause seems to be entirely mechanical, and such patients often exhibit an abnormal gait with excessive heel strike. High-impact aerobic exercise has also been implicated in the development of calcaneal spur syndrome (Fig. 122-2).

SIGNS AND SYMPTOMS

The pain of calcaneal spurs is most severe when first walking after a period of non–weight bearing and is made worse by prolonged standing or walking. On physical examination, patients exhibit

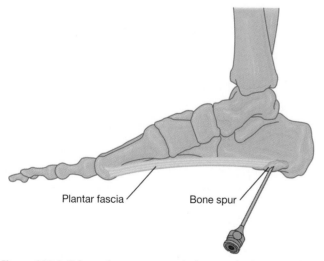

Figure 122-1 Calcaneal spurs commonly form at the insertion of the plantar fascia on the medial calcaneal tuberosity. *(From Waldman SD: Atlas of pain management injection techniques, ed 2, Philadelphia, 2007, Saunders, p 554.)*

Plantar fascia   Bone spur

380

point tenderness over the plantar medial calcaneal tuberosity; they may also have tenderness along the plantar fascia as it moves anteriorly. The pain of calcaneal spurs is increased by weight bearing and is relieved by padding of the affected heel.

TESTING

Plain radiographs are indicated in all patients who present with pain thought to be caused by calcaneal spurs, to confirm the diagnosis, as well as to rule out fracture of the spur, occult bony disorders, and tumor. Characteristic radiographic changes are lacking, but radionuclide bone scanning may show increased uptake at the point of attachment of the plantar fascia to the medial calcaneal tuberosity (Fig. 122-3). Magnetic resonance imaging (MRI) of the foot is indicated if calcaneal spurs, an occult mass, or a tumor is suspected (Fig. 122-4). MRI and radionuclide bone scanning may also be useful to exclude stress fractures not visible on plain radiographs (Fig. 122-5). Based on the patient's clinical presentation, additional testing may be warranted, including a complete blood count, prostate-specific antigen level, erythrocyte sedimentation rate, and antinuclear antibody testing. The injection technique described later serves as both a diagnostic and a therapeutic maneuver.

DIFFERENTIAL DIAGNOSIS

The pain of calcaneal spurs is often confused with that of plantar fasciitis, although the characteristic pain on dorsiflexion of the toes associated with plantar fasciitis should distinguish between these conditions. Stress fractures of the calcaneus, bursitis, and tendinitis can also confuse the clinical picture.

TREATMENT

Initial treatment of the pain and functional disability associated with calcaneal spur syndrome includes a combination of nonsteroidal antiinflammatory drugs or cyclooxygenase-2 inhibitors and physical therapy. The local application of heat and cold may also be beneficial. Avoidance of repetitive activities that aggravate the patient's symptoms, combined with short-term immobilization of the affected heel, may provide relief. For patients who do not respond to these treatment modalities, injection with local anesthetic and steroid is a reasonable next step.

To inject the calcaneal spur, the patient is placed in the supine position. The painful area of the heel overlying the calcaneal spur is identified by palpation, and the skin overlying this point is prepared with antiseptic solution. A syringe containing 2 mL of 0.25% preservative-free bupivacaine and 40 mg methylprednisolone is attached to a 1½-inch, 25-gauge needle. The needle is slowly advanced through the previously identified point at a right angle

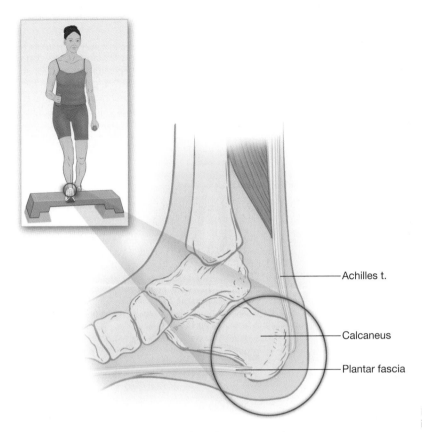

Achilles t.

Calcaneus

Plantar fascia

Figure 122-2 High-impact aerobic exercise has been implicated in the development of calcaneal spurs.

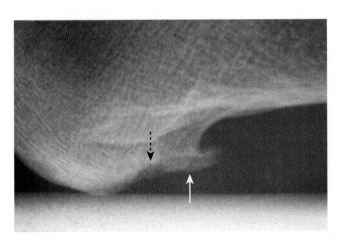

Figure 122-3 Close-up view of a heel spur demonstrated on a lateral weight-bearing radiograph. The *dashed arrow* indicates a small "saddle injury." The *solid arrow* indicates a subtle fracture line. *(From Smith S, Tinley P, Gilheany M, et al: The inferior calcaneal spur: anatomical and histological considerations,* Foot *17[1]:25–31, 2007.)*

to the skin, directly toward the center of the painful area, until it impinges on bone. The needle is then withdrawn slightly out of the periosteum, and the contents of the syringe are gently injected as the needle is slowly withdrawn. The operator should feel slight resistance to injection, given the closed nature of the heel.

Physical modalities, including local heat and gentle range-of-motion exercises, should be introduced several days after the patient undergoes injection.

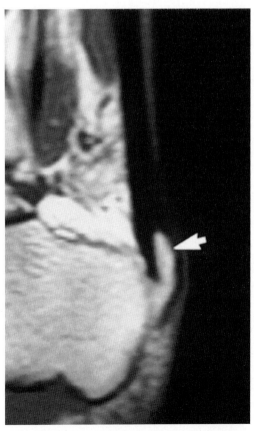

Figure 122-4 Sagittal T1-weighted spin-echo magnetic resonance image shows a large marrow-containing calcaneal enthesophyte arising at the insertion of the Achilles tendon *(arrow)*. *(From Resnick D: Diagnosis of bone and joint disorders, ed 4, Philadelphia, 2002, Saunders, p 555.)*

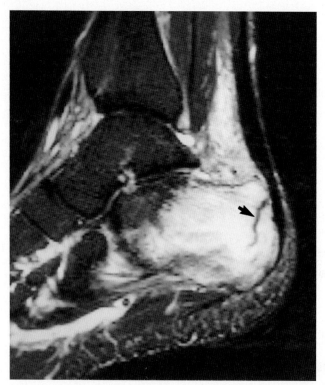

Figure 122-5 Calcaneal stress fracture. In a marathon runner, a sagittal short tau inversion recovery magnetic resonance image shows a fatigue fracture *(arrow)* of the calcaneus, with extensive marrow edema and slight thickening of the Achilles tendon. Abnormal high signal intensity anterior to this tendon indicates peritendinitis. *(From Resnick D: Diagnosis of bone and joint disorders, ed 4, Philadelphia, 2002, Saunders, p 2661.)*

COMPLICATIONS AND PITFALLS

Failure to identify primary or metastatic tumor of the foot that is causing the patient's pain can have disastrous results. The major complication of injection is infection, although this should be exceedingly rare if strict aseptic technique is followed. Approximately 25% of patients complain of a transient increase in pain after injection, and patients should be warned of this possibility.

Clinical Pearls

Coexistent bursitis, plantar fasciitis, and tendinitis may contribute to the patient's foot pain, thus necessitating additional treatment with more localized injection of local anesthetic and methylprednisolone. The injection technique described is extremely effective in treating the pain of calcaneal spur syndrome, and it is safe if careful attention is paid to the clinically relevant anatomy.

SUGGESTED READINGS

Kenny NW, Sylvester BS: The calcaneal spur fracture, *Foot* 1(4):211, 1992.
Onwuanyi ON: Calcaneal spurs and plantar heel pad pain, *Foot* 10(4):182–185, 2000.
Smith S, Tinley P, Gilheany M, et al: The inferior calcaneal spur: anatomical and histological considerations, *Foot* 17(1):25–31, 2007.
Wainwright AM, Kelly AJ, Winson IG: Calcaneal spurs and plantar fasciitis, *Foot* 5(3):123–126, 1995.
Waldman SD: Calcaneal spurs. In *Atlas of pain management injection techniques,* ed 2, Philadelphia, 2007, Saunders, pp 553–556.
Waldman SD: Functional anatomy of the ankle and foot. In *Pain review,* Philadelphia, 2009, Saunders, pp 155–156.

Chapter **123**

MALLET TOE

ICD-9 CODE **735.4**

ICD-10 CODE **M20.40**

THE CLINICAL SYNDROME

Mallet toe is a painful flexion deformity of the distal interphalangeal joint (Fig. 123-1). The second toe is affected most commonly, although the deformity may occur in all toes (Fig. 123-2). Mallet toe is usually the result of a jamming injury to the toe. However, as with bunion and hammer toe, the wearing of tight, narrow-toed shoes has also been implicated (Fig. 123-3); also like bunion, mallet toe occurs more commonly in female patients than in male patients. An inflamed adventitious bursa may accompany mallet toe and contribute to the patient's pain. A callus or ulcer overlying the tip of the affected toe may be present as well. High-heeled shoes may exacerbate the problem.

SIGNS AND SYMPTOMS

Most patients complain of pain localized to the distal interphalangeal joint and an inability to get shoes to fit. Walking makes the pain worse, whereas rest and heat provide some relief. The pain is constant and is characterized as aching. Some patients complain of a grating or popping sensation with use of the joint, and crepitus may be present on physical examination. In addition to pain, patients with mallet toe develop a characteristic flexion deformity of the distal interphalangeal joint. Unlike with bunion, alignment of the toes is relatively normal.

TESTING

Plain radiographs are indicated in all patients who present with mallet toe. Magnetic resonance imaging of the toe is indicated if joint instability, an occult mass, or a tumor is suspected. Based on the patient's clinical presentation, additional testing may be warranted, including a complete blood count, erythrocyte sedimentation rate, and antinuclear antibody testing.

DIFFERENTIAL DIAGNOSIS

The diagnosis of mallet toe is usually obvious on clinical grounds alone. Bursitis and tendinitis of the foot and ankle frequently coexist with mallet toe. In addition, stress fractures of the metatarsals, phalanges, or sesamoid bones may confuse the clinical diagnosis and require specific treatment.

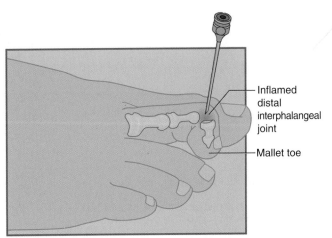

Figure 123-1 Mallet toe is a painful flexion deformity of the distal interphalangeal joint. *(From Waldman SD:* Atlas of pain management injection techniques, *Philadelphia, 2000, Saunders, p 357.)*

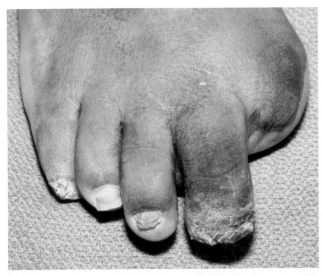

Figure 123-2 Foot of a diabetic patient with osteomyelitis of the distal phalanx of an insensate second mallet toe (distal interphalangeal [DIP] joint contracture). Disarticulation at the DIP joint removed the infective focus and shortened the prominent toe. Previous metatarsophalangeal joint disarticulation of the great toe had exposed the second toe to distal trauma from a shoe. *(From Bowker JH, Pfeifer MA, editors:* Levin and O'Neal's the diabetic foot, *ed 7, Philadelphia, 2008, Mosby, pp 403–428.)*

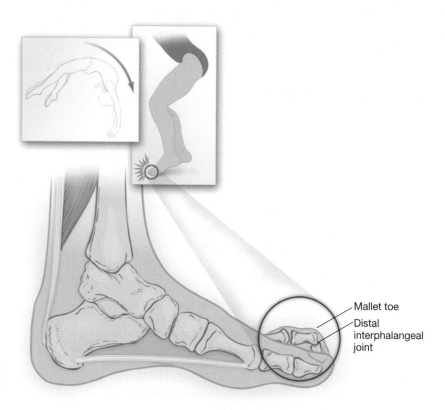

Figure 123-3 Mallet toe is usually the result of a jamming injury to the second toe. It is often seen in gymnasts, although the wearing of tight, narrow-toed shoes has also been implicated in its development.

TREATMENT

Initial treatment of the pain and functional disability associated with mallet toe includes a combination of nonsteroidal antiinflammatory drugs or cyclooxygenase-2 inhibitors and physical therapy. The local application of heat and cold may also be beneficial. Avoidance of repetitive activities that aggravate the patient's symptoms, avoidance of narrow-toed or high-heeled shoes, and short-term immobilization of the affected toes may provide relief. For patients who do not respond to these treatment modalities, injection with local anesthetic and steroid is a reasonable next step.

To inject mallet toe, the patient is placed in the supine position, and the skin overlying the affected toe is prepared with antiseptic solution. A sterile syringe containing 1.5 mL of 0.25% preservative-free bupivacaine and 40 mg methylprednisolone is attached to a ⅝-inch, 25-gauge needle by using strict aseptic technique. The mallet toe is identified, and the needle is carefully advanced against the affected distal phalanges (see Fig. 123-1). The needle is then withdrawn slightly out of the periosteum, and the contents of the syringe are gently injected. The operator should feel little resistance to injection. If resistance is encountered, the needle is probably in a ligament or tendon and should be advanced or withdrawn slightly until the injection can proceed without significant resistance. The needle is removed, and a sterile pressure dressing and ice pack are applied to the injection site.

COMPLICATIONS AND PITFALLS

Failure to identify primary or metastatic tumor of the foot that is causing the patient's pain can have disastrous results. The major complication of injection is infection, although this should be

exceedingly rare if strict aseptic technique is followed. Approximately 25% of patients complain of a transient increase in pain after injection, and patients should be warned of this possibility.

Physical modalities, including local heat and gentle range-of-motion exercises, should be introduced several days after the patient undergoes injection.

Clinical Pearls

Coexistent bursitis and tendinitis may contribute to the patient's foot pain, thus necessitating additional treatment with more localized injection of local anesthetic and methylprednisolone. The injection technique described is extremely effective in treating the pain of mallet toe, and it is safe if careful attention is paid to the clinically relevant anatomy. Narrow-toed and high-heeled shoes should be avoided, because they will exacerbate the patient's symptoms.

SUGGESTED READINGS

Barakat MJ, Gargan MF: Deformities of the lesser toes: how should we describe them? *Foot* 16(1):16–18, 2006.

Coughlin MJ, Grimes JS, Schenck RC Jr: Lesser-toe disorders. In Porter DA, Schon LC, editors: *Baxter's the foot and ankle in sport,* ed 2, St Louis, 2008, Mosby, pp 383–409.

Menz HB: Disorders of the toes. In *Foot problems in older people: assessment and management,* New York, 2004, Churchill Livingstone, pp 149–177.

Waldman SD: Mallet toe pain syndrome. In *Atlas of pain management injection techniques,* ed 2, Philadelphia, 2007, Saunders, pp 569–571.

Waldman SD: Functional anatomy of the ankle and foot. In *Pain review,* Philadelphia, 2009, Saunders, pp 155–156.

Chapter **124**

HAMMER TOE

ICD-9 CODE **735.3**

ICD-10 CODE **M20.40**

THE CLINICAL SYNDROME

Hammer toe is a painful flexion deformity of the proximal interphalangeal joint in which the middle and distal phalanges are flexed down onto the proximal phalange (Fig. 124-1). The second toe is affected most often, and the condition is usually bilateral. Like hallux valgus deformity, hammer toe is usually the result of wearing shoes that are too tight in the toe box, although trauma has also been implicated (Fig. 124-2). As with bunion, hammer toe deformity occurs more commonly in females than in males. An inflamed adventitious bursa may accompany hammer toe and contribute to the patient's pain. A callus overlying the plantar surface of these bony prominences is usually present as well. High-heeled shoes may exacerbate the problem.

SIGNS AND SYMPTOMS

Most patients complain of pain localized to the proximal interphalangeal joint and an inability to get shoes to fit. Walking makes the pain worse, whereas rest and heat provide some relief. The pain is constant and is characterized as aching; it may interfere with sleep. Some patients complain of a grating or popping sensation with use of the joint, and crepitus may be present on physical examination. In addition to pain, patients with hammer toe develop a characteristic flexion deformity of the proximal interphalangeal joint.

TESTING

Plain radiographs are indicated in all patients who present with hammer toe. Magnetic resonance imaging of the toe is indicated if joint instability, an occult mass, or a tumor is suspected. Based on the patient's clinical presentation, additional testing may be warranted, including a complete blood count, erythrocyte sedimentation rate, and antinuclear antibody testing.

DIFFERENTIAL DIAGNOSIS

The diagnosis of hammer toe is usually obvious on clinical grounds alone. Bursitis and tendinitis of the foot and ankle frequently coexist with hammer toe. In addition, stress fractures of the metatarsals, phalanges, or sesamoid bones may confuse the clinical diagnosis and require specific treatment.

TREATMENT

Initial treatment of the pain and functional disability associated with hammer toe includes a combination of nonsteroidal antiinflammatory drugs or cyclooxygenase-2 inhibitors and physical therapy. The local application of heat and cold may also be beneficial. Avoidance of repetitive activities that aggravate the patient's symptoms, avoidance of narrow-toed or high-heeled shoes, and short-term immobilization of the affected toes may provide relief. For patients who do not respond to these treatment modalities, injection with local anesthetic and steroid is a reasonable next step.

To inject hammer toe, the patient is placed in the supine position, and the skin overlying the affected toe is prepared with antiseptic solution. A sterile syringe containing 1.5 mL of 0.25% preservative-free bupivacaine and 40 mg methylprednisolone is attached to a ⅝-inch, 25-gauge needle by using strict aseptic technique. The hammer toe is identified, and the needle is carefully advanced against the second metatarsal head (see Fig. 124-1). The needle is then withdrawn slightly out of the periosteum, and the contents of the syringe are gently injected. The operator should feel little resistance to injection. If resistance is encountered, the needle is probably in a ligament or tendon and should be advanced or withdrawn slightly until the injection can proceed without significant resistance. The needle is removed, and a sterile pressure dressing and ice pack are applied to the injection site.

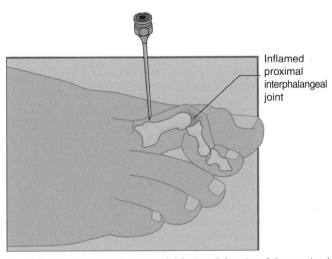

Inflamed proximal interphalangeal joint

Figure 124-1 Hammer toe is a painful flexion deformity of the proximal interphalangeal joint in which the middle and distal phalanges are flexed down onto the proximal phalanx. *(From Waldman SD:* Atlas of pain management injection techniques, *Philadelphia, 2000, Saunders, p 359.)*

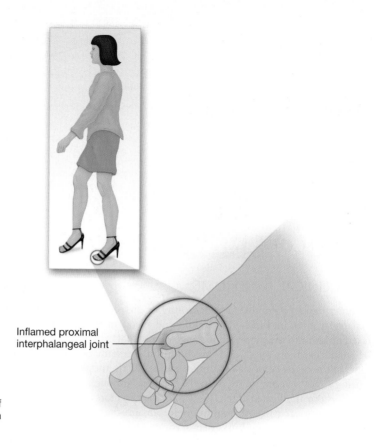

Inflamed proximal interphalangeal joint

Figure 124-2 Hammer toe deformity is usually the result of wearing shoes that are too tight in the toe box, although trauma has also been implicated.

Physical modalities, including local heat and gentle range-of-motion exercises, should be introduced several days after the patient undergoes injection.

COMPLICATIONS AND PITFALLS

Failure to identify primary or metastatic tumor of the foot that is causing the patient's pain can have disastrous results. The major complication of injection is infection, although this should be exceedingly rare if strict aseptic technique is followed. Approximately 25% of patients complain of a transient increase in pain after injection, and patients should be warned of this possibility.

Clinical Pearls

Coexistent bursitis and tendinitis may contribute to the patient's foot pain, thus necessitating additional treatment with more localized injection of local anesthetic and methyl-prednisolone. The injection technique described is extremely effective in treating the pain of hammer toe, and it is safe if careful attention is paid to the clinically relevant anatomy. Narrow-toed and high-heeled shoes should be avoided, because they will exacerbate the patient's symptoms.

SUGGESTED READINGS

Bade H, Tsikaras P, Koebke J: Pathomorphology of the hammer toe, *Foot Ankle Surg* 4(3):139–143, 1998.

Barakat MJ, Gargan MF: Deformities of the lesser toes: how should we describe them? *Foot* 16(1):16–18, 2006.

Coughlin MJ, Grimes JS, Schenck RC Jr: Lesser-toe disorders. In Porter DA, Schon LC, editors: *Baxter's the foot and ankle in sport*, ed 2, St Louis, 2008, Mosby, pp 383–409.

Menz HB: Disorders of the toes. In *Foot problems in older people: assessment and management*, New York, 2004, Churchill Livingstone, pp 149–177.

Schuberth JM: Hammer toe syndrome, *J Foot Ankle Surg* 38(2):166–178, 1999.

Waldman SD: Hammer toe pain syndrome. In *Atlas of pain management injection techniques*, ed 2, Philadelphia, 2007, Saunders, pp 572–574.

Waldman SD: Functional anatomy of the ankle and foot. In *Pain review*, Philadelphia, 2009, Saunders, pp 155–156.

INDEX

Note: Page numbers followed by *f* indicate figures and *t* indicate tables.

A

Abortive therapy
    for migraine headache, 7
    for tension-type headache, 9
Acceleration-deceleration injuries, 204
Acetaminophen, 17, 202, 348
Acetazolamide, 24
Achilles tendon
    rupture of, 365–367, 365*f*, 365*t*, 366*f*
    tendinitis of, 362–364, 362*f*, 363*f*
ACL. *See* Anterior cruciate ligament
Acquired immunodeficiency syndrome
        (AIDS), 2, 63
Acromioclavicular joint, 82–84, 82*f*, 83*f*
Active radiocapitellar compression
        test, 133*f*
Acute cholecystitis, 228, 230–232
Acute intermittent porphyria, 201
Acute pancreatitis, 227–229, 227*f*, 228*f*,
        228*t*, 229*f*
    chronic pancreatitis and, 230
Acyclovir, 3, 217
Adhesive capsulitis, 94–97, 94*f*, 300, 349
Adson test, 69*f*, 77
AIDS. *See* Acquired immunodeficiency
        syndrome
Alcohol
    acute pancreatitis and, 227, 227*f*
    chronic pancreatitis and, 230
    diabetic truncal neuropathy and, 201
    Dupuytren's contracture and, 188
    knee avascular necrosis and, 303
    SAH and, 25
    ulnar nerve entrapment and, 146
Allodynia, 221*f*
Aluminum sulfate, 3, 217
Amitriptyline, 10, 19–20, 198, 213–214
Amyloidosis
    carpal tunnel syndrome and, 160
    diabetic truncal neuropathy and, 201
Analgesics. *See also specific analgesics*
    for acute pancreatitis, 228–229
    for diabetic truncal neuropathy, 200
    for hyoid syndrome, 40
    for phantom limb syndrome, 295
    for postherpetic neuralgia, 222
    for tension-type headache, 9
    for VZV
        of thoracic dermatome, 217
        of trigeminal nerve, 3
Analgesic rebound headache, 17–18
Anconeus syndrome, 137–139, 137*f*, 138*f*
Anesthetic
    for gluteus maximus syndrome, 265
    for iliopectineal bursitis, 286
    for latissimus dorsi syndrome, 244
    for snapping hip syndrome, 284
Angiosarcoma of ribs, 198*f*

Ankle. *See also specific diseases*
    arthritis of, 349–350, 350*f*
        anterior tarsal tunnel syndrome and, 357
        deltoid ligament strain and, 353
        posterior tarsal tunnel syndrome and, 360
    bursitis of
        ankle arthritis and, 349
        deltoid ligament strain and, 353
        hammer toe and, 385
    stress fractures of
        Achilles tendinitis and, 363
        Achilles tendon rupture and, 366
    tendinitis of, hammer toe and, 385
Ankylosing spondylitis, 326*f*
    costosternal syndrome and, 191
    costovertebral joint syndrome and, 218
    manubriosternal syndrome and, 194
    osteitis pubis and, 262
    precordial catch syndrome and, 207
    sacroiliac joint pain and, 256, 258
    Tietze's syndrome and, 204
Anterior cruciate ligament (ACL), 313–316,
        313*f*, 314*f*, 316*f*
Anterior drawer test, 315*f*
Anterior tarsal tunnel syndrome, 356–358,
        356*f*, 357*f*
Antiarrhythmics
    for Baker's cyst of knee, 341
    for diabetic truncal neuropathy, 201
Antibiotics
    for diskitis, 253, 255*f*
    for olecranon bursa, 154
    for retropharyngeal abscess, 63
    for wrist arthritis, 158
Anticonvulsants
    for diabetic truncal neuropathy, 201
    for phantom limb syndrome, 295
    for postherpetic neuralgia, 222
    for VZV of thoracic dermatome, 217
Antidepressants. *See also* Tricyclic
        antidepressants
    for atypical facial pain, 38
    for brachioradialis syndrome, 145
    for deltoid syndrome, 111
    for diabetic truncal neuropathy, 201
    for fibromyalgia of cervical musculature, 53
    for hyoid syndrome, 40
    for latissimus dorsi syndrome, 244
    for levator ani syndrome, 273–274
    for lumbar radiculopathy, 239–240
    occipital neuralgia and, 19–20
    for phantom limb syndrome, 295
    for postherpetic neuralgia, 222
    for scapulocostal syndrome, 119
    for tension-type headache, 10
    for VZV
        of thoracic dermatome, 217
        of trigeminal nerve, 3

Antimyotonic agents, 66
Antivirals, for VZV
    of thoracic dermatome, 217
    of trigeminal nerve, 3
Apley grinding test, 309
Arachnoiditis, 248–251, 248*t*, 249*f*, 250*f*
Arnold-Chiari malformations
    cervical strain and, 55–56
    cervicothoracic bursitis and, 66
    pseudotumor cerebri and, 23–24
    tension-type headache and, 9, 9*f*
Arthritis. *See also specific types and locations*
    ACL and, 315
    carpal boss syndrome and, 185–186
    de Quervain's tenosynovitis and, 164
    Dupuytren's contracture and, 188–189
    Freiberg's disease and, 375
    golfer's elbow and, 126, 127*f*
    lumbar radiculopathy and, 239
    MCL and, 306
    medial meniscal tear and, 309
    osteochondritis dissecans of elbow and, 152
    plastic bag palsy and, 183–184
    posterior tarsal tunnel syndrome and, 360
    prepatellar bursitis and, 328
    runner's knee and, 321
    sacroiliac joint pain and, 258
    sesamoiditis of hand and, 181
    spinal stenosis and, 246
    supinator syndrome and, 141
    tennis elbow and, 123
    thrower's elbow and, 133–135
    trigger finger and, 178
    trigger thumb and, 176
    of wrist, 157–159, 157*f*
Aspirin, 17, 348
Atelectasis, 224
Atlanto-occipital block, 46, 56
Atypical facial pain, 30–31, 37*t*
Avascular necrosis, of knee, 303–305, 303*f*,
        304*f*, 304*t*
Avulsion fractures
    deltoid ligament strain and, 353
    thrower's elbow and, 132

B

Babinski's sign, 252
Baclofen
    for brachial plexopathy, 70
    for Pancoast's tumor syndrome, 74–75
    for thoracic outlet syndrome, 79
    for trigeminal neuralgia, 31
Baker's cyst, of knee, 341–343, 341*f*, 342*f*
Barbiturates, 7, 9, 188
Benzodiazepines, 43
Berry aneurysm, 25*f*, 25*t*
Biceps tendon tear, 98–101, 98*f*, 100*f*

Bicipital tendinitis, 88–90
Biofeedback, 10
Birth control pills, 5
β-blockers, 7
Bone scan. *See* Radionuclide bone scanning
Bornholm disease
  costosternal syndrome and, 191
  costovertebral joint syndrome and, 219
  intercostal neuralgia and, 197
  manubriosternal syndrome and, 195
  post-thoracotomy pain syndrome and, 213
Botulinum toxin type A
  for anconeus syndrome, 139
  for brachioradialis syndrome, 145
  for deltoid syndrome, 111
  for gluteus maximus syndrome, 265
  for latissimus dorsi syndrome, 244
  for levator ani syndrome, 273–274
  for scapulocostal syndrome, 119
  for supinator syndrome, 141
  for supraspinatus syndrome, 103–104
Bowel obstruction, 228
Brachial plexopathy, 68–71, 69*f*
Brachial plexus block
  for Pancoast's tumor syndrome, 75
  for thoracic outlet syndrome, 79
Brachioradialis syndrome, 143–145, 143*f*, 144*f*
Brain abscess
  cluster headache and, 12–13
  migraine headache and, 6
Bunions, 370–371, 370*f*
Bupivacaine
  for Achilles tendinitis, 363
  for ankle arthritis, 349–350
  for anterior cruciate ligament syndrome, 315
  for Baker's cyst of knee, 342
  for bunions, 370–371
  for distal biceps tendon tear, 130
  for ischiogluteal bursitis, 270
  for jumper's knee, 319
  for knee arthritis, 301
  for mallet toe, 384
  for medial meniscal tear, 311–312
  for Osgood-Schlatter disease, 338–339
  for plantar fasciitis, 378
  for sacroiliac joint pain, 258
  for superficial infrapatellar bursitis, 332
  for suprapatellar bursitis, 327
  for toe arthritis, 369
  for trochanteric bursitis, 298
Bursitis. *See also specific locations*
  Achilles tendinitis and, 363
  Achilles tendon rupture and, 366
  ACL and, 315
  brachioradialis syndrome and, 144–145
  calcaneal spur syndrome and, 380
  elbow arthritis and, 120
  Freiberg's disease and, 375
  golfer's elbow and, 126, 127*f*
  MCL and, 306
  medial meniscal tear and, 309
  osteitis pubis and, 260
  osteochondritis dissecans of elbow and, 151–152
  runner's knee and, 321
  shoulder osteoarthritis and, 81
  supinator syndrome and, 141

Bursitis *(Continued)*
  tennis elbow and, 123
  thrower's elbow and, 133–135
Butalbital (Fiorinal), 17

C

C6-7 radiculopathy
  de Quervain's tenosynovitis and, 165
  golfer's elbow and, 127*f*
  tennis elbow and, 124
Caffeine, 7, 17
Calcaneal spur syndrome, 380–382, 380*f*, 381*f*, 382*f*
Calcium channel blockers, 7
Capsaicin, 201
Carbamazepine
  for brachial plexopathy, 70
  for diabetic truncal neuropathy, 201
  for Pancoast's tumor syndrome, 74
  for phantom limb syndrome, 295
  for postherpetic neuralgia, 222
  for thoracic outlet syndrome, 79
  for trigeminal neuralgia, 31
  for VZV
    of thoracic dermatome, 217
    of trigeminal nerve, 3
Carcinoid syndrome, 201
Carpal boss syndrome, 185–187, 185*f*, 186*f*
  ganglion cysts of wrist and, 171, 186*f*
Carpal tunnel syndrome, 160–163, 160*f*, 161*f*, 162*f*, 163*f*
  cervical radiculopathy and, 51
  ulnar nerve entrapment and, 146–148
Carpometacarpal joint arthritis, 167–169, 167*f*, 168*f*, 169*f*
  carpal tunnel syndrome and, 162
Catching tendon sign, 179*f*
Cauda equina syndrome, 246, 248
Celiac plexus block, 228–229, 229*f*, 232
Cerebrospinal fluid (CSF), 22
Cervical arthritis, 49, 56, 66
Cervical bursitis, 49, 56
Cervical epidural nerve block, 10, 66
Cervical facet syndrome, 45–47
Cervical fibromyositisis, 49, 56, 66
Cervical radiculopathy, 48–51
  carpal tunnel syndrome and, 161–162, 163
  de Quervain's tenosynovitis and, 164–165
  lateral antebrachial cutaneous nerve entrapment and, 149–150
  osteochondritis dissecans of elbow and, 152
  thrower's elbow and, 133–135
  ulnar nerve entrapment and, 146–148
Cervical spondylosis, 69
Cervical strain, 55–57, 66
Cervicalgia, 49
Cervicothoracic bursitis, 66*f*
Cervicothoracic interspinous bursitis, 65–67, 65*f*
Charcot-Marie-Tooth disease, 201
Cheiralgia paresthetica, 164–165
Chemotherapy, VZV and, 1, 215
Chlorthalidone, 24
Chondroid metaplasia, 176*f*
Chondroma, 182*f*
Chondromatosis, 299*f*
Chondrosarcoma of sternum, 195*f*

Chronic pancreatitis, 230–232, 230*f*, 231*f*, 232*f*
Chronic subdural hematoma
  cluster headache and, 12–13
  migraine headache and, 6
  tension-type headache and, 9
Chvostek's sign, 228
Clonidine, 7
Cluster headache, 11–13, 11*t*
Cocaine, 25
Coccydynia, 275–278, 275*f*, 276*f*
Collagen vascular disease
  adhesive capsulitis and, 95
  anconeus syndrome and, 138
  ankle arthritis and, 349
  carpometacarpal joint arthritis and, 167
  chronic pancreatitis and, 230–232
  elbow arthritis and, 121
  fibromyalgia of cervical musculature and, 53
  hip arthritis and, 279
  iliopectineal bursitis and, 286
  knee arthritis and, 300
  knee avascular necrosis and, 303
  latissimus dorsi syndrome and, 243
  midtarsal joint arthritis and, 351
  postherpetic neuralgia and, 221
  sacroiliac joint pain and, 256
  SAH and, 26
  scapulocostal syndrome and, 119
  shoulder osteoarthritis and, 81
  subdeltoid bursitis and, 85
  supinator syndrome and, 141
  supraspinatus syndrome and, 103
  teres major syndrome and, 115
  toe arthritis and, 368
  wrist arthritis and, 158
Colloids, 232
Compartment syndrome, 138
Compression. *See also* Spinal cord compression
  of median nerve, 160
  plastic bag palsy and, 183, 183*f*
Compression test, 150*f*
  active radiocapitellar, 133*f*
Computed tomography (CT)
  for acute pancreatitis, 228, 228*f*
  for arachnoiditis, 248
  for brachial plexopathy, 68
  of chondroma, 182*f*
  for chronic pancreatitis, 230, 232, 232*f*
  for diskitis, 253
  for intercostal neuralgia, 197
  for longus colli tendinitis, 58–59, 59*f*
  for lumbar radiculopathy, 238
  for manubriosternal syndrome, 195
  for Pancoast's tumor syndrome, 72
  for post-thoracotomy pain syndrome, 213, 213*f*, 214*f*
  for pseudotumor cerebri, 22
  for retropharyngeal abscess, 62–63, 62*f*
  for rib fractures, 209–210, 210*f*
  for sacroiliac joint pain, 258, 258*f*
  for SAH, 26
  for spinal stenosis, 246
  for swimmer's headache, 15
  for thoracic vertebral compression fractures, 224
Costosternal syndrome, 191–193, 192*f*, 193*f*

Costovertebral joint syndrome, 218–220, 218f
C-reactive protein, 63
Creak sign, 363f
Crystal deposition diseases, 141, 144–145
Crystalloids, 232
CSF. *See* Cerebrospinal fluid
CT. *See* Computed tomography
Cubital tunnel syndrome, 144, 146–148, 147f
Cushing's disease, 303
Cystic fibrosis, 230

D

de Quervain's tenosynovitis, 164–166, 164f, 165f
  carpometacarpal joint arthritis and, 168
  trigger thumb and, 175–176
Deep infrapatellar bursitis, 334–336, 334f, 335f
Deltoid ligament strain, 353–355, 353f, 354f
Deltoid syndrome, 109–112, 110f
Demyelinating disease, 254
Depression
  brachioradialis syndrome and, 143
  myofascial pain syndrome and, 114
  scapulocostal syndrome and, 117
  supinator syndrome and, 140
  tension-type headache and, 8
Desipramine, 198, 213–214
Devil's grip, 207
Diabetes
  Achilles tendon rupture and, 365
  anterior tarsal tunnel syndrome and, 357
  carpal tunnel syndrome and, 162
  Dupuytren's contracture and, 188
  Freiberg's disease and, 374
  ulnar nerve entrapment and, 146
Diabetic femoral neuropathy, 246
Diabetic ketoacidosis, 228, 230–232
Diabetic polyneuropathy
  anterior tarsal tunnel syndrome and, 357
  carpal tunnel syndrome and, 161–162
  for costosternal syndrome, 191
  costovertebral joint syndrome and, 219
  genitofemoral neuralgia and, 236
  ilioinguinal neuralgia and, 233–234
  intercostal neuralgia and, 197
  manubriosternal syndrome and, 195
  posterior tarsal tunnel syndrome and, 360
  post-thoracotomy pain syndrome and, 213
Diabetic truncal neuropathy, 200–202, 200f
Diffuse idiopathic skeletal hyperostosis (DISH), 40f
DISH. *See* Diffuse idiopathic skeletal hyperostosis
Diskitis, 252–255, 252f, 253f, 255f, 255t
Distal biceps tendon tear, 129–131, 129f, 130f
Distal patella tendinopathy, 335f
Dorsal root entry zone lesioning, 70, 75
Double-crush syndrome
  carpal tunnel syndrome and, 162
  lateral antebrachial cutaneous nerve entrapment and, 149–150
  meralgia paresthetica and, 292
  piriformis syndrome and, 267–268
  posterior tarsal tunnel syndrome and, 360
  ulnar nerve entrapment and, 146–148

Drop arm test, 107f
Dupuytren's contracture, 188–190, 188f, 189f
Dysesthesia, 221f

E

Ecchymosis
  Achilles tendon rupture and, 365
  adhesive capsulitis and, 96
  anconeus syndrome and, 139
  anterior tarsal tunnel syndrome and, 357
  bicipital tendinitis and, 89
  brachioradialis syndrome and, 145
  carpal boss syndrome and, 185
  coccydynia and, 277
  de Quervain's tenosynovitis and, 165–166
  distal biceps tendon tear and, 131
  hip arthritis and, 280
  latissimus dorsi syndrome and, 244
  olecranon bursa and, 155
  osteochondritis dissecans of elbow and, 151–152
  posterior tarsal tunnel syndrome and, 360
  scapulocostal syndrome and, 119
  sesamoiditis of hand and, 181–182
  snapping hip syndrome and, 284
  supinator syndrome and, 141–142
  teres major syndrome and, 115
  thoracic vertebral compression fracture and, 224
  trigger finger and, 179
Elbow. *See also specific diseases*
  arthritis of, 120–122, 120f
  synovial cysts of, 154
Electrocardiography
  for rib fractures, 209–210
  for thoracic vertebral compression fractures, 224
Electromyography (EMG), 68
  for anterior tarsal tunnel syndrome, 356
  for arachnoiditis, 248
  for carpal tunnel syndrome, 161–162
  for de Quervain's tenosynovitis, 164–165
  for deep infrapatellar bursitis, 334–335
  for diabetic truncal neuropathy, 200
  for Dupuytren's contracture, 189
  for Freiberg's disease, 374–375
  for genitofemoral neuralgia, 236
  for glenohumeral joint avascular necrosis, 91–92
  for golfer's elbow, 127f
  for ilioinguinal neuralgia, 233
  for knee avascular necrosis, 303
  for lateral antebrachial cutaneous nerve entrapment, 149
  for lumbar radiculopathy, 238
  for meralgia paresthetica, 291–292
  for osteochondritis dissecans of elbow, 152
  for Pancoast's tumor syndrome, 72
  for pes anserine bursitis, 344–345
  for piriformis syndrome, 266–267
  for plastic bag palsy, 183–184
  for posterior tarsal tunnel syndrome, 360
  for prepatellar bursitis, 328–329
  for runner's knee, 321
  for spinal stenosis, 246
  for superficial infrapatellar bursitis, 331–332

Electromyography (EMG) *(Continued)*
  for supinator syndrome, 141
  for suprapatellar bursitis, 326
  for tennis elbow, 124
  for thrower's elbow, 133
  for trochanteric bursitis, 298
  for ulnar nerve entrapment, 146
Elixir, 3
EMG. *See* Electromyography
Endotracheal intubation, 63
Ependymoma, 276f
Ergot alkaloids, 7
Ergotamines, 7, 17
Eversion test, 354f

F

Famciclovir, 3, 217
Femoral neuropathy, 328–329
Fiber
  for postherpetic neuralgia, 222
  for VZV
    of thoracic dermatome, 216
    of trigeminal nerve, 3
Fibromyalgia
  anconeus syndrome and, 139
  of cervical musculature, 52–54
  scapulocostal syndrome and, 119
  supinator syndrome and, 141
  teres major syndrome and, 115
Fibrous xanthoma, 184f
Finkelstein test, 164, 165f
Fiorinal. *See* Butalbital
Flexion, abduction, external rotation, extension test (Patrick-FABERE), 279, 280f
Fluoroquinolones, 365
Fluoroscopy, 258
Fluoxetine
  for diabetic truncal neuropathy, 201
  for tension-type headache, 10
Foot. *See also specific diseases*
  bursitis of
    hammer toe and, 385
    mallet toe and, 383
    midtarsal joint arthritis and, 351
    Morton's neuroma and, 373
    toe arthritis and, 368
  stress fractures of, 373
  tendinitis of
    hammer toe and, 385
    mallet toe and, 383
    Morton's neuroma and, 373
    toe arthritis and, 368
Fractures. *See also specific types and locations*
  glenohumeral joint avascular necrosis and, 92
Freiberg's disease, 374–376, 374f, 375f
Froment sign, 146, 147f
Frontal sinusitis, 9
Frozen ankle, 349
Frozen shoulder, 212–213
Furosemide, 24

G

Gabapentin
  for brachial plexopathy, 69
  for brachioradialis syndrome, 145

Gabapentin *(Continued)*
  for diabetic truncal neuropathy, 201
  for intercostal neuralgia, 198–199
  for Pancoast's tumor syndrome, 72–74
  for phantom limb syndrome, 295
  for piriformis syndrome, 268
  for plastic bag palsy, 184
  for postherpetic neuralgia, 222
  for post-thoracotomy pain syndrome, 214
  for scapulocostal syndrome, 119
  for supinator syndrome, 141
  for swimmer's headache, 15
  for teres major syndrome, 115
  for thoracic outlet syndrome, 78–79
  for trigeminal neuralgia, 31
  for VZV
    of thoracic dermatome, 217
    of trigeminal nerve, 3
Gadolinium, 374–375
Gallbladder disease
  chronic pancreatitis and, 230
  intercostal neuralgia and, 197
  post-thoracotomy pain syndrome
      and, 213
  rib fractures and, 210
  thoracic vertebral compression fracture and,
      224–225
Gallstones, 227
Gamekeeper's thumb, 177*f*
Ganglion cysts of wrist, 170–174, 170*f*, 171*f*,
      172*f*, 173*f*
  carpal boss syndrome and, 186*f*
Ganglionitis, VZV and
  of thoracic dermatome, 215–216
  of trigeminal nerve, 1–2
Gasserian ganglion, 31–32
Genitofemoral neuralgia, 235–237, 235*f*
Giant cell tumor, 179*f*
Glaucoma
  cluster headache and, 12–13
  VZV of trigeminal nerve and, 2
Glenohumeral joint avascular necrosis, 91–93,
      91*f*, 91*t*, 92*f*
Glioblastoma multiforme, 6*f*
Glossopharyngeal neuralgia, 39
Gluteal bursitis
  gluteus maximus syndrome and, 264
  levator ani syndrome and, 273
Gluteus maximus syndrome, 260*f*, 263–265,
      264*f*, 265*f*
Glycerol, 31
Golfer's elbow, 126–128, 127*f*
  thrower's elbow and, 132
  ulnar nerve entrapment and, 146–148
Gout
  Achilles tendon rupture and, 365
  calcaneal spur syndrome and, 380
  carpal boss syndrome and, 186
  de Quervain's tenosynovitis and,
      164, 165
  Dupuytren's contracture and, 188–189
  Freiberg's disease and, 375
  glenohumeral joint avascular necrosis and,
      91, 93
  golfer's elbow and, 126, 127*f*
  knee avascular necrosis and, 303
  midtarsal joint arthritis and, 351
  olecranon bursitis and, 154

Gout *(Continued)*
  osteochondritis dissecans of elbow and,
      152
  plastic bag palsy and, 183–184
  sesamoiditis of hand and, 181
  thrower's elbow and, 133–135
  trigger finger and, 178
  trigger thumb and, 176
Guillain-Barré syndrome, 201

H
Hallux valgus deformity, 370, 371*f*
Hammer toe, 385–386, 385*f*, 386*f*
Hansen's disease, 201
Headache. *See also* Cluster headache; Migraine
      headache; Tension-type headache
  analgesic rebound, 17–18
  with atypical facial pain, 36
  with SAH, 26*f*
Hematoma. *See also* Chronic subdural
      hematoma
  Achilles tendon rupture and, 365
  adhesive capsulitis and, 96
  anconeus syndrome and, 139
  anterior tarsal tunnel syndrome and, 357
  bicipital tendinitis and, 89
  brachioradialis syndrome and, 145
  coccydynia and, 277
  de Quervain's tenosynovitis and, 165–166
  distal biceps tendon tear and, 131
  genitofemoral neuralgia and, 236
  hip arthritis and, 280
  ilioinguinal neuralgia and, 233–234
  latissimus dorsi syndrome and, 244
  olecranon bursa and, 155
  posterior tarsal tunnel syndrome and, 360
  scapulocostal syndrome and, 119
  snapping hip syndrome and, 284
  supinator syndrome and, 141–142
  tennis leg and, 347
  teres major syndrome and, 115
  thoracic vertebral compression fracture
      and, 224
  trigger finger and, 179
Herniated disk
  arachnoiditis and, 248
  lumbar radiculopathy and, 238
  meralgia paresthetica and, 291–292
Herpes zoster. *See* Varicella-zoster virus
Hip
  arthritis of, 279–281, 279*f*, 281*t*
    iliopectineal bursitis and, 285
    trochanteric bursitis and, 297
  snapping hip syndrome, 282–284, 282*f*,
      283*f*, 284*f*
HLA. *See* Human leukocyte antigen
Hoffa's disease, 332, 338
Homans' sign, 341
Horner syndrome, 11*f*
Housemaid's knee. *See* Prepatellar bursitis
Human immunodeficiency virus
  diabetic truncal neuropathy and, 201
  Freiberg's disease and, 374
  glenohumeral joint avascular necrosis and, 91
  knee avascular necrosis and, 303
  postherpetic neuralgia and, 221
  VZV and, 216

Human leukocyte antigen (HLA), 45–46
  for arachnoiditis, 248
  for cervical radiculopathy, 49
  for cervical strain, 55–56
  for costovertebral joint syndrome, 219
  for lumbar radiculopathy, 238–239
  for sacroiliac joint pain, 257–258
  for spinal stenosis, 246
Hunchback sign, 185, 186*f*
Hydrocephalus, 6, 12–13
Hydrocodone
  for Achilles tendon rupture, 366
  for acute pancreatitis, 228–229
  for rib fractures, 210
  for tennis leg, 348
  for thoracic vertebral compression fracture,
      225
Hyoid syndrome, 39–41
Hyperesthesia, 2
Hyperlipidemia
  Achilles tendon rupture and, 365
  glenohumeral joint avascular necrosis and, 91
  knee avascular necrosis and, 303
Hyperparathyroidism, 209–210
Hypertension, 25
Hypertensive crisis, 26
Hypopigmentation, 1–2
Hypotension, 228
Hypothyroidism
  diabetic truncal neuropathy and, 201
  fibromyalgia of cervical musculature and, 53
Hypoventilation, 224
Hypovolemia
  acute pancreatitis and, 228
  chronic pancreatitis and, 232
  colloids for, 232
  crystalloids for, 232

I
Idiopathic intracranial hypertension.
      See Pseudotumor cerebri
Idiopathic synovial osteochondromatosis, 142*f*
Ilioinguinal neuralgia, 233–234, 233*f*, 234*f*
Iliopectineal bursitis, 285–287, 285*f*, 286*f*
Iliotibial band friction syndrome, 323*f*
Iliotibial bursitis, 321–322
Immunosuppressive therapy, 1
Infrapatellar bursitis, 337–338
Infraspinatus musculotendinous unit, 119, 119*f*
Insufficiency fractures
  coccydynia and, 275
  iliopectineal bursitis and, 286*f*
  ischiogluteal bursitis and, 270
Intercostal neuralgia, 197–199, 197*f*, 198*f*
Intraarticular injection
  for Achilles tendinitis, 363
  for anconeus syndrome, 139
  for ankle arthritis, 349–350
  for anterior cruciate ligament syndrome,
      315
  for anterior tarsal tunnel syndrome, 357
  for Baker's cyst of knee, 342, 342*f*
  for brachioradialis syndrome, 145
  for bunions, 370–371
  for calcaneal spur syndrome, 380–381
  for carpal boss syndrome, 186
  for carpal tunnel syndrome, 162–163, 163*f*

Intraarticular injection *(Continued)*
  for carpometacarpal joint arthritis, 167, 168, 169*f*
  for coccydynia, 275–277
  for costosternal syndrome, 191–192, 193*f*
  for costovertebral joint syndrome, 219–220, 220*f*
  for de Quervain's tenosynovitis, 165
  for deep infrapatellar bursitis, 335–336
  for deltoid ligament strain, 354
  for distal biceps tendon tear, 130
  for Dupuytren's contracture, 189–190
  for elbow arthritis, 121–122
  for ganglion cysts of wrist, 171, 173*f*
  for golfer's elbow, 127*f*, 127–128
  for hammer toe, 385
  for hip arthritis, 280
  for iliopectineal bursitis, 286–287
  for intercostal neuralgia, 199
  for ischial bursitis, 289–290, 289*f*
  for jumper's knee, 319, 319*f*
  for knee arthritis, 301
  for lateral antebrachial cutaneous nerve entrapment, 150
  for mallet toe, 384
  for manubriosternal syndrome, 195, 196*f*
  for MCL, 307–308, 308*f*
  for medial meniscal tear, 311–312
  for meralgia paresthetica, 292, 292*f*
  for midtarsal joint arthritis, 352
  for Morton's neuroma, 373, 373*f*
  for olecranon bursa, 155
  for Osgood-Schlatter disease, 338–339
  for osteitis pubis, 262
  for osteochondritis dissecans of elbow, 152–153
  for pes anserine bursitis, 345
  for plantar fasciitis, 378
  for plastic bag palsy, 184
  for posterior tarsal tunnel syndrome, 360
  for post-thoracotomy pain syndrome, 214
  for prepatellar bursitis, 329, 329*f*
  for rib fractures, 210
  for runner's knee, 322
  for sacroiliac joint pain, 258, 258*f*
  for sesamoiditis of hand, 181–182
  for snapping hip syndrome, 284
  for superficial infrapatellar bursitis, 332
  for supinator syndrome, 141
  for suprapatellar bursitis, 326–327
  for tennis elbow, 124, 125*f*
  for thrower's elbow, 133, 135, 135*f*
  for Tietze's syndrome, 204
  for toe arthritis, 369
  for trigger finger, 179
  for trigger thumb, 175–176
  for trochanteric bursitis, 298, 299*f*
  for ulnar nerve entrapment, 148
  for wrist arthritis, 158–159
Ischial bursitis, 288–290, 288*f*, 289*f*
Ischiogluteal bursitis, 269–270, 269*f*, 270*f*
Isometheptene mucate (Midrin), 7

J
Jannetta's procedure, 32
Jump sign
  anconeus syndrome and, 137
  brachioradialis syndrome and, 143–144

Jump sign *(Continued)*
  gluteus maximus syndrome and, 264
  latissimus dorsi syndrome and, 243
  levator ani syndrome and, 273
  plantar fasciitis and, 377*f*
  teres major syndrome and, 113, 115
Jumper's knee, 317–320, 317*f*, 318*f*, 319*f*

K
Kaposi's sarcoma, 2, 216
Keratitis, 3
Klippel-Feil syndrome, 66, 66*f*
Knee
  arthritis of, 300–302, 300*f*
    deep infrapatellar bursitis and, 334
    Osgood-Schlatter disease and, 337–338
    superficial infrapatellar bursitis and, 331
    tennis leg and, 347
  avascular necrosis of, 303–305, 303*f*, 304*f*, 304*t*, 305*f*
  Baker's cyst of, 341–343, 341*f*, 342*f*
  bursitis of, 301, 347
  tendinitis of
    deep infrapatellar bursitis and, 334
    Osgood-Schlatter disease and, 337–338
    superficial infrapatellar bursitis and, 331
Kyphoplasty, 225

L
Labrum tears, 92
Lasègue's straight leg raising sign, 238, 239*f*
Lateral antebrachial cutaneous nerve entrapment, 149–150, 149*f*, 150*f*
  de Quervain's tenosynovitis and, 165
Lateral epicondylitis. *See* Tennis elbow
Latissimus dorsi syndrome, 242–244, 242*f*, 243*f*
Levator ani syndrome, 271–274, 271*f*, 272*f*
Lidocaine, 7
  for anterior tarsal tunnel syndrome, 357
  for diabetic truncal neuropathy, 201
  for genitofemoral neuralgia, 236
  for ilioinguinal neuralgia, 234
  for rib fractures, 210
Lipomas, 171, 172*f*
List, 238
Lithium carbonate, 13
Longus colli tendinitis, 58–60, 59*f*
Ludington test, 99*f*
Lumbar bursitis
  lumbar radiculopathy and, 239
  posterior tarsal tunnel syndrome and, 360
  sacroiliac joint pain and, 258
  spinal stenosis and, 246
Lumbar dermatome, 216*f*
Lumbar fibromyositis
  lumbar radiculopathy and, 239
  sacroiliac joint pain and, 258
  spinal stenosis and, 246
Lumbar myelopathy
  arachnoiditis and, 249*f*
  spinal stenosis and, 246
Lumbar plexus, 233–234
Lumbar puncture, 26
Lumbar radiculopathy, 238–241, 238*t*, 239*f*
  ankle arthritis and, 349
  anterior tarsal tunnel syndrome and, 357

Lumbar radiculopathy *(Continued)*
  deep infrapatellar bursitis and, 334–335
  hip arthritis and, 280
  ischiogluteal bursitis and, 270
  knee arthritis and, 301
  meralgia paresthetica and, 292
  MRI for, 240*f*
  pes anserine bursitis and, 344–345
  piriformis syndrome and, 266–268
  posterior tarsal tunnel syndrome and, 360
  prepatellar bursitis and, 328–329
  trochanteric bursitis and, 297*f*
Lyme disease
  adhesive capsulitis and, 95
  ankle arthritis and, 349
  carpometacarpal joint arthritis and, 167
  diabetic truncal neuropathy and, 201
  fibromyalgia of cervical musculature and, 53
  hip arthritis and, 279
  iliopectineal bursitis and, 286
  knee arthritis and, 300
  sacroiliac joint pain and, 256
  shoulder osteoarthritis and, 81
  toe arthritis and, 368
  wrist arthritis and, 158
Lymphoma, 1, 295

M
Magnetic resonance imaging (MRI)
  for Achilles tendinitis, 362, 363*f*
  for Achilles tendon rupture, 366, 366*f*
  for acromioclavicular joint, 82, 83*f*
  for analgesic rebound headache, 17
  for anconeus syndrome, 138*f*
  for ankle arthritis, 349
  for anterior cruciate ligament syndrome, 314–315, 314*f*
  for anterior tarsal tunnel syndrome, 356
  for arachnoiditis, 248, 249*f*
  for atypical facial pain, 37
  for Baker's cyst of knee, 341
  for biceps tendon tear, 99
  for brachial plexopathy, 68, 69*f*
  for bunions, 370
  for calcaneal spur syndrome, 380, 381*f*
  for carpal boss syndrome, 185–186
  for carpometacarpal joint arthritis, 168, 168*f*
  for cervical facet syndrome, 45–46
  for cervical radiculopathy, 49
  for cervical strain, 55–56
  for cervicothoracic bursitis, 66*f*
  for cluster headache, 12
  for coccydynia, 275
  for costosternal syndrome, 191
  for costovertebral joint syndrome, 219
  for de Quervain's tenosynovitis, 164–165, 165*f*
  for deep infrapatellar bursitis, 334–335
  for deltoid ligament strain, 353
  for diabetic truncal neuropathy, 200
  for diskitis, 253
  for distal biceps tendon tear, 130*f*
  for elbow arthritis, 121
  for Freiberg's disease, 374–375, 375*f*
  for ganglion cysts of wrist, 171, 172*f*
  for genitofemoral neuralgia, 236
  for glenohumeral joint avascular necrosis, 91–92

Magnetic resonance imaging (MRI) *(Continued)*
  for golfer's elbow, 127*f*
  for hammer toe, 385
  for hip arthritis, 279
  for ilioinguinal neuralgia, 233
  for iliopectineal bursitis, 286
  for ischiogluteal bursitis, 270
  for knee arthritis, 300
  for knee avascular necrosis, 303
  of knee avascular necrosis, 305*f*
  for lateral antebrachial cutaneous nerve
    entrapment, 149
  for lumbar radiculopathy, 238, 240*f*
  for mallet toe, 383
  for manubriosternal syndrome, 195
  for MCL, 306
  for medial meniscal tear, 309, 311*f*
  for meralgia paresthetica, 291–292
  for midtarsal joint arthritis, 351
  for migraine headache, 6
  for Morton's neuroma, 372, 373*f*
  for occipital neuralgia, 19
  for olecranon bursa, 154
  for Osgood-Schlatter disease, 338*f*
  for osteochondritis dissecans of elbow, 152*f*
  for Pancoast's tumor syndrome, 72, 73*f*
  for pes anserine bursitis, 344–345
  of piriformis syndrome, 267*f*, 268,
    268*f*
  for posterior tarsal tunnel syndrome, 360
  for precordial catch syndrome, 207*f*
  for prepatellar bursitis, 328–329, 329*f*
  for pseudotumor cerebri, 22
  for retropharyngeal abscess, 62–63
  for rotator cuff tear, 105
  for runner's knee, 321
  for sacroiliac joint pain, 257*f*
  for SAH, 26
  for sesamoiditis of hand, 181
  for shoulder osteoarthritis, 80
  for snapping hip syndrome, 282, 284*f*
  for spinal stenosis, 246
  for superficial infrapatellar bursitis,
    331–332, 332*f*
  for suprapatellar bursitis, 326
  for swimmer's headache, 15
  for tennis elbow, 124
  for tennis leg, 347, 348*f*
  for tension-type headache, 8–9, 9*f*
  for teres major syndrome, 114*f*
  for thoracic outlet syndrome, 77–78
  for thoracic vertebral compression fractures,
    224
  for thrower's elbow, 135*f*
  for Tietze's syndrome, 204
  for TMJ, 34
  for toe arthritis, 368
  for trigeminal neuralgia, 30
  for trigger finger, 178
  for trochanteric bursitis, 298*f*
  for ulnar nerve entrapment, 146
  for wrist arthritis, 158, 158*f*
Malignant melanoma, 173*f*
Mallet toe, 383–384, 383*f*, 384*f*
Manubriosternal syndrome, 194–196, 194*f*,
  196*f*
MCL. *See* Medial collateral ligament
McMurray test, 309

Medial collateral ligament (MCL), 121*f*,
  306–308, 306*f*, 307*f*, 308*f*
  thrower's elbow and, 132
Medial epicondylar apophysis, 132
Medial epicondyle, 126*f*
  tennis elbow and, 127*f*
  thrower's elbow and, 132
Medial meniscal tear, 309–312, 309*t*, 310*f*,
  311*f*, 345
  Baker's cyst of knee and, 341, 342
Menstruation, 5
Meperidine, 228–229
Meralgia paresthetica, 291–293, 291*f*, 292*f*,
  293*f*
  knee arthritis and, 301
  trochanteric bursitis and, 298
Mesenteric infarction, 230–232
Metastases
  Freiberg's disease and, 375
  ganglion cysts of wrist and, 171
  hip arthritis and, 280
  knee avascular necrosis and, 304
  manubriosternal syndrome and, 194
  osteitis pubis and, 262
  thoracic vertebral compression fracture and,
    225*f*
  toe arthritis and, 368
Metastatic renal carcinoma, 219*f*
Methadone, 3, 72
Methylprednisolone
  for Achilles tendinitis, 363
  for acromioclavicular joint, 83–84
  for adhesive capsulitis, 95–96
  for ankle arthritis, 349–350
  for anterior cruciate ligament syndrome,
    315
  for anterior tarsal tunnel syndrome, 357
  arachnoiditis and, 248
  for Baker's cyst of knee, 342
  for bunions, 370–371
  for carpal tunnel syndrome, 162
  for carpometacarpal joint arthritis, 168
  for costosternal syndrome, 192
  for de Quervain's tenosynovitis, 165
  for deep infrapatellar bursitis, 335–336
  for Dupuytren's contracture, 189–190
  for elbow arthritis, 121–122
  for genitofemoral neuralgia, 236
  for golfer's elbow, 127–128
  for ilioinguinal neuralgia, 234
  for intercostal neuralgia, 199
  for ischiogluteal bursitis, 270
  for jumper's knee, 319
  for mallet toe, 384
  for manubriosternal syndrome, 195
  for Morton's neuroma, 373
  for Osgood-Schlatter disease, 338–339
  for osteitis pubis, 262
  for piriformis syndrome, 268
  for plantar fasciitis, 378
  for rotator cuff tear, 107
  for sesamoiditis of hand, 181–182
  for shoulder osteoarthritis, 81
  for superficial infrapatellar bursitis, 332
  for suprapatellar bursitis, 327
  for thrower's elbow, 135
  for Tietze's syndrome, 204
  for TMJ, 35

Methylprednisolone *(Continued)*
  for toe arthritis, 369
  for trigger finger, 179
  for trigger thumb, 176
Mexiletine, 201
Microvascular decompression, 32
Midrin. *See* Isometheptene mucate
Midtarsal joint, 353
  arthritis of, 351–352, 351*f*
Migraine headache, 5–7, 6*f*
  cluster headache and, 11*t*, 12
  swimmer's headache and, 15*t*
  tension-type headache and, 9*t*
Migraine with aura, 5
Milk of Magnesia
  for postherpetic neuralgia, 222
  for VZV
    of thoracic dermatome, 216
    of trigeminal nerve, 3
Milking maneuver of Veltri, 132
Monoamine oxidase inhibitors, 10
Morphine, 3, 72
Morton's neuroma, 372–373, 372*f*, 373*f*
  Freiberg's disease and, 375
  plantar fasciitis and, 377–378
MRI. *See* Magnetic resonance imaging
Mulder's sign, 372, 372*f*
Müller's muscles, 23*f*
Multiple myeloma, 262
Multiple sclerosis
  anconeus syndrome and, 138
  fibromyalgia of cervical musculature and, 53
  latissimus dorsi syndrome and, 243
  scapulocostal syndrome and, 119
  supraspinatus syndrome and, 103
  teres major syndrome and, 115
  trigeminal neuralgia and, 30–31
Muscle relaxants, 66
Myelitis
  postherpetic neuralgia and, 222
  VZV of trigeminal nerve and, 2–3
Myocardial infarction, 228, 230–232
Myofascial pain syndrome
  anconeus syndrome and, 137, 137*f*
  brachioradialis syndrome and, 143
  deltoid syndrome and, 109
  depression and, 114
  gluteus maximus syndrome and, 263, 264*f*
  latissimus dorsi syndrome and, 242
  levator ani syndrome and, 271, 272*f*
  osteochondritis dissecans of elbow and, 151–152
  posture and, 140
  scapulocostal syndrome and, 117
  stress and, 114
  supinator syndrome and, 140
  supraspinatus syndrome and, 102
  teres major syndrome and, 113
  trigger points and, 113

N
Naproxen, 7
Nerve block. *See also* Intraarticular injection.
  specific agents and locations
  for brachial plexopathy, 70
  for cervical facet syndrome, 46
  for cervical radiculopathy, 49
  for cervical strain, 56

Nerve block *(Continued)*
  for coccydynia, 275–277
  for diabetic truncal neuropathy, 202
  for genitofemoral neuralgia, 236
  for ilioinguinal neuralgia, 234, 234*f*
  for intercostal neuralgia, 198
  for occipital neuralgia, 19–20
  for phantom limb syndrome, 295
  for postherpetic neuralgia, 222
  for post-thoracotomy pain syndrome, 214
  for spinal stenosis, 246
  for swimmer's headache, 15–16, 16*f*
  for trigeminal neuralgia, 31
  for VZV
    of thoracic dermatome, 216
    of trigeminal nerve, 3
Nerve entrapment
  ACL and, 315
  anterior tarsal tunnel syndrome and, 356
  carpal tunnel syndrome and, 160
  diabetic truncal neuropathy and, 201
  gluteus maximus syndrome and, 264, 265*f*
  hip arthritis and, 280
  ilioinguinal neuralgia and, 234
  knee arthritis and, 301
  lateral antebrachial cutaneous, 149–150,
    149*f*, 150*f*
    de Quervain's tenosynovitis and, 165
  levator ani syndrome and, 273
  MCL and, 306
  medial meniscal tear and, 309
  midtarsal joint arthritis and, 351
  osteochondritis dissecans of elbow and, 151–152
  piriformis syndrome and, 266
  plastic bag palsy and, 183
  tennis leg and, 347
  thrower's elbow and, 132
  ulnar, 146–148, 146*f*
    plastic bag palsy and, 183
    ultrasound for, 147*f*
Neurofibromatosis, 254
Nortriptyline
  for atypical facial pain, 38
  for cervical facet syndrome, 46
  for cervical radiculopathy, 49
  for cervicothoracic bursitis, 66
  for hyoid syndrome, 40
  for intercostal neuralgia, 198
  for lumbar radiculopathy, 239–240
  for post-thoracotomy pain syndrome,
    213–214
  for spinal stenosis, 246
  for TMJ, 35

O
Occipital neuralgia, 19–21
Occult fractures
  ankle arthritis and, 349
  carpal boss syndrome and, 186
  intercostal neuralgia and, 197
  midtarsal joint arthritis and, 351
  sesamoiditis of hand and, 181
  toe arthritis and, 368
  trigger finger and, 178
Olecranon bursa, 135*f*, 154–156, 154*f*, 155*f*
  osteochondritis dissecans of elbow and, 152
  thrower's elbow and, 133–135

Opioids
  for Achilles tendon rupture, 366
  for acute pancreatitis, 228–229
  analgesic rebound headache and, 17
  for chronic pancreatitis, 232
  for migraine headache, 7
  for Pancoast's tumor syndrome, 72
  for phantom limb syndrome, 295
  for postherpetic neuralgia, 222
  for rib fractures, 210
  for RSD, 43
  SAH and, 26
  for tennis leg, 348
  for tension-type headache, 9
  for thoracic vertebral compression fracture,
    225
  for VZV
    of thoracic dermatome, 216
    of trigeminal nerve, 3
Opponens weakness test, 161*f*
Orthotics
  for anterior cruciate ligament syndrome, 315
  for atypical facial pain, 38
  for diskitis, 253
  for thoracic vertebral compression fracture,
    225
  for TMJ, 35
Os styloideum. *See* Carpal boss syndrome
Osgood-Schlatter disease, 337–340, 337*f*,
    337*t*, 338*f*, 339*f*
Osseous neoplasm, 181
Osteitis pubis, 260–262, 260*f*, 261*f*
Osteoarthritis, 37*f*, 46*f*, 369*f*
  ankle arthritis and, 349
  carpometacarpal joint arthritis and, 167
  costosternal syndrome and, 191
  costovertebral joint syndrome and, 218
  hallux valgus deformity and, 371*f*
  hip arthritis and, 279
  iliopectineal bursitis and, 286
  knee arthritis and, 300
  manubriosternal syndrome and, 194
  precordial catch syndrome and, 207
  Tietze's syndrome and, 204
  wrist arthritis and, 158
Osteochondritis dissecans of elbow, 151–153,
    151*f*, 152*f*
Osteochondrosis, thrower's elbow and, 132
Osteomyelitis
  hyoid syndrome and, 39
  knee avascular necrosis and, 303
  mallet toe and, 383*f*
  phantom limb syndrome and, 295
Osteoporosis
  rib fractures and, 209–210
  thoracic vertebral compression fracture and,
    224–225, 224*f*
Osteosarcoma, 37*f*

P
Paget's disease, 254
Pancoast's tumor syndrome, 72–76, 73*f*, 74*f*
  lateral antebrachial cutaneous nerve
    entrapment and, 149
Pancreas. *See also* Acute pancreatitis; Chronic
    pancreatitis
  cancer of, 231*f*

Paragangliomas, 207*f*
Paraneoplastic syndromes, 201
Patella
  tendinosis of, 318, 318*f*
  tuberculosis of, 332*f*
Patrick-FABERE. *See* Flexion, abduction,
    external rotation, extension test
Peptic ulcer, 228, 230–232
Peripheral neuritis
  diabetic truncal neuropathy and, 200
  phantom limb syndrome and, 295
  postherpetic neuralgia and, 222
  VZV and
    of thoracic dermatome, 215–216
    of trigeminal nerve, 1–2
Pernicious anemia, 201
Pes anserine bursitis, 344–346, 344*f*
Pes anserine spurs, 345, 345*f*
Phalen's maneuver, 160–161, 161*f*
Phantom limb pain, 294–296, 294*f*
Phenytoin
  for diabetic truncal neuropathy, 201
  lymphoma and, 295
  for phantom limb syndrome, 295
  for VZV of trigeminal nerve, 3
Photophobia, 3
Piriformis syndrome, 266–268, 266*f*, 267*f*,
    268*f*
  sacroiliac joint pain and, 258
Pisotriquetral joint osteoarthritis, 158*f*
Plantar fasciitis, 377–379, 377*f*, 378*f*
  midtarsal joint arthritis and, 351
Plastic bag palsy, 183–184, 183*f*
Pleomorphic adenoma, 41*f*
Pleurisy, 207
Plexopathy
  brachial, 68–71, 69*f*
  deep infrapatellar bursitis and, 334–335
  pes anserine bursitis and, 344–345
Pneumonia
  acute pancreatitis and, 228
  chronic pancreatitis and, 230–232
  precordial catch syndrome and, 207
  thoracic vertebral compression fracture and,
    224
Pneumothorax
  costosternal syndrome and, 192–193
  deltoid syndrome and, 111
  manubriosternal syndrome and, 196
  scapulocostal syndrome and, 119
Polyarteritis nodosa, 230–232
Polymethyl methacrylate, 225*f*
Popliteal artery aneurysm, 342
Posterior tarsal tunnel syndrome, 359–361,
    359*f*, 360*f*
Postherpetic neuralgia, 2, 216, 221–223,
    221*f*
Post-thoracotomy pain syndrome, 212–214,
    212*f*, 212*t*, 213*f*, 214*f*
Posttraumatic arthritis
  ankle arthritis and, 349
  carpometacarpal joint arthritis and, 167
  of elbow, 121
  hip arthritis and, 279
  iliopectineal bursitis and, 286
  knee arthritis and, 300
  toe arthritis and, 368
  wrist arthritis and, 157–158

Posture
    brachioradialis syndrome and, 143
    myofascial pain syndrome and, 140
Precordial catch syndrome, 206–208, 206f, 207f
Prednisone, 13
Pregabalin
    for brachial plexopathy, 70
    for brachioradialis syndrome, 145
    for deltoid syndrome, 111
    for diabetic truncal neuropathy, 201
    for fibromyalgia of cervical musculature, 53
    knee avascular necrosis and, 303
    for Pancoast's tumor syndrome, 74
    for postherpetic neuralgia, 222
    for post-thoracotomy pain syndrome, 214
    for RSD, 43
    for scapulocostal syndrome, 119
    for supinator syndrome, 141
    for supraspinatus syndrome, 103–104
    for teres major syndrome, 115
    for thoracic outlet syndrome, 79
    for VZV
        of thoracic dermatome, 217
        of trigeminal nerve, 3
Pregnancy
    carpal tunnel syndrome and, 160
    glenohumeral joint avascular necrosis and, 91
    osteitis pubis and, 260f
Prepatellar bursitis, 328–330, 328f, 329f
Primary inflammatory muscle disease
    anconeus syndrome and, 138
    brachioradialis syndrome and, 144–145
    latissimus dorsi syndrome and, 243
    levator ani syndrome and, 273
    supinator syndrome and, 141
Proctalgia fugax, 275
Pronator teres, 126, 126f
Propranolol, 7
Pseudoclaudication, 245, 245f
Pseudocyst, 230, 231f
Pseudotumor cerebri, 22–24
    cluster headache and, 12–13
    costosternal syndrome and, 191
    costovertebral joint syndrome and, 218
    diagnostic criteria for, 23t
    migraine headache and, 6
Psoriatic arthritis
    carpometacarpal joint arthritis and, 167
    of elbow, 121
    manubriosternal syndrome and, 194
    precordial catch syndrome and, 207
    sesamoiditis of hand and, 181
    wrist arthritis and, 157
Pulmonary embolus
    for costosternal syndrome, 191
    costovertebral joint syndrome and, 219
    manubriosternal syndrome and, 195
    post-thoracotomy pain syndrome and, 213
    precordial catch syndrome and, 207

Q
Quadriceps expansion syndrome, 318, 338

R
Radial tunnel syndrome
    brachioradialis syndrome and, 144–145
    supinator syndrome and, 141
    tennis elbow and, 124

Radiation therapy
    glenohumeral joint avascular necrosis and, 91
    knee avascular necrosis and, 303
    VZV and, 1, 215
Radiocapitellar joint, 151–152
Radiofrequency destruction
    of brachial plexopathy, 70
    for cervical facet syndrome, 46
    of gasserian ganglion, 31–32
    for Pancoast's tumor syndrome, 75
Radionuclide bone scanning
    for Achilles tendinitis, 362
    for Achilles tendon rupture, 366
    for adhesive capsulitis, 95
    for carpal boss syndrome, 185–186
    for coccydynia, 275
    for costosternal syndrome, 191
    for costovertebral joint syndrome, 219
    for deltoid ligament strain, 353
    for iliopectineal bursitis, 286
    for intercostal neuralgia, 197
    for ischial bursitis, 289
    for manubriosternal syndrome, 195
    for MCL, 306
    for Morton's neuroma, 372
    for Osgood-Schlatter disease, 338
    for osteitis pubis, 260–262
    for phantom limb syndrome, 295
    for post-thoracotomy pain syndrome,
        213
    for rib fractures, 209–210
    for sacroiliac joint pain, 257–258
Rectal cancer, 273f
Reflex sympathetic dystrophy
    carpal tunnel syndrome and, 163
    phantom limb syndrome and, 294
    postherpetic neuralgia and, 221
Reflex sympathetic dystrophy of the face
        (RSD), 34–35, 42f
    atypical facial pain and, 37
Reiter's syndrome
    calcaneal spur syndrome and, 380
    costosternal syndrome and, 191
    costovertebral joint syndrome and, 218
    manubriosternal syndrome and, 194
    precordial catch syndrome and, 207
    Tietze's syndrome and, 204
Renal failure
    glenohumeral joint avascular necrosis and, 91
    knee avascular necrosis and, 303
Resisted abduction release test, 298f
Resisted hip extension test
    for ischial bursitis, 289f
    for ischiogluteal bursitis, 270f
Retro-orbital tumor, 2
Retropharyngeal abscess, 61–64, 62f, 63t
Rheumatoid arthritis, 192f
    Achilles tendon rupture and, 365
    ankle arthritis and, 349
    Baker's cyst of knee and, 341
    calcaneal spur syndrome and, 380
    carpal tunnel syndrome and, 160
    carpometacarpal joint arthritis and, 167
    costosternal syndrome and, 191
    costovertebral joint syndrome and, 218
    of elbow, 121
    iliopectineal bursitis and, 286
    manubriosternal syndrome and, 194

Rheumatoid arthritis (Continued)
    midtarsal joint arthritis and, 351
    olecranon bursitis and, 154
    osteitis pubis and, 262
    posterior tarsal tunnel syndrome and, 359
    precordial catch syndrome and, 207
    Tietze's syndrome and, 204
    toe arthritis and, 368
    wrist arthritis and, 157, 158
Ribs
    angiosarcoma of, 198f
    fractures of, 209–211, 209f
        costosternal syndrome and, 191
        costovertebral joint syndrome and, 219
        CT for, 209–210, 210f
        intercostal neuralgia and, 197
        mortality rate for, 211f
        nonunion of, 209f
        post-thoracotomy pain syndrome and, 213
Rotator cuff tear, 105–108, 106f, 107f
    biceps tendon tear and, 99
    bicipital tendinitis and, 88
    deltoid syndrome and, 110–111
    supraspinatus syndrome and, 103
RSD. See Reflex sympathetic dystrophy
    of the face
Runner's knee, 321–324, 321f, 322f

S
Sacroiliac joint pain, 256–259, 256f, 257f,
        258f
    trochanteric bursitis and, 297
SAH. See Subarachnoid hemorrhage
Sarcoidosis
    cluster headache and, 12–13
    diabetic truncal neuropathy and, 201
    migraine headache and, 6
Sarcomas, 171
Scapulocostal syndrome, 117–119, 117f,
        118f
Schwannoma
    brachial plexopathy and, 69
    thoracic outlet syndrome and, 78
    of trigeminal nerve, 30f
Sciatica. See Lumbar radiculopathy
Selective serotonin reuptake inhibitors, 201
Sesamoiditis
    of hand, 181–182, 181f
    plantar fasciitis and, 377–378
Sever's disease, 377–378
Shingles. See Varicella-zoster virus
Shoulder. See also specific diseases
    bursitis of
        rotator cuff tear and, 105
        supraspinatus syndrome and, 103
    osteoarthritis of, 80–81, 81f
        acromioclavicular joint and, 83
        adhesive capsulitis and, 95
        glenohumeral joint avascular necrosis and,
            93
Sickle cell disease, 91, 303
Sinusitis, 6, 12–13
SLAP. See Superior labral tear from
    anterior to posterior
Smoking
    Pancoast's tumor syndrome and, 74f
    thoracic outlet syndrome and, 78

Snapping hip syndrome, 282–284, 282*f*, 283*f*, 284*f*
Sphenopalatine, 13
Spinal cord compression
  diskitis and, 253–254, 255*t*
  retropharyngeal abscess and, 63*t*
Spinal stenosis, 245–247, 246*f*, 247*f*
  meralgia paresthetica and, 291–292
  pseudoclaudication and, 245, 245*f*
  stoop test for, 246*f*
Squat test, 309, 311*f*
Staphylococcus aureus, 63, 253
Stellate ganglion block, 37, 43
Steroids. *See also* Methylprednisolone
  Achilles tendon rupture and, 365
  for adhesive capsulitis, 95
  for arachnoiditis, 248
  for carpal tunnel syndrome, 162
  for cervical radiculopathy, 49
  for hyoid syndrome, 40
  for iliopectineal bursitis, 286
  for intercostal neuralgia, 199
  for ischial bursitis, 289
  for longus colli tendinitis, 59
  for Morton's neuroma, 373
  for postherpetic neuralgia, 222
  for post-thoracotomy pain syndrome, 214
  SAH and, 26
  for sesamoiditis of hand, 181
  for snapping hip syndrome, 284
  for tennis elbow, 124
  for VZV, 1, 215
    of thoracic dermatome, 216
  for wrist arthritis, 158
Stoop test, 246*f*
Stress
  brachioradialis syndrome and, 143
  myofascial pain syndrome and, 114
  scapulocostal syndrome and, 117
  supinator syndrome and, 140
  TMJ and, 33*f*
Stress fractures
  calcaneal spur syndrome and, 380, 382*f*
  jumper's knee and, 318
  mallet toe and, 383
  thrower's elbow and, 132
Stroke, 26
Stylohyoid ligament, 39
Subarachnoid hemorrhage (SAH), 25–28, 26*f*
Subdeltoid bursitis, 85–87, 86*f*, 87*f*
Sumatriptan, 7, 17
Superficial infrapatellar bursitis, 331–333, 331*f*, 332*f*
Superior labral tear from anterior to posterior (SLAP), 95*f*
Supinator syndrome, 140–142, 141*f*
Suprapatellar bursitis, 325–327, 325*f*
  Osgood-Schlatter disease and, 337–338
Supraspinatus syndrome, 102–104
Supratentorial ependymoma, 20*f*
Swimmer's headache, 14–16, 15*t*, 16*f*
Synovial cysts of elbow, 154
Synovial osteochondromatosis, 299*f*
Synovial sarcoma, 378*f*
Synovitis, 375. *See also* De Quervain's tenosynovitis; Tenosynovitis; Villonodular synovitis
Syringohydromyelia, 56*f*

Syringomyelia
  brachial plexopathy and, 69
  diskitis and, 254
  thoracic outlet syndrome and, 78
Systemic lupus erythematosus
  Achilles tendon rupture and, 365
  chronic pancreatitis and, 230–232
  glenohumeral joint avascular necrosis and, 91
  knee avascular necrosis and, 303

T
Tachycardia, 228
Tarsal tunnel syndrome
  deltoid ligament strain and, 353
  midtarsal joint arthritis and, 351
Temporal arteritis
  atypical facial pain and, 37
  cluster headache and, 12–13
  migraine headache and, 6
  swimmer's headache and, 15
  tension-type headache and, 9
Temporomandibular joint (TMJ), 33–35, 33*f*
Tendinitis
  Baker's cyst of knee and, 342
  brachioradialis syndrome and, 144–145
  calcaneal spur syndrome and, 380
  carpometacarpal joint arthritis and, 168
  Dupuytren's contracture and, 189
  elbow arthritis and, 120
  Freiberg's disease and, 375
  ischiogluteal bursitis and, 270
  MCL and, 306
  olecranon bursitis and, 154
  osteitis pubis and, 260
  osteochondritis dissecans of elbow and, 151–152
  prepatellar bursitis and, 328
  runner's knee and, 321
  shoulder osteoarthritis and, 81
  supinator syndrome and, 141
  suprapatellar bursitis and, 326–327
Tennis elbow, 123–125, 123*f*, 124*f*, 125*f*
  lateral antebrachial cutaneous nerve entrapment and, 149–150
  medial epicondyle and, 127*f*
  supinator syndrome and, 141
Tennis leg, 347–348, 348*f*
Tenosynovitis
  carpal boss syndrome and, 186
  ganglion cysts of wrist and, 171
  plastic bag palsy and, 183–184
  posterior tarsal tunnel syndrome and, 359
  sesamoiditis of hand and, 181
Tension-type headache, 6*t*, 8–10, 9*t*
  migraine headache and, 6
Teres major syndrome, 113–116, 113*f*, 114*f*, 115*f*
Thompson squeeze test, 365, 365*f*
Thoracic aorta, 197, 198*f*
Thoracic dermatomes, 215–217, 215*f*
Thoracic outlet syndrome, 77–79, 78*f*
Thoracic radiculopathy
  postherpetic neuralgia and, 222
  VZV of thoracic dermatome, 216
Thoracic vertebral compression fracture, 224–226
  metastases and, 225*f*
  osteoporosis and, 224–225, 224*f*

Thrombophlebitis
  Baker's cyst of knee and, 341–342
  posterior tarsal tunnel syndrome and, 359
Thrower's elbow, 132–136, 132*t*, 135*f*
  osteochondritis dissecans of elbow and, 151–152
Thymoma, 194, 207
Tibial collateral ligament. *See* Medial collateral ligament
Tietze's syndrome, 203–205, 203*f*, 204*f*
  costosternal syndrome and, 191
  intercostal neuralgia and, 197
  manubriosternal syndrome and, 195
  post-thoracotomy pain syndrome and, 213
  rib fractures and, 210
Tinel sign, 146
  anterior tarsal tunnel syndrome and, 356, 357*f*
  carpal tunnel syndrome and, 160–161, 161*f*
  meralgia paresthetica and, 291
Tizanidine, 66
TMJ. *See* Temporomandibular joint
Toe arthritis, 368–369, 368*f*
Tolosa-Hunt syndrome, 2
Tramadol, 202
Transcutaneous electrical nerve stimulation
  for anconeus syndrome, 139
  for brachioradialis syndrome, 145
  for deltoid syndrome, 111
  for gluteus maximus syndrome, 265
  for latissimus dorsi syndrome, 244
  for levator ani syndrome, 273–274
  for supinator syndrome, 141
  for supraspinatus syndrome, 103–104
  for VZV of trigeminal nerve, 3
Transplantation
  Achilles tendon rupture and, 365
  glenohumeral joint avascular necrosis and, 91
  knee avascular necrosis and, 303
Traveling salesman's shoulder. *See* Scapulocostal syndrome
Trazodone, 10
Tricyclic antidepressants
  for atypical facial pain, 38
  for cervical facet syndrome, 46
  for cervical radiculopathy, 49
  for cervical strain, 56
  for cervicothoracic bursitis, 66
  for intercostal neuralgia, 198
  for migraine headache, 7
  for post-thoracotomy pain syndrome, 213–214
  for RSD, 43
  for spinal stenosis, 246
  for TMJ, 35
Trigeminal nerve, 29–32
  atypical facial pain and, 37*t*
  microvascular decompression of, 32
  nerve block for, 38
  postherpetic neuralgia and, 222
  schwannoma of, 30*f*
  VZV of, 1–4
Trigger finger, 178–180, 178*f*, 179*f*
  Dupuytren's contracture and, 188–189
Trigger points
  anconeus syndrome and, 137–139, 138*f*
  brachioradialis syndrome and, 143–145, 144*f*

Trigger points *(Continued)*
  deltoid syndrome and, 109, 110*f*, 111
  gluteus maximus syndrome and, 263, 264
  latissimus dorsi syndrome and, 242–243,
    243*f*
  levator ani syndrome and, 271–273
  myofascial pain syndrome and, 113
  scapulocostal syndrome and, 117–119
  supinator syndrome and, 140–141, 141*f*
  supraspinatus syndrome and, 102, 102*f*
  teres major syndrome and, 115, 115*f*
Trigger thumb, 175–177, 175*f*, 176*f*
Triptans, 7, 17
Trochanteric bursitis, 297–299, 297*f*, 298*f*,
    299*f*
  meralgia paresthetica and, 292
  snapping hip syndrome and, 282
Trousseau's sign, 228
Tuberculosis, 332*f*
Turner's sign, 228

U

Ulnar collateral ligament, 134*f*
Ulnar nerve entrapment, 146–148, 146*f*
  plastic bag palsy and, 183
  ultrasound for, 147*f*
Ulnar nerve subluxation, 132
Ultrasound
  for Achilles tendon rupture, 366, 366*f*
  for acromioclavicular joint, 82
  for carpal tunnel syndrome, 161–162, 162*f*

Ultrasound *(Continued)*
  for iliopectineal bursitis, 286
  for jumper's knee, 318
  of levator ani syndrome, 272*f*
  of meralgia paresthetica, 293*f*
  for Morton's neuroma, 372
  for Osgood-Schlatter disease, 339*f*
  for prepatellar bursitis, 328–329
  for runner's knee, 321
  for sacroiliac joint pain, 258
  for tennis leg, 347, 348*f*
  for ulnar nerve entrapment, 147*f*
Uremia, 201
Uric acid
  anterior tarsal tunnel syndrome and, 356
  Freiberg's disease and, 374–375
  for meralgia paresthetica, 291–292

V

Valacyclovir, 3
Valgus stress test, 307*f*
Valproic acid, 7
Valsalva maneuver, 26
Vancomycin, 253
Varicella-zoster virus (VZV), 215. *See also*
    Postherpetic neuralgia
  biceps tendon tear and, 99
  bicipital tendinitis and, 88
  chronic pancreatitis and, 230–232
  costovertebral joint syndrome and, 219
  intercostal neuralgia and, 197

Varicella-zoster virus (VZV) *(Continued)*
  of lumbar dermatome, 216*f*
  manubriosternal syndrome and, 195
  post-thoracotomy pain syndrome and, 213
  of thoracic dermatomes, 215–217, 215*f*
  thoracic vertebral compression fracture and,
    224–225
  of trigeminal nerve, 1–4
Vasculitis, 374
Verapamil, 7
Villonodular synovitis
  adhesive capsulitis and, 95
  ankle arthritis and, 349
  iliopectineal bursitis and, 286
  knee arthritis and, 300
  shoulder osteoarthritis and, 81
  wrist arthritis and, 158
VZV. *See* Varicella-zoster virus

W

Waldman method, 366*f*
Wartenberg sign, 146
Watson test, 162
Wrist arthritis, 157–159, 157*f*, 158*f*

Y

Yergason's test, 89*f*

Z

Zinc oxide, 3